Behavior Change Contract

Choose a health behavior that you would like to change, starting this quarter or semester. Sign the contract at the bottom to affirm your commitment to making a healthy change and ask a friend to witness it.

My behavior change will be:

_____

My long-term goal for this behavior change is:

_____

Barriers that I must overcome to make this behavior change are   (things that I am currently doing or situations that contribute to this behavior or make it harder to change):

    1. _____
    2. _____
    3. _____

The strategies I will use to overcome these barriers are:

    1. _____
    2. _____
    3. _____

Resources I will use to help me change this behavior include:

    a friend/partner/relative: _____
    a school-based resource: _____
    a community-based resource: _____
    a book or reputable website: _____

In order to make my goal more attainable, I have devised these short-term goals

short-term goal	target date	reward
short-term goal	target date	reward
short-term goal	target date	reward

When I make the long-term behavior change described above, my reward will be:

_____ target date: _____

I intend to make the behavior change described above. I will use the strategies and rewards to achieve the goals that will contribute to a healthy behavior change.

Signed: _____   Witness: _____

Behavior Change Contract

Choose a health behavior that you would like to change, starting this quarter or semester. Sign the contract at the bottom to affirm your commitment to making a healthy change and ask a friend to witness it.

My behavior change will be:

_____

My long-term goal for this behavior change is:

_____

Barriers that I must overcome to make this behavior change are   (things that I am currently doing or situations that contribute to this behavior or make it harder to change):

1. _____
2. _____
3. _____

The strategies I will use to overcome these barriers are:

1. _____
2. _____
3. _____

Resources I will use to help me change this behavior include:

a friend/partner/relative: _____

a school-based resource: _____

a community-based resource: _____

a book or reputable website: _____

In order to make my goal more attainable, I have devised these short-term goals

short-term goal	target date	reward
short-term goal	target date	reward
short-term goal	target date	reward

When I make the long-term behavior change described above, my reward will be:

_____ target date: _____

I intend to make the behavior change described above. I will use the strategies and rewards to achieve the goals that will contribute to a healthy behavior change.

Signed: _____   Witness: _____

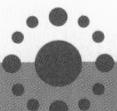

FOURTH EDITION

Total Fitness and Wellness

SCOTT K. POWERS
University of Florida

STEPHEN L. DODD
University of Florida

VIRGINIA J. NOLAND
University of Florida

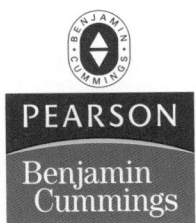

PEARSON

Benjamin Cummings

San Francisco   Boston   New York
Cape Town   Hong Kong   London   Madrid   Mexico City
Montreal   Munich   Paris   Singapore   Sydney   Tokyo   Toronto

Publisher: Daryl Fox
Senior Acquisitions Editor: Deirdre Espinoza
Development Manager: Claire Alexander
Assistant Editor: Alison Rodal
Managing Editor: Wendy Earl
Production Editor: Sharon Montooth
Art Coordinator: Linda Jupiter
Photo Researcher: Kristin Piljay
Cover and Text Design: tani hasegawa
Copyeditor: Lori Cavanaugh
Compositor: The Left Coast Group
Senior Manufacturing Buyer: Stacey Weinberger
Senior Marketing Manager: Sandy Lindelof

Photography and illustration credits appear on p. CR-1.

Library of Congress Cataloging-in-Publication Data
Powers, Scott K. (Scott Kline), 1950–
   Total fitness and wellness/Scott K. Powers, Stephen L. Dodd,
Virginia J.
Noland.—4th ed.
    p. cm.
   Includes index.
   ISBN 0-8053-7967-3
1. Exercise. 2. Nutrition. 3. Health. I. Dodd, Stephen L. II. Noland,
Virginia J. III. Title.
RA781 .P66 2005
613.7—dc21

2004065525

Many of the designations used by manufacturers and sellers to distinguish their products are claimed as trademarks. Where those designations appear in this book, and the publisher was aware of a trademark claim, the designations have been printed in initial caps or all caps.

The Author(s) and Publisher believe that the activities and methods described in this publication, when conducted according to the descriptions herein, are reasonably safe for the students to whom this publication is directed. Nonetheless, many of the described activities and methods are accompanied by some degree of risk, including human error. The Author(s) and Publisher disclaim any liability arising from such risks in connection with any of the activities and methods contained in this publication. If students have any questions or problems with the activities and methods, they should always ask their instructor for help before proceeding.

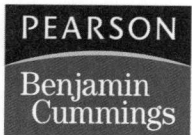

ISBN 0-8053-7967-3
1 2 3 4 5 6 7 8 9 10—CRK—09 08 07 06 05

www.aw-bc.com

☀ To Jen, Haney, and Will. Your love and encouragement have always meant more than you will ever know.
  Stephen L. Dodd

☀ To my mother who encouraged me to pursue academic endeavors.
  Scott K. Powers

☀ To my husband and children for making my life complete. And to my parents for your ever-present love and support.
  Virginia J. Noland

☀ Brief Contents

⊙ Contents

Chapter 5: Improving Muscular Strength and Endurance   121

❂ Preface

Good health is our most precious possession. Although it is usually only in times of illness or injury that we really appreciate good health, more and more people are realizing that health is not simply the lack of disease. Indeed, there are degrees of health, or wellness, on which lifestyle can have a major impact.

Intended for an introductory college course in physical fitness and wellness, *Total Fitness and Wellness* focuses on how lifestyle can be altered to achieve a high degree of physical fitness and wellness. Two major aspects of daily life that most affect our level of wellness are exercise and diet. Hence, the interaction of exercise and diet and the essential role of regular exercise and good nutrition in achieving total fitness and wellness are major themes of the text.

Total Fitness and Wellness, Fourth Edition, was built on a strong foundation of both exercise physiology and nutrition. The text provides clear and objective research-based information to college students during their first course in physical fitness and wellness. By offering a research-based text, we hope to dispel many myths associated with exercise, nutrition, weight loss, and wellness. For the evaluation of various wellness components such as fitness levels and nutritional status, a how-to approach is used. Ways to change your lifestyle that will improve wellness (e.g., designing a fitness program, altering food choices) are described. Indeed, the title of the book, "Total Fitness and Wellness," reflects our goals.

Numerous physical fitness and wellness texts are available today. Our motivation in writing *Total Fitness and Wellness,* Fourth Edition, was to create a unique physical fitness and well balanced text, one that not only covers primary concepts of physical fitness and wellness but also addresses important issues such as behavior change, exercise-related injuries, exercise and the environment, and exercise for special populations.

FOUNDATION IN EXERCISE PHYSIOLOGY

We believe it is imperative that students develop an understanding of the basic physiological adaptations that occur in response to both acute exercise and regular exercise training. Without this understanding, it is impossible to plan, modify, and properly execute a lifetime exercise program.

STRONG EMPHASIS ON NUTRITION

Because we feel so strongly about the important interaction between nutrition and exercise, a nutritional theme is incorporated throughout the text. Each chapter includes Nutritional Links to Fitness boxes, which

explain how nutrition affects health and wellness in areas such as cardiorespiratory fitness, muscular strength and endurance, and prevention of cardiovascular disease. We put major emphasis on and provide comprehensive coverage of basic nutrition and weight control by dedicating separate chapters to each topic: Chapter 7, Nutrition, Health, and Fitness (includes new information on popular "low-carb" diets) and Chapter 8, Exercise, Diet, and Weight Control.

COVERAGE OF THE LATEST SCIENTIFIC RESEARCH ON PHYSICAL FITNESS, NUTRITION, AND WELLNESS

We firmly believe that college physical fitness and wellness texts should contain the latest scientific information and include references for scientific studies to support key information about physical fitness, nutrition, and wellness. Our approach is to provide current scientific references that document the validity of facts presented. Accordingly, source information and suggested readings are placed at the end of each chapter.

The most current research in the arena of fitness and wellness is offered in *Total Fitness and Wellness,* Fourth Edition. For example, it is now clear that exercise plays a role in reducing the risk of some cancers and can contribute to a longer life. While there has long been speculation about the health benefits of exercise, evidence that supports the exercise and wellness connection has only recently become available. In the area of nutrition, scientific data now suggest that vitamins may play a new role in preventing certain diseases and combating the aging process. In addition, while it is well accepted that fat in the diet increases our risk of heart disease, it has just lately been shown that dietary fat plays a greater role than other nutrients in weight gain.

With any attempt to present the most current information, there is always the danger of presenting ideas that are not fully substantiated by good research. We have made a concerted effort to avoid such a risk by using information from the most highly respected scientific journals and consulting with experts in the field.

Layout and Features

While many topic and organization options have to be considered when developing a text, the best way to determine content and order is to ask instructors. Therefore, with input from instructors across the country, we have included the following coverage, layout, and features:

- **Coverage:** By design, *Total Fitness and Wellness, Fourth Edition* contains more material than can be covered in a typical 15-week semester. The text is comprehensive in order to afford instructors a large degree of freedom in selecting concepts to be covered in their course. (The text is also available in a Brief Edition, which contains Chapters 1–10 and 17.)

- **Unique Topics:** Several unique chapters are offered in the fourth edition, which are not contained in other introductory fitness and wellness texts. For example, this book includes chapters on exercise and the environment, exercise for special populations, and prevention and rehabilitation of exercise-related injuries. Further, in several chapters we have incorporated an elementary discussion of the physiology of exercise to improve students' knowledge of how the body operates and responds to regular exercise.

- **Informational Boxes:** Each chapter contains informational boxes. **A Closer Look** boxes offer extended coverage of concepts discussed in the body of the text with suggestions for practical application. **Nutritional Links to Health and Fitness** boxes emphasize the importance of nutrition to physical fitness. **Ask an Expert** boxes provide the latest information from internationally known experts in the fields of resistance training, exercise and nutrition, obesity and weight loss, exercise and the environment, and adherence to regular exercise. **Fitness and Wellness for All** boxes contain fitness, wellness, and nutritional information with respect to diversity. **Fitness-Wellness Consumer** boxes provide exercise and wellness information related to consumer issues.

- **Lab Exercises:** Most chapters contain easy-to-follow, application-based lab exercises such as fitness testing, nutritional evaluation, and cardiovascular risk assessment.

- **Healthy People 2010 Objectives:** National health promotion and disease prevention initiatives are reflected in selected Healthy People 2010 goals listed in Appendix A.

- **Food Appendices:** To assist students in tracking and modifying food intake, caloric and nutrient content of common foods and fast foods is offered in Appendices B and C.

- **Pedagogical Aids:** To stimulate students' interest and alert them to the significance of the material to be covered, Learning Objectives open each chapter. In Summary lists, found throughout the text, recapitulate the more difficult sections, prompting students to recall and process main concepts covered. To emphasize and support understanding of material, important terms are boldfaced in the text and defined in a running glossary at the bottom of text pages. Also, several features are offered at the end of each chapter to reinforce learning. For students' review, the Chapter Summary sections succinctly restate the most significant ideas presented in the chapter. Study Questions encourage analysis of chapter discussions and prepare students for tests. Suggested Readings and References offer quality information sources for further study of fitness and wellness.

Instructor Supplements

A complete resource package accompanies *Total Fitness and Wellness* to assist the instructor with classroom preparation and presentation.

INSTRUCTOR'S GUIDE AND TEST BANK

The Instructor's Guide and Test Bank supplement includes suggestions for class discussion, student activities, readings, lecture outlines, learning objectives, chapter summaries, web references, and media resources. The Test Bank includes over 1,000 multiple choice, true or false, short answer, and matching questions to use for student review or testing.

COMPUTERIZED TEST BANK

This cross-platform CD-ROM includes over 1,000 multiple choice, true or false, short answer, and matching questions in a format that allows instructors to incorporate these questions into their exams.

MyHealthLab

This online standard course management system is loaded with valuable free teaching resources that make giving assignments and tracking student progress easy. With the convenience of all the resources for the course in one location, MyHealthLab, powered by CourseCompass™, features a wealth of preloaded content for instructors, including PowerPoint® slides, an interactive e-book, Test Bank questions, Instructor's Manual material, and more. URL: http://www.aw-bc.com/myhealthlab

DISCOVERY HEALTH CHANNEL HEALTH AND WELLNESS LECTURE LAUNCHER VIDEOS AND CD-ROM

(VOLUME 1, 0-8053-5369-0; VOLUME II, 0-8053-6001-8; CD-ROM, 0-8053-7830-8)

Created in partnership between Discovery Health Channel and Benjamin Cummings, these VHS tapes and

CD-ROM feature a series of quick lecture-launcher clips on topics from nutrition and stress management to substance abuse. There are 24 clips in all, each one 5–10 minutes in length. An excellent way to engage your students and enliven your lectures.

BENJAMIN CUMMINGS HEALTH VIDEO SERIES

In addition to the Discovery Lecture Launcher series, additional videos are available to qualified adopters on a variety of topics. Contact your local Benjamin Cummings Sales Representative for a complete list of videos.

FILMS FOR THE HUMANITIES

More than 80 videos from respected sources available for qualified adopters. For ordering information, sales representatives should contact Linda Gallegos at (415) 402-2366.

INSTRUCTOR RESOURCE CD-ROM

This multi-platform CD-ROM includes PowerPoint® Presentation Slides to provide instructors with a multimedia presentation for their classroom or a lecture hall. Presented on a CD-ROM, the presentation is easily run and allows instructors to download lecture notes and images from over 200 slides. New to this edition is all of the art and tables from the text.

TRANSPARENCY ACETATES

Over 140 transparency acetates contain all figures, graphs, and tables from the main text. The transparencies are excellent for presentation of information in a clear manner consistent with that of the text.

Student Supplements

BEHAVIOR CHANGE LOG BOOK AND WELLNESS JOURNAL

This assessment tool helps students track daily exercise and nutritional intake and create a long-term nutritional and fitness prescription plan. It also includes a Behavior Change Contract and topics for journal-based activities. Packaged with each new copy of the text.

STAND-ALONE EvaluEat WINDOWS-ONLY CD-ROM

EvaluEat diet analysis software helps students track their eating habits and evaluate the nutritional content of their diets. Available for individual purchase or packaged with the alternate edition of the text, this software features a database of more than 6,200 food items

and can report on dozens of different nutrients. Students can do a single or multi-day diet analysis, create a variety of reports, and determine whether they are meeting the DRIs for various vitamins and minerals. This program also allows users to input their activity levels to create expenditure reports.

MyHealthLab

MyHealthLab features online access to a selection of the print and media supplements for students, and makes studying convenient and fun. The preloaded content on this interactive Website includes an interactive e-book, self-assessment worksheets, Behavior Change Log Book and Wellness Journal, Research Navigator™, the Discovery Channel Lecture Launcher clips, links to e-themes from the *New York Times,* and more.

COMPANION WEBSITE

This student resource site offers approximately 500 practice quiz questions, interactive activities, web links to sites for further information, and e-themes from the *New York Times* containing 17 *New York Times* articles reporting on the latest in health and wellness news and research. For the instructor, the site includes PowerPoint® presentations and lecture outlines.

Changes in the Fourth Edition

Each chapter of the fourth edition has been revised to include the newest research developments in exercise, wellness, and health-related nutrition. In addition to the changes listed in the paragraphs above, several other features have been added. These include

- expanded wellness and behavior change coverage and the addition of a third author who brings an expertise in the area of behavior change practices and stress management;
- new and improved art and photos throughout the text;
- new and updated references in every chapter;
- coverage of sexually transmitted infections and addictive substances (drug abuse) now split into two new chapters.

Acknowledgments

The publication of this edition of *Total Fitness and Wellness* was accomplished by an enormous number of people at Benjamin Cummings. From the campus sales representatives to the president of the company, they are truly "first rate" and our interaction with them is always delightful.

There were several key people in the process. Our Acquisitions Editor, Deirdre Espinoza, has worked with us for the last two editions and her insight and organization continue to be key to the success of the text. Several new additions to the team have been important in both the revisions of the text as well as the production process. Christina Pierson coordinated reviews for this edition and organized the original editorial schedule. Alison Rodal has been a major contributor, as she took over the editorial process from Christina. Alison has truly played a significant role in the production of this edition. Sharon Montooth, Production Editor, expertly guided the manuscript through each stage of production. Finally, Linda Jupiter coordinated the artwork for this edition. Her efforts certainly added to the "look" but more importantly, helped convey a message.

Melissa Deering and Jenna Jones at the University of Florida have made major contributions to both the text and ancillaries. Their technical and editing work was important but their personal interest in fitness and wellness has made their contributions even greater.

Finally, there is a long list of professionals whose reviews of the content and style or participation in a fitness and wellness forum have helped to shape this book. We owe these individuals a tremendous debt of gratitude:

Robert Axtell	Southern Connecticut State University
Jeff Burnett	Fort Hays State University
Charlie Chatterton	Eastern Connecticut State University
Donna Cobb	University of Central Oklahoma
Trey Cone	University of Central Oklahoma
Kathryn Davis	Slippery Rock University
Forest Dolgener	University of Northern Iowa
Bill Eliziuk	Broward Community College
Marisha Fortner	Notre Dame University
David Harackiewicz	Central Connecticut State University
John Hammett	Jacksonville State University
Virginia Hicks	University of Wisconsin-Whitewater
Amy Howton	Kennesaw State University
Erica Jackson	Auburn University
Daniel Keefer	Millersville University
Lynn Maska	Fort Hays State University
Glen McNeil	Fort Hays State University
Marilyn Miller	Bloomsburg University
Rochel Rittgers	Augustana College
Russell Robinson	Greensboro College
Jeff Schlicht	Western Connecticut State University
Jan Schroeder	California State University, Long Beach
Steve Sedbrook	Fort Hays State University
Deonna Shake	Abilene Christian University
Phil Sparling	Georgia Tech
Jiri Stelzer	Valdosta State University
Scott Swanson	Ohio Northern University
Lynn Spadine Taylor	Slippery Rock University
John Todorovich	University of Florida
Nanette Tummers	Eastern Connecticut State University

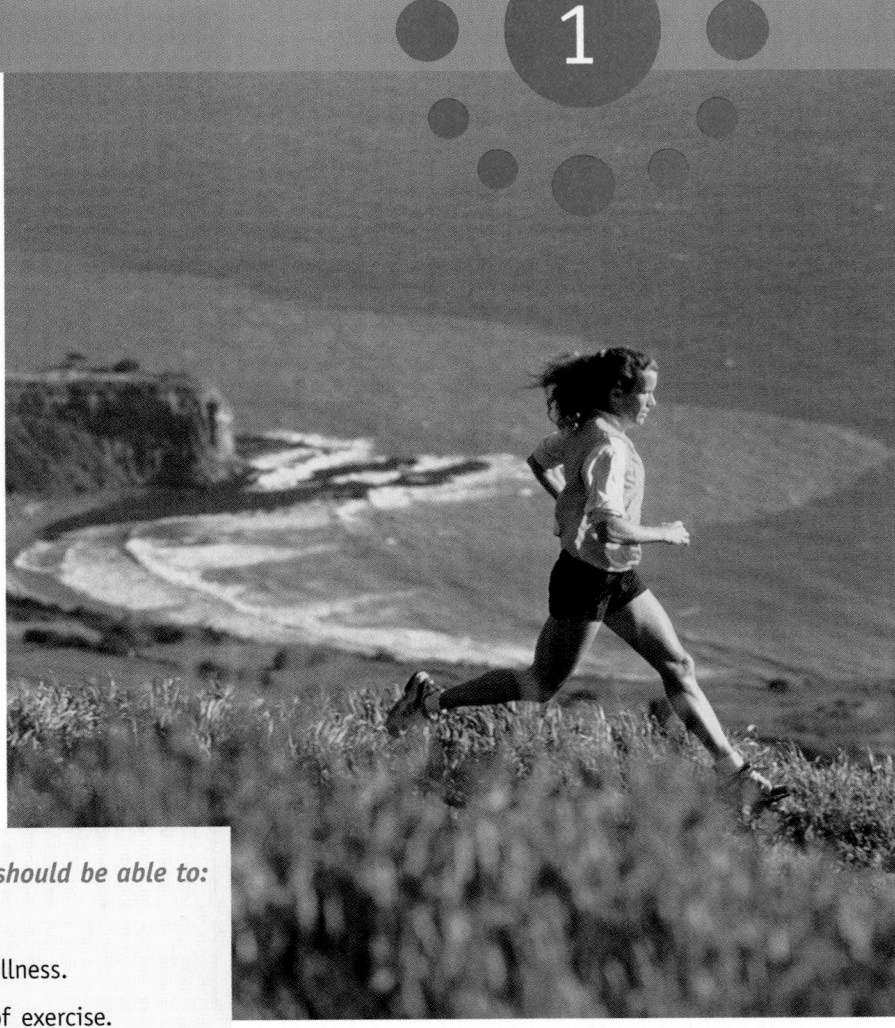

1

After studying this chapter, you should be able to:

1. Discuss the wellness concept.

2. Outline the components of wellness.

3. Describe the health benefits of exercise.

4. Define the terms coronary artery disease and myocardial infarction.

5. Compare the goals of health-related fitness programs and sport performance conditioning programs.

6. Describe the components of health-related physical fitness.

Understanding Health-Related Fitness and Wellness

Congratulations! By reading this chapter, you are taking the first step toward improving your physical fitness and maintaining good health. By deciding to improve your personal fitness, you will join millions of people worldwide who are becoming interested in maintaining good health through daily exercise, improved health behaviors, and proper diet.

This book contains the latest scientific information on health and wellness. Moreover, this book provides detailed information on how to develop and maintain a physical fitness program. A major theme of the text is that good nutrition and exercise work together to improve health and overall well-being. Additional chapters discuss issues such as preventing and treating exercise-related injuries, environmental effects on exercise, stress reduction, and modifying unhealthy behavior. Careful reading of the material throughout will provide answers to hundreds of diet- and exercise-related questions.

In this first chapter, we present the concept of wellness, discuss the health benefits of exercise, outline the major components of physical fitness, and introduce exercise goal setting. Understanding the role that exercise plays in the maintenance of good health and wellness is a strong motivation for developing and sustaining a lifetime physical fitness program.

☀ Wellness Concept

Good health was once defined as the absence of disease. In the 1970s and 1980s many exercise scientists and health educators became dissatisfied with this limited definition of good health. These futuristic thinkers believed that health was not only an absence of disease but included physical fitness and emotional and spiritual health as well. This new concept of good health is called **wellness** (2). In a broad sense, the term wellness means "healthy living." This state of healthy living is achieved by the practice of a healthy lifestyle that includes regular physical activity, proper nutrition (Nutritional Links to Health and Fitness), eliminating unhealthy behaviors (avoiding high-risk activities such as reckless driving, smoking, and drug use), and maintain-

---

Nutritional Links
TO HEALTH AND FITNESS

Good Nutrition Is Essential to Achieving Physical Fitness and Wellness

A major theme of this book is that good nutrition is essential for developing and maintaining physical fitness and a state of wellness. Good nutrition means that an individual's diet provides all of the components of food (called nutrients) needed to promote growth and repair body tissues. Additionally, a proper diet supplies the energy required to meet the body's daily needs.

Consuming too little of any nutrient can impair physical fitness and potentially result in disease (32). Therefore, achieving good nutrition should be a goal for everyone. In many of the chapters that follow, we provide nutritional information in the form of informational boxes such as this one. In addition, Chapter 7 is devoted entirely to nutrition.

Although consuming inadequate nutrients increases your risk of disease, consuming too much food energy (overeating) can be problematic as well. Overeating on a regular basis can result in large amounts of fat gain, resulting in obesity. As mentioned earlier, obesity increases your risk of heart disease and type II diabetes. Chapter 8 discusses the relationship among nutrition, exercise, and weight loss.

---

ing good emotional and spiritual health (2). Given the importance of wellness, let's discuss wellness and a healthy lifestyle in more detail.

☀ Wellness: A Healthy Lifestyle

A healthy lifestyle refers to health behaviors aimed at reducing one's risk of disease and accidents, achieving optimal physical health, and maximizing emotional, social, intellectual, and spiritual health (2, 3, 7). A healthy lifestyle can be achieved by eliminating unhealthy behavior to reach a state of wellness. Wellness is defined specifically as a state of optimal health that includes physical, emotional, intellectual, spiritual, social health, and environmental health (Figure 1.1).

---

wellness   A state of healthy living. This state is achieved by the practice of a healthy lifestyle, which includes regular physical activity, proper nutrition, eliminating unhealthy behaviors, and maintaining good emotional and spiritual health.

PHYSICAL HEALTH

Physical health means not only freedom from disease but includes physical fitness as well. Physical fitness can positively affect your health by reducing your risk of disease and improving your quality of life.

EMOTIONAL HEALTH

Emotions play an important role in how you feel about yourself and others. Emotional health (also called mental health) includes your social skills and interpersonal relationships. Also included are your levels of self-esteem and your ability to cope with the routine stress of daily living.

The cornerstone of emotional health is emotional stability, which describes how well you deal with the day-to-day stresses of personal interactions and the physical environment. Although it is normal to experience some range of emotional highs and lows, the objective of achieving emotional wellness is to maintain emotional stability somewhere between an extreme high and an extreme low.

INTELLECTUAL HEALTH

Intellectual health can be maintained by keeping your mind active through life-long learning. Although there are many ways to maintain an active mind, attending lectures, engaging in thoughtful discussions with friends or teachers, and reading are obvious ways to promote intellectual health. Maintaining good intellectual health can improve your quality of life by increasing your ability to define and solve problems. Further, continuous learning and thinking can provide you with a sense of fulfillment that accompanies an active mind.

SPIRITUAL HEALTH

Spiritual health is often called the glue that holds an individual together. The term spiritual means different things to different people, but regardless of whether you define spiritual health as religious beliefs or the establishment of personal values, it is an important aspect of wellness and is closely linked to emotional health (34).

Optimal spiritual health is often described as the development of spiritual makeup to its fullest potential. This includes the ability to understand the basic purpose in life and to experience love, joy, pain, peace, and sorrow, and to care for and respect all living things (34). Anyone who has experienced a beautiful sunset or smelled the first scents of spring can appreciate the pleasure of maintaining optimal spiritual health (34).

SOCIAL HEALTH

Social health is defined as the development and maintenance of meaningful interpersonal relationships. This results in the creation of a support network of friends and family. Good social health results in feelings of confidence in social interactions and provides you with a feeling of emotional security.

ENVIRONMENTAL HEALTH

Our environment can negatively influence our ability to achieve total wellness. For example, air pollution and water contamination are two important environmental factors that can harm physical health. Undeniably, breathing air polluted with particulate matter and other contaminants can lead to a variety of respiratory disorders (e.g., asthma). Air pollution can have multiple origins, including second-hand smoke and pollutant discharge from cars and factories.

Contaminated drinking water can also contribute to numerous health problems. For instance, water that contains bacteria can lead to infection. Also, drinking water that contains carcinogens (cancer-producing agents) can increase the risk of certain types of cancers (e.g., stomach, colon, and rectal cancer). Other examples of environmental problems that can negatively impact health are the safety of our food supply, overexposure to ultraviolet radiation, and household factors such as lead paint.

To summarize, it is clear that the environment plays an important role in our ability to achieve total wellness. Hence, achieving total wellness requires learning about the environment and protecting yourself against environmental hazards that threaten your health and well-being.

☀ Interaction of Wellness Components

None of the components of wellness work in isolation; a strong interaction must occur among the five. For example, poor physical health can lead to poor emotional health. Similarly, a lack of spiritual health can contribute to poor emotional health as well as poor physical and intellectual health. These mind–body interactions are illustrated in Figure 1.1. Total wellness can be achieved only by a balance of physical, intellectual, social, emotional, spiritual, and environmental health.

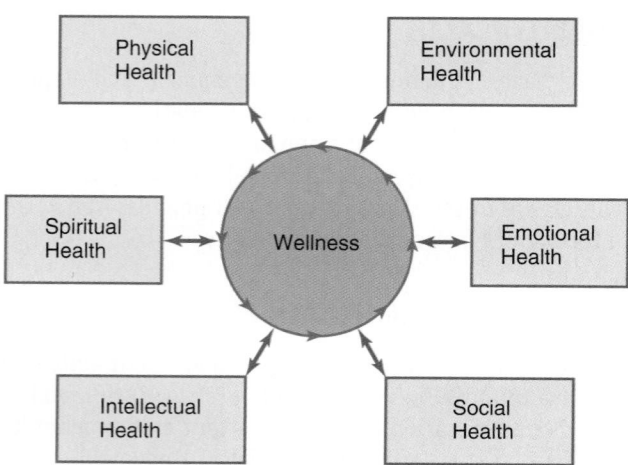

FIGURE 1.1
The wellness components and their interactions.

⊙ Achieving Wellness Through a Healthy Lifestyle

The key to achieving wellness is a healthy lifestyle. Accomplishing a healthy lifestyle requires an understanding of the components of a healthy life and how your current lifestyle deviates from the desired life habits. Indeed, before you can start changing a wellness-related behavior, you must know that the behavior is unhealthy and that you can make changes. A good place to begin is with a personal assessment of your health risk status. Laboratory 1.1 is a lifestyle assessment inventory designed to increase your awareness of factors that affect your health. As you work on Laboratory 1.1, develop a list of your behaviors that are less than optimal. Importantly, keep in mind that you have control over each of these health behaviors, but awareness alone does not bring about change.

To achieve total wellness, a decision to alter unhealthy behavior in your lifestyle is necessary and is a decision that only you can make. So, make a commitment today to improve the quality of your life by practicing a healthy lifestyle. This can be accomplished by modification of your behavior to eliminate unhealthy activities. A key point to remember is, don't try to change all of your bad behaviors at once. Develop your list of unhealthy behaviors from Laboratory 1.1 and concentrate on changing one unhealthy behavior at a time. Attacking one behavior at a time is a good strategy because it is difficult to change everything at once. A good suggestion is to start with a simple behavior change and achieve success. Achievement of one healthy behavior goal will provide motivation for you to pursue another objective.

Once you make the decision to make lifestyle changes, you should devise a strategy to achieve your goals one at a time. Your key to success will be a good plan of action that will require attacking one target behavior at a time. Complete details for modifying unhealthy behavior will be presented later in this book (Chapter 10). Nonetheless, a good foundation for changing any unhealthy behavior is to develop a personal behavior contract. Studies have revealed that a serious personal contract can increase your chances of successfully changing behavior as opposed to a casual, offhand statement to make changes. An example of a personal behavior change contract can be found in the front of your textbook. After identifying your first behavior change goal, take a few minutes to complete your personal contract to modify this unhealthy behavior. Completion of this written contract serves several important purposes. First, the contract provides a clear statement of your goal and the start date to take action. Second, this contract should contain details of

---

FITNESS AND WELLNESS FOR ALL

Wellness Issues Across the Population

The steps required to achieve wellness are the same across all populations. However, some individuals may experience difficulties in achieving wellness due to factors related to ethnicity, gender, age, and socioeconomic status. For example, compared to the U.S. population as a whole, the risk of developing hypertension (high blood pressure) is greater among African Americans. Similarly, diabetes is more common in Native Americans or people with a Latino heritage. Further, men and women differ in their risk for heart disease, osteoporosis, and certain types of cancer. Aging can also affect the ability of people to fulfill wellness. For instance, the risk of many diseases (e.g., heart disease and cancer) increases with age. Finally, people earning low incomes experience a higher incidence of obesity, heart disease, and drug abuse. Therefore, although wellness goals are similar across all populations, individual differences among people can present special challenges in achieving wellness. This important issue will be discussed throughout this book.

your plan and the steps you will take to measure your success. Further, this contract should list potential rewards for obtaining goals and identify dates for complete elimination of the selected behavior.

☀ Wellness Goals for the Nation

Healthy people are one of a nation's greatest resources. Poor health drains national resources by reducing worker productivity and increasing the amount of government money spent on health care. Because of this fact, the U.S. government has established wellness goals for the nation. The government's nationwide Healthy People Initiative seeks to prevent unnecessary disease and to improve the quality of life for all Americans. The wellness goals for the nation are discussed in Healthy People reports first published in 1980 and revised every 10 years. Each report includes a broad range of health and wellness objectives based on 10-year agendas. For example, major objectives contained in the current report (*Healthy People 2010*) include increasing the span of healthy life of all Americans and reducing health disparities across special populations of our society (Fitness and Wellness for All). For more details on the goals and objectives of *Healthy People 2010,* see Table 1.1 or visit the Healthy People Web site listed at the end of this chapter.

☀ IN SUMMARY

- Wellness is defined as a state of optimal health achieved by living a healthy lifestyle.
- Wellness is composed of six interacting components: physical health, emotional health, intellectual health, spiritual health, social health, and environmental health.

☀ Physical Activity vs. Exercise: What's the Difference?

Before we begin our discussion of the health benefits of exercise, a definition of both physical activity and exercise is necessary. Although the terms "physical activity" and "exercise" are often used interchangeably in newspapers and magazines, these terms do not mean the same thing. For example, physical activity is defined as any movement of the body produced by a skeletal muscle that results in exercise expenditure (39, 41). So, physical activity includes all physical movement regardless of the level of energy expenditure. Examples of physical activity include activities such as housework, gardening, or getting out of bed in the morning. By contrast, exercise is defined as a planned,

---

| **TABLE 1.1**
Healthy People 2010 |
| --- |
| Healthy People is a national health promotion and disease prevention initiative developed and coordinated by U.S. Department of Health and Human Services, Office of Diseases Prevention and Health Promotion. The goal of *Healthy People 2010* is to improve the health of all Americans, eliminate disparities in health across populations, and improve years and quality of healthy life. This goal is to be achieved by meeting numerous health-related objectives. Selected *Healthy People 2010* objectives are listed below.
• Increase the proportion of people who engage in daily physical activity.
• Reduce activity limitation due to chronic back conditions.
• Reduce the prevalence of cigarette smoking among people.
• Increase the consumption of fruits and vegetables.
• Reduce the lung cancer death rate.
• Reduce the prostate cancer death rate.
• Reduce the melanoma death rate.
• Reduce the number of college students engaging in heavy drinking of alcoholic beverages.
• Reduce the proportion of people who experience adverse health effects from stress each year.
• Reduce the prevalence of overweight people (age 20 and older). |

structured, and repetitive bodily movement done to improve or maintain one or more components of physical fitness (39, 41). Therefore, exercise is a subcategory of physical activity. That is, exercise is physical activity that is planned, structured, and designed to contribute to physical fitness. It follows that virtually all conditioning activities and sports are considered exercise because they are planned and contribute to the maintenance or improvement of physical fitness. A primary focus of this book is on the application of regular exercise as a means of improving physical fitness and maintaining good health. Let's begin our discussion with an introduction to the health benefits of exercise.

HEALTH BENEFITS OF EXERCISE

Why exercise? Almost all of us ask this question at some time in our lives. The answer is simple: Exercise is good for you. Indeed, regular exercise makes us feel better and look better, and provides added vitality and energy to achieve everyday tasks. And perhaps more importantly, it can improve your health and assist in achieving total wellness (1–7, 40–43). The importance of regular exercise in promoting good health and

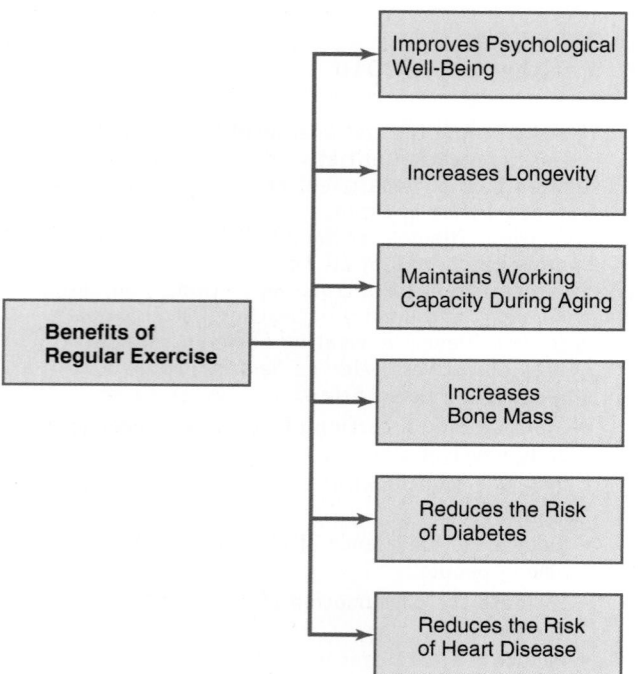

FIGURE 1.2
Benefits of regular exercise.

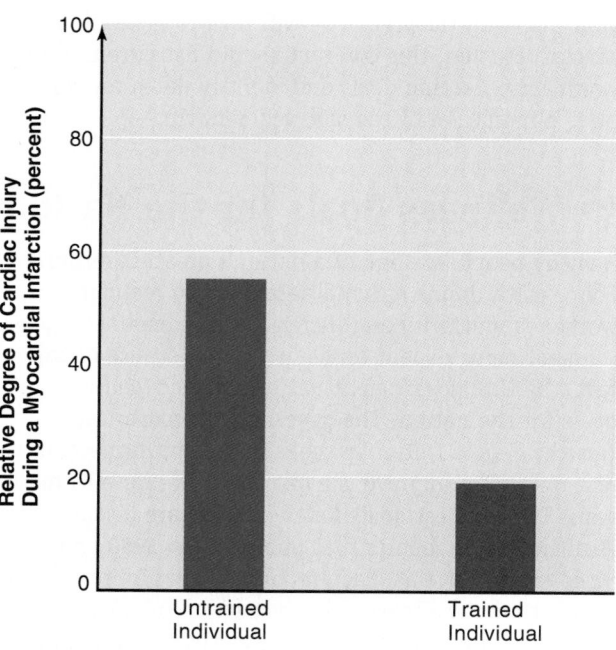

FIGURE 1.3
Regular endurance exercise protects the heart against injury during a heart attack. This figure illustrates that during a myocardial infarction (i.e., heart attack), exercise-trained individuals suffer less cardiac (i.e., heart) injury compared to the untrained individuals.
Source: Data from Yamashita et al., "Exercise provides direct biphasic cardioprotection via manganese superoxide dismutase activation," *Journal of Experimental Medicine* 189:1699–1706, 1999.

wellness is emphasized in a report by the Surgeon General. This report concludes that a lack of physical activity is a major public health problem in the United States, and that all Americans can improve their health by engaging in regular exercise. The Surgeon General's report recognizes numerous health benefits of exercise as illustrated in Figure 1.2. A discussion of the health benefits of exercise follows.

EXERCISE REDUCES THE RISK OF HEART DISEASE
Cardiovascular diseases (i.e., ailments of the heart and blood vessels) are a major cause of death in the United States (A Closer Look). In fact, one of every two Americans dies of cardiovascular disease (8). It is well established, however, that regular exercise can significantly reduce your risk of developing cardiovascular disease (1–4, 6–13). Further, strong evidence suggests that regular physical activity reduces the risk of death during a heart attack (14–17). The protective effect of exercise training during a heart attack is illustrated in

Figure 1.3. Notice that exercise training can reduce the magnitude of cardiac injury during a heart attack by 66% (15, 16). Many preventive medicine specialists argue that these facts alone are reason enough to exercise regularly (3, 9, 18). Chapter 9 provides a detailed discussion of exercise and cardiovascular disease.

EXERCISE REDUCES THE RISK OF DIABETES
Diabetes is a disease characterized by high blood sugar (glucose) levels. Untreated diabetes can result in numerous health problems, including blindness and kidney dysfunction. Regular exercise can reduce the risk of a specific type of diabetes, called type II (or "adult-onset" diabetes). Specifically, exercise reduces the risk of type II diabetes by improving the regulation of blood glucose (5, 19, 20). More is said about diabetes in Chapters 9 and 12.

EXERCISE INCREASES BONE MASS   The primary
functions of the skeleton are to provide a mechanical lever system of interconnected bones to permit movement, and to protect internal organs. Given these roles, it is important to maintain strong and healthy bones. The loss of bone mass and strength (called **osteoporosis**) increases the risk of bone fractures. Although osteoporosis can occur in men and women of all ages, it is more common in the elderly, particularly among women.

diabetes   A metabolic disorder characterized by high blood glucose levels. Chronic elevation of blood glucose is associated with increased incidence of heart disease, kidney disease, nerve dysfunction, and eye damage.

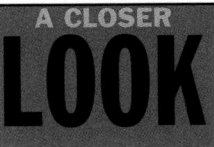

Coronary Heart Disease and Heart Attacks

Coronary heart disease (CHD) is a form of cardiovascular disease that results from a blockage of one or more of the arteries in the heart. The most common cause of coronary artery blockage is the formation of a fatty deposit (called plaque) composed of cholesterol, calcium, and fibrous tissue (9). Narrowing of coronary arteries due to plaque buildup can vary from a partial to a severe blockage.

Numerous influences contribute to the development of CHD. Damage to

the interior of a coronary artery creates an area that is vulnerable to the collection of cholesterol, and the formation of plaque begins. The factor(s) that create the original damage to the artery continue to be debated; stress and high blood pressure are potential causes (9). Once the plaque collection begins, elevated blood cholesterol increases the buildup and therefore accelerates the progress of disease.

Blockage of coronary arteries by plaque can reduce the blood flow to the working heart muscle during

heavy exercise, thereby depriving the heart of needed oxygen and nutrients. Inadequate heart blood flow can result in chest pain (called angina), and advanced CHD can result in complete blockage of a coronary artery. When the heart is deprived of blood flow for several minutes, a heart attack or **myocardial infarction (MI)** occurs, resulting in the death of heart muscle cells. Mild MIs result in the death of only a few heart cells, while severe MIs can destroy hundreds or even thousands of heart cells. Damage to a large portion of the heart reduces its effectiveness as a pump, and in severe cases can result in death.

Is there a link between exercise and maintenance of good bone health? Yes! A key factor in regulating bone mass and strength is mechanical force applied by muscular activity. Indeed, numerous studies have demonstrated that regular exercise increases bone mass and strength in young adults (21–23). Further, research on osteoporosis suggests that regular exercise can prevent bone loss in the elderly and is also useful in the treatment of the osteoporotic patient (21).

EXERCISE MAINTAINS PHYSICAL WORKING CAPACITY DURING AGING
Human aging is characterized by a gradual loss of physical working capacity. As we grow older, there is a progressive decline in our ability to perform strenuous activities (e.g., running, cycling, or swimming). Although this process may begin as early as the 20s, the most dramatic changes occur after approximately 60 years of age (1, 24–26). It is well established that regular exercise training can reduce the rate of decline in physical working capacity during aging (24, 27, 28). This fact is illustrated in Figure 1.4. Notice the differences in physical working capacity among highly trained, moderately trained, and inactive individuals during the aging process. The key point is that, although a natural decline of physical working capacity occurs with age, regular exercise can reduce the rate of this decline, resulting in an increased ability to enjoy a lifetime of physical recreation. Indeed, perhaps the most important benefit of regular exercise may be the improved quality of life associated with being physically fit.

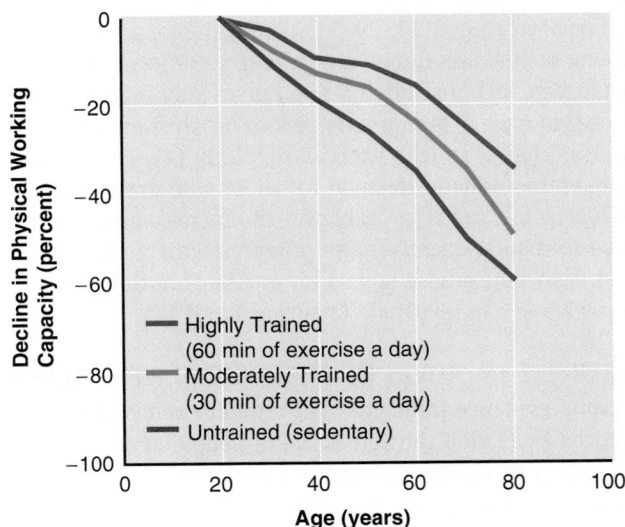

FIGURE 1.4
The relationship among age, physical activity, and decline in physical working capacity.

myocardial infarction (MI)   Damage to the heart due to a reduction in blood flow, resulting in the death of heart muscle cells.
osteoporosis   The loss of bone mass and strength, which increases the risk of bone fractures.

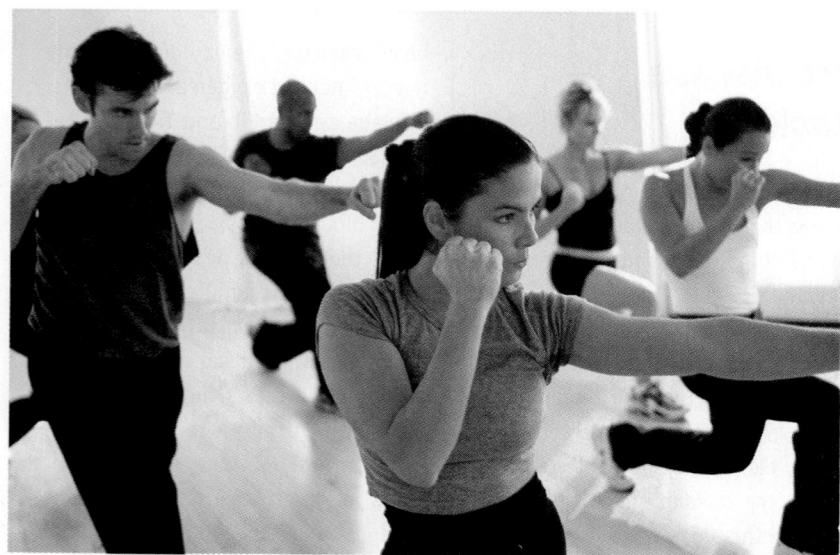

Regular exercise can prevent loss of bone mass.

EXERCISE INCREASES LONGEVITY Although it is controversial, growing evidence suggests that regular exercise (combined with a healthy lifestyle) increases longevity (1, 3, 4, 17, 29–31). For example, a classic study of Harvard alumni over the past 30 years reported that men with a sedentary (i.e., physically inactive) lifestyle have a 31% greater risk of death from all causes than men who exercise regularly (4). This translates into a longer life span for those who exercise. What factors are responsible for the increased longevity due to regular exercise? The primary factor is that individuals who exercise have a lower risk of both heart attack and cancer (3, 4) (Chapters 9 and 14).

EXERCISE IMPROVES PSYCHOLOGICAL WELL-BEING Strong evidence indicates that regular exercise improves psychological well-being in people of all ages. Specifically, the mental health benefits of regular exercise include a reduction in anxiety, depression, and reactivity to stress (1). These mental benefits of exercise lead to an improved sense of well-being in the physically active individual. We will further discuss the role of exercise as a method for reducing psychological stress in Chapter 10.

☀ IN SUMMARY

- Regular exercise reduces the risk of both heart disease and diabetes.
- Exercise increases bone mass in young people and reduces bone loss in the elderly.
- Systematic physical activity maintains physical working capacity during aging.
- Regular exercise has been shown to increase longevity and improve quality of life.
- Exercise promotes psychological well-being and reduces feelings of depression and anxiety.

☀ Exercise Does Not Guarantee Good Health

We have seen that there are many good reasons for engaging in regular exercise. While it is well established that exercise can lower risk of coronary heart disease (CHD), reduce the loss in physical working capacity due to aging, and generally improve the quality of life, exercise alone does not guarantee good health. Indeed, good health is the complex interaction of many variables. Factors such as age, gender, genetics, diet, lifestyle, smoking habits, and environment all contribute to the risk of disease (1, 3–7). The interaction among exercise, nutrition, and factors that increase the risk of disease is discussed throughout this text.

☀ Exercise Training for Health-Related Fitness

In general, exercise conditioning programs can be divided into two broad categories defined by their goals: exercise training to improve sport performance and health-related physical fitness. This textbook focuses on health-related fitness. The overall goal of a total health-related physical fitness program is to optimize

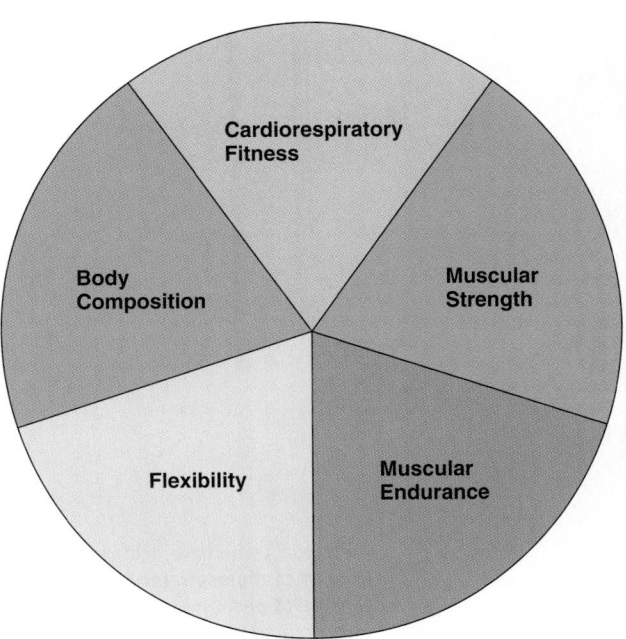

FIGURE 1.5
Components of health-related physical fitness.

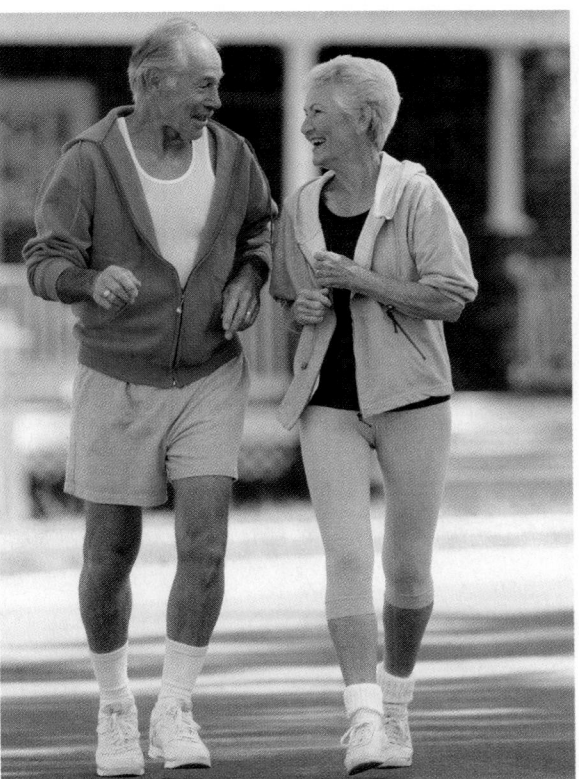

Regular physical activity has been shown to improve longevity.

the quality of life (1, 2, 10). The specific goals of this type of fitness program are to reduce the risk of disease and to improve total physical fitness so that daily tasks can be completed with less effort and fatigue.

Although some conditioning programs aimed at improving sport performance may reduce the risk of disease, this is not their primary purpose. By contrast, the single goal of sport conditioning is to improve physical performance in a specific sport. However, the "weekend" athlete who engages in a total health-related physical fitness program could also improve his or her physical performance in many sports. Specifically, a health-related fitness program improves sport performance by increasing **muscular strength** and **endurance**, improving flexibility, and reducing the risk of injury, as we see in the chapters that follow.

COMPONENTS OF HEALTH-RELATED PHYSICAL FITNESS

Exercise scientists (i.e., experts in exercise and physical fitness) do not always agree on all of the basic components of physical fitness. However, most do agree that the five major components of total health-related physical fitness (Figure 1.5) are

1. cardiorespiratory endurance
2. muscular strength
3. muscular endurance
4. flexibility
5. body composition

In addition to these, many people also include motor skill performance as a sixth component. Motor skills are those movement qualities, such as agility and coordination, that are required to achieve success in athletics. Although motor skills are important to sport performance, they are not directly linked to improvement of health in young adults and are therefore not considered a major component of health-related physical fitness.

CARDIORESPIRATORY FITNESS   Cardiorespiratory fitness (sometimes called aerobic fitness or cardiorespiratory endurance) is considered a key component of health-related physical fitness. It is a measure of the heart's ability to pump oxygen-rich blood to the working muscles during exercise. It is also a measure of the muscles' ability to take up and use the delivered oxygen to produce the energy needed to continue exercising. In practical terms, cardiorespiratory endurance is

---

muscular strength   The maximal ability of a muscle to generate force.
muscular endurance   The ability of a muscle to generate force over and over again.

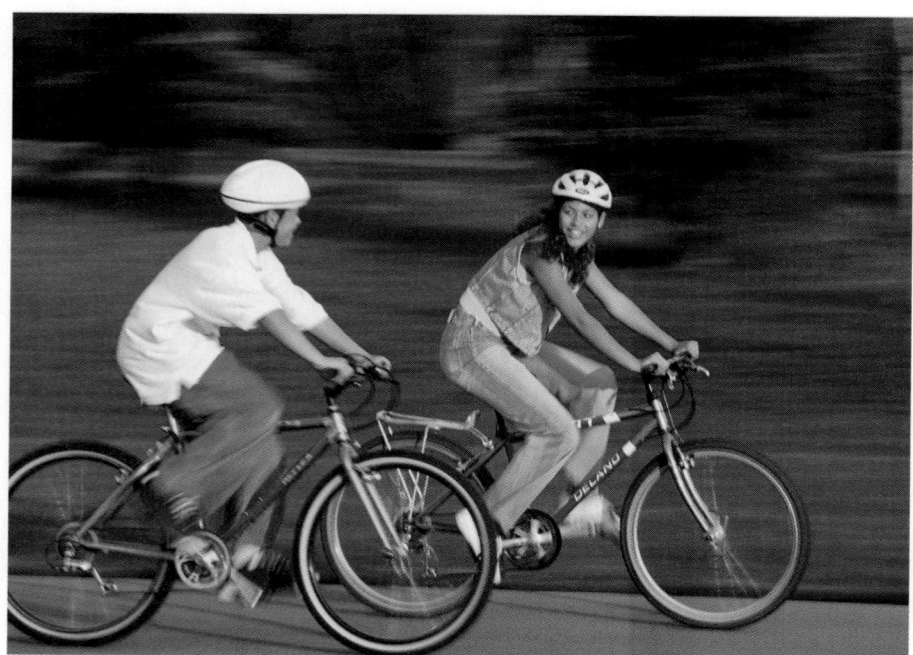

Individuals who have achieved a high level of cardiorespiratory fitness are capable of performing 30 to 60 minutes of vigorous exercise without undue fatigue.

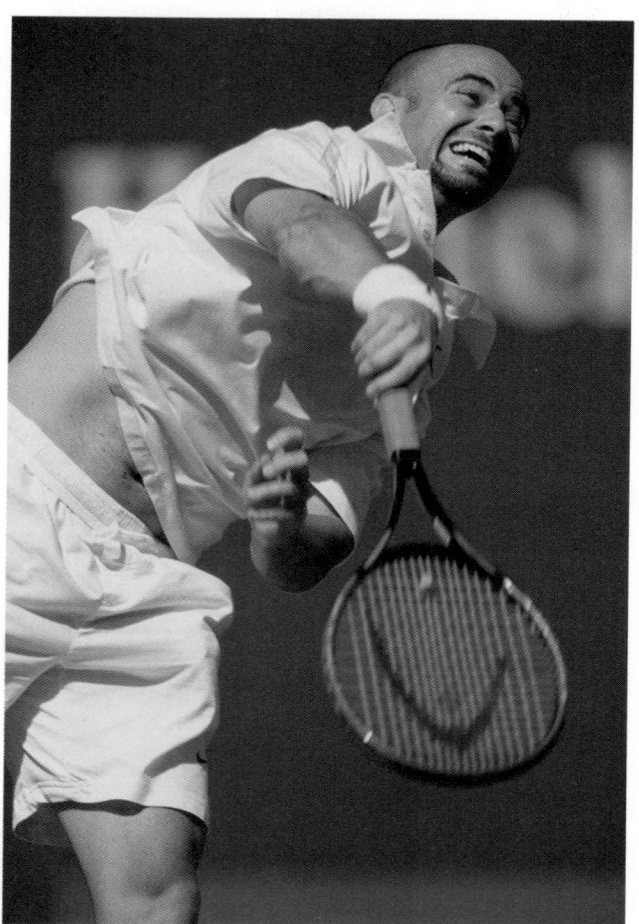

Professional tennis players require a high level of muscular endurance to play long matches.

the ability to perform endurance-type exercises (distance running, cycling, swimming, etc.). The individual that has achieved a high measure of cardiorespiratory endurance is generally capable of performing 30 to 60 minutes of vigorous exercise without undue fatigue. Chapter 4 discusses the details of exercise training designed to improve cardiorespiratory fitness.

MUSCULAR STRENGTH   Muscular strength is the maximal ability of a muscle to generate force (32–34). It is evaluated by how much force a muscle (or muscle group) can generate during a single maximal contraction. Practically, this means how much weight an individual can lift during one maximal effort.

Muscular strength is important in almost all sports. Sports such as football, basketball, and events in track and field require a high level of muscular strength. Even nonathletes require some degree of muscular strength to function in everyday life. For example, routine tasks around the home, such as lifting bags of groceries and moving furniture, require muscular strength. Weight training (also called strength training) results in an increase in the size and strength of muscles. The principles of developing muscular strength are presented in Chapter 5.

MUSCULAR ENDURANCE   Muscular endurance is defined as the ability of a muscle to generate force over and over again. Although muscular strength and muscular endurance are related, they are not the same. These two terms can be best distinguished by examples. An excellent example of muscular strength is a person lifting a heavy barbell during one maximal muscular

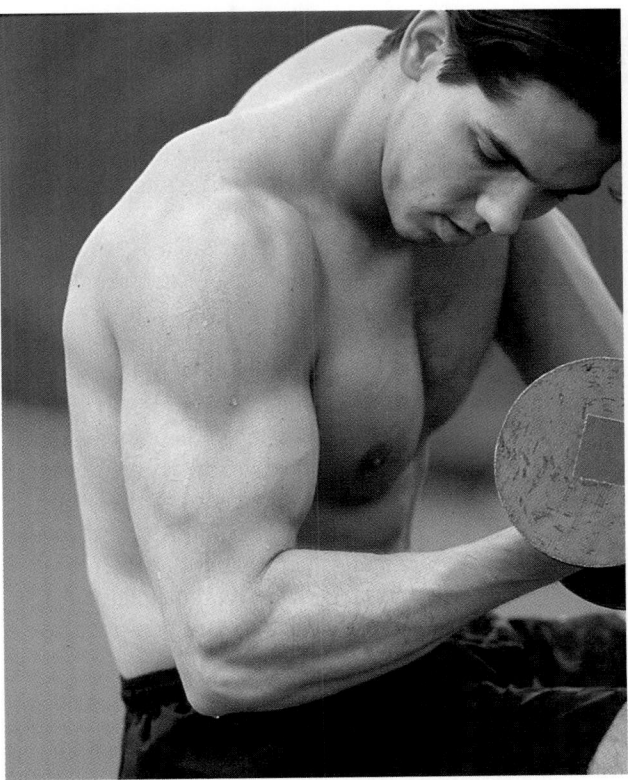

Weight training results in an increase in muscular strength.

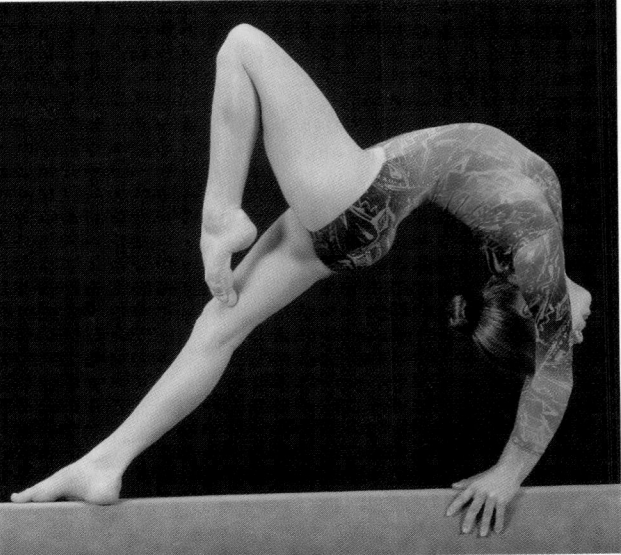

Gymnasts require great flexibility to be successful.

effort. In contrast, muscular endurance is illustrated by a weight lifter performing multiple lifts or repetitions of a lighter weight.

Most successfully played sports require muscular endurance. For instance, tennis players, who must repeatedly swing their racquets during a match, require a high level of muscular endurance. Many everyday activities (e.g., waxing your car) also require some level of muscular endurance. Techniques of developing muscular endurance are discussed in Chapter 5.

FLEXIBILITY   Flexibility is the ability to move joints freely through their full range of motion. Flexible individuals can bend and twist at their joints with ease. Without routine stretching, muscles and tendons shorten and become tight; this can retard the range of motion around joints and impair flexibility.

Individual needs for flexibility vary. Certain athletes (such as gymnasts and divers) require great flexibility in order to accomplish complex movements. The average individual requires less flexibility than an athlete; however, everyone needs some flexibility in order to perform activities of daily living. Research suggests that flexibility is useful in preventing some types of muscle–tendon injuries and may be useful in reducing low back pain (35, 36). Techniques for improving flexibility are discussed in Chapter 6.

BODY COMPOSITION   The term body composition refers to the relative amounts of fat and lean body tissue (muscle, organs, bone) found in your body. The rationale for including body composition as a component of health-related physical fitness is that having a high percentage of body fat (a condition known as obesity) is associated with an increased risk of CHD. Obesity increases the risk of development of type II diabetes and contributes to joint stress during movement. In general, being "over-fat" elevates the risk of medical problems.

Lack of physical activity has been shown to play a major role in gaining body fat. Conversely, regular exercise is an important factor in promoting the loss of body fat. Assessment of body composition is discussed in Chapter 2, and the relationship between exercise and weight loss is discussed in Chapter 8.

☀ IN SUMMARY
Health-related physical fitness comprises five components:

- cardiorespiratory fitness
- muscular strength
- muscular endurance
- flexibility
- body composition

> **flexibility**   The ability to move joints freely through their full range of motion.
> **body composition**   The relative amounts of fat and lean body tissue (muscle, organs, bone) found in the body.

> **TABLE 1.2**
> **Strategies for Setting Exercise Goals**
>
> - Establish achievable goals.
> - Put goals in writing and in a place where you can see them every day.
> - Establish both short-term and long-term goals.
> - Establish goals that are measurable.
> - Set target dates for achieving goals.
> - After you achieve a goal, establish another achievable goal.
> - Reward yourself after achieving each goal.

Motivation and Setting Exercise Goals

Achieving physical fitness requires time and effort. Unfortunately, many people who begin an exercise program stop before much progress has been achieved. Fitness cannot be achieved in a matter of a few days. In general, 3 to 6 weeks of regular exercise is required for noticeable improvements in muscle tone or muscular endurance. After beginning your personal fitness program, be patient; improvement will come, and you will like the changes.

The key to maintaining a long-term exercise program is personal motivation. Motivation, in this case, can be viewed as the energy required to maintain your drive to engage in daily exercise (33). The motivation to change from a sedentary lifestyle to an active lifestyle requires behavior modification and establishing goals. Without question, goal-setting is the cornerstone of any successful exercise program. Establishing realistic goals provides a target for your fitness efforts.

Table 1.2 contains some helpful information concerning exercise goal-setting. Note, it is important to establish both short-term and long-term goals. Short-term goals permit you to achieve a goal in a few weeks or months, whereas long-term goals are designed to provide motivation for years to come. Achievement of a short-term goal delivers great personal satisfaction and provides the needed incentive to pursue another fitness goal.

An additional point to notice in Table 1.2 is that goals should be written down. Putting exercise goals on paper is an excellent means of establishing a "contract" with yourself to maintain regular exercise habits. Another important aspect of goal-setting is that goals should be measurable. For example, your short-term goal for weight loss might be to lose 5 pounds during a period of 6 weeks. Because body weight is easily measured, you can assess your progress toward the attainment of your goal by periodic weighing. After achieving a fitness goal, it is important to set new goals to provide the incentive and motivation to continue your fitness program. More guidance in exercise goal-setting is provided in Chapters 3 and 16.

Physical Fitness and Wellness: A Final Word

In this chapter we discussed the benefits of regular exercise and the importance of a healthy lifestyle to achieve wellness. The remainder of this book will present information that will help you set goals to increase your physical fitness, enrich your diet, and improve your health. Simply reading this book, however, will not accomplish these goals. Achieving physical fitness and wellness requires a personal commitment to regular exercise and wise lifestyle choices. Indeed, there is no "magic pill" that you can take to make you healthy or improve your physical fitness. Start today and become an exercise convert; your body will love you for it!

Summary

1. The term wellness means "healthy living." This state is achieved by the practice of a positive healthy lifestyle, which includes regular physical activity, proper nutrition, eliminating unhealthy behaviors (avoiding high-risk activities such as reckless driving, smoking, and drug use), and maintaining good emotional and spiritual health.

2. Total wellness can be achieved only by a balance of physical, emotional, intellectual, spiritual, social, and environmental health. The components of wellness do not work in isolation; the six components interact strongly. For example, poor physical health can lead to poor emotional health. Similarly, a lack of spiritual health can contribute to poor emotional health as well as poor physical health. Finally, achieving total wellness also requires learning about the environment and protecting yourself against environmental hazards such as air pollution and contaminated water.

3. Exercise offers many health benefits. Regular exercise has been shown to reduce risk of CHD and diabetes, increase bone mass, and maintain physical working capacity during normal aging.

4. The five major components of "total" health-related physical fitness are:
cardiorespiratory endurance
muscular strength
muscular endurance
flexibility
body composition

5. Setting exercise goals is a key component in the maintenance of a lifetime fitness program.

Study Questions

1. Define the wellness concept.

2. List and discuss the six components of wellness.

3. Define the term body composition.

4. What is cardiorespiratory endurance?

5. Define osteoporosis.

6. List and discuss four major health benefits of regular exercise.

7. Discuss fitness training for sport performance versus training for health-related fitness.

8. List and discuss the five components of health-related fitness.

9. Outline the seven strategies for setting exercise goals.

Suggested Reading

Blair, S. N., M. LaMonte, and M. Nichaman. The evolution of physical activity recommendations: How much is enough? *American Journal of Clinical Nutrition* 79:913S–920S, 2004.

Blair, S., and M. Moore. Surgeon General's report on physical fitness. The inside story. *ACSM's Health and Physical Journal* 1:14–18, 1997.

Brooks, G. A., N. Butte, W. Rand, J. Flatt, and B. Caballero. Chronicle of the Institute of Medicine physical activity recommendation: How a physical activity recommendation came to be among dietary recommendations. *American Journal of Clinical Nutrition* 79:921S–930S, 2004.

Brown, D., D. Brown, G. Heath, L. Balluz, W. Giles, E. Ward, and A. Mokdad. Associations between physical activity dose and health-related quality of life. *Medicine and Science in Sports and Exercise* 36:890–896, 2004.

Franklin, B. Improved fitness = Increased longevity. *ACSM's Health and Fitness Journal* 5:32–33, 2001.

Howley, E., and D. Franks. *Health Fitness Instructor's Handbook.* 4th edition. Human Kinetics Publishers. Champaign, IL. 2003

Powers, S. and E. Howley. *Exercise Physiology: Theory and Application to Fitness and Performance.* 5th edition. McGraw Hill, St. Louis, MO. 2004.

Powers, S., S. Lennon, J. Quindry, and J. Mehta. Exercise and cardioprotection. *Current Opinion in Cardiology.* 17:495–502, 2002.

Thompson, P., et al. Exercise and physical activity in the prevention and treatment of atherosclerotic cardiovascular disease. *Circulation* 107:3109–3116, 2003.

For links to the web sites below visit The Total Fitness and Wellness Website at www.aw-bc.com/powers.

American Heart Association

Contains latest information about ways to reduce your risk of heart and vascular diseases. Site includes information about exercise, diet, and heart disease.

American College of Sports Medicine

Contains information about exercise, health, and fitness.

WebMD

Contains the latest information on a variety of health-related topics including diet, exercise, and stress. Links to nutrition, fitness, and wellness topics.

Healthy People

Contains information about the U.S. government's initiative to improve health and wellness for the American people.

References

1. Bouchard, C., R. Shephard, T. Stephens, J. Sutton, and B. McPherson, eds. *Exercise, Fitness, and Health: A Consensus of Current Knowledge.* Champaign, IL: Human Kinetics, 1990.

2. Margen, S., et al., eds. *The Wellness Encyclopedia.* Boston: Houghton Mifflin, 1995.

3. Paffenbarger, R., J. Kampert, I-Min Lee, R. Hyde, R. Leung, and A. Wing. Changes in physical activity and other lifeway patterns influencing longevity. *Medicine and Science in Sports and Exercise* 26:857–865, 1994.

4. Paffenbarger, R., R. Hyde, A. Wing, and C. Hsieh. Physical activity, all cause mortality, longevity of college alumni. *New England Journal of Medicine* 314:605–613, 1986.

5. Helmrich, S., D. Ragland, and R. Paffenbarger. Prevention of non-insulin-dependent diabetes mellitus with physical activity. *Medicine and Science in Sports and Exercise* 26:824–830, 1994.

6. Wood, P. Physical activity, diet, and health: Independent and interactive effects. *Medicine and Science in Sports and Exercise* 26:838–843, 1994.

7. Morris, J. Exercise in the prevention of coronary heart disease: Today's best buy in public health. *Medicine and Science in Sports and Exercise* 26:807–814, 1994.

8. American Heart Association. *Heart and Stroke Facts.* Dallas, TX. 2004.

9. Barrow, M. *Heart Talk: Understanding Cardiovascular Diseases.* Gainesville, FL: Cor-Ed Publishing, 1992.

10. Pollock, M., and J. Wilmore. *Exercise in Health and Disease.* Philadelphia: W. B. Saunders, 1990.

11. Williams, P. T. Relationship between distance run per week to coronary heart disease risk factors in 8283 male runners. The National Runners Health Study. *Archives of Internal Medicine* 157:191–198, 1997.

12. Fagard, R. Physical activity in the prevention and treatment of hypertension in the obese. *Medicine and Science in Sports and Exercise* 31:S624–S630, 1999.

13. Williams, P. Physical fitness and activity as separate heart disease risk factors: A meta-analysis. *Medicine and Science in Sports and Exercise* 33:754–761, 2001.

14. Lennon, S., J. Quindry, K. Hamilton, J. French, J. Staib, J. Mehta, and S. K. Powers. Loss of cardioprotection after cessation of exercise. *Journal of Applied Physiology* 96:1299–1305, 2004.

15. Powers, S., M. Locke, and H. Demirel. Exercise, heat shock proteins, and myocardial protection from I-R injury. *Medicine and Science in Sports and Exercise* 33:386–392, 2001.

16. Hamilton, K., J. Staib, T. Phillips, A. Hess, S. Lennon, and S. Powers. Exercise, antioxidants, and HSP72: Protection against myocardial ischemia-reperfusion. *Free Radicals in Biology and Medicine* 34:800–809, 2003.

17. Lee, I. M., and R. Paffenbarger. Associations of light, moderate, and vigorous intensity physical activity with longevity: The Harvard Alumni Health Study. *American Journal of Epidemiology* 151:293–299, 2000.

18. Powell, K., and S. Blair. The public health burdens of sedentary living habits: Theoretical but realistic estimates. *Medicine and Science in Sports and Exercise* 26:851–856, 1994.

19. Rodnick, K., J. Holloszy, C. Mondon, and D. James. Effects of exercise training on insulin-regulatable glucose-transporter protein levels in rat skeletal muscle. *Diabetes* 39:1425–1429, 1990.

20. Pan, X. R., et al. Effects of diet and exercise in preventing NIDDM in people with impaired glucose tolerance. *Diabetes Care* 20:537–544, 1997.

21. Rankin, J. Diet, exercise, and osteoporosis. *Certified News* (American College of Sports Medicine) 3:1–4, 1993.

22. Wheeler, D., J. Graves, G. Miller, R. Vander Griend, T. Wronski, S. K. Powers, and H. Park. Effects of running on the torsional strength, morphometry, and bone mass on the rat skeleton. *Medicine and Science in Sports and Exercise* 27:520–529, 1995.

23. Taaffe, D., T. Robinson, C. Snow, and R. Marcus. High impact exercise promotes bone gain in well-trained female athletes. *Journal of Bone and Mineral Research* 12:255–260, 1997.

24. Hagberg, J. Effect of training in the decline of VO_{2max} with aging. *Federation Proceedings* 46:1830–1833, 1987.

25. Fleg, J., and E. Lakatta. Role of muscle loss in the age-associated reduction in VO2max. *Journal of Applied Physiology* 65:1147–1151, 1988.

26. Nakamura, E., T. Moritani, and A. Kanetaka. Effects of habitual physical exercise on physiological age in men and women aged 20–85 years as estimated using principal component analysis. *European Journal of Applied Physiology* 73:410–418, 1996.

27. Hammeren, J., S. Powers, J. Lawler, D. Criswell, D. Martin, D. Lowenthal, and M. Pollock. Exercise training–induced alterations in skeletal muscle oxidative and antioxidant enzyme activity in senescent rats. *International Journal of Sports Medicine* 13:412–416, 1992.

28. Powers, S., J. Lawler, D. Criswell, Fu-Kong Lieu, and D. Martin. Aging and respiratory muscle metabolic plasticity: Effects of endurance training. *Journal of Applied Physiology* 72:1068–1073, 1992.

29. Holloszy, J. Exercise increases average longevity of female rats despite increased food intake and no growth retardation. *Journal of Gerontology* 48:B97–B100, 1993.

30. Lee, I., R. Paffenbarger, and C. Hennekens. Physical activity, physical fitness, and longevity. *Aging-Milano* 9:2–11, 1997.

31. Franklin, B. Improved fitness 5 increased longevity. *ACSM's Health and Fitness Journal* 5:32–33, 2001.

32. Powers, S., and E. Howley. *Exercise Physiology: Theory and Application to Fitness and Performance,* 4th ed. St. Louis: McGraw-Hill, 2001.

33. Roberts, R., and S. Keteyian. *Fundamental Principles of Exercise Physiology: For Fitness, Performance, and Health.* St. Louis: McGraw-Hill, 2002.

34. Williams, M. *Lifetime Fitness and Wellness.* Dubuque, IA: Wm. C. Brown, 1996.

35. Cady, L., D. Bischoff, E. O'Connell, P. Thomas, and J. Allan. Strength and fitness and subsequent back injuries in fire-fighters. *Journal of Occupational Medicine* 4:269–272, 1979.

36. Cady, L., P. Thomas, and R. Karasky. Programs for increasing health and physical fitness of fire-fighters. *Journal of Occupational Medicine* 2:111–114, 1985.

37. U.S. Department of Health and Human Services. Physical activity and health: A report of the Surgeon General. U.S. Department of Health and Human Services, Centers for Disease Control and Prevention, National Center for Chronic Disease Prevention and Health Promotion, Atlanta, GA, 1996.

38. Armbruster, B., and L. Gladwin. More than fitness for older adults. *ACSM's Health and Fitness Journal* 5:6–12, 2001.

39. Nieman, D. *Exercise Testing and Prescription: A Health-related Approach.* 5th edition. McGraw Hill, St. Louis, MO. 2002.

40. Blair, S. N., M. LaMonte, and M. Nichaman. The evolution of physical activity recommendations: How much is enough? *American Journal of Clinical Nutrition* 79:913–920S, 2004.

41. Thompson, P., et al. Exercise and physical activity in the prevention and treatment of atherosclerotic cardiovascular disease. *Circulation* 107:3109–3116, 2003.

42. Brooks, G. A., N. Butte, W. Rand, J. Flatt, and B. Caballero. Chronicle of the Institute of Medicine. Physical activity recommendation: How a physical activity recommendation came to be among dietary recommendations. *American Journal of Clinical Nutrition* 79:921S–930S, 2004.

43. Brown, D., D. Brown, G. Heath, L. Balluz, W. Giles, E. Ward, and A. Mokdad. Associations between physical activity dose and health-related quality of life. *Medicine and Science in Sports and Exercise* 36:890–896, 2004.

Lifestyle Assessment Inventory

NAME _____ DATE _____

The purpose of this lifestyle assessment inventory is to increase your awareness of areas in your life that increase your risk of disease, injury, and possibly premature death. A key point to remember is that you have control over each of the lifestyle areas discussed.

Awareness is the first step in making change. After identifying the areas that require modification, you will be able to use the behavior modification techniques presented in Chapter 10 to bring about positive lifestyle changes.

DIRECTIONS

Put a check by each statement that applies to you. You may select more than one choice per category.

A. PHYSICAL FITNESS

_____ I exercise for a minimum of 20 to 30 minutes at least 3 days per week.

_____ I play sports routinely (2 to 3 times per week).

_____ I walk for 15 to 30 minutes (3 to 7 days per week).

B. BODY FAT

_____ There is no place on my body where I can pinch more than 1 inch of fat.

_____ I am satisfied with the way my body appears.

C. STRESS LEVEL

_____ I find it easy to relax.

_____ I rarely feel tense or anxious.

_____ I am able to cope with daily stresses without undue emotional stress.

D. CAR SAFETY

_____ I have not had an auto accident in the past 4 years.

_____ I always use a seat belt when I drive.

_____ I rarely drive above the speed limit.

E. SLEEP

_____ I always get 7 to 9 hours of sleep.

_____ I do not have trouble going to sleep.

_____ I generally do not wake up during the night.

(continued on next page)

F. RELATIONSHIPS

_____ I have a happy and satisfying relationship with my spouse or boy/girl friend.

_____ I have a lot of close friends.

_____ I get a great deal of love and support from my family.

G. DIET

_____ I generally eat three balanced meals per day.

_____ I rarely overeat.

_____ I rarely eat large quantities of fatty foods and sweets.

H. ALCOHOL USE

_____ I consume fewer than two drinks per day.

_____ I never get intoxicated.

_____ I never drink and drive.

I. TOBACCO USE

_____ I never smoke (cigarettes, pipe, cigars, etc.).

_____ I am not exposed to second-hand smoke on a regular basis.

_____ I do not use smokeless tobacco.

J. DRUG USE

_____ I never use illicit drugs.

_____ I never abuse legal drugs such as diet or sleeping pills.

K. SEXUAL PRACTICES

_____ I always practice safe sex (e.g., always using condoms or being involved in a monogamous relationship).

SCORING

1. Individual areas: If there are any unchecked areas in categories A through K, you can improve those aspects of your lifestyle.

2. Overall lifestyle: Add up your total number of checks. Scoring can be interpreted as follows:

23–29	Very healthy lifestyle
17–22	Average healthy lifestyle
≤16	Unhealthy lifestyle (needs improvement)

Fitness and Wellness Survey

NAME _____ DATE _____

Answer the following questions in the spaces provided.

1. List the previous fitness/wellness activities in which you have participated, or are currently participating in. Examples include recreational tennis, high school basketball, or yoga classes. Use extra paper if necessary.

_____

_____

_____

2. Which of these activities did you enjoy the most? Why?

_____

_____

_____

3. Which activity did you enjoy the least? Why?

_____

_____

_____

4. What components of physical fitness did these activities affect? For instance, jogging improves cardiovascular fitness, while weight lifting increases muscular strength.

_____

_____

_____

5. What areas of physical and mental health would you like to improve? Can you think of any physical activities that would aid in this goal?

_____

_____

_____

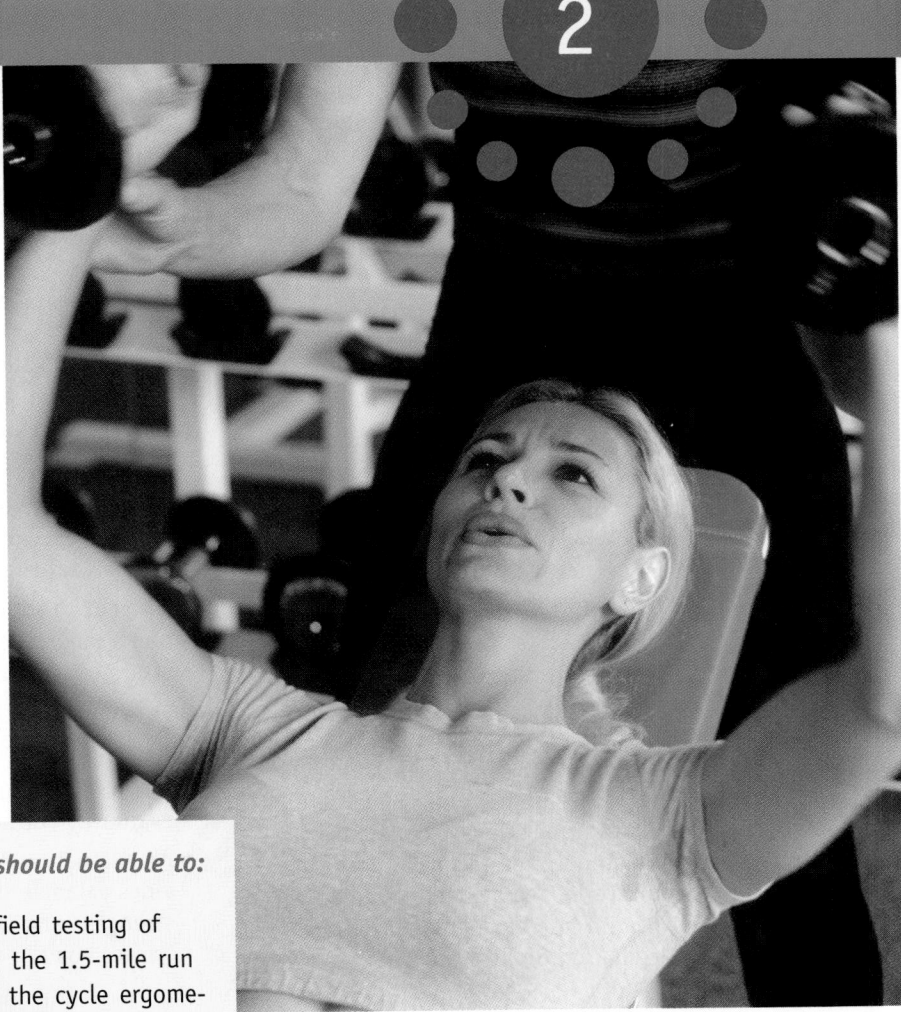

After studying this chapter, you should be able to:

1. Explain the principle behind field testing of cardiorespiratory fitness using the 1.5-mile run test, the 1-mile walking test, the cycle ergometer exercise test, and the step test.

2. Outline the design of the one-repetition maximum test for measurement of muscular strength.

3. Compare the push-up and sit-up tests as a means of evaluating muscular endurance.

4. Define the term *flexibility* and discuss two field tests used to assess it.

5. Discuss why assessment of body composition is important in health-related fitness testing.

6. Explain how body composition is assessed using hydrostatic weighing, the skinfold test, body mass index, and waist-to-hip circumference ratio.

Fitness Evaluation: Self-Testing

An objective evaluation of your current fitness status is important prior to beginning an exercise training program (1–7). This evaluation provides valuable information concerning your fitness strengths and weaknesses and enables you to set reasonable fitness goals. Further, testing your initial fitness level also provides a benchmark against which you can compare future evaluations. Periodic re-testing (e.g., every three to six months) provides motivating feedback as your fitness program progresses.

This chapter presents a battery of physical fitness tests you can use to assess your fitness level. These tests are designed to evaluate each of the major components of health-related physical fitness: cardiorespiratory fitness, muscular strength, muscular endurance, flexibility, and body composition.

Although the risks associated with regular exercise are generally less than the risks associated with living a sedentary lifestyle, it is important to evaluate your health status before engaging in any physical fitness test. A brief discussion of the need for medical clearance prior to beginning an exercise program follows.

☀ Evaluating Health Status

Is a medical exam required before beginning a fitness program? The answer is probably "no" for healthy college-age individuals (1, 2). Although regular medical exams are encouraged for everyone, most people under 29 years of age generally do not require special medical clearance before beginning a low-to-moderate intensity exercise program. However, if you have any concerns about your health, an examination by a physician is prudent prior to starting an exercise program. Laboratory 2.1 on p. 49 is a useful screening questionnaire for people of all ages who are beginning an exercise program. An answer of "yes" to any of the questions in Laboratory 2.1 suggests that a medical problem may exist and that a complete medical exam is required.

Should individuals over 30 years old have a medical exam at the beginning of an exercise program? The most conservative answer is "yes." This is particularly true for obese and/or sedentary individuals. The following general guidelines apply:

18–29 years (men and women): You should have had a medical checkup within the last 2 years and completed Laboratory 2.1.

30–39 years (men) and 30–44 years (women): You should have had a medical checkup within the last year and completed Laboratory 2.1.

40 years and above (men): You should have had a medical checkup and a physician-supervised stress test within the last year (A Closer Look).

45 years and above (women): You should have had a medical checkup and a physician-supervised stress test within the last year (A Closer Look).

☀ IN SUMMARY

- Prior to beginning a fitness program you should evaluate your health status.
- An evaluation of your current fitness status provides valuable information regarding fitness strengths and weaknesses and enables you to set fitness goals.

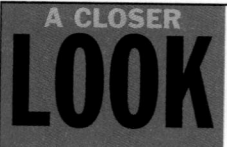

A CLOSER LOOK

The Exercise ECG

The electrocardiogram (ECG, or sometimes EKG) is a common medical test that measures the electrical activity of the heart and can be used to diagnose several types of heart disease (7, 8). Although a resting ECG is useful for determining the heart's function, ECG monitoring during exercise is particularly useful in diagnosing hidden heart problems, because heart abnormalities often appear during periods of emotional or exercise stress (7). An exercise ECG, commonly called an **exercise stress test,** is generally performed on a treadmill while a physician monitors heart rate, blood pressure, and ECG. The test begins with a brief warm-up period followed by a progressive increase in exercise intensity until the patient cannot continue or the physician stops the test for medical reasons. In general, the duration of the test varies as a function of the subject's fitness level. For example, poorly conditioned people may exercise for only a few minutes, whereas well-conditioned subjects may work for much longer periods. Therefore, the exercise stress test not only provides data about your cardiovascular health, but also provides information about cardiorespiratory fitness.

TABLE 2.1
Fitness Categories for Cooper's 1.5-Mile Run Test to Determine Cardiorespiratory Fitness

Fitness Category	Age (years)					
	13–19	**20–29**	**30–39**	**40–49**	**50–59**	**60+**
Men						
Very poor	>15:30	>16:00	>16:30	>17:30	>19:00	>20:00
Poor	12:11–15:30	14:01–16:00	14:46–16:30	15:36–17:30	17:01–19:00	19:01–20:00
Average	10:49–12:10	12:01–14:00	12:31–14:45	13:01–15:35	14:31–17:00	16:16–19:00
Good	9:41–10:48	10:46–12:00	11:01–12:30	11:31–13:00	12:31–14:30	14:00–16:15
Excellent	8:37–9:40	9:45–10:45	10:00–11:00	10:30–11:30	11:00–12:30	11:15–13:59
Superior	<8:37	<9:45	<10:00	<10:30	<11:00	<11:15
Women						
Very poor	>18:30	>19:00	>19:30	>20:00	>20:30	>21:00
Poor	16:55–18:30	18:31–19:00	19:01–19:30	19:31–20:00	20:01–20:30	20:31–21:31
Average	14:31–16:54	15:55–18:30	16:31–19:00	17:31–19:30	19:01–20:00	19:31–20:30
Good	12:30–14:30	13:31–15:54	14:31–16:30	15:56–17:30	16:31–19:00	17:31–19:30
Excellent	11:50–12:29	12:30–13:30	13:00–14:30	13:45–15:55	14:30–16:30	16:30–18:00
Superior	<11:50	<12:30	<13:00	<13:45	<14:30	<16:30

Times are given in minutes and seconds. (> = greater than; < = less than)

Source: From Cooper, K. The aerobics program for total well-being. Bantam Books, New York, 1982. Copyright © 1982 by Kenneth H. Cooper. Used by permission of Bantam Books, a division of Random House, Inc.

☀ Measuring Cardiorespiratory Fitness

As we saw in Chapter 1, cardiorespiratory fitness is the ability to perform endurance-type exercises (e.g., running, cycling, swimming) and is considered a key component of health-related physical fitness. The most accurate means of measuring cardiorespiratory fitness is the laboratory assessment of maximal oxygen consumption (9, 10) (called $\dot{V}O_{2max}$). In simple terms, $\dot{V}O_{2max}$ is a measure of the endurance capacity of both the cardiorespiratory system and exercising skeletal muscles. Because direct measurement of $\dot{V}O_{2max}$ requires expensive laboratory equipment and is very time consuming, it is impractical for general use. Fortunately, researchers have developed numerous methods for estimating $\dot{V}O_{2max}$ using simple field tests (11–13, 3). Although each of these of these tests is subject to error, the practical advantages of these field tests outweigh the disadvantages. In the following paragraphs we describe several types of field exercise tests designed to evaluate cardiorespiratory fitness.

THE 1.5-MILE RUN TEST

One of the simplest and most accurate means of evaluating cardiorespiratory fitness is the **1.5-mile run test**. This test, popularized by Dr. Kenneth Cooper, works on the physiological principle that people with a high level of cardiorespiratory fitness can run 1.5 miles in less time than less-fit individuals (11, 12).

The 1.5-mile run test is excellent for physically active college-age individuals. Due to its intensity, however, the 1.5-mile run test is not well suited for sedentary people over 30 years of age, severely deconditioned people, individuals with joint problems, and obese individuals.

exercise stress test   A diagnostic text designed to determine if a patient's cardiovascular system has a normal response to exercise. The test is generally performed on a treadmill while a physician monitors heart rate, blood pressure, and ECG.
1.5-mile run test   A fitness test designed to evaluate cardiorespiratory fitness. The objective of the test is to complete a 1.5-mile distance (preferably on a track) in the shortest possible time.

TABLE 2.2
Fitness Classification for 1-Mile Walk Test

Fitness Category	Age (years)			
	13–19	20–29	30–39	40+
Men				
Very poor	>17:30	>18:00	>19:00	>21:30
Poor	16:01–17:30	16:31–18:00	17:31–19:00	18:31–21:30
Average	14:01–16:00	14:31–16:30	15:31–17:30	16:01–18:30
Good	12:30–14:00	13:00–14:30	13:30–15:30	14:00–16:00
Excellent	<12:30	<13:00	<13:30	<14:00
Women				
Very poor	>18:01	>18:31	>19:31	>20:01
Poor	16:31–18:00	17:01–18:30	18:01–19:30	19:31–20:00
Average	14:31–16:30	15:01–17:00	16:01–18:00	18:01–19:30
Good	13:31–14:30	13:31–15:00	14:01–16:00	14:31–18:00
Excellent	<13:30	<13:30	<14:00	<14:30

Because the 1-mile walk test is designed primarily for older or less conditioned individuals, the fitness categories listed here do not include a "superior" category.

Source: Modified from Rockport Fitness Walking Test. *Copyright © 1993. The Rockport Company, Inc. All rights reserved. Reprinted by permission of The Rockport Company, Inc.*

The objective of the test is to complete a 1.5-mile distance (flat measured distance, preferably on a track) in the shortest possible time. The test is best conducted in moderate weather conditions (avoiding very hot or very cold days). For a reasonably physically fit individual, the 1.5-mile distance can be covered by running or jogging. For less fit individuals, the test becomes a run/walk test. A good strategy is to try to keep a steady pace during the entire distance. In this regard, it is essential to perform a practice test in order to determine the optimal pace that you can maintain. Accurate timing of the test is essential, and use of a stop watch is best. Laboratory 2.2 on p. 51 provides instructions for performing the test and recording the score.

Interpreting your test results is simple. Table 2.1 contains norms for cardiorespiratory fitness using the 1.5-mile run test. Find your sex, age group, and finish time in the table and then locate your fitness category on the left side of the table. Consider the following example: Johnny Jones is 21 years old and completes the 1.5-mile run in 13 minutes and 25 seconds (13:25). Us-

ing Table 2.1 on p. 21, locate Johnny's age group and time column. Note that a finish time of 13:25 for the 1.5-mile run would place Johnny in the "average" fitness category.

THE 1-MILE WALK TEST

Another field test to determine cardiorespiratory fitness is the **1-mile walk test**, which is particularly useful for sedentary individuals (14–16). It is a weight-bearing test, however, so individuals with joint problems should not participate.

The 1-mile walk test works on the same principle as the 1.5-mile run test. That is, individuals with high levels of cardiorespiratory fitness will complete a 1-mile walk in a shorter time than those who are less conditioned. This test is also best conducted in moderate weather conditions, preferably on a track. Subjects should try to maintain a steady pace over the distance. Again, because test scores are based on time, accurate timing is essential.

Laboratory 2.3 on p. 53 provides instructions for performing the test and for recording your score. Table 2.2 contains norms for scoring cardiorespiratory fitness using the 1-mile walk test. Find your age group and finish time in the table and then locate your fitness category on the left side of it.

1-mile walk test   A fitness test designed to evaluate cardiorespiratory fitness. The objective of the test is to complete a 1-mile walk (preferably on a track) in the shortest possible time.

TABLE 2.3
Work Rates for Submaximal Cycle Ergometer Fitness Test

Gender	Age (years)	Pedal Speed (RPM)	Load	(watts)
Male				
	Up to 29	60	150	(900 KPM)
	30 and up	60	50	(300 KPM)
Female				
	Up to 29 (or poorly conditioned)	60	100	(600 KPM)
	30 and up (or poorly conditioned)	60	50	(300 KPM)

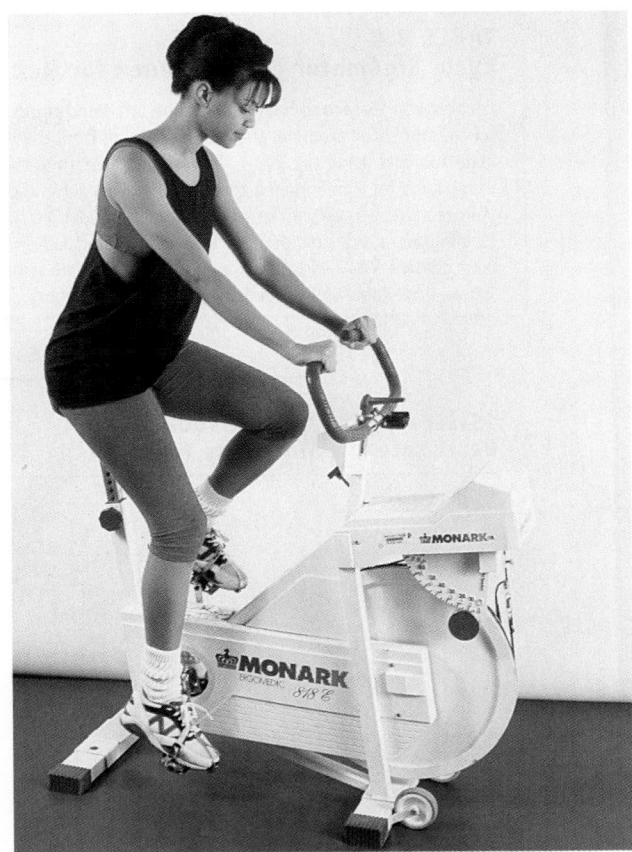

Friction-braked cycle ergometer (exercise cycle) can be used to evaluate cardiorespiratory fitness.

THE CYCLE ERGOMETER FITNESS TEST

For those with access to a cycle ergometer (a stationary exercise bicycle that provides pedaling resistance via friction applied to the wheel), a **cycle ergometer fitness test** is an excellent means of evaluating cardiorespiratory fitness. It offers advantages over running or walking tests for individuals with joint problems due to the non-weight-bearing nature of cycling. Further, because this type of test can be performed indoors, it has advantages over outdoor fitness tests during very cold or hot weather.

Although numerous types of cycle ergometers exist, the most common type is friction braked, which incorporates a belt wrapped around the wheel. The belt can be loosened or tightened to provide a change in resistance (pedaling difficulty). The work performed on a cycle ergometer is commonly expressed either in units called *kilopond meters per minute (KPM)* or in watts. It is not important that you understand the details of these units, but you should recognize that KPMs and watts are measurement units that represent how much work is performed. For example, a workload of 300 KPM (50 watts) on the cycle ergometer would be considered a submaximal (involving a light load) work rate for almost everyone, whereas a load of 3000 KPM (500 watts) would represent a high work rate for even highly conditioned individuals.

In addition to friction-braked ergometers, electronic cycle ergometers are also available for fitness testing. These cycles are similar to friction-braked cycles but adjust the workload using an electronic brake on the cycle flywheel. An electronic gauge, located near the handlebars, displays both the pedal speed and workload.

The cycle ergometer fitness test is conducted as follows:

1. Warm up for 3 minutes while pedaling the cycle at 60 revolutions per minute (RPM) with no load against the pedals.

2. After completion of the warm-up, begin the fitness test. Set the load on the cycle ergometer using Table 2.3 and perform 5 minutes of exercise.

3. During the last minute of exercise, measure your heart rate for 15 seconds. This can be achieved by palpation of the pulse in your wrist (radial artery) or by gentle palpation of the pulse in your neck (carotid artery) (Figure 2.1). Note that accurate measurement of heart rate is critical for this test to be a valid assessment of cardiorespiratory fitness.

This type of submaximal cycle test works on the principle that individuals with high cardiorespiratory fitness levels have a lower exercise heart rate at a standard workload than less fit individuals (8, 13).

cycle ergometer fitness test A submaximal exercise test designed to evaluate cardiorespiratory fitness.

TABLE 2.4
Cycle Ergometer Fitness Index for Men and Women

Locate your 15-second heart rate in the left-hand column; then find your estimated $\dot{V}O_{2max}$ in the appropriate column on the right. For example, the second column from the left contains the absolute $\dot{V}O_{2max}$ (expressed in ml/min) for male subjects using the 900-KPM work rate. The third column from the left contains the absolute $\dot{V}O_{2max}$ (expressed in ml/min) for women using the 600-KPM work rate, and so on. After determination of your absolute $\dot{V}O_{2max}$, calculate your relative $\dot{V}O_{2max}$ (ml/kg/min) by dividing your $\dot{V}O_{2max}$ expressed in ml/min by your body weight in kilograms (1 kilogram = 2.2 pounds). For example, if your body weight is 70 kilograms and your absolute $\dot{V}O_{2max}$ is 2631 ml/min, your relative $\dot{V}O_{2max}$ is approximately 38 ml/kg/min (i.e., 2631 divided by 70 = 37.6). After computing your relative $\dot{V}O_{2max}$, use Table 2.5 to identify your fitness category.

	Estimated Absolute $\dot{V}O_{2max}$ (ml/min)		
15-Second Heart Rate	Men: 900-KPM Work Rate (ml/min)	Women: 600-KPM Work Rate (ml/min)	Men or Women: 300-KPM Work Rate (ml/min)
28	3560	2541	1525
29	3442	2459	1475
30	3333	2376	1425
31	3216	2293	1375
32	3099	2210	1325
33	2982	2127	1275
34	2865	2044	1225
35	2748	1961	1175
36	2631	1878	1125
37	2514	1795	1075
38	2397	1712	1025
39	2280	1629	—
40	2163	1546	—
41	2046	1463	—
42	1929	1380	—
43	1812	1297	—
44	1695	1214	—
45	1578	1131	—

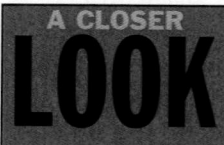

A CLOSER LOOK

Maximum Oxygen Uptake ($\dot{V}O_{2max}$)

As discussed earlier, $\dot{V}O_{2max}$ is the maximal capacity to transport and utilize oxygen during exercise, and it is considered to be the most valid measurement of cardiorespiratory fitness (9, 10). In cardiorespiratory fitness testing, it is common to express $\dot{V}O_{2max}$ as a function of body weight (called relative $\dot{V}O_{2max}$). This means that the "absolute" $\dot{V}O_{2max}$ (expressed in milliliters per minute; commonly written as ml/min) is divided by the subject's body weight in kilograms (1 kilogram = 2.2 pounds). Therefore, relative $\dot{V}O_{2max}$ is expressed in milliliters (ml) of oxygen consumed per minute per kilogram of body weight (ml/kg/min). Expressing $\dot{V}O_{2max}$ relative to body weight is particularly appropriate when describing an individual's fitness status during weight-bearing activities such as running, walking, climbing steps, or ice skating (9).

The higher the relative $\dot{V}O_{2max}$, the greater the cardiorespiratory fitness. For example, a 20-year-old female college student with a relative $\dot{V}O_{2max}$ of 53 ml/kg/min would be classified in the "superior" cardiorespiratory fitness category. In contrast, a 20-year-old woman with a $\dot{V}O_{2max}$ of 29 ml/kg/min would be classified in the "very poor" fitness category (17) (Table 2.5).

TABLE 2.5
Cardiorespiratory Fitness Norms for Men and Women Based on Estimated $\dot{V}O_{2max}$ Values Determined by the Bicycle Ergometer Fitness Test

After determining your relative $\dot{V}O_{2max}$ (ml/kg/min) in Table 2.4, find your appropriate fitness category.

Age Group (years)	Fitness Categories Based on $\dot{V}O_{2max}$ (ml/kg/min)					
	Very Poor	Poor	Average	Good	Excellent	Superior
Men						
18–25	<30	30–39	40–45	46–60	61–64	>64
26–35	<29	29–38	39–43	44–55	56–59	>59
36–45	<27	27–35	36–40	41–49	50–55	>55
46–55	<25	25–31	32–35	36–45	46–49	>49
56–65	<22	22–28	29–33	34–40	41–43	>43
>65	<20	20–25	26–28	29–34	35–38	>38
Women						
18–25	<30	30–38	39–43	44–54	55–58	>58
26–35	<28	28–33	34–41	42–53	54–58	>58
36–45	<24	24–32	33–36	37–46	47–50	>50
46–55	<22	22–28	29–31	32–41	42–45	>45
56–65	<19	19–25	26–29	30–36	37–40	>40
>65	<17	17–21	22–25	26–30	31–34	>34

Source: Data reprinted from Golding, L., (ed.). YMCA Fitness testing and assessment manual. 4th Edition, with permission of the YMCA of the USA, Chicago IL. Copyright © 2000.

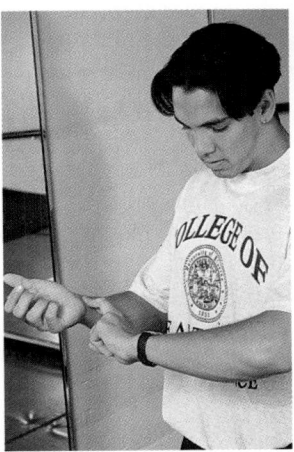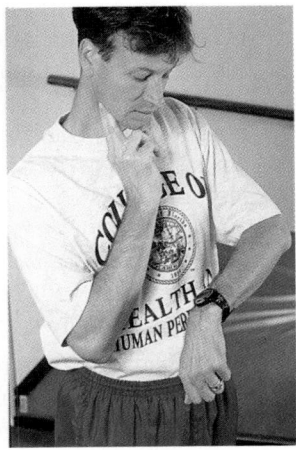

FIGURE 2.1
Subjects counting heart rate for 15 seconds using the radial or carotid artery. Palpation of the radial artery (wrist) or carotid artery (neck) is a simple means of determining heart rate. The procedure is performed as follows. Locate your radial or carotid artery using your index finger. After finding your radial or carotid pulse, count the number of heart beats (pulses) that occur during a 15-second period. Heart rate for one minute is computed by multiplying the number of heart beats counted in 15 seconds by four. For example, a 15-second heart rate count of 30 beats would indicate that the heart rate was 120 beats/min (i.e., 30 × 4 = 120). When palpating the carotid artery, take care to apply limited pressure on the neck. Application of too much force on the carotid artery will result in a reflexic lowering of your heart rate and will therefore bias heart rate measurement.

After completing the test, use your 15-second heart rate count to find your estimated $\dot{V}O_{2max}$ as instructed in Table 2.4. For example, a 21-year-old woman with a 15-second heart rate of 36 would have an estimated $\dot{V}O_{2max}$ of 27 ml/kg/min. (See A Closer Look on facing page for a discussion of $\dot{V}O_2$ units.) Now use Table 2.5 to find the corresponding fitness category. A $\dot{V}O_{2max}$ of 27 ml/kg/min for a 21-year-old woman would place her in the "very poor" cardiorespiratory fitness category. Laboratory 2.4 on p. 55 permits recording of your score on this test.

THE STEP TEST

An alternative test to determine your cardiorespiratory fitness level is the **step test**. The step test works on

step test   A submaximal exercise test designed to evaluate cardiorespiratory fitness. The step test works on the principle that individuals with a high level of cardiorespiratory fitness will have a lower heart rate during recovery from 3 minutes of standardized exercise (bench stepping) than less-conditioned individuals.

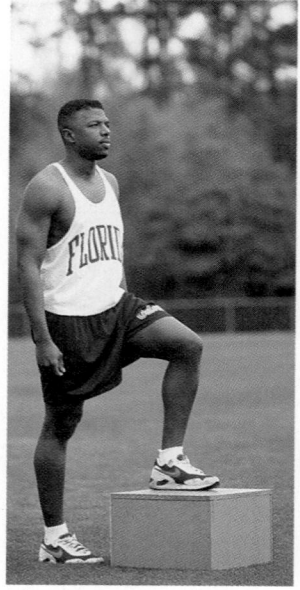 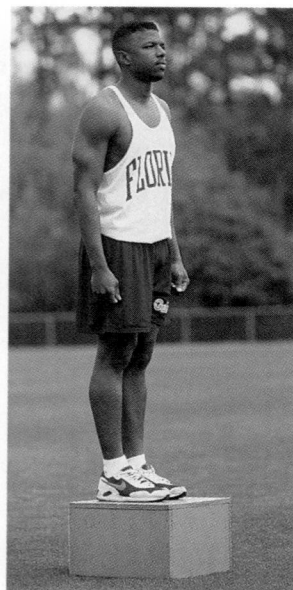

(a)   (b)

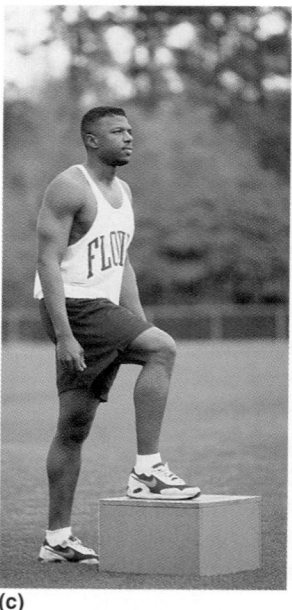 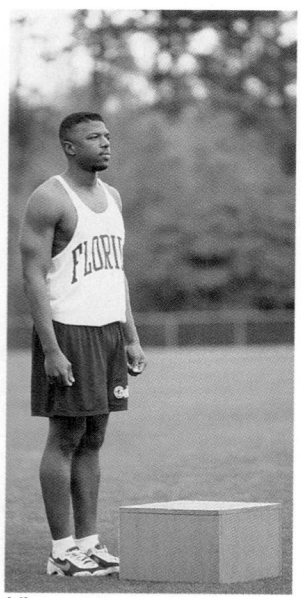

(c)   (d)

FIGURE 2.2
Step test to evaluate cardiorespiratory fitness. Subjects step up onto an 18-inch surface (a), (b), and then down (c), (d) once every 2 seconds.

the principle that individuals with a high level of cardiorespiratory fitness will have a lower heart rate during recovery from 3 minutes of standardized exercise (bench stepping) than less conditioned individuals (4, 9). Although the step test is not considered the best field method to estimate cardiorespiratory fitness, it does have advantages in that it can be performed indoors and can be used by people at all fitness levels. Further, the step test does not require expensive equipment and can be performed in a short amount of time.

TABLE 2.6
Norms for Cardiorespiratory Fitness Using the Sum of Three Recovery Heart Rates Obtained Following the Step Test

	3-Minute Step Test Recovery Index	
Fitness Category	**Women**	**Men**
Superior	95–120	95–117
Excellent	121–135	118–132
Good	136–153	133–147
Average	154–174	148–165
Poor	175–204	166–192
Very poor	205–233	193–217

Fitness categories are for college-age men and women (ages 18–25 years) at the University of Florida who performed the test on an 18-inch bench.

Step height for both men and women should be approximately 18 inches. In general, locker room benches or sturdy chairs can be used as stepping devices. The test is conducted as follows:

1. Select a partner to assist you in the step test. Your partner is responsible for timing the test and assisting you in maintaining the proper stepping cadence. The exercise cadence is 30 complete steps (up and down) per minute during a 3-minute exercise period, which can be maintained by a metronome or voice cues from your friend ("up, up, down, down"). Thus you need to make one complete step cycle every 2 seconds (i.e., set the metronome at 60 tones/min and step up and down with each sound). Note that it is important that you straighten your knees during the "up" phase of the test (Figure 2.2).

2. After completing the test, sit quietly in a chair or on the step bench. Find your pulse and count your heart rate for 30-second periods during the following recovery times:

   1 to 1.5 minutes post exercise
   2 to 2.5 minutes post exercise
   3 to 3.5 minutes post exercise

Your partner should assist you in timing the recovery period and recording your recovery heart rates. Note that the accuracy of this test depends on both the faithful execution of 30 steps per minute during the test and the valid measurement of heart rate during the appropriate recovery times.

> # Nutritional Links
> ## TO HEALTH AND FITNESS
>
> ## Dehydration Can Negatively Impact a Cardiorespiratory Fitness Test
>
> Approximately 60–70% of the body is water. Heavy sweating and/or the failure to drink enough fluids during the day can lower body water levels and result in dehydration. Water is involved in every vital process of the body, so dehydration can impair exercise performance. For example, dehydration results in reduced blood volume and elevated heart rates during submaximal exercise. This dehydration-induced high heart rate during submaximal exercise will result in an underestimation of $\dot{V}O_{2max}$ during submaximal fitness tests (e.g., a cycle ergometer or step fitness test) (9). Further, dehydration can negatively impact endurance performance during field tests of $\dot{V}O_{2max}$ (e.g., 1.5-mile run) (9, 19). Therefore, because dehydration can impair exercise performance, cardiorespiratory fitness tests should be performed only when the test subjects are adequately hydrated. See Chapter 7 for more details on the maintenance of normal body water levels.

Laboratory 2.5 on p. 57 provides a place to record your recovery heart rates and fitness category. To determine your fitness category, add the three 30-second heart rates obtained during recovery; this is called the **recovery index**. Table 2.6 contains norms for step test results in a college-age population (18–25 years). For example, a male student with a recovery index of 165 beats would be classified as having average cardiorespiratory fitness.

CARDIORESPIRATORY FITNESS: HOW DO YOU RATE?

After completing the cardiorespiratory fitness test of your choice, the next step is to interpret your results and set goals for improvement. If your cardiorespiratory fitness test score placed you in the "very poor" or "poor" classification, your current fitness level is below average compared with that of other healthy men or women of similar age in North America. On the other hand, a fitness test score in the "good" category means that your current cardiorespiratory fitness level is above average for your gender and age group. The fitness category "excellent" means that your level of cardiorespiratory conditioning is well above average. The "superior" rating is reserved for those individuals whose cardiorespiratory fitness level ranks in the top 15% of people in their age group. A key point here is that regardless of how low your current cardiorespiratory fitness level may be, you can improve by adherence to a regular exercise training program.

As mentioned earlier, testing your initial cardiorespiratory fitness level provides a benchmark against which you can compare future evaluations. Performing additional fitness tests as your fitness level improves is important because this type of positive feedback provides motivation to maintain regular exercise habits (3–5, 18).

☀ IN SUMMARY

- Cardiorespiratory fitness is the ability to perform endurance exercises (e.g., running, cycling) and is a key component of health-related physical fitness.
- Individuals with superior cardiorespiratory fitness have the ability to perform high levels of endurance-type activities.
- Field tests to evaluate cardiorespiratory fitness include the 1.5-mile run test, the 1-mile walk test, the cycle ergometer fitness test, and the step test.
- All cardiorespiratory fitness tests are subject to error and therefore these tests may over- or underpredict your "true" fitness level (see A Closer Look on p. 28 for details).

Muscular strength can be measured using either free weights or any one of several commercial "weight machines." Nonetheless, it is important to make ongoing strength measures using the same weight apparatus since strength measurements using free weights may differ from the same assessment (e.g., bench press) using a commercial weight machine.

> **recovery index** Measurement of heart rate during three 30-second recovery periods following a submaximal step test. (See the text for complete details.)

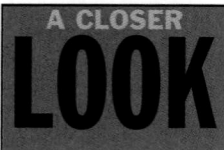

Error in Estimating V̇O₂max from Field Tests

Note that the estimation of $\dot{V}O_{2max}$ using any of the methods described in this chapter is subject to error compared to laboratory tests that directly measure $\dot{V}O_{2max}$. These errors can come from many of sources so that the predicted $\dot{V}O_{2max}$ will not be equal to the "true" value. The size of the error is described using a term called the standard error. The standard error describes how far off (higher or lower) the predicted value might be from the "true" value. Specifically, one standard error describes where 68% of the test estimates are compared to the true value. In simple terms, the standard error explains the range of error that exists for the estimation of a "true" value.

Here's an example of the standard error associated with two cardiorespiratory fitness tests. If $\dot{V}O_{2max}$ is estimated by heart rates during the cycle ergometer fitness test or by the time required to complete the 1.5-mile run test, the standard error is approximately 5 ml/kg/min (9). This means that if your predicted $\dot{V}O_{2max}$ was 45 ml/kg/min, then your "true" $\dot{V}O_{2max}$ is likely between 40 and 50 ml/kg/min. The relatively large standard errors for estimation of $\dot{V}O_{2max}$ do not indicate that these tests have no value. Indeed, each of the cardiorespiratory tests described in this chapter are very useful "field" tests that can be used to measure

improvements in cardiorespiratory fitness during a training program. This information can be used as both an educational and motivational tool for individuals engaged in a regular exercise program.

What testing factors diminish the accuracy of a cardiovascular fitness test? Obviously, error in the measurement of heart rates (i.e., cycle ergometer test) or timing of the 1.5-mile run will have a negative impact on the accuracy of the test. Moreover, performing the test on a hot and humid day can also diminish the accuracy of any cardiorespiratory fitness test. Other factors that could impact test accuracy include the use of prescription medications or eating a large meal immediately prior to participating in the test.

☀ Evaluation of Muscular Strength

As discussed in Chapter 1, muscular strength is defined as the maximum amount of force you can produce during one contraction (19). Muscular strength not only is important for success in athletics, but also is useful for the average person in performing routine tasks at work or home. Strength can be measured by the **one-repetition maximum (1 RM) test**, which measures the maximum amount of weight that can be lifted one time. It is also possible to estimate the 1 RM by performing multiple repetitions using a submaximal weight. Methods for directly measuring and for estimating the 1 RM are discussed in the following sections.

THE 1 RM TEST

Although the 1 RM test for muscular strength is widely accepted (7), it has been criticized as unsuitable for use with older individuals or highly deconditioned people. The major concern is the risk of injury. The 1 RM test should therefore be attempted only after several weeks of strength training, which will result in improvements in both skill and strength and reduce the risk of injury during the test. An older or sedentary individual would probably require 6 weeks of exercise training prior to the 1 RM test, whereas a physically active college-age student could probably perform the 1 RM test after 1 to 2 weeks of training.

The 1 RM test is designed to test muscular strength in selected muscle groups and is performed in the following manner. Begin with a 5- to 10-minute warm-up using the muscles to be tested. For each muscle group, select an initial weight that you can lift without undue stress. Then gradually add weight until you reach the maximum weight that you can lift one time. If you can lift the weight more than once, add additional weight until you reach a level of resistance such that you can perform only one repetition. Remember that a true 1 RM is the maximum amount of weight that you can lift one time.

Figures 2.3 through 2.6 illustrate four common lifts used to measure strength. Three of these (bench press, biceps curl, and shoulder press) use upper body muscle groups; the fourth lift (leg press) measures leg strength. Your muscle strength score is your percentage of body

---

one-repetition maximum (1 RM) test Measurement of the maximum amount of weight that can be lifted one time.

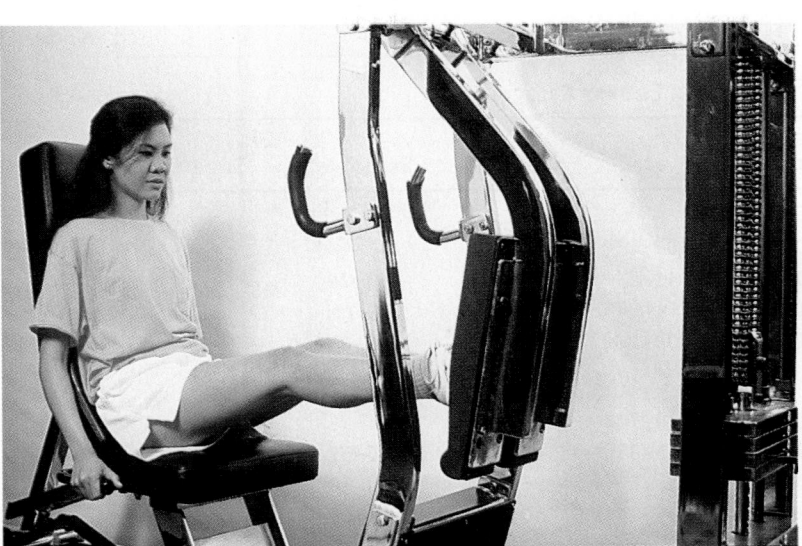

FIGURE 2.3
A leg press to evaluate muscular strength.

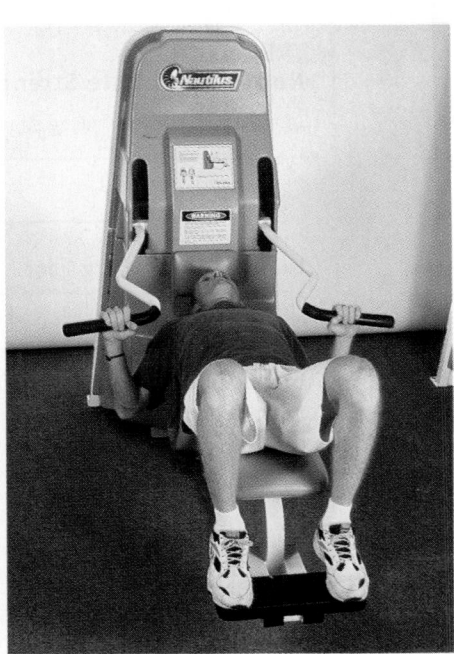

FIGURE 2.4
The bench press to evaluate muscular strength.

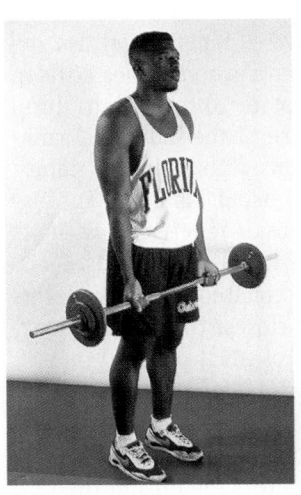 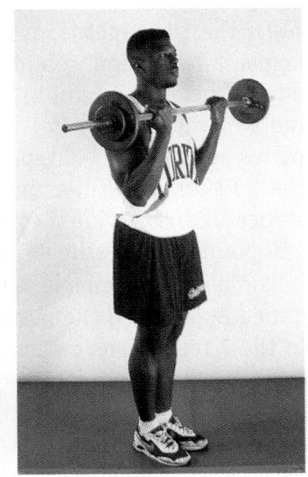

FIGURE 2.5
A biceps curl to evaluate muscular strength.

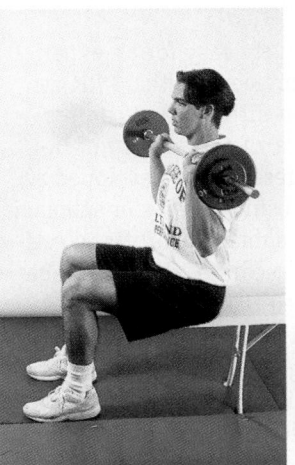 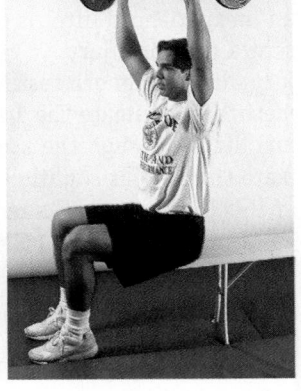

FIGURE 2.6
The shoulder or "military" press to evaluate muscular strength.

weight lifted in each exercise. To compute your strength score in each lift, divide your 1 RM weight in pounds by your body weight in pounds and then multiply by 100. For example, suppose a 150-pound man has a bench press 1 RM of 180 pounds. This individual's muscle strength score for the bench press is computed as

$$\frac{1 \text{ RM weight}}{\text{body weight}} \times 100 = \text{muscle strength score}$$

Therefore,

$$\text{muscle strength score} = \frac{180 \text{ pounds}}{150 \text{ pounds}} \times 100 = 120$$

Table 2.7 contains strength score norms for college-age men and women in each of these lifts. Using Table 2.7, a muscle strength score of 120 on the bench press places a college-age man in the "good" category. You can record your muscle strength scores in Laboratory 2.6 on p. 59.

TABLE 2.7
Norms for Muscle Strength Scores Using a 1 RM Test

In this table, use your muscle strength score to locate your fitness level.

	Fitness Category					
Exercise	Very Poor	Poor	Average	Good	Excellent	Superior
Men						
Bench press	< 50	50–99	100–110	111–130	131–149	>149
Biceps curl	< 30	30–40	41–54	55–60	61–79	> 79
Shoulder press	< 40	41–50	51–67	68–80	81–110	>110
Leg press	<160	161–199	200–209	210–229	230–239	>239
Women						
Bench press	< 40	41–69	70–74	75–80	81–99	> 99
Biceps curl	< 15	15–34	35–39	40–55	56–59	> 59
Shoulder press	< 20	20–46	47–54	55–59	60–79	> 79
Leg press	<100	100–130	131–144	145–174	175–189	>189

Norms are from ref. 7.

ESTIMATING THE 1 RM USING A 10 RM TEST

Determining the 1 RM is relatively easy for an experienced weight lifter, but measurement of the 1 RM for an inexperienced lifter is often difficult and can present a risk for injury. To reduce the possibility of injury during strength testing, researchers developed a method to estimate the 1 RM using a series of submaximal lifts. Although the use of submaximal lifts to estimate the 1 RM is slightly less accurate, the advantage of this technique is the reduced risk of injury.

Estimation of the 1 RM in any particular lift (e.g., bench press) is achieved using the following procedure (19). Testing begins with the individual performing a set of 10 repetitions using a light weight. Depending on the ease with which these repetitions are completed, the instructor then adds additional weight, and the individual performs another set of 10 repetitions. This process continues until a weight is reached that can only be lifted 10 times (called the 10 RM). In general, an experienced instructor can aid the individual by supervising the process so that the 10 RM weight can be discovered in fewer than five trials (19). Note that a rest period of approximately 5 minutes should separate these trials to permit adequate time for recovery.

After determining the 10 RM, the 1 RM can be estimated using Table 2.8. For example, if an individual's 10 RM for a particular lift is 100 pounds, then the estimate for the 1 RM would be 135 pounds. This was determined by locating the number closest to 100 pounds in the 10 repetitions column (i.e., 99.2 pounds) in Table 2.8 and then locating the 1 RM weight in the left-hand column for this row.

Note that the 1 RM can also be estimated using fewer than 10 repetitions (i.e., 7–9 repetitions). For example, a beginning weight lifter can sometimes develop muscle fatigue and fail to complete 10 repetitions during a testing period. In this case, if the individual completes as many as 7–9 repetitions with a given weight, the 1 RM can be still estimated using Table 2.8. For instance, if an individual completes 7 repetitions with 110 pounds, the estimate for 1 RM is 135 pounds. As in the previous example, the estimated 1 RM was determined by locating the number closest to 110 pounds in the 7 repetitions column (i.e., 109.4 pounds) in Table 2.8, and then locating the 1 RM weight in the left-hand column for this row.

After determining the estimated 1 RM, the individual's muscle strength score is determined using the formula discussed in the previous section. That is,

$$\text{muscle strength score} = \frac{1 \text{ RM weight}}{\text{body weight}} \times 100$$

After calculating your muscle strength score, record your strength scores in Laboratory 2.6 on p. 59.

MUSCULAR STRENGTH: HOW DO YOU RATE?

When you have completed your muscular strength test, the next step is to interpret your results (Table 2.7) and set goals for improvement. Similar to the fitness categories used for cardiorespiratory fitness, the fitness categories for muscular strength range from very poor (lowest) to superior (highest). If your current strength level is classified as average or below, don't be discour-

TABLE 2.8
Estimating the 1 RM from the 10 RM

Estimated 1 RM (pounds)	Weight (pounds) Lifted During 7 Repetitions	Weight (pounds) Lifted During 8 Repetitions	Weight (pounds) Lifted During 9 Repetitions	Weight (pounds) Lifted During 10 Repetitions
5.0	4.1	3.9	3.8	3.7
10.0	8.2	7.9	7.6	7.4
15.0	12.2	11.8	11.4	11.0
20.0	16.2	15.7	15.2	14.7
25.0	20.2	19.6	19.0	18.4
30.0	24.3	23.6	22.8	22.1
35.0	28.4	27.5	26.6	25.7
40.0	32.4	31.4	30.4	29.4
45.0	36.5	35.3	34.2	33.1
50.0	40.5	39.3	38.0	36.8
55.0	44.6	43.2	41.8	40.4
60.0	48.6	47.1	45.6	44.1
65.0	52.7	51.0	49.4	47.8
70.0	56.7	55.0	53.2	51.5
75.0	60.8	58.9	57.0	55.1
80.0	64.8	62.8	60.8	58.8
85.0	68.9	66.7	64.6	62.5
90.0	72.9	70.7	68.4	66.2
95.0	77.0	74.6	72.2	69.8
100.0	81.0	78.5	76.0	73.5
105.0	85.1	82.4	79.8	77.2
110.0	89.1	86.4	83.6	80.9
115.0	93.2	90.3	87.4	84.5
120.0	97.2	94.2	91.2	88.2
125.0	101.3	98.1	95.0	91.9
130.0	105.3	102.1	98.8	95.6
135.0	109.4	106.0	102.6	99.2
140.0	113.4	109.9	106.4	102.9
145.0	117.5	113.8	110.2	106.6
150.0	121.5	117.8	114.0	110.3
155.0	125.6	121.7	117.8	113.9
160.0	129.6	125.6	121.6	117.6
165.0	133.7	129.5	125.4	121.3
170.0	137.7	133.5	129.2	125.0
175.0	141.8	137.4	133.0	128.6
180.0	145.8	141.3	136.8	132.3
185.0	149.9	145.2	140.6	136.0
190.0	153.9	149.2	144.4	139.7
195.0	158.0	153.1	148.2	143.3
200.0	162.0	157.0	152.0	147.0
205.0	166.1	160.9	155.8	150.7
210.0	170.1	164.9	159.6	154.4
215.0	174.2	168.8	163.4	158.0
220.0	178.2	182.7	167.2	161.7
225.0	182.3	176.6	171.0	165.4

(continued)

TABLE 2.8
Estimating the 1 RM from the 10 RM (continued)

Estimated 1 RM (pounds)	Weight (pounds) Lifted During 7 Repetitions	Weight (pounds) Lifted During 8 Repetitions	Weight (pounds) Lifted During 9 Repetitions	Weight (pounds) Lifted During 10 Repetitions
230.0	186.3	180.6	174.8	169.1
235.0	190.4	184.5	178.6	172.7
240.0	194.4	188.4	182.4	176.4
245.0	198.5	192.3	186.2	180.1
250.0	202.5	196.3	190.0	183.8
255.0	206.6	200.2	193.8	187.4
260.0	210.6	204.1	197.6	191.2
265.0	214.7	208.1	201.4	194.8
270.0	218.7	212.0	205.2	198.5
275.0	222.8	215.9	209.0	202.1
280.0	226.8	219.8	212.8	205.8
285.0	230.9	223.7	216.6	209.5
290.0	234.9	227.7	220.4	213.2
295.0	239.0	231.6	224.2	216.8
300.0	243.0	235.5	228.0	220.5
305.0	247.1	239.4	231.8	224.2
310.0	251.1	243.4	235.6	227.9
315.0	255.2	247.3	239.4	231.5
320.0	259.2	251.2	243.2	235.2
325.0	263.3	255.1	247.0	238.9
330.0	267.3	259.1	250.8	242.6
335.0	271.4	263.0	254.6	246.2
340.0	275.4	266.9	258.4	249.9
345.0	279.5	270.8	262.2	253.6
350.0	283.6	274.8	266.0	257.3
355.0	287.6	278.7	269.8	260.9
360.0	291.6	282.6	273.6	264.6
365.0	295.7	286.5	277.4	268.3
370.0	299.7	290.5	281.2	272.0
375.0	303.8	294.4	285.0	275.6
380.0	307.8	298.3	288.8	279.3
385.0	311.9	302.0	292.6	283.0
390.0	315.9	306.2	296.4	286.7
395.0	320.0	310.1	300.2	290.3
400.0	324.0	314.0	304.0	294.0
405.0	328.1	317.9	307.8	297.7
410.0	332.1	321.9	311.6	301.4
415.0	336.2	325.8	315.4	305.0
420.0	340.2	329.7	319.2	308.7
425.0	344.3	333.6	323.0	312.4
430.0	348.3	337.6	326.8	316.1
435.0	352.4	341.5	330.6	319.7
440.0	356.4	345.4	334.4	323.4
445.0	360.5	349.3	338.2	327.1
450.0	364.5	353.3	342.0	330.8
455.0	368.6	357.2	345.8	334.4

Source: Data are from ref. 20.

aged; you can improve! A key point in maintaining your motivation to exercise regularly is the establishment of goals. Record both short-term and long-term goals for improvement. After 6 to 12 weeks of training, perform a retest to evaluate your progress. Reaching a short-term goal provides added incentive to continue your exercise program.

☀ IN SUMMARY

- Muscular strength is the maximum amount of force you can produce during one contraction.
- A common method of evaluating muscular strength is the one-repetition maximum (1 RM) test. However, it is possible to estimate the 1 RM by using the 10 RM (submaximal) test. Compared to the 1 RM test, the 10 RM poses less risk of injury to an inexperienced weight lifter.

☀ Measurement of Muscular Endurance

Muscular endurance is the ability of a muscle or muscle group to generate force over and over again. Although an individual might have sufficient strength to lift a heavy box from the ground to the back of a truck, he or she might not have sufficient muscular endurance to perform this task multiple times. Because many everyday tasks require submaximal but repeated muscular contractions, muscular endurance is an important facet of health-related physical fitness.

Although numerous methods exist to evaluate muscular strength, two simple tests to assess muscular endurance involve the performance of push-ups and either sit-ups or curl-ups. Push-ups are a measure of muscular endurance using the shoulder, arm, and chest muscles, whereas sit-ups and curl-ups primarily evaluate abdominal muscle endurance.

THE PUSH-UP TEST

The standard **push-up test** to evaluate muscular endurance is performed in the following way. Start by positioning yourself on the ground in push-up position (Figure 2.7A). Your hands should be approximately shoulder width, and your legs should be extended in a straight line with your weight placed on your toes. Lower your body until your chest is within 1 to 2 inches of the ground and raise yourself back to the up position. It is important to keep your back straight and to lower your entire body to the ground as a unit.

The push-up test is performed as follows:

1. Select a partner to count your push-ups and assist in the timing of the test (test duration is 60 seconds).

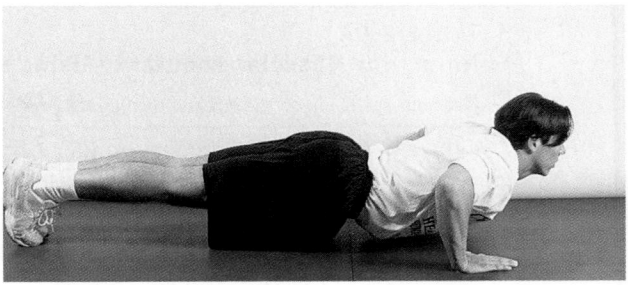

FIGURE 2.7a
The standard push-up.

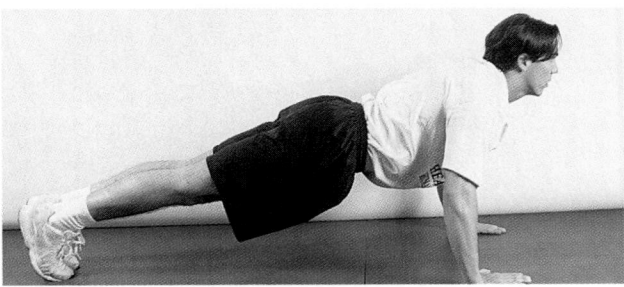

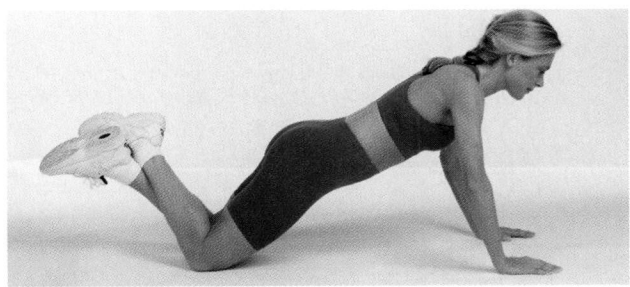

FIGURE 2.7b
The modified push-up.

Warm up with a few push-ups. Give yourself a 2- to 3-minute recovery period after the warm-up and prepare to start the test.

2. On the command "go," start performing push-ups. Your partner counts your push-ups aloud and informs you of the amount of time remaining in the test period (e.g., at 15-second intervals). Remember only those push-ups that are performed correctly will be counted toward your total; therefore, use the proper form and make every push-up count.

3. After completion of the push-up test, use Table 2.9 on p. 34 to determine your fitness classification, and then record your scores in Laboratory 2.7A on p. 61.

---

push-up test A fitness test designed to evaluate muscular endurance of shoulder and arm muscles.

TABLE 2.9A
Norms for Muscular Endurance Using the Push-Up Test

Find your age group on the left and then locate your fitness category in the appropriate column to the right.

Fitness Category Based on Push-Ups (1 min)

Age Group (years)	Very Poor	Poor	Average	Good	Excellent	Superior
Men						
15–19	<20	20–24	25–34	35–44	45–53	>53
20–29	<19	19–23	24–33	34–43	44–52	>52
30–39	<15	15–20	21–24	25–34	35–44	>44
40–49	<12	12–14	15–19	20–29	30–39	>39
50–59	<8	8–11	12–15	16–24	25–34	>34
601	<5	5–7	8–9	10–19	20–29	>29
Women						
15–19	<5	5–9	10–12	13–14	15–19	>19
20–29	<4	4–8	9–10	11–12	13–18	>18
30–39	<3	3–7	8–11	12–13	14–16	>16
40–49	<2	2–5	6–9	10–12	13–15	>15
50–59	1	2–3	4–5	6–9	10–11	>11
60+	0	1–2	2–3	4–5	6–8	>8

Sources: Men's norms are modified from Pollock, M., J. Wilmore, and S. Fox. Health and fitness through physical activity. John Wiley and Sons, New York, 1978. Women's norms are unpublished data from the University of Florida.

TABLE 2.9B
Norms* for Testing Muscular Endurance in Females Using the Modified Push-Up Test

Locate your age group in the left column and then determine your fitness category in the appropriate column to the right.

Fitness Category Based on Modified Push-Ups

Age Group (Years)	Very poor	Poor	Average	Good	Excellent	Superior
18–29	<17	17–22	23–29	30–35	36–44	>44
30–39	<11	11–18	19–23	24–30	31–38	>38
40–49	<6	6–10	13–17	18–23	24–32	>32
50–59	<5	5–9	12–16	17–20	21–27	>27
60+	<2	2–4	5–11	12–14	15–19	>19

*Norms are a modification of norms obtained from the Cooper Institute for Aerobic Research, Dallas, Texas.

MODIFIED PUSH-UP TEST

Biologically, men tend to be stronger than women. Therefore, in some cases, the modified push-up test is superior to the standard push-up test to determine muscular endurance in females. Therefore, when appropriate, the modified push-up test can be substituted for the standard push-up for fitness testing in females. The modified push-up test is performed in the following way.

1. Begin in the modified push-up position with your body supported by your hands and knees (Figure 2.7B). Identical to the standard push-up position, your arms and back should be straight in the starting position (Figure 2.7B).

2. Start the test by lowering your chest to the floor with your back straight and then return to the upward starting position. Complete as many push-ups as you can without stopping. Note that this test is not timed and the test is completed when you cannot complete another push-up without a rest period.

3. After completion of the test, go to Table 2.9B on p. 34 to determine your fitness classification and then record your scores in Laboratory 2.7B on p. 63.

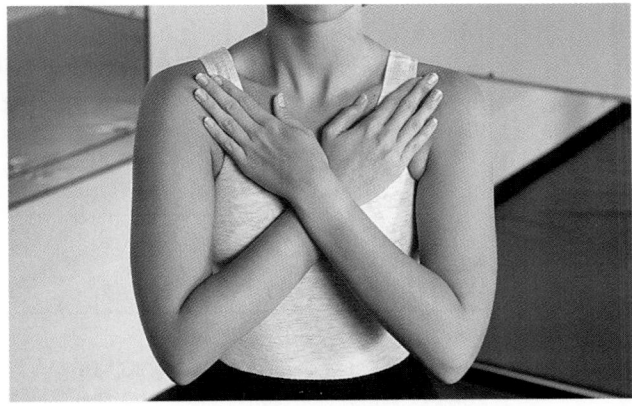
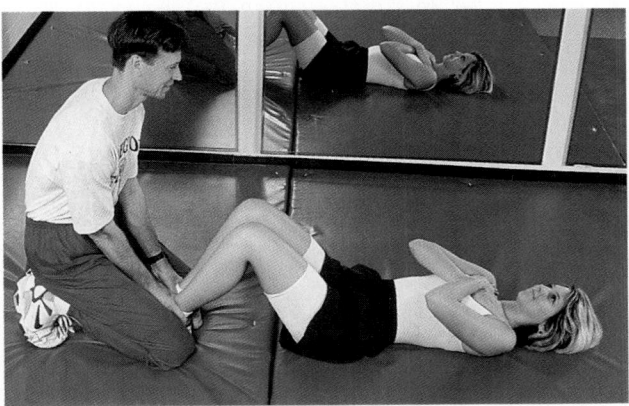
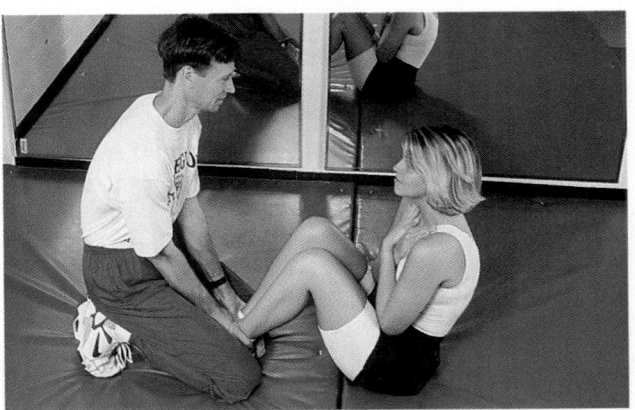

FIGURE 2.8
The proper position for the performance of sit-ups.

FITNESS-WELLNESS
CONSUMER

Fitness-Testing Software

A quick search of the Internet using the search term "physical fitness" reveals hundreds of fitness-related sites and products. Included in this long list of fitness items are numerous advertisements for "fitness-testing" software. While many fitness-testing software packages contain useful information and step-by-step approaches to evaluating various aspects of physical fitness, these packages do not provide advantages over the information contained in the current fitness literature (e.g., fitness textbooks). Therefore, there is no advantage in obtaining fitness-testing information via a computer software program compared to an up-to-date textbook. Nonetheless, if you are considering the purchase of a commercial fitness-testing software package, please take the following two steps before making your purchase. First, check the academic credentials of the software author(s). The author(s) should have a graduate degree in exercise science or exercise physiology. Second, preview a sample of the software to determine if the software package is "user friendly" and meets your fitness needs.

THE SIT-UP TEST

The bent-knee **sit-up test** is probably the best-known field test available to evaluate abdominal muscle endurance (4, 6). Figure 2.8 illustrates the correct position for performance of bent-knee sit-ups. Begin by lying on your back with your arms crossed on your chest. Your knees should be bent at approximately 90-degree

sit-up test A field test to evaluate abdominal and hip muscle endurance.

TABLE 2.10
Norms for Muscular Endurance Using the 1-Minute Sit-Up Test
Find your gender and age group on the left and then locate your fitness category in the appropriate column to the right.

Age Group (years)	Fitness Category Based on Sit-Ups (1 min)					
	Very Poor	Poor	Average	Good	Excellent	Superior
Men						
17–29	<17	17–35	36–41	42–47	48–50	>50
30–39	<13	13–26	27–32	33–38	39–48	>48
40–49	<12	12–22	23–27	28–33	34–43	>43
50–59	<8	8–16	17–21	22–28	29–38	>38
60+	<6	6–12	13–17	18–24	25–35	>35
Women						
20–29	<14	14–28	29–32	33–35	36–47	>47
30–39	<11	11–22	23–28	29–34	35–45	>45
40–49	<9	9–18	19–23	24–30	31–40	>40
50–59	<6	6–12	13–17	18–24	25–35	>35
60+	<5	5–10	11–14	15–20	21–30	>30

Source: Modified from Pollock, M., J. Wilmore, and S. Fox. Health and fitness through physical activity. Reprinted by permission of Jack Wilmore.

angles, with your feet flat on the floor. The complete sit-up is performed by bringing your chest up to touch your knees and returning to the original lying position.

Note that although the abdominal muscles are very active during the performance of a bent-leg sit-up, leg muscles such as hip flexors also play a role. Therefore, this test evaluates not only abdominal muscle endurance but hip muscle endurance as well (21).

Sit-up tests are generally considered to be relatively safe fitness tests, but two precautions should be mentioned. First, avoid undue stress on your neck during the "up" phase of the exercise. That is, let your abdominal muscles do the work; do not whip your neck during the sit-up movement. Second, avoid hitting the back of your head on the floor during the "down" phase of the sit-up. Performance of the test on a padded mat is helpful.

The protocol for the sit-up test is as follows:

1. Select a partner to count your sit-ups, to hold your feet on the floor by grasping your ankles, and to assist in the timing of the test.

2. Warm up with a few sit-ups. Give yourself a 2- to 3-minute recovery period after the warm-up and prepare to start the test.

3. On the command "go," start performing sit-ups and continue for 60 seconds. Your partner should count

your sit-ups aloud and inform you of the time remaining in the test period (perhaps by called-out 15-second intervals). Remember that only sits-ups performed correctly will be counted toward your total.

4. After completing the sit-up test, use Table 2.10 to determine your fitness classification. Record your scores in Laboratory 2.7A on p. 61.

THE CURL-UP TEST

As mentioned earlier, although sit-up tests utilize abdominal muscles, leg muscles are also recruited to move the trunk upward. Use of these leg muscles can be eliminated by performing a partial sit-up or a curl-up. The curl-up differs from the sit-up in that the trunk is not raised more than 30 to 40 degrees above the mat (attained when the shoulders are lifted approximately 6–10 inches above the mat; Figure 2.9) (21, 22). There are two advantages of the curl-up over the sit-up. First, the curl-up recruits only abdominal muscles, whereas the sit-up test involves both abdominal muscles and hip flexors. Second, research suggests that the curl-up provides less stress on the lower back than the conventional sit-up (20). For these reasons, the **curl-up test** is growing in popularity and is often used instead of the

TABLE 2.11
Norms for Muscular Endurance Using the Curl-Up Test

Find your gender and age group on the left and locate the fitness category closest to your score in the columns to the right.

	Fitness Category Based on Curl-Ups Performed				
Age Group (years)	**Poor**	**Average**	**Good**	**Excellent**	**Superior**
Men					
<35	15	30	45	60	75
35–44	10	25	40	50	60
>44	5	15	25	40	50
Women					
<35	10	25	40	50	60
35–44	6	15	25	40	50
>44	4	10	15	30	40

Modified from Faulkner, R. A., et al. A partial curl-up protocol for adults based on two procedures. Canadian Journal of Sports Sciences *14:135–141, 1989.*

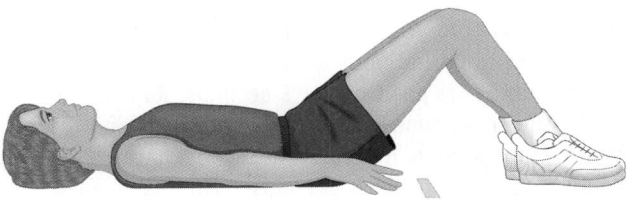

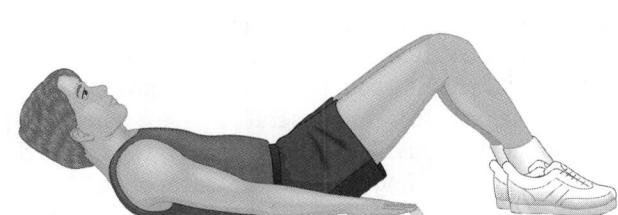

FIGURE 2.9
The proper position and movement pattern for the performance of a curl-up.

sit-up test to evaluate abdominal muscle endurance. The protocol for the curl-up test is as follows:

1. Select a partner to count your curl-ups; lie on your back with knees bent 90 degrees.

2. Extend your arms so that your fingertips touch a strip of tape perpendicular to the body (Figure 2.9). A second strip of tape is located toward the feet and parallel to the first (8 centimeters or 3 inches apart). The curl-up is accomplished by raising your trunk (i.e., curling upward) until your fingertips touch the second strip of tape and then returning to the starting position.

3. The curl-up test is not timed and is performed at a slow and controlled cadence of 20 curl-ups per minute. This cadence is guided by the aid of a metronome set at 40 beats per minute (curl up on one beat and down on the second).

4. On the command "go," start performing curl-ups in cadence with the metronome. Perform as many curl-ups as you can to a maximum of 75 without missing a beat. See Table 2.11 to determine your fitness category, and then record your score in Laboratory 2.7A on p. 61.

MUSCULAR ENDURANCE: HOW DO YOU RATE?

The fitness categories for muscular endurance range from very poor (lowest) to superior (highest). If your muscular endurance test score placed you in the "very poor" or "poor" classification, your present muscular

curl-up test   A field test to evaluate abdominal muscle endurance.

endurance level is below average compared with other men or women of your age group. On the other hand, a fitness test score in the "good" category means that your current muscular endurance is above average. The fitness category "excellent" means that your muscular endurance level is well above average. Finally, the fitness category labeled "superior" is reserved for those individuals whose muscular endurance ranks in the top 15% of men or women in your age group.

If you scored poorly on either the push-up or sit-up test, do not be discouraged. Establish your goals and begin doing sit-ups and push-ups on a regular basis (see Chapter 5 for the exercise prescription for muscular strength). Your ability to perform both sit-ups and push-ups will increase within the first 3 to 4 weeks of training and will continue to improve for weeks to come.

☀ IN SUMMARY

- Muscular endurance is the ability of a muscle or muscle group to generate force over and over again during repeated contractions.
- Two common methods to evaluate muscular endurance are the push-up and sit-up tests.

☀ Assessment of Flexibility

Flexibility, the ability to move joints freely through their full range of motion, can decrease over time due to tightening of muscles and/or tendons. Loss of flexibility can occur due to both muscle disuse and muscular training. The key to maintaining flexibility is a program of regular stretching exercises (Chapter 6).

Individual needs for flexibility are variable. Some athletes, such as gymnasts, require great flexibility in order to perform complex movements in competition (3, 5, 10, 18). In general, the nonathlete requires less flexibility than the athlete. Some flexibility, however, is required for everyone in order to perform common activities of daily living or recreational pursuits.

It is important to understand that flexibility is joint specific. That is, a person might be flexible in one joint but lack flexibility in another. Although no single test is representative of total body flexibility, measurements of trunk and shoulder flexibility are commonly evaluated.

---

sit and reach test   A fitness test that measures the ability to flex the trunk (i.e., stretching the lower back muscles and the muscles in the back of the thigh).

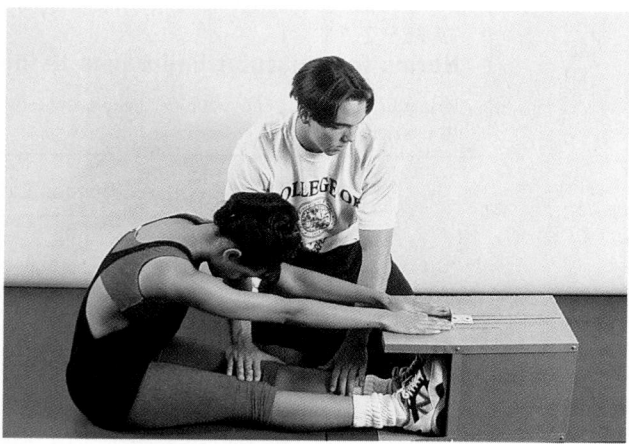

FIGURE 2.10
The sit and reach test to evaluate trunk flexibility.

TRUNK FLEXIBILITY

The **sit and reach test** measures the ability to flex the trunk, which means stretching the lower back muscles and the muscles in the back of the thigh (hamstrings). Figure 2.10 illustrates the sit and reach test using a sit and reach box. The test is performed in the following manner.

Start by sitting upright with your feet flat against the box. Keeping your feet flat on the box and your legs straight, extend your hands as far forward as possible and hold this position for 3 seconds. Repeat this procedure three times. Your score on the sit and reach test is the distance, measured in inches, between the edge of the sit and reach box closest to you and the tips of your fingers during the best of your three stretching efforts.

Note that a brief warm-up period consisting of a few minutes of stretching is recommended prior to performance of the test. To reduce the possibility of injury, participants should avoid rapid or jerky movements during the test. It is often useful to have a partner help by holding your legs straight during the test and to assist in measuring the distance. After completing the test, consult Table 2.12 to locate your flexibility fitness category, and record your scores in Laboratory 2.8 on p. 65.

SHOULDER FLEXIBILITY

As the name implies, the shoulder flexibility test evaluates shoulder range of motion (flexibility). The test is performed in the following manner. While standing, raise your right arm and reach down your back as far as possible (Figure 2.11). At the same time, extend your left arm behind your back and reach upward toward your right hand. The objective is to try to overlap your fingers as much as possible. Your score on the shoulder flexibility test is the distance, measured in inches, of finger overlap.

<table>
<tr><td colspan="4">

TABLE 2.12
Physical Fitness Norms for Trunk Flexion

Note that these norms are from the YMCA's sit and reach test. Units for the sit and reach score are in inches.

</td></tr>
</table>

Fitness Category Based on Sit and Reach

Age Group	Excellent	Average	Poor
Men			
18–25	22	16	13
26–35	21	15	12
36–45	21	15	11
Women			
18–25	24	19	16
26–35	23	18	14
36–45	22	17	13

Source: Modified from Golding, L., ed. YMCA Fitness Testing and Assessment Manual. 4th Edition, with permission of the YMCA of the USA, Chicago, IL. Copyright © 2000.

TABLE 2.13
Physical Fitness Norms for Shoulder Flexibility

Note that these norms are for both men and women of all ages. Units for the shoulder flexibility test score are inches and indicate the distance between the fingers of your right and left hands.

Right Hand Up Score	Left Hand Up Score	Fitness Classification
<0	<0	Very poor
0	0	Poor
+1	+1	Average
+2	+2	Good
+3	+3	Excellent
+4	+4	Superior

Source: From Fox, E. L., Kirby, T. E., and Fox, A. R. Bases of fitness. Copyright © 1987. All rights reserved. Adapted by permission of Allyn and Bacon. Norms from ref. 4.

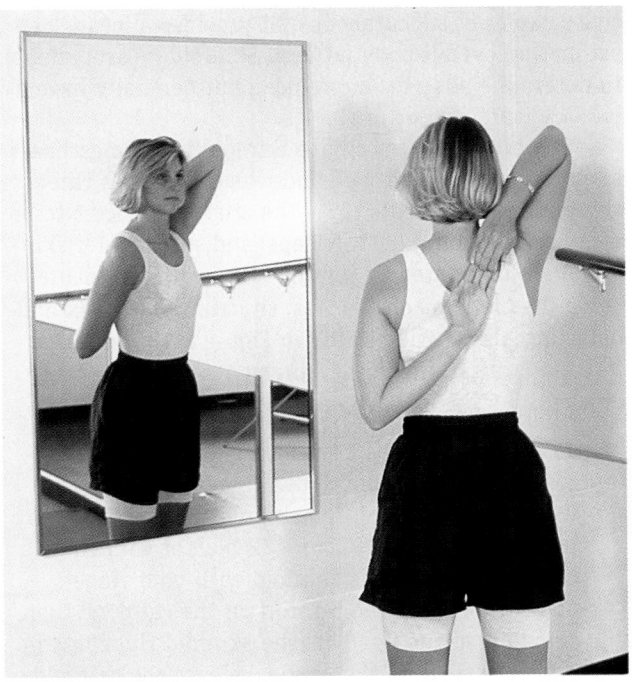

FIGURE 2.11
The shoulder flexibility test.

Measure the distance of finger overlap to the nearest inch. For example, an overlap of 3/4 inch would be recorded as 1 inch. If your fingers fail to overlap, record this score as minus one (−1). Finally, if your fingertips barely touch, record this score as zero (0).

After completing the test with the right hand up, repeat the test in the opposite direction (left hand up). Note that it is common to be more flexible on one side than on the other.

A brief warm-up period consisting of a few minutes of stretching is recommended prior to performance of the shoulder flexibility test. Again, to prevent injury, avoid rapid or jerky movements during the test. After completion of the test, consult Table 2.13 to locate your shoulder flexibility category, and record your scores in Laboratory 2.8 on p. 65.

FLEXIBILITY: HOW DO YOU RATE?

It is not uncommon for both active and inactive individuals to be classified as average or below for both trunk and shoulder flexibility. In fact, only individuals who regularly perform stretching exercises are likely to possess flexibility levels that exceed the average. Regardless of your current flexibility classification, your flexibility goal should be to reach a classification of above average (i.e., good, excellent, or superior).

✦ IN SUMMARY

- Flexibility is defined as the ability to move joints freely through their full range of motion.
- Flexibility measurements are joint specific.
- Two popular tests to evaluate flexibility are the sit and reach test and the shoulder flexibility test.

Nutritional Links

Can the Content of a Pre-Exercise Meal Improve the Results of a Fitness Test?

Many manufacturers of "quick energy" candy bars claim that consumption of their products prior to exercise can improve performance. There is no scientific evidence, however, to support the idea that any type of meal eaten before exercise can improve physical performance (see ref. 23 for a review on this topic). In fact, consumption of high volumes of fluid or large solid meals immediately before exercising can negatively impact performance by creating abdominal discomfort (23). To avoid stomach cramps or other forms of abdominal discomfort during exercise, the pre-exercise meal should be relatively small and eaten at least 2 to 3 hours before exercise. This pre-exercise meal should contain primarily complex carbohydrates (complex sugars such as fruits and breads) and be low in fat. The rationale for this recommendation is based on the fact that carbohydrates are digested rapidly, whereas fat is broken down and absorbed slowly (9). See Cooper (1999) in the suggested reading list for details, and Chapter 7 for a complete discussion of nutrition and physical fitness.

☀ Assessment of Body Composition

Body composition refers to the relative amounts of fat and lean tissue (e.g., muscle) in the body. Recall that a high percentage of body fat is associated with an increased risk of heart disease and other diseases. It is therefore not surprising that several methods of assessing body composition have been developed. A technique considered to be the gold standard for laboratory assessment of body fat in humans is **hydrostatic weighing**, which involves weighing the individual both on land and in a tank of water (7, 9, 24). The two body weights are then entered into a simple formula to calculate percent body fat. Unfortunately, underwater weighing is very time consuming and requires expensive equipment. Thus, this procedure is rarely employed to assess body composition in collegiate physical fitness courses. A rapid and inexpensive method to assess body composition involves measuring subcutaneous (beneath the skin) fat or fat and is called the *skinfold test*.

hydrostatic weighing A method of determining body composition that involves weighing an individual both on land and in a tank of water.

skinfold test A field test to estimate body composition. The test works on the principle that over 50% of body fat lies just beneath the skin. Therefore, measurement of representative samples of subcutaneous fat provides a means of estimating overall body fatness.

THE SKINFOLD TEST

Subcutaneous fat is measured using an instrument called a skinfold caliper. The **skinfold test** relies on the fact that over 50% of body fat lies just beneath the skin (7, 9, 25). Therefore, measurement of representative samples of subcutaneous fat provides a means of estimating overall body fatness. Skinfold measurements to determine body fat are reliable but generally have a ±3–4% margin of error (7, 9).

One of the most accurate skinfold tests to estimate body fatness for both men and women requires three skinfold measurements (25). The anatomical sites to be measured in men (chest, triceps, and subscapular skinfolds) are illustrated in Figure 2.12, and the measurement sites for women (triceps, suprailium, and abdominal skinfolds) are illustrated in Figure 2.13. Note that for standardization, all measurements should be made on the right side of the body.

1. To make each measurement, hold the skinfold between the thumb and index finger and slowly release the tension on the skinfold calipers so as to pinch the skinfold within 1/2 inch of your fingers. Continue to hold the skinfold with your fingers and fully release the tension on the calipers; then, simply read the number (the skinfold thickness in millimeters) from the gauge. Release the skinfold and allow the tissue to relax. Repeat this procedure three times and average the three measurements.

2. After completing the three skinfold measurements, total the measurements and use Tables 2.14 and 2.15 on pgs. 42 and 43 to determine the percent body fat for women and men, respectively. After obtaining your percent body fat, refer to Table 2.16 (26) on p. 44 to determine the body composition fitness category, and record your score in Laboratory 2.9 on p. 67.

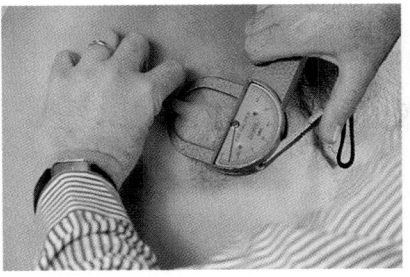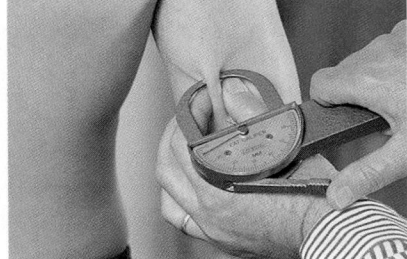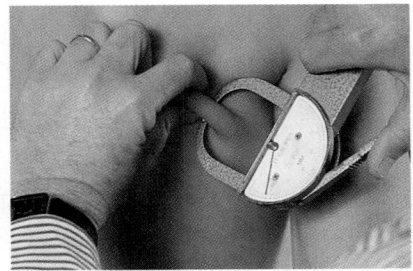

FIGURE 2.12
Skinfold measurement sites for men.

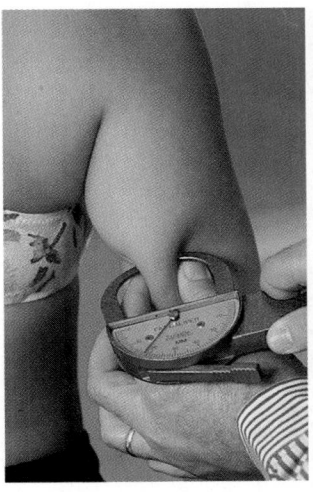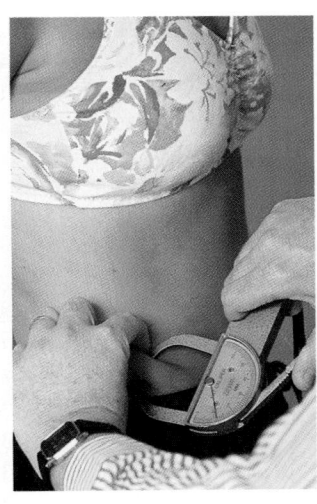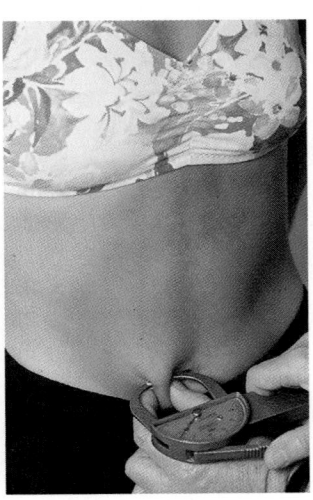

FIGURE 2.13
Skinfold measurement sites for women.

ESTIMATION OF BODY COMPOSITION: FIELD TECHNIQUES

Several quick and inexpensive field techniques exist to evaluate body composition and the risk of heart disease associated with over-fatness (18, 27, 28). Next we describe some of the more popular procedures currently in use.

WAIST-TO-HIP CIRCUMFERENCE RATIO   Recent evidence suggests that the waist-to-hip circumference ratio is an excellent index for determining the risk of disease associated with high body fat (28). The rationale for this technique is that a high percentage of fat in the abdominal region is associated with an increased risk of disease (such as heart disease or hypertension). Therefore, an individual with a large fat deposit in the abdominal region would have a high waist-to-hip ratio and would have a higher risk of disease than someone with a lower waist-to-hip ratio. The procedure for assessing the **waist-to-hip circumference ratio** is as follows:

1. Both waist and hip circumference measurements should be made while standing, using a nonelastic tape. It is important that bulky clothing not be worn during the measurement, because it could bias the circumference measurement. During measurement, the tape should be placed snugly around the body but should not press into the skin. Record your measurements to the nearest millimeter or sixteenth of an inch.

> **waist-to-hip circumference ratio**   An index for determining the risk of disease associated with high body fat. The rationale for this technique is that a high percentage of fat in the abdominal region is associated with an increased risk of disease (e.g., heart disease or hypertension). Therefore, an individual with a large fat deposit in the abdominal region would have a high waist-to-hip ratio and would have a higher risk of disease than someone with a lower waist-to-hip ratio.

TABLE 2.14
Percent Fat Estimate for Women

Sum of Triceps, Abdominal, and Suprailium Skinfolds

Sum of Skinfolds (mm)	Age (years)								
	18–22	23–27	28–32	33–37	38–42	43–47	48–52	53–57	>57
8–12	8.8	9.0	9.2	9.4	9.5	9.7	9.9	10.1	10.3
13–17	10.8	10.9	11.1	11.3	11.5	11.7	11.8	12.0	12.2
18–22	12.6	12.8	13.0	13.2	13.4	13.5	13.7	13.9	14.1
23–27	14.5	14.6	14.8	15.0	15.2	15.4	15.6	15.7	15.9
28–32	16.2	16.4	16.6	16.8	17.0	17.1	17.3	17.5	17.7
33–37	17.9	18.1	18.3	18.5	18.7	18.9	19.0	19.2	19.4
38–42	19.6	19.8	20.0	20.2	20.3	20.5	20.7	20.9	21.1
43–47	21.2	21.4	21.6	21.8	21.9	22.1	22.3	22.5	22.7
48–52	22.8	22.9	23.1	23.3	23.5	23.7	23.8	24.0	24.2
53–57	24.2	24.4	24.6	24.8	25.0	25.2	25.3	25.5	25.7
58–62	25.7	25.9	26.0	26.2	26.4	26.6	26.8	27.0	27.1
63–67	27.1	27.2	27.4	27.6	27.8	28.0	28.2	28.3	28.5
68–72	28.4	28.6	28.7	28.9	29.1	29.3	29.5	29.7	29.8
73–77	29.6	29.8	30.0	30.2	30.4	30.6	30.7	30.9	31.1
78–82	30.9	31.0	31.2	31.4	31.6	31.8	31.9	32.1	32.3
83–87	32.0	32.2	32.4	32.6	32.7	32.9	33.1	33.3	33.5
88–92	33.1	33.3	33.5	33.7	33.8	34.0	34.2	34.4	34.6
93–97	34.1	34.3	34.5	34.7	34.9	35.1	35.2	35.4	35.6
98–102	35.1	35.3	35.5	35.7	35.9	36.0	36.2	36.4	36.6
103–107	36.1	36.2	36.4	36.6	36.8	37.0	37.2	37.3	37.5
108–112	36.9	37.1	37.3	37.5	37.7	37.9	38.0	38.2	38.4
113–117	37.8	37.9	38.1	38.3	39.2	39.4	39.6	39.8	39.2
118–122	38.5	38.7	38.9	39.1	39.4	39.6	39.8	40.0	40.0
123–127	39.2	39.4	39.6	39.8	40.0	40.1	40.3	40.5	40.7
128–132	39.9	40.1	40.2	40.4	40.6	40.8	41.0	41.2	41.3
133–137	40.5	40.7	40.8	41.0	41.2	41.4	41.6	41.7	41.9
138–142	41.0	41.2	41.4	41.6	41.7	41.9	42.1	42.3	42.5
143–147	41.5	41.7	41.9	42.0	42.2	42.4	42.6	42.8	43.0
148–152	41.9	42.1	42.3	42.4	42.6	42.8	43.0	43.2	43.4
153–157	42.3	42.5	42.6	42.8	43.0	43.2	43.4	43.6	43.7
158–162	42.6	42.8	43.0	43.1	43.3	43.5	43.7	43.9	44.1
163–167	42.9	43.0	43.2	43.4	43.6	43.8	44.0	44.1	44.3
168–172	43.1	43.2	43.4	43.6	43.8	44.0	44.2	44.3	44.5
173–177	43.2	43.4	43.6	43.8	43.9	44.1	44.3	44.5	44.7
178–182	43.3	43.5	43.7	43.8	44.0	44.2	44.4	44.6	44.8

Source: From Jackson, A., and M. Pollock. Practical assessment of body composition. Physician and Sports Medicine *13:76–90, 1985.* The McGraw Hill Companies.

TABLE 2.15
Percent Fat Estimate for Men

Sum of Triceps, Chest, and Subscapular Skinfolds

Sum of Skinfolds (mm)	Age (years)								
	<22	23–27	28–32	33–37	38–42	43–47	48–52	53–57	>57
8–10	1.5	2.0	2.5	3.1	3.6	4.1	4.6	5.1	5.6
11–13	3.0	3.5	4.0	4.5	5.1	5.6	6.1	6.6	7.1
14–16	4.5	5.0	5.5	6.0	6.5	7.0	7.6	8.1	8.6
17–19	5.9	6.4	6.9	7.4	8.0	8.5	9.0	9.5	10.0
20–22	7.3	7.8	8.3	8.8	9.4	9.9	10.4	10.9	11.4
23–25	8.6	9.2	9.7	10.2	10.7	11.2	11.8	12.3	12.8
26–28	10.0	10.5	11.0	11.5	12.1	12.6	13.1	13.6	14.2
29–31	11.2	11.8	12.3	12.8	13.4	13.9	14.4	14.9	15.5
32–34	12.5	13.0	13.5	14.1	14.6	15.1	15.7	16.2	16.7
35–37	13.7	14.2	14.8	15.3	15.8	16.4	16.9	17.4	18.0
38–40	14.9	15.4	15.9	16.5	17.0	17.6	18.1	18.6	19.2
41–43	16.0	16.6	17.1	17.6	18.2	18.7	19.3	19.8	20.3
44–46	17.1	17.7	18.2	18.7	19.3	19.8	20.4	20.9	21.5
47–49	18.2	18.7	19.3	19.8	20.4	20.9	21.4	22.0	22.5
50–52	19.2	19.7	20.3	20.8	21.4	21.9	22.5	23.0	23.6
53–55	20.2	20.7	21.3	21.8	22.4	22.9	23.5	24.0	24.6
56–58	21.1	21.7	22.2	22.8	23.3	23.9	24.4	25.0	25.5
59–61	22.0	22.6	23.1	23.7	24.2	24.8	25.3	25.9	26.5
62–64	22.9	23.4	24.0	24.5	25.1	25.7	26.2	26.8	27.3
65–67	23.7	24.3	24.8	25.4	25.9	26.5	27.1	27.6	28.2
68–70	24.5	25.0	25.6	26.2	26.7	27.3	27.8	28.4	29.0
71–73	25.2	25.8	26.3	26.9	27.5	28.0	28.6	29.1	29.7
74–76	25.9	26.5	27.0	27.6	28.2	28.7	29.3	29.9	30.4
77–79	26.6	27.1	27.7	28.2	28.8	29.4	29.9	30.5	31.1
80–82	27.2	27.7	28.3	28.9	29.4	30.0	30.6	31.1	31.7
83–85	27.7	28.3	28.8	29.4	30.0	30.5	31.1	31.7	32.3
86–88	28.2	28.8	29.4	29.9	30.5	31.1	31.6	32.2	32.8
89–91	28.7	29.3	29.8	30.4	31.0	31.5	32.1	32.7	33.3
92–94	29.1	29.7	30.3	30.8	31.4	32.0	32.6	33.1	33.4
95–97	29.5	30.1	30.6	31.2	31.8	32.4	32.9	33.5	34.1
98–100	29.8	30.4	31.0	31.6	32.1	32.7	33.3	33.9	34.4
101–103	30.1	30.7	31.3	31.8	32.4	33.0	33.6	34.1	34.7
104–106	30.4	30.9	31.5	32.1	32.7	33.2	33.8	34.4	35.0
107–109	30.6	31.1	31.7	32.3	32.9	33.4	34.0	34.6	35.2
110–112	30.7	31.3	31.9	32.4	33.0	33.6	34.2	34.7	35.3
113–115	30.8	31.4	32.0	32.5	33.1	33.7	34.3	34.9	35.4
116–118	30.9	31.5	32.0	32.6	33.2	33.8	34.3	34.9	35.5

Source: From Jackson, A., and M. Pollock. Practical assessment of body composition. Physician and Sports Medicine 13:76–90, 1985. The McGraw Hill Companies.

TABLE 2.16
Body Composition Fitness Categories for Men and Women

Percent Body Fat	Body Composition Fitness Category
Men	
<10%	Low body fat
10–20%	Optimal range of body fat
21–25%	Moderately high body fat
26–31%	High body fat
>31%	Very high body fat
Women	
<15%	Low body fat
15–25%	Optimal range of body fat
26–30%	Moderately high body fat
31–35%	High body fat
>35%	Very high body fat

Source: Data from T. Lohman, The use of skinfold to estimate body fatness in children and youth, Journal of Physical Education, Recreation and Dance *58(9): 98–102, 1987.*

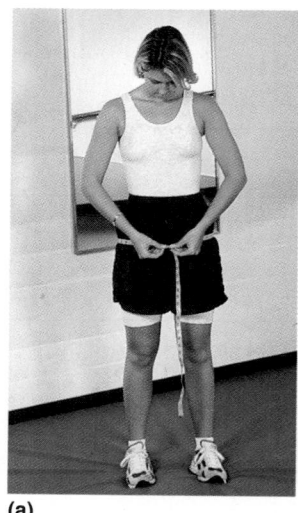 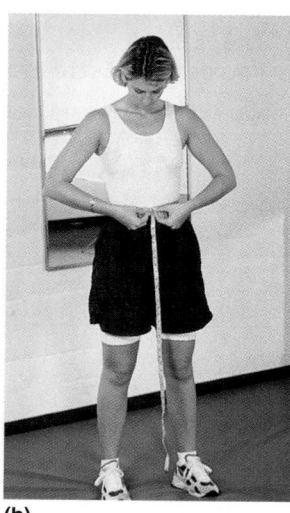

(a) (b)

FIGURE 2.14
Illustration of the waist-to-hip circumference measurements.

2. Perform the waist measurement first. Begin by placing the tape at the level of the umbilicus (navel; Figure 2.14 (a)). Make your measurement at the end of a normal expiration.

3. To make the hip measurement, place the tape around the maximum circumference of the buttocks (Figure 2.14 (b)).

4. After completing the measurements, divide the waist circumference by the hip circumference to determine the waist-to-hip ratio. Use Table 2.17 to determine the waist-to-hip ratio rating. Your goal in terms of waist-to-hip ratio classification should be to reach the optimal classification that places you in the lowest risk category for heart disease.

BODY MASS INDEX Research has shown that the **body mass index** (BMI), despite its many limitations, is a useful technique for placing people into categories of normal or too much body fat (27, 28). The BMI is simply the ratio of the body weight (kilograms; kg) divided by height (in meters) squared (m2):

$$\text{BMI} = \text{weight (kg)}/\text{height (m)}^2$$

(Note: 1 kg = 2.2 pounds, and 1 m = 39.25 inches.)

body mass index (BMI) A useful technique for categorizing people with respect to their degree of body fat. The BMI is simply the ratio of body weight (kilograms; kg) divided by height squared (meters^2).

For example, if an individual weighs 64.5 kg and is 1.72 m tall, the BMI would be computed as follows:

$$64.5 \text{ kg}/(1.72 \text{ m})^2 = 64.5/2.96 = 21.8$$

After calculating your BMI, use Table 2.18 to determine your degree of body fatness. The concept behind the BMI is that individuals with low percent body fat will have a low BMI. For example, men and women with a BMI of less than 25 and 27, respectively, are classified as having optimal body fat. In contrast, men and women with a BMI of greater than 40 are considered to be extremely obese.

Although BMI is a simple and inexpensive method for estimating body composition, this technique has limitations. Indeed, in some cases this method can over- or underestimate body fatness. For example, an individual with a low percentage of body fat but a high level of muscularity would typically have a relatively high BMI, which would incorrectly suggest a high percentage of body fat. Therefore, this technique should be used only when other more sensitive techniques (i.e., hydrostatic weighing and skinfold measurements) are not available.

HEIGHT/WEIGHT TABLES The Metropolitan Life Insurance Company has published a height/weight table designed to determine whether a person is overweight due to too much body fat. Although the idea that a simple table could be used to determine an individual's ideal body weight is attractive, several problems affect this procedure. The major problem with this approach is that the tables do not indicate how much of the body weight is fat. For example, an individual can exceed the ideal body weight on such a chart by being either heavily muscled or overfat. Therefore, this approach to a determination of an "ideal body weight" is not recommended.

TABLE 2.17
Waist-to-Hip Circumference Ratio Rating Scale

Men	Women	Classification (risk of disease)
>1.0	>0.85	High risk
0.90–1.0	0.80–0.85	Moderately high risk
<0.90	<0.80	Optimal low risk of disease

Source: Modified from Van Itallie, T. Topography of body fat: Relationship to risk of cardiovascular and other diseases. In T. Lohman, et al., eds. Anthropometric standardization reference manual. Human Kinetics, Champaign, IL, 1988.

TABLE 2.18
Body Mass Index Classification of the Degree of Body Fatness

Body Fat Category	BMI (weight/height^2) Men	Women
Optimal body fat	<25	<27
Moderately high body fat	25–30	27–30
High body fat	31–40	31–40
Very high body fat	>40	>40

Source: Adapted from DiGirolamo, M. Body composition—roundtable. Physician and Sports Medicine (March):144–162, 1986.

BODY COMPOSITION: HOW DO YOU RATE?

The fitness categories presented for body composition differ from those earlier for the other components of health-related physical fitness. While "superior" was the highest fitness level presented that could be achieved for cardiorespiratory, strength, and muscular endurance fitness, the classification of "optimal" is the highest standard for body composition. Regardless of the body composition test employed to assess body fat, any category other than optimal is considered unsatisfactory for health-related fitness. Therefore, your goal should be to reach and maintain an optimal body composition.

The rationale for the concept of optimal body composition is as follows. Research suggests that a range of 10% to 20% body fat is an optimal health and fitness goal for men; the optimal range for women is 15% to 25%. These ranges in body fat provide little risk of disease associated with body fatness and permit individual differences in physical activity patterns and diet. Body fat levels above the optimal range are associated with an increased risk of disease and are therefore undesirable.

What is less obvious is that a body fat percentage that is lower than the recommended optimal range is also undesirable. Indeed, percentages of body fat below the optimal range may also increase the risk of health problems. This is because extremely low percentages of body fat are often associated with poor nutrition and a loss of muscle mass. This is clearly undesirable. The relationships among diet, exercise, and body composition are discussed in detail in Chapter 8.

☀ IN SUMMARY

- Body composition is an important part of health-related physical fitness because a high percentage of body fat is associated with an increased risk of disease.

- Field tests for estimating body composition include skinfold measurements, assessment of the body mass index, and/or examination of the waist-to-hip circumference ratio.

Summary

1. Prior to beginning a fitness program (or performing a fitness evaluation), you should have your health status evaluated by a physician.

2. An objective evaluation of your current fitness status is important before beginning an exercise training program. Further, periodic retesting can provide feedback about your training progress.

3. Cardiorespiratory fitness is the ability of the heart to pump oxygen-rich blood to exercising muscles; this translates into the ability to perform endurance-type exercise. Field tests to evaluate cardiorespiratory fitness include the 1.5-mile run test, the 1-mile walk test, the cycle ergometer fitness test, and the step test.

4. Muscular strength is the maximum amount of force you can produce during one contraction. The most popular method of evaluating muscular strength is the one-repetition maximum (1 RM) test.

5. Muscular endurance is the ability of a muscle group to generate force over and over again. Two commonly used methods of evaluating muscular endurance are the push-up and sit-up tests.

6. Flexibility is defined as the ability to move joints freely through their full range of motion. Although flexibility is joint specific, two popular means of evaluating flexibility are the sit and reach test and the shoulder flexibility test.

7. Body composition is an important component of health-related physical fitness because a high percentage of body fat is associated with an increased risk of disease. In the field, the amount of body fat can be estimated using skinfold measurements, assessment of the body mass index, or examination of the waist-to-hip circumference ratio.

Study Questions

1. Describe the following field tests used to evaluate cardiorespiratory fitness: the 1.5-mile run test, the 1-mile walk test, the cycle ergometer fitness test, and the step test.

2. Discuss the one-repetition maximum (1 RM) test for measuring muscular strength. What safety concerns are associated with this test?

3. Explain how the push-up and sit-up tests are used to evaluate muscular endurance.

4. Discuss the concept that flexibility is joint specific.

5. Identify two field tests used to examine flexibility.

6. Define the term *recovery index*.

7. Discuss the following techniques for assessing body composition: hydrostatic weighing and the skinfold test.

8. How can measurement of the waist-to-hip circumference ratio and body mass index be used to assess body composition?

Suggested Reading

American College of Sports Medicine. *Guidelines for Exercise Testing,* 6th ed. Philadelphia: Lea and Febiger, 2000.

Howley, E., and D. Franks. *Health Fitness Instructor's Handbook,* 4th edition. Champaign, IL: Human Kinetics Publishers, 2003.

Nieman, D. *Exercise Testing and Prescription: A Health-related Approach,* 5th edition. St. Louis, MO: McGraw Hill, 2002.

Powers, S., and E. Howley. *Exercise Physiology: Theory and Application to Fitness and Performance,* 5th edition. St. Louis, MO: McGraw Hill, 2004.

Roitman, J. (Editor). *ACSM'S Resource Manual for Guidelines for Exercise Testing and Prescription.* Philadelphia: Lippincott Williams and Williams, 2001.

For links to the web sites below visit The Total Fitness and Wellness Website at www.aw-bc.com/powers.

American Heart Association

Contains latest information about ways to reduce your risk of heart and vascular diseases. Site includes information about exercise, diet, and heart disease.

American College of Sports Medicine

Contains information about exercise, health, and fitness.

Fitness Tests

Describes tests for aerobic power, anaerobic power, flexibility, and body composition.

References

1. American College of Sports Medicine. *Guidelines for Exercise Testing,* 6th ed. Philadelphia: Lea and Febiger, 2000.

2. American College of Sports Medicine. *Resource Manual for Exercise Testing and Prescription.* Philadelphia: Lea and Febiger, 1998.

3. Corbin, C., G. Welk, R. Lindsey, and W. Corbin. *Concepts of Physical Fitness.* St. Louis, MO: McGraw-Hill, 2003.

4. Getchell, B. *Physical Fitness: A Way of Life,* 5th ed. Needham Heights, MA: Allyn and Bacon, 1998.

5. Barrow, M. *Heart Talk: Understanding Cardiovascular Diseases.* Gainesville, FL: Cor-Ed Publishing, 1992.

6. McGlynn, G. *Dynamics of Fitness: A Practical Approach,* 5th ed. Dubuque, IA: Wm. C. Brown, 1998.

7. Pollock, M., and J. Wilmore. *Exercise in Health and Disease,* 3rd ed. Philadelphia: W. B. Saunders, 1990.

8. Pollock, M., J. Wilmore, and S. Fox. *Health and Fitness Through Physical Activity.* New York: John Wiley and Sons, 1978.

9. Powers, S., and E. Howley *Exercise Physiology: Theory and Application to Fitness and Performance,* 4th ed. St. Louis, MO: McGraw Hill, 2004.

10. Robergs, R., and S. Keteyian. *Fundamental Principles of Exercise Physiology: For Fitness, Performance, and Health.* St. Louis, MO: McGraw Hill, 2002.

11. Cooper, K. *The Aerobics Program for Total Well-Being.* New York: M. Evans, 1982.

12. Cooper, K. *The Aerobics Way.* New York: Bantam Books, 1977.

13. Fox, E. A simple technique for predicting maximal aerobic power. *Journal of Applied Physiology* 35:914–916, 1973.

14. Rippe, J., A. Ward., J. Porcari, and P. Freedson. Walking for fitness and health. *Journal of the American Medical Association* 259:2720–2724, 1988.

15. Rippe, J. Walking for fitness: A roundtable. *Physician and Sports Medicine* 14:144–159, 1986.

16. Ward, A., and J. Rippe. *Walking for Health and Fitness.* Philadelphia: J. B. Lippincott, 1988.

17. Golding, L., C. Myers, and W. Sinning. *Y's Way to Physical Fitness: The Complete Guide to Fitness Testing and Instruction,* 3rd ed. Champaign, IL: Human Kinetics, 1989.

18. Howley, E., and D. Franks. *Health Fitness Instructor's Handbook,* 4th edition. Champaign, IL: Human Kinetics Publishers, 2003.

19. Roitman, J., ed. *ACSM's Resource Manual for Guidelines for Exercise Testing and Prescription.* Philadelphia: Lippincott Williams & Wilkins, 2001.

20. Axler, C., and S. McGill. Low back loads over a variety of abdominal exercises: Searching for the safest abdominal challenge. *Medicine and Science in Sports and Exercise* 29:804–810, 1997.

21. Sparling, P. Field testing for abdominal muscular fitness; speed versus cadence sit-ups. *ACSM's Health and Fitness Journal* 1(4):30–33, 1997.

22. Faulkner, R., et al. A partial curl-up protocol for adults based on two procedures. *Canadian Journal of Sports Sciences* 14:135–141, 1989.

23. Lamb, D., and M. Williams. *Ergogenics: Enhancement of Performance in Exercise and Sport.* Vol. 4. Dubuque, IA: Brown and Benchmark, 1991.

24. Lohman, T., et al. Body fat measurement goes high-tech: Not all are created equal. *ACSM's Health and Fitness Journal* 1(1):30–35, 1997.

25. Williams, M. *Lifetime Fitness and Wellness.* Dubuque, IA: Wm. C. Brown, 1996.

26. Jackson, A., and M. Pollock. Practical assessment of body composition. *Physician and Sports Medicine* 13:76–90, 1985.

27. DiGirolamo, M. Body composition—roundtable. *Physician and Sports Medicine* (March):144–162, 1986.

28. Van Itallie, T. Topography of body fat: Relationship to risk of cardiovascular and other diseases. In T. Lohman et al., eds. *Anthropometric Standardization Reference Manual.* Champaign, IL: Human Kinetics, 1988.

29. Lohman, T. The use of skinfold to estimate body fatness in children and youth. *Journal of Alliance for Health, Physical Education, Recreation, and Dance* 58:98–102, 1987.

30. Gardiner, P. F. *Neuromuscular Aspects of Physical Activity.* Champaign, IL: Human Kinetics, 2001.

31. Larsen, G., J. George, J. Alexander, G. Fellingham, S. Aldana, and A. Parcel. Prediction of maximum oxygen consumption from walking, jogging, or running. *Research Quarterly for Exercise and Sport* 73: 66–72, 2002.

Health Status Questionnaire

NAME _____ DATE _____

The following questions are part of an exercise screening questionnaire originally developed by the Connecticut Mutual Life Insurance Company and modified by the authors. If you answer "yes" to any of the following questions, you should have a thorough medical exam prior to beginning an exercise program.

1. Have you ever had chest pains or a sensation of pressure in your chest that occurred during or immediately following exercise?

2. Do you have chest discomfort when climbing stairs or walking against a cold wind, or during any physical activity?

3. Does your heart ever beat unevenly or irregularly or seem to flutter or skip beats?

4. Do you ever experience sudden bursts of very rapid heart action or periods of slow heart action without apparent cause?

5. Do you take any prescription medicine on a regular basis?

6. Has your doctor ever told you that you have heart problems?

7. Do you have any respiratory problems such as asthma, or do you experience shortness of breath during light physical activity?

8. Do you have arthritis or any condition affecting your joints or back that makes exercise painful?

9. Do you have any of the following risk factors for heart disease: (a) high blood pressure*; (b) high blood cholesterol; (c) overweight by more than 30%; (d) smoking; or (e) any close relatives (father, mother, brother, etc.) that have had a history of heart disease prior to age 55?

*High blood pressure is generally defined as systolic blood pressure $\geq$ 140 mmHg and diastolic blood pressure $\geq$ 90 mmHg.

Measurement of Cardiorespiratory Fitness:
The 1.5-Mile Run Test

NAME _____ DATE _____

DIRECTIONS

The objective of the test is to complete the 1.5-mile distance as quickly as possible. The run can be completed on an oval track or any properly measured course. You should attempt this test only if you have met the medical clearance criteria discussed in Chapter 2 of this text.

Prior to beginning the test, perform a 5- to 10-minute warm-up. If you become extremely fatigued during the test, slow your pace—do not overstress yourself! If you feel faint or nauseated, or experience any unusual pains in your upper body, stop and notify your instructor!

On completion of the test, cool down and record your time and fitness category (Table 2.1).

TEST 1 DATE _____

Ambient conditions:

*Temperature: _____ *Relative humidity: _____

Finish time: _____ Fitness category: _____

TEST 2 DATE _____

Ambient conditions:

*Temperature: _____ *Relative humidity: _____

Finish time: _____ Fitness category: _____

TEST 3 DATE _____

Ambient conditions:

*Temperature: _____ *Relative humidity: _____

Finish time: _____ Fitness category: _____

*The purpose of recording the temperature and relative humidity is to provide a record of the amount of heat stress during the test. High heat and relative humidity could have a negative impact on your test score.

Measurement of Cardiorespiratory Fitness:
The 1-Mile Walk Test

NAME _____ DATE _____

DIRECTIONS

The objective of the test is to walk the 1-mile distance as quickly as possible. The walk can be completed on an oval track or any properly measured course. You should attempt this test only if you have met the medical clearance criteria discussed in Chapter 2 of this text.

Prior to beginning the test, perform a 5- to 10-minute warm-up. If you become extremely fatigued during the test, slow your pace—do not overstress yourself! If you feel faint or nauseated, or experience any unusual pains in your upper body, stop and notify your instructor!

On completion of the test, cool down and record your time and fitness category (Table 2.2).

TEST 1 DATE _____

Ambient conditions:

*Temperature: _____ *Relative humidity: _____

Finish time: _____ Fitness category: _____

TEST 2 DATE _____

Ambient conditions:

*Temperature: _____ *Relative humidity: _____

Finish time: _____ Fitness category: _____

TEST 3 DATE _____

Ambient conditions:

*Temperature: _____ *Relative humidity: _____

Finish time: _____ Fitness category: _____

*The purpose of recording the temperature and relative humidity is to provide a record of the amount of heat stress during the test. High heat and relative humidity could have a negative impact on your test score.

Submaximal Cycle Test to Determine Cardiorespiratory Fitness

NAME _____ DATE _____

DIRECTIONS

Warm up for 3 minutes using unloaded pedaling. Set the appropriate load for your age and gender and begin. (See p. 23 for load-setting instructions.) Exercise for a 5-minute period. Count your pulse during a 15-second period between minutes 4.5 and 5 of the test.

Cool down for 3 to 5 minutes using unloaded pedaling. Record your heart rate (15-second count) below and compute your relative $\dot{V}O_{2max}$ using Table 2.4. After calculating your relative $\dot{V}O_{2max}$, locate your fitness category in Table 2.5.

TEST 1 DATE _____

Heart rate (15-second count) during minute 5 of test: _____

Fitness category: _____

TEST 2 DATE _____

Heart rate (15-second count) during minute 5 of test: _____

Fitness category: _____

TEST 3 DATE _____

Heart rate (15-second count) during minute 5 of test: _____

Fitness category: _____

Step Test to Determine Cardiorespiratory Fitness

NAME _____ DATE _____

DIRECTIONS

Perform 30 complete step ups and downs per minute using an 18-inch step over a 3-minute period. On completion of 3 minutes of exercise, sit quietly and count the number of heart beats in 30 seconds during the following time periods: 1 to 1.5 minutes post exercise; 2 to 2.5 minutes post exercise; and 3 to 3.5 minutes post exercise. Record your heart rates below and use Table 2.6 to determine your fitness category.

TEST 1 DATE _____

Recovery heart rate post exercise (beats)

1–1.5 min: _____

2–2.5 min: _____

3–3.5 min: _____

Total: _____ (recovery index)

Fitness category: _____

TEST 2 DATE _____

Recovery heart rate post exercise (beats)

1–1.5 min: _____

2–2.5 min: _____

3–3.5 min: _____

Total: _____ (recovery index)

Fitness category: _____

TEST 3 DATE _____

Recovery heart rate post exercise (beats)

1–1.5 min: _____

2–2.5 min: _____

3–3.5 min: _____

Total: _____ (recovery index)

Fitness category: _____

Measurement of Muscular Strength:
The 1 RM Test

NAME _____ DATE _____

DIRECTIONS

After performance of your 1 RM test, compute your muscular strength scores as follows:

$$\frac{\text{1 RM weight}}{\text{body weight}} \times 100 = \text{muscle strength score}$$

Record your muscular strength scores below and use Table 2.7 to determine your fitness category.

Age: _____ **Body weight:** _____ **pounds**

TEST 1 DATE _____

Exercise	1 RM (lbs)	Muscular Strength	Fitness Category
Bench press	_____	_____	_____
Biceps curl	_____	_____	_____
Shoulder press	_____	_____	_____
Leg press	_____	_____	_____

TEST 2 DATE _____

Exercise	1 RM (lbs)	Muscular Strength	Fitness Category
Bench press	_____	_____	_____
Biceps curl	_____	_____	_____
Shoulder press	_____	_____	_____
Leg press	_____	_____	_____

Measurement of Muscular Endurance:
The Regular Push-Up, Sit-Up, and Curl-Up Tests

NAME _____ **DATE** _____

DIRECTIONS

After completion of the regular push-up, sit-up, and curl-up tests, record your scores and fitness classifications (Tables 2.9A, 2.10, and 2.11).

Age: _____

TEST 1 **DATE** _____

Number of push-ups (1 min): _____   Fitness category: _____

Number of sit-ups (1 min): _____   Fitness category: _____

Number of curl-ups: _____   Fitness category: _____

TEST 2 **DATE** _____

Number of push-ups (1 min): _____   Fitness category: _____

Number of sit-ups (1 min): _____   Fitness category: _____

Number of curl-ups: _____   Fitness category: _____

Measurement of Muscular Endurance Using the Modified Push-Up Test

NAME _____ DATE _____

DIRECTIONS

After completion of the modified push-up test, record your scores and fitness classification (use Table 2.9B for fitness classification).

TEST 1 DATE _____

Number of modified push-ups _____ Fitness category _____

TEST 2 DATE _____

Number of modified push-ups _____ Fitness category _____

Assessment of Flexibility: Trunk Flexion (Sit and Reach Test) and the Shoulder Flexibility Test

NAME _____ **DATE** _____

DIRECTIONS

After completion of the sit and reach test and the shoulder flexibility test, record your scores and fitness classifications (Tables 2.12 and 2.13).

TEST 1 DATE _____

Sit and reach score (inches): _____   Fitness category: _____

Shoulder flexibility (inches): _____   Fitness category: _____

TEST 2 DATE _____

Sit and reach score (inches): _____   Fitness category: _____

Shoulder flexibility (inches): _____   Fitness category: _____

Assessment of Body Composition

NAME _____ DATE _____

DIRECTIONS

In the spaces below, record your body composition raw data and fitness categories obtained using the skinfold test, body mass index, and/or the waist-to-hip circumference ratio (Tables 2.14–2.17).

TEST 1   DATE _____

Skinfold Test

Sum of three skinfolds (mm): _____

Percent body fat: _____

Fitness category: _____

Body Mass Index

Body mass index score: _____

Fitness category: _____

Waist-to-Hip Circumference Ratio

Waist-to-hip circumference ratio: _____

Fitness category: _____

TEST 2   DATE _____

Skinfold Test

Sum of three skinfolds (mm): _____

Percent body fat: _____

Fitness category: _____

Body Mass Index

Body mass index score: _____

Fitness category: _____

Waist-to-Hip Circumference Ratio

Waist-to-hip circumference ratio: _____

Fitness category: _____

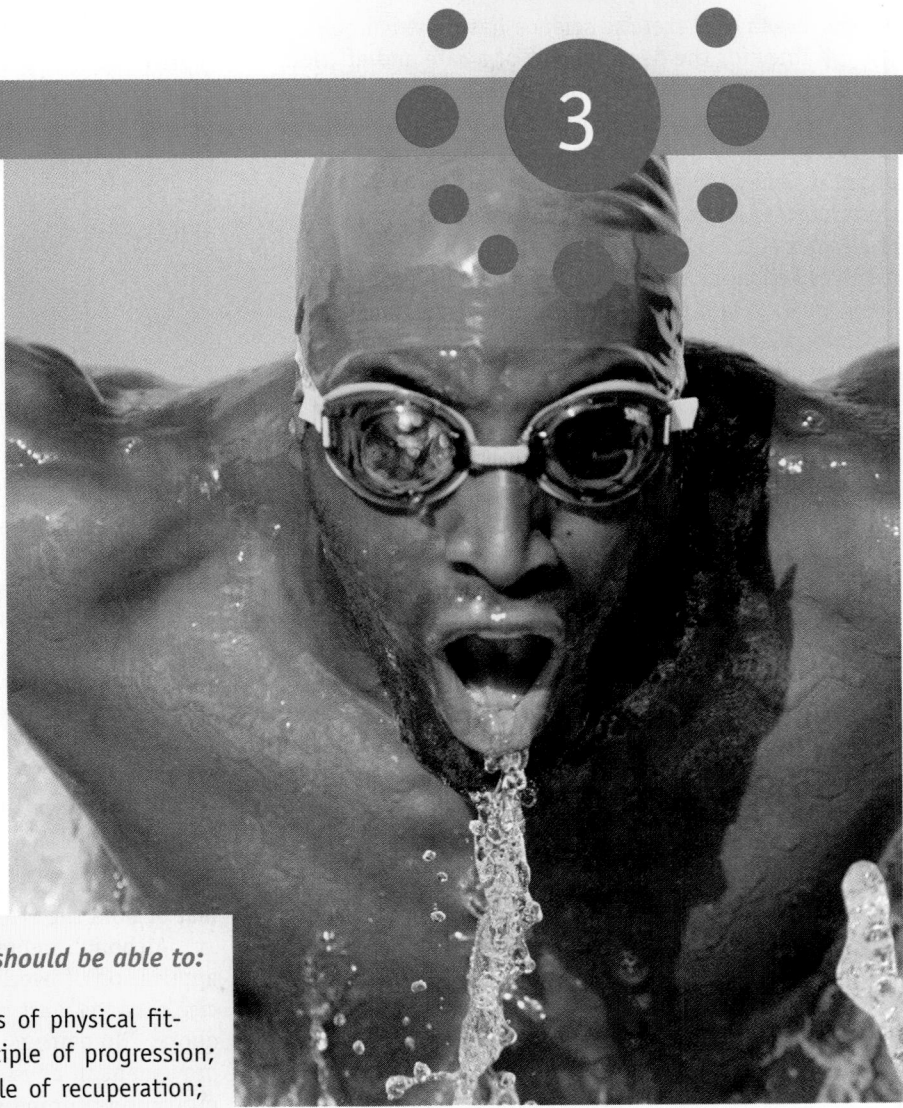

General Principles of Exercise for Health and Fitness

After studying this chapter, you should be able to:

1. Discuss the following concepts of physical fitness: overload principle; principle of progression; specificity of exercise; principle of recuperation; and reversibility of training effects.

2. Outline the physiological objectives of a warm-up and cool-down.

3. Identify the general principles of exercise prescription.

4. Discuss the concepts of progression and maintenance of exercise training.

5. Explain why individualizing the workout is an important concept for the development of an exercise prescription.

6. Discuss how much exercise is required to reach the "threshold for health benefits."

Research in exercise science has provided guidelines for the development of a safe and efficient program to improve personal fitness (1–9). The purpose of this chapter is to provide you with an overview of general principles for improving your physical fitness. The basic concepts contained within this chapter can be applied to both men and women of all ages and fitness levels. The individual components of health-related physical fitness are covered in Chapters 4, 5, and 6, which detail the development of cardiorespiratory fitness, muscular strength/endurance, and flexibility, respectively.

☀ Principles of Exercise Training to Improve Physical Fitness

Although the specifics of exercise training programs should be tailored to the individual, the general principles of physical fitness are the same for everyone. In the following sections we describe the training concepts of overload, progression, specificity, recuperation, and reversibility.

OVERLOAD PRINCIPLE

The **overload principle** is a key component of all conditioning programs (1–9). In order to improve physical fitness, the body or specific muscles must be stressed. For example, for a skeletal muscle to increase in strength, the muscle must work against a heavier load than normal. We achieve an overload by increasing the intensity of exercise (i.e., by using heavier weights). Note, however, that overload can also be achieved by increasing the duration of exercise. For instance, to increase muscular endurance, a muscle must be worked over a longer duration than normal (by performing a higher number of exercise repetitions). Another practical example of the overload principle applied to health-related physical fitness is the improvement of flexibility. To increase the range of motion at a joint, we must

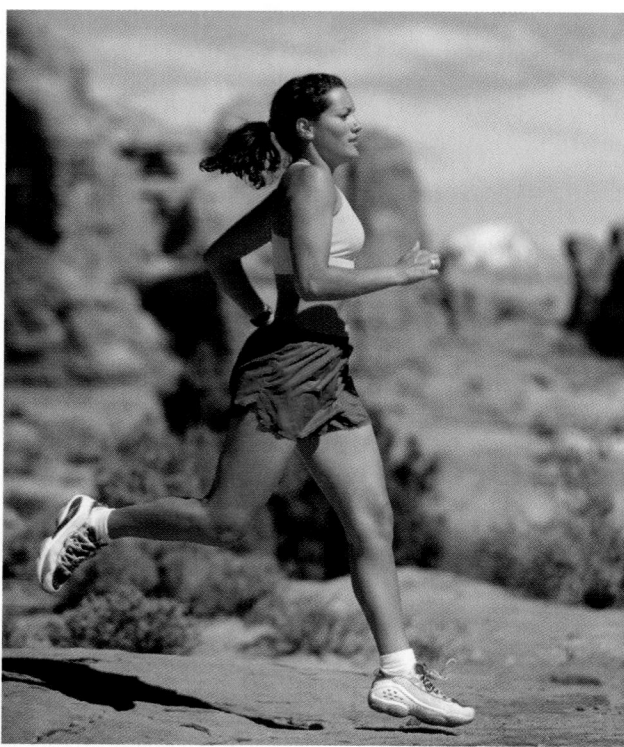

Running illustrates the concept of specificity because it promotes improvements in muscular endurance in the legs.

either stretch the muscle to a longer length than normal or hold the stretch for a longer time.

Although improvement in physical fitness requires application of overload, this does not mean that exercise sessions must be exhausting. The often-heard quote, "No pain, no gain," is not accurate. In fact, improvement in physical fitness can be achieved without punishing training sessions (5).

PRINCIPLE OF PROGRESSION

The **principle of progression** is an extension of the overload principle. It states that overload should be increased gradually during the course of a physical fitness program. This concept is illustrated in Figure 3.1. Note that the overload of a training program should generally be increased slowly during the first 4 to 6 weeks of the exercise program. After this initial period, the overload can be increased at a steady but progressive rate during the next 18 to 20 weeks of training. It is important that the overload not be increased too slowly or too rapidly if optimum fitness improvement is to result. Progression that is too slow will result in limited improvement in physical fitness. Increasing the exercise overload too rapidly may result in chronic fatigue and injury.

Muscle or joint injuries that occur because of too much exercise are called *overuse injuries*. Exercise-induced injuries can come from either short bouts of

---

overload principle A basic principle of physical conditioning that states that in order to improve physical fitness, the body or specific muscles must be stressed. For example, for a skeletal muscle to increase in strength, the muscle must work against a heavier load than normal.

principle of progression A principle of training that dictates that overload should be increased gradually during the course of a physical fitness program.

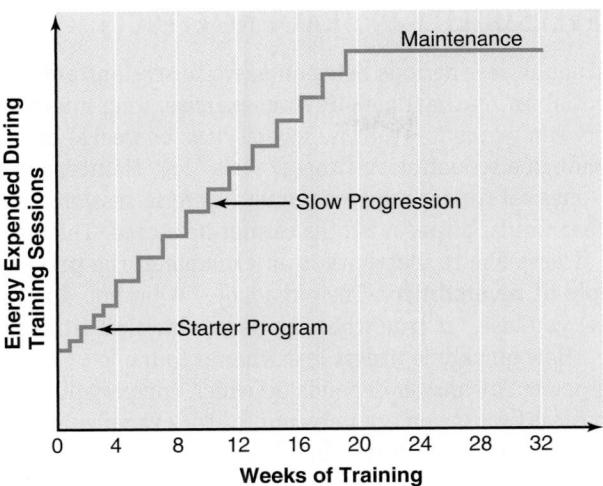

FIGURE 3.1
The progression and maintenance of exercise training during the first several months after beginning an exercise training program.
Source: From Pollack, Wilmore, and Fox, *Health and Fitness through Physical Activity.* Copyright © 1978. Reprinted by permission of Pearson Education, Inc.

high-intensity exercise or long bouts of low-intensity exercise. (See Chapter 13 for information on the care and prevention of injuries.)

What is a safe rate of progression during an exercise training program? A definitive answer to this question is not possible because individuals vary in their tolerance for exercise overload. However, a commonsense guideline for improving physical fitness and avoiding overuse injuries is the **ten percent rule** (6). In short, this rule says that the training intensity or duration of exercise should not be increased more than 10% per week. For example, a runner running 20 minutes per day could increase his or her daily exercise duration to 22 minutes per day (10% of 20 = 2) the following week.

When an individual reaches his or her desired level of physical fitness (that is, you have reached your goal as defined by one of the fitness tests described in Chapter 2), it is no longer necessary to increase the training intensity or duration. Indeed, once a desired level of fitness has been achieved, physical fitness can be maintained by regular exercise at a constant level (Figure 3.1). Exercising to sustain a certain level of physical fitness is referred to as a *maintenance program.*

SPECIFICITY OF EXERCISE

Another key concept of training is the **principle of specificity,** which states that the exercise training effect is specific to those muscles involved in the activity (10). You would not expect your arms to become trained following a 10-week jogging program!

Specificity of training also applies to the types of adaptations that occur in the muscle. For example, strength training results in an increase in muscle

Principle of Recuperation

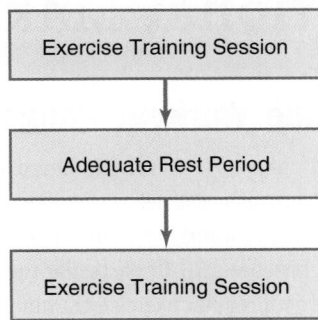

FIGURE 3.2
Principle of recuperation. This principle of training requires that adequate rest periods separate exercise training sessions.

strength but does not greatly improve the endurance of the muscle. Therefore, strength training is specific to improving muscular strength (11). Similarly, endurance exercise training results in an improvement in muscular endurance without altering muscular strength much (12).

Consider the following simple illustration of exercise specificity. Suppose you want to improve your ability to run a distance of 3 miles. In this case, specific training should include running 3 or more miles several times a week. This type of training would improve muscular endurance in your legs but would not result in large improvements in leg strength (10).

PRINCIPLE OF RECUPERATION

Because the principle of overload requires exercise stress to improve physical fitness, it follows that exercise training places a stress on the body. During the recovery period between exercise training sessions, the body adapts to the exercise stress by increasing endurance or becoming stronger. Therefore, a period of rest is essential for achieving maximal benefit from exercise. This needed rest period between exercise training sessions is called the **principle of recuperation** (Figure 3.2).

ten percent rule   The training intensity or duration of exercise should not be increased more than 10% per week.
principle of specificity   The effect of exercise training is specific to those muscles involved in the activity.
principle of recuperation   The body requires recovery periods between exercise training sessions in order to adapt to the exercise stress. Therefore, a period of rest is essential for achieving maximal benefit from exercise.

Nutritional Links
TO HEALTH AND FITNESS

Diet and the Workout Hangover

Can a poor diet contribute to fatigue and overtraining? Yes! Failure to consume the recommended amounts of carbohydrates, fats, proteins, vitamins, and minerals can lead to chronic fatigue (15). Of particular importance to people engaged in a regular exercise training program is dietary carbohydrates. Because heavy exercise uses carbohydrates as a primary fuel source (6), diets low in carbohydrates can result in a depletion of muscle carbohydrate stores and can lead to a feeling of chronic fatigue. To maintain muscle carbohydrate stores, these nutrients should make up 60% of the total energy contained in your diet (6, 15). See Chapter 7 for a complete discussion of diet and nutrition for physical fitness.

How much rest is required between heavy exercise training sessions? One or two days is adequate for most individuals (6). Failure to get enough rest between sessions may result in a fatigue syndrome referred to as **overtraining.** Overtraining may lead to chronic fatigue and/or injuries. A key question is, How do you diagnose overtraining? Sore and stiff muscles or a feeling of general fatigue the morning after an exercise training session, sometimes called a "workout hangover," is a common symptom. The cure is to increase the duration of rest between workouts, reduce the intensity of workouts, or both. Although too much exercise is the primary cause of the overtraining syndrome, failure to consume a well-balanced diet can contribute to the feeling of a workout hangover (Nutritional Links to Health and Fitness).

overtraining   The result of failure to get enough rest between exercise training sessions. Overtraining may lead to chronic fatigue and/or injuries.
principle of reversibility   The loss of fitness due to inactivity.
exercise prescription   The dosage of exercise to effectively promote physical fitness. Exercise prescriptions should be tailored to meet the needs of the individual and include fitness goals, mode of exercise, a warm-up, a primary conditioning period, and a cool-down.

REVERSIBILITY OF TRAINING EFFECTS

Although rest periods between exercise sessions are essential for maximal benefit from exercise, long intervals between workouts (that is, several days or weeks) can result in a reduction in fitness levels (13). Maintenance of physical fitness requires regular exercise sessions. In other words, physical fitness cannot be stored. The loss of fitness due to inactivity is an example of the **principle of reversibility.** The old adage, "What you don't use, you lose," is true when applied to physical fitness.

How quickly is fitness lost when training is stopped? The answer depends on which component of physical fitness you are referring to. For example, after cessation of strength training, the loss of muscular strength is relatively slow (11, 14). In contrast, after you stop performing endurance exercise, the loss of muscular endurance is relatively rapid (13). Figure 3.3 illustrates this point. Note that 8 weeks after stopping strength training, only 10% of muscular strength is lost (14). In contrast, 8 weeks after cessation of endurance training, 30% to 40% of muscular endurance is lost (13).

☀ IN SUMMARY

- Five key principles of exercise training are: (1) overload principle; (2) principle of progression; (3) specificity of exercise; (4) principle of recuperation; and (5) reversibility of training effects.
- The overload principle refers to the fact that in order to improve physical fitness, the body or the specific muscle group used during exercise must be stressed.
- The principle of progression is an extension of the overload principle and states that overload should be increased gradually over the course of a physical fitness training program.
- The principle of specificity refers to the fact that exercise training is specific to those muscles involved in the activity.
- The requirement for a rest period between training sessions is called "the principle of recuperation."
- Loss of physical fitness due to inactivity is referred to as "the principle of reversibility."

☀ General Principles of Exercise Prescription

Doctors often prescribe medications to treat certain diseases, and for every individual there is an appropriate dosage of medicine to treat an illness. Similarly, for each individual there is a correct "dosage" of exercise to effectively promote physical fitness, called an **exercise prescription** (5, 8). Exercise prescriptions should

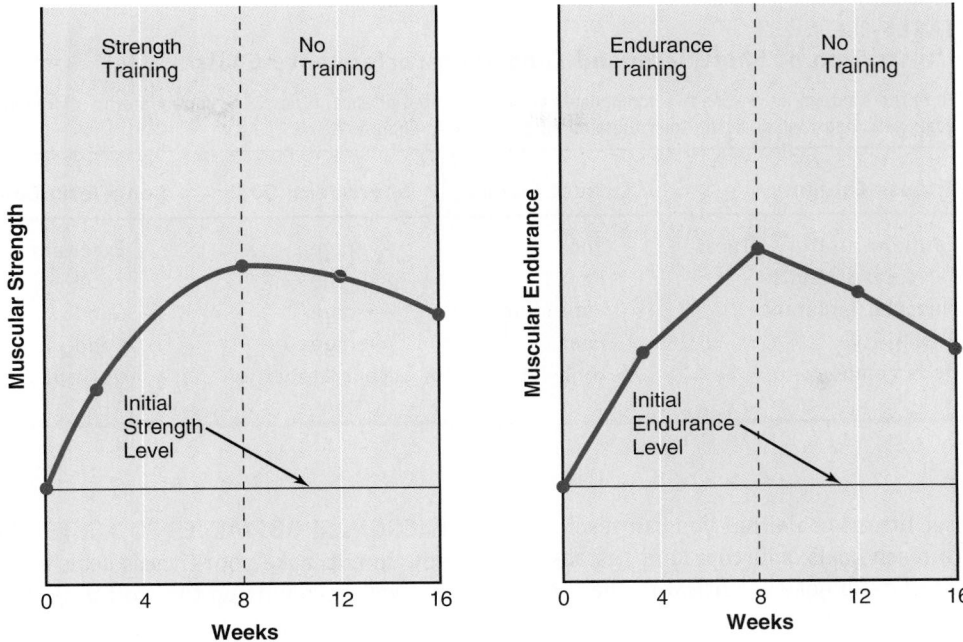

FIGURE 3.3
Retention of muscular strength and muscular endurance after training is stopped.

be tailored to meet the needs of the individual (1–9, 16). They should include fitness goals, mode of exercise, a warm-up, a primary conditioning period, and a cool-down (Figure 3.4). The following sections provide a general introduction to each of these components.

FITNESS GOALS

As mentioned in Chapter 1, establishing short-term and long-term fitness goals is an important part of an exercise prescription. Goals serve as motivation to start an exercise program. Further, attaining your fitness goals improves self-esteem and provides the incentive needed to make a lifetime commitment to regular exercise.

A logical and common type of fitness goal is a performance goal. You can establish performance goals in each component of health-related physical fitness. Table 3.1 on p. 74 illustrates a hypothetical example of how Susie Jones might establish short-term and long-term performance goals using fitness testing (Chapter 2) to determine when she has reached her objective. The column labeled "current status" contains Susie's fitness ratings based on tests performed prior to starting her exercise program. After consultation with her instructor, Susie has established short-term goals that she hopes to achieve within the first 8 weeks of training. Note that the short-term goals are not "fixed in stone" and can be modified if the need arises. Susie's long-term goals are fitness levels that she hopes to reach within the first 18 months of training. Similar to short-term goals, long-term goals can be modified to meet changing needs or circumstances.

In addition to performance goals, consider establishing exercise adherence goals. That is, set a goal to exercise a specific number of days per week. Exercise adherence goals are important because fitness will improve only if you exercise regularly!

In writing your personal fitness goals, consider the following guidelines:

SET REALISTIC GOALS   The most important rule in setting goals is that you must establish realistic ones. After a thorough self-evaluation and consultation with

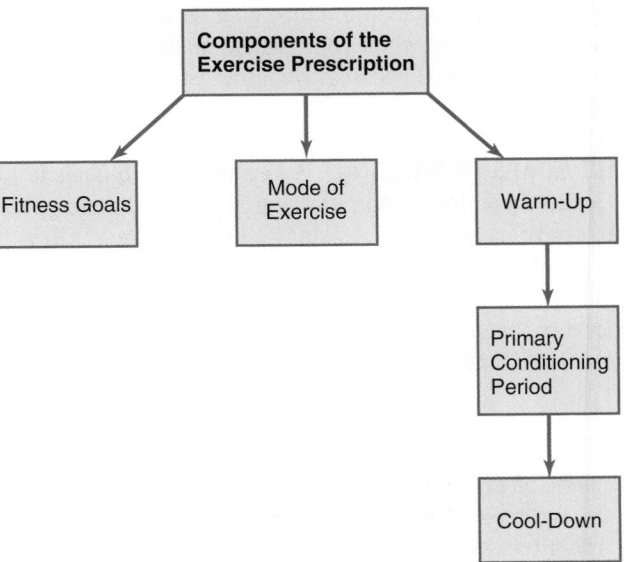

FIGURE 3.4
Components of the exercise prescription.

TABLE 3.1
Illustration of Short-Term and Long-Term Performance Goals

The fitness categories are the five components of health-related physical fitness. The current status, short-term goals, and long-term goals are the fitness norms presented in Chapter 2.

Fitness Category	Current Status	Short-Term Goal	Long-Term Goal
Cardiorespiratory fitness	Poor	Average	Excellent
Muscular strength	Poor	Average	Excellent
Muscular endurance	Very poor	Average	Good
Flexibility	Poor	Average	Good
Body composition	High fat	Moderately high	Optimal

your instructor, set fitness goals that you can reach. Because failure to reach goals is discouraging, establishing realistic short-term goals is critical to the success of your exercise program.

ESTABLISH SHORT-TERM GOALS FIRST Reaching short-term fitness goals is a great motivation to continue exercising. Therefore, establishing realistic short-term goals is critical. After reaching a short-term goal, establish a new one.

SET REALISTIC LONG-TERM GOALS In establishing long-term goals, consider your physical limitations. Heredity plays an important role in determining our fitness limits. Therefore, in establishing long-term goals, set goals that are realistic for you and not based on performance scores of other people.

ESTABLISH LIFETIME MAINTENANCE GOALS In addition to short-term and long-term goals, consider establishing a fitness maintenance goal. A maintenance goal is established when your fitness goals have been met and your focus becomes remaining physically active and fit.

LIST GOALS IN WRITING A key to meeting goals is to write them down and put them in a place where you can see them every day. Goals can be forgotten if they are not verifiable in writing. Further, remember that all goals should be periodically reevaluated and modified if necessary. Just because goals are in writing does not mean that they cannot be changed.

mode of exercise The specific type of exercise to be performed. For example, to improve cardiorespiratory fitness, one could select from a wide variety of exercise modes, including running, swimming, or cycling.

RECOGNIZE OBSTACLES TO ACHIEVING GOALS If you do not make your fitness goals a serious priority, you will keep putting them off until they no longer exist. Once you begin your fitness program, be prepared for setbacks (such as skipping workouts and losing motivation) and to backslide some (and have your fitness level decline temporarily). This is normal. However, once you realize that you have stopped making progress toward your goals, you must get back on track and start making progress again as soon as you can.

The importance of fitness goals cannot be overemphasized. Goals provide structure and motivation for a personal fitness program. Keys to maintaining a lifelong fitness program are discussed again in Chapter 16.

MODE OF EXERCISE

Every exercise prescription includes at least one **mode of exercise**—that is, a specific type of exercise to be performed. For example, to improve cardiorespiratory fitness, you could select from a wide variety of exercise modes, such as running, swimming, or cycling. Key factors to consider when selecting an exercise mode are enjoyment, availability of the activity, and risk of injury.

Physical activities can be classified as being either high impact or low impact based on the amount of stress placed on joints during the activity. Activities that place a large amount of pressure on joints are called high-impact activities, whereas low-impact activities are less stressful. Because of the strong correlation between high-impact modes of exercise and injuries, many fitness experts recommend low-impact activities for fitness beginners or for those individuals susceptible to injury (such as participants who are older or overweight). Examples of some high-impact activities include running, basketball, and high-impact aerobic dance. Low-impact activities include walking, cycling, swimming, and low-impact aerobic dance.

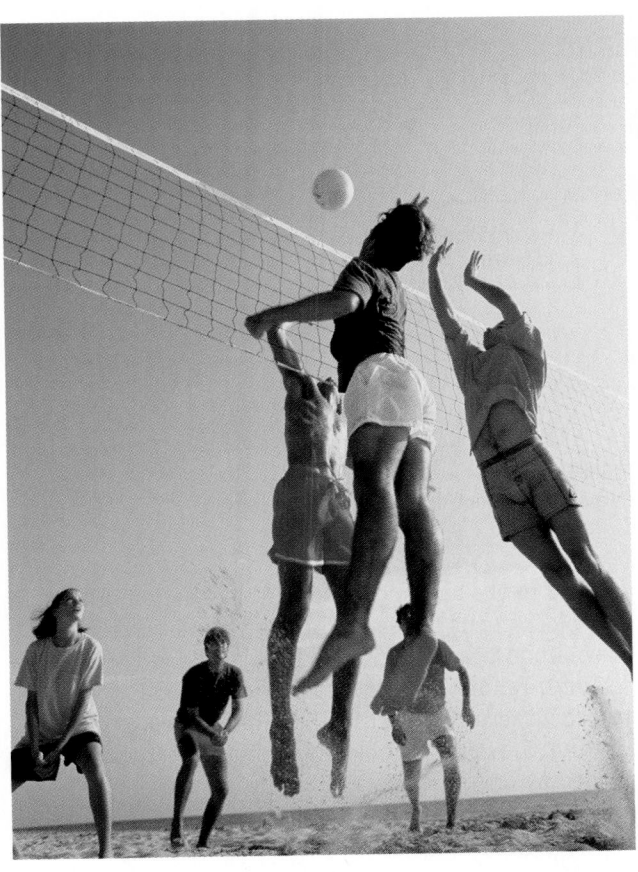

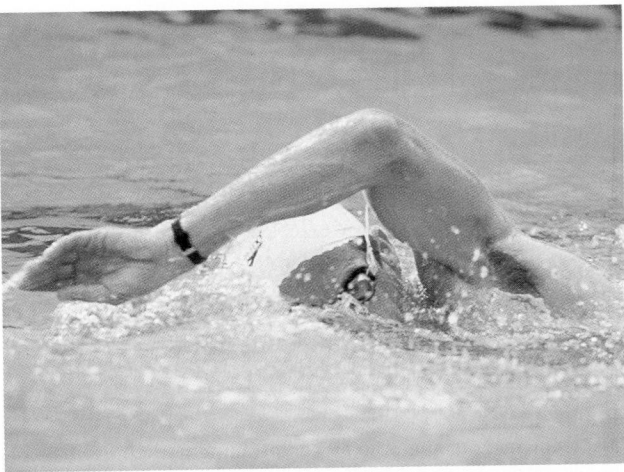

Whereas swimming is considered a low-impact activity, volleyball is considered a high-impact activity.

WARM-UP

A **warm-up** is a brief (5- to 15-minute) period of exercise that precedes a workout. It generally involves light calisthenics or a low-intensity form of the actual mode of exercise and often includes stretching exercises as well (Chapter 6). The purpose of a warm-up is to elevate muscle temperature and increase blood flow to those muscles that will be engaged in the workout (3, 6, 17). A warm-up can also reduce the strain on the heart imposed by rapidly engaging in heavy exercise and may reduce the risk of muscle and tendon injuries (17).

THE WORKOUT

Regardless of the mode of exercise, the major components of the exercise prescription that make up the workout (also called the primary conditioning period) are frequency, intensity, and duration of exercise (Figure 3.5). The **frequency of exercise** is the number of times per week that you intend to exercise. The recommended frequency of exercise to improve most components of health-related physical fitness is three to five times per week (5, 18–20).

The **intensity of exercise** is the amount of physiological stress or overload placed on the body during the

exercise. The method for determining the intensity of exercise varies with the type of exercise performed. For example, because heart rate increases linearly with energy expenditure during exercise, measurement of heart rate has become a standard means of determining exercise intensity during training to improve cardiorespiratory fitness. Although heart rate can also be used to gauge exercise intensity during strength training, the number of exercise repetitions that can be performed before muscular fatigue occurs is more useful for monitoring intensity during weight lifting. For instance, a load that can be lifted only five to eight times before complete muscular fatigue is an example of high-intensity weight lifting. In contrast, a load that

warm-up A brief (5- to 15-minute) period of exercise that precedes a workout. The purpose of a warm-up is to elevate muscle temperature and increase blood flow to those muscles that will be engaged in the workout.
frequency of exercise The number of times per week that one intends to exercise.
intensity of exercise The amount of physiological stress or overload placed on the body during exercise.

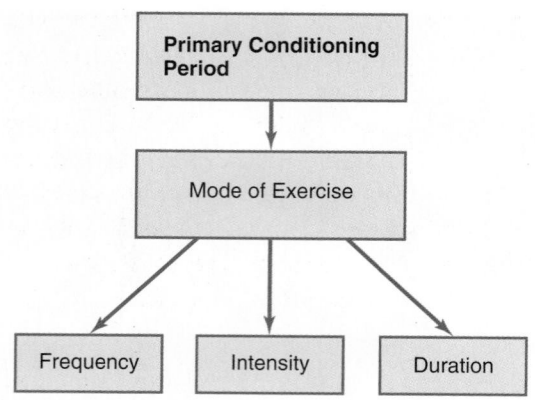

FIGURE 3.5
The components of the primary conditioning period: the frequency, intensity, and duration of exercise.

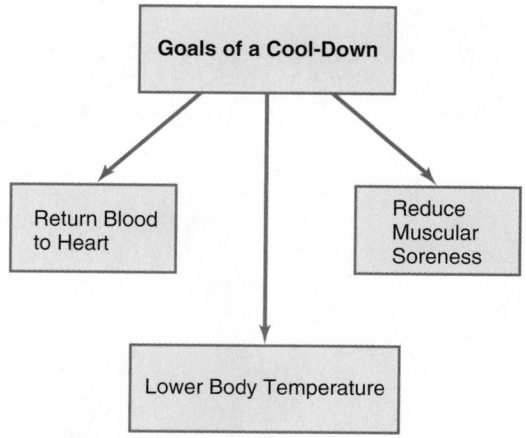

FIGURE 3.6
Purposes of a cool-down.

can be lifted 50 to 60 times without resulting in muscular fatigue is an illustration of low-intensity weight training.

Finally, flexibility is improved by stretching muscles beyond their normal lengths. Intensity of stretching is monitored by the degree of tension felt during the stretch. Low-intensity stretching results in only minor tension on the muscles and tendons. In contrast, high-intensity stretching places great tension or moderate discomfort on the muscle groups being stretched.

A key aspect of the primary conditioning period is the **duration of exercise**—that is, the amount of time invested in performing the primary workout. Note that the duration of exercise does not include the warm-up or cool-down. Research has shown that 30 minutes per exercise session (performed three or more times per week) is the minimum amount of time required to significantly improve physical fitness.

COOL-DOWN

The **cool-down** (sometimes called a *warm-down*) is a 5- to 15-minute period of low-intensity exercise that immediately follows the primary conditioning period. For instance, a period of slow walking might be used as a cool-down following a running workout. A cool-down period accomplishes several goals (Figure 3.6). In addition to its goal of lowering body temperature after exercise, one primary purpose of a cool-down is to allow blood to be returned from the muscles back toward the heart (3–6). During exercise, large amounts of blood are

pumped to the working muscles. On cessation of exercise, blood tends to remain in large blood vessels located around the exercised muscles (a process called *pooling*). Failure to redistribute pooled blood after exercise could result in your feeling lightheaded or even fainting. Prevention of blood pooling is best accomplished by low-intensity exercise using those muscles utilized during the workout.

Finally, some fitness experts believe that post-exercise muscle soreness may be reduced as a result of a cool-down (21). Although a cool-down period may not eliminate muscular soreness entirely, it seems possible that the severity of exercise-induced muscle soreness may be reduced in people who perform a proper cool-down (21).

INDIVIDUALIZING THE WORKOUT

A key point to remember about exercise prescriptions is that each should be tailored to the needs and objectives of the individual. Although the same general principles of exercise training apply to everyone, no two people are the same. Therefore, the exercise prescription should consider such factors as the individual's general health, age, fitness status, musculoskeletal condition, and body composition. More will be said about individualizing workouts in later chapters.

☀ IN SUMMARY

- The "dosage" of exercise required to effectively promote physical fitness is called the exercise prescription.
- The components of the exercise prescription include fitness goals, mode of exercise, the warm-up, the workout, and the cool-down.
- Exercise training programs should be individualized by considering such factors as age, health, and fitness status of the individual.

---

duration of exercise The amount of time invested in performing the primary workout.
cool-down A 5- to 15-minute period of low-intensity exercise that immediately follows the primary conditioning period; sometimes called a *warm-down*.

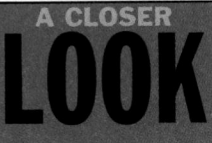

Too Much Exercise Increases Your Risk of Illness

Recent research indicates that intense exercise training (i.e., overtraining) reduces the body's immunity to disease (22). In contrast, light to moderate exercise training boosts the immune system and reduces the risk of infections (23). The relationship between exercise training and the risk of developing an upper respiratory tract infection (i.e., a cold) is shown in the figure in this box. The J-shaped curve in the figure indicates that moderate exercise training reduces the risk of infection, whereas high-intensity and long-duration exercise training increase the risk of infection.

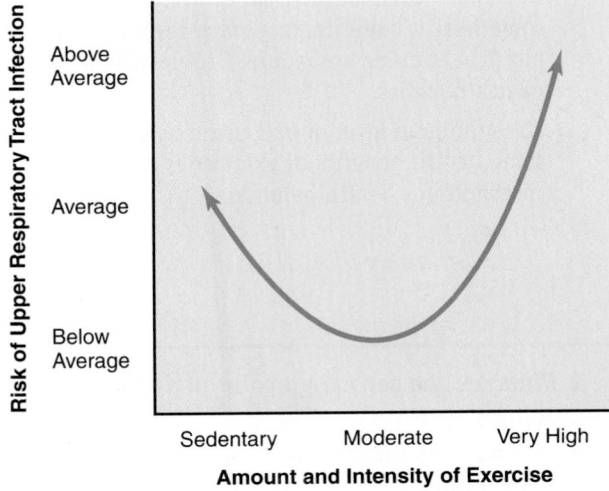

This J-shaped curve illustrates the relationship between physical activity and colds. Note that moderate physical activity reduces your risk of infection, whereas long-duration or high-intensity exercise increases your risk of disease.

Source: Redrawn from Nieman, D., Moderate exercise boosts the immune system: Too much exercise can have the opposite effect. ACSM's *Health and Fitness Journal* 1(5):14–18, 1997. Reprinted by permission of Lippincott Williams & Wilkins, http://lww.com.

⚙ Health Benefits of Exercise: How Much Exercise Is Enough

As discussed earlier (Chapter 1), exercise training to improve physical fitness for sport performance differs from exercise performed to achieve health benefits. For example, the single goal of exercise for sport performance is to improve physical performance in a specific sport. This form of exercise training typically includes long workouts (i.e., 60–180 minutes/day) involving high-intensity exercise. In contrast, the objective of health-related exercise is to obtain health benefits such as a reduced risk of heart disease, cancer, and diabetes. Exercise performed to achieve health benefits does not require high-intensity exercise lasting several hours daily.

The critical question related to exercising to achieve health benefits is, how much exercise is required to provide health benefits? Although even low levels of physical activity can provide some health benefits, evidence indicates that moderate-to-high levels of physical activity are required to provide major health benefits (18, 20, 22, 27, 28, 30). The theoretical relationship between physical activity and health benefits is illustrated in Figure 3.7. Note that the minimum level of exercise required to achieve some of the health benefits of exercise is often called the "**threshold for**

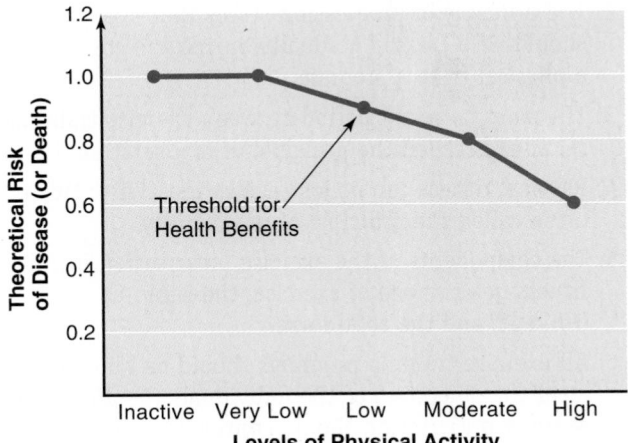

FIGURE 3.7
The relationship between physical activity and improved health benefits. Note that as the level of regular physical activity is increased, the theoretical risk of disease (or death) is decreased.
Source: Data are from References 25–27.

threshold for health benefits   The minimum level of physical activity required to achieve some of the health benefits of exercise.

health benefits." Most experts believe that 30–60 minutes of moderate-to-high intensity exercise performed 3–5 days per week will surpass the threshold for health benefits and will reduce all cause mortality (i.e., all causes of death) (27–29, 31–35). More specifically, current public health recommendations for physical activity are for a minimum of 30 minutes of moderate-intensity activity each day (31–34). This level of physical activity provides substantial health benefits for sedentary people and can be divided into 2–3 segments of exercise throughout the day (e.g., 15 minutes of exercise twice per day) (32). However, this dose of exercise may be insufficient to prevent weight gain in some individuals who may need additional exercise and caloric restriction to prevent weight gain (32) (see Chapter 8 for more details). Further, people who get 30 minutes of moderate intensity exercise per day are likely to achieve additional health benefits if they exercise for longer periods of time (32).

What modality of physical activity is optimal to obtain health benefits? A definitive answer to this question is not available. Nonetheless, it is clear that any one of many exercise modalities (e.g., running, swimming, cycling, walking, etc.) can be used to achieve exercise-related health benefits. Details on how to achieve health-related aspects of physical fitness will be discussed in Chapters 4 through 6.

☀ IN SUMMARY

- While low levels of physical activity can provide some health benefits, moderate-to-high levels of physical activity are required to provide major health benefits.
- The minimum level of exercise required to achieve some health benefits of exercise is called the threshold for health benefits.

Summary

1. The overload principle, which is the most important principle of exercise training, states that in order to improve physical fitness, the body or muscle group used during exercise must be overloaded.

2. The principle of progression states that overload should be increased gradually during the course of a physical fitness program.

3. The need for a rest period between exercise training sessions is called the principle of recuperation.

4. Physical fitness can be lost due to inactivity; this is often called the principle of reversibility.

5. The components of the exercise prescription include fitness goals, mode of exercise, the warm-up, the workout, and the cool-down.

6. All exercise training programs should be tailored to meet the objectives of the individual. Therefore, the exercise prescription should consider the individual's age, health, fitness status, musculoskeletal condition, and body composition.

7. The minimum level of physical activity required to achieve some of the health benefits of exercise is called the threshold for health benefits.

Study Questions

1. Define the following terms: *overtraining* and *principle of recuperation*.

2. What are the general purposes of a cool-down and a warm-up?

3. Describe and discuss the components of the exercise prescription.

4. How does the principle of progression apply to the exercise prescription?

5. Discuss the overload principle.

6. Define the term *threshold for health benefits*.

7. What happens to physical fitness if you stop training?

8. Explain why the exercise prescription should be individualized.

Suggested Reading

Blair, S., M. LaMonte, and M. Nichman. The evolution of physical activity recommendations: How much exercise is enough? *American Journal of Clinical Nutrition* 79: 913S–920S, 2004.

Howley, E. T. You asked for it: Is rigorous exercise better than moderate activity in achieving health-related goals? *ACSM Health and Fitness Journal* 4(2): 6, 2000.

Powers, S., and E. Howley. *Exercise Physiology: Theory and Application to Fitness and Performance.* 4th edition. St. Louis, MO: McGraw Hill, 2004.

Roitman, J. *ACSM's Resource Manual for Exercise Testing and Prescription.* Philadelphia: Lippicott Williams and Williams, 2001.

Thompson, P. et al. Exercise and physical activity in the prevention and treatment of atherosclerotic cardiovascular disease. *Circulation* 107:3109–3116, 2003.

For links to the web sites below visit **The Total Fitness and Wellness Website** at www.aw-bc.com/powers.

American Heart Association

Contains the latest information about ways to reduce your risk of heart and vascular diseases. Site includes information about exercise, diet, and heart disease.

American College of Sports Medicine

Contains information about exercise, health, and fitness.

WebMD

Contains the latest information on a variety of health-related topics, including diet, exercise, and stress. Includes links to nutrition, fitness, and wellness topics.

References

1. Getchell, B. *Physical Fitness: A Way of Life.* Needham Heights, MA: Allyn and Bacon, 1997.

2. Hockey, R. *Physical Fitness: The Pathway to Healthful Living.* St. Louis: Times Mirror/Mosby, 1996.

3. Howley, E., and B. D. Franks. *Health Fitness: Instructors Handbook.* Champaign, IL: Human Kinetics, 1997.

4. Fleck, S. and W. Kraemer. *Designing Resistance Training Programs.* Champaign, Il: Human Kinetics, 1997.

5. Pollock, M., and J. Wilmore. *Exercise in Health and Disease.* Philadelphia: W. B. Saunders, 1990.

6. Powers, S., and E. Howley. *Exercise Physiology: Theory and Application to Fitness and Performance,* 4th ed. St. Louis: McGraw-Hill, 2004.

7. Williams, M. *Lifetime Fitness and Wellness.* Dubuque, IA: Wm. C. Brown, 1996.

8. American College of Sports Medicine. *Guidelines for Exercise Testing and Prescription.* Philadelphia: Lea and Febiger, 1991.

9. Corbin, C., and R. Lindsey. *Concepts of Physical Fitness and Wellness.* Dubuque, IA: Brown and Benchmark, 1997.

10. Roberts, J., and J. Alspaugh. Specificity of training effects resulting from programs of treadmill running and bicycle ergometer riding. *Medicine and Science in Sports* 4:6–10, 1972.

11. Abernethy, P., J. Jurimae, P. Logan, A. Taylor, and R. Thayer. Acute and chronic response of skeletal muscle to resistance exercise. *Sports Medicine* 17:22–28, 1994.

12. Powers, S., D. Criswell, J. Lawler, L. Ji, D. Martin, R. Herb, and G. Dudley. Influence of exercise and fiber type on antioxidant enzyme activity in rat skeletal muscle. *American Journal of Physiology* 266:R375–R380, 1994.

13. Coyle, E., W. Martin, D. Sinacore, M. Joyner, J. Hagberg, and J. Holloszy. Time course of loss of adaptations after stopping prolonged intense endurance training. *Journal of Applied Physiology* 57:1857–1864, 1984.

14. Costill, D., and A. Richardson. *Handbook of Sports Medicine: Swimming.* London: Blackwell Publishing, 1993.

15. Lamb, D., and M. Williams. *Ergogenics: Enhancement of Performance in Exercise and Sport.* Vol. 4. Madison, WI: Brown and Benchmark, 1991.

16. McGlynn, G. *Dynamics of Fitness: A Practical Approach.* Dubuque, IA: Wm. C. Brown, 1996.

17. DeVries, H., and T. Housh. *Exercise Physiology,* 5th ed. Dubuque, IA: Brown and Benchmark, 1994.

18. Bouchard, C., R. Shephard, T. Stephens, J. Sutton, and B. McPherson, eds. *Exercise, Fitness, and Health: A Consensus of Current Knowledge.* Champaign, IL: Human Kinetics, 1990.

19. Barrow, M. *Heart Talk: Understanding Cardiovascular Diseases.* Gainesville, FL: Cor-Ed Publishing, 1992.

20. Morris, J. Exercise in the prevention of coronary heart disease: Today's best buy in public health. *Medicine and Science in Sports and Exercise* 26:807–814, 1994.

21. Robergs, R., and S. Roberts. *Fundamental Principles of Exercise Physiology: For Fitness, Performance, and Health.* St. Louis, MO: McGraw-Hill, 2001.

22. Nieman, D. Immune response to heavy exertion. *Journal of Applied Physiology* 82:1385–1394, 1997.

23. Nieman, D. Moderate exercise boosts the immune system: Too much exercise can have the opposite effect. *ACSM's Health and Fitness Journal* 1(5):14–18, 1997.

24. Paffenbarger, R., J. Kampert, I-Min Lee, R. Hyde, R. Leung, and A. Wing. Changes in physical activity and other lifeway patterns influencing longevity. *Medicine and Science in Sports and Exercise* 26:857–865, 1994.

25. Blair, S., H. W. Kohl, N. Gordon, and R. Paffenbarger. How much physical activity is good for health? *Annual Review of Public Health* 13:99–126, 1992.

26. Lee, I., and R. Paffenbarger. Associations of light, moderate, and vigorous intensity physical activity with longevity. *American Journal of Epidemiology* 151:293–299, 2000.

27. Williams, P. Physical fitness and activity as separate heart disease risk factors: A meta-analysis. *Medicine and Science in Sports and Exercise* 33:754–761, 2001.

28. Pollock, M., G. Gaesser, J. Butcher, J. P. Despres, R. Dishman, B. Franklin, and C. Garber. The recommended quantity and quality of exercise for developing and maintaining cardiorespiratory fitness and muscular fitness, and flexibility in healthy adults. *Medicine and Science in Sports and Exercise* 30:975–991, 1998.

29. Howley, E. T. You asked for it: Is rigorous exercise better than moderate activity in achieving health-related goals? *ACSM's Health and Fitness Journal* 4(2):6, 2000.

30. Roitman, J. *ACSM's Resource Manual for Exercise Testing and Prescription.* Philadelphia: Lippincott Williams & Wilkins, 2001.

31. Thompson, P. et al. Exercise and physical activity in the prevention and treatment of atherosclerotic cardiovascular disease. *Circulation* 107:3109–3116, 2003.

32. Blair, S., M. LaMonte, and M. Nichman. The evolution of physical activity recommendations: How much exercise is enough? *American Journal of Clinical Nutrition* 79: 913S–920S, 2004.

33. Brooks, G., N. Butte, W. Rand, J.P. Flatt, and B. Caballero. Chronicle of the institute of medicine physical activity recommendation: How a physical activity recommendation came to be among dietary recommendations. *American Journal of Clinical Nutrition* 79:921S–930S, 2004.

34. Ishikawa-Takata, K., T. Ohta, and H. Tanaka. How much exercise is required to reduce blood pressure in essential hypertensive: A dose-response study. *American Journal of Hypertension* 16:629–633, 2003.

35. Brown, D., D. Brown, G. Heath, L. Balluz, W. Giles, E. Ford, and A. Mokdad. Associations between physical activity dose and health-related quality of life. *Medicine and Science in Sports and Exercise* 36:890–896, 2004.

Warming Up and Cooling Down

NAME _____ DATE _____

Use the following activities to warm up your body for aerobic exercise. This general program is intended for activities such as jogging, walking, or cycling. Perform the exercises slowly, holding each stretch for 20 to 30 seconds. Do not bounce or jerk the muscle. Each stretch should be done at least once and up to three times.

CARDIOVASCULAR WARM-UP

Walk briskly or jog slowly for 5 minutes.

STRETCHES:

CALF STRETCH FOR GASTROCNEMIUS AND SOLEUS

Stand with your right foot about 1 to 2 feet in front of your left foot, with both feet pointing forward. Keeping your left leg straight, lunge forward by bending your right knee and pushing your left heel backward. Hold this position. Then pull your left foot in slightly and bend your left knee. Shift your weight to your left leg and hold. Repeat this entire sequence with the left leg forward.

SITTING TOE TOUCH FOR HAMSTRINGS

Sit on the ground with your right leg straight and your left leg tucked close to your body. Reach toward your outstretched right foot as far as possible with both hands. Repeat with the left leg.

STEP STRETCH FOR QUADRICEPS AND HIP

Step forward and bend your front knee about 90°, keeping your knee directly above your ankle. Stretch the opposite leg back so that it is parallel to the floor. Rotate your hips forward and slightly down to stretch. Your arms can be at your sides or resting on top of your forward thigh. Repeat on the other side.

LEG HUG FOR THE HIP AND BACK EXTENSORS

Lie flat on your back with both legs straight. Bending your knees, bring your legs up to your torso and grasp both legs behind the thighs. Pull both legs in to your chest and hold.

SIDE STRETCH FOR THE TORSO

Stand with feet shoulder width apart, knees slightly bent, and pelvis tucked under. Raise one arm over your head and bend sideways from the waist. Support your torso by placing the hand of your resting arm on your hip or thigh for support. Repeat on the other side.

These same exercises can also be repeated after a workout to cool down.

   1. Did you notice an increase in heart rate during the cardiovascular warm-up?

(continued on next page)

2. In which stretch did you feel the most tightness?

3. Do you think the sample warm-up and cool-down program is adequate for the activities you plan to do as part of your exercise program? If not, what exercises would you add?

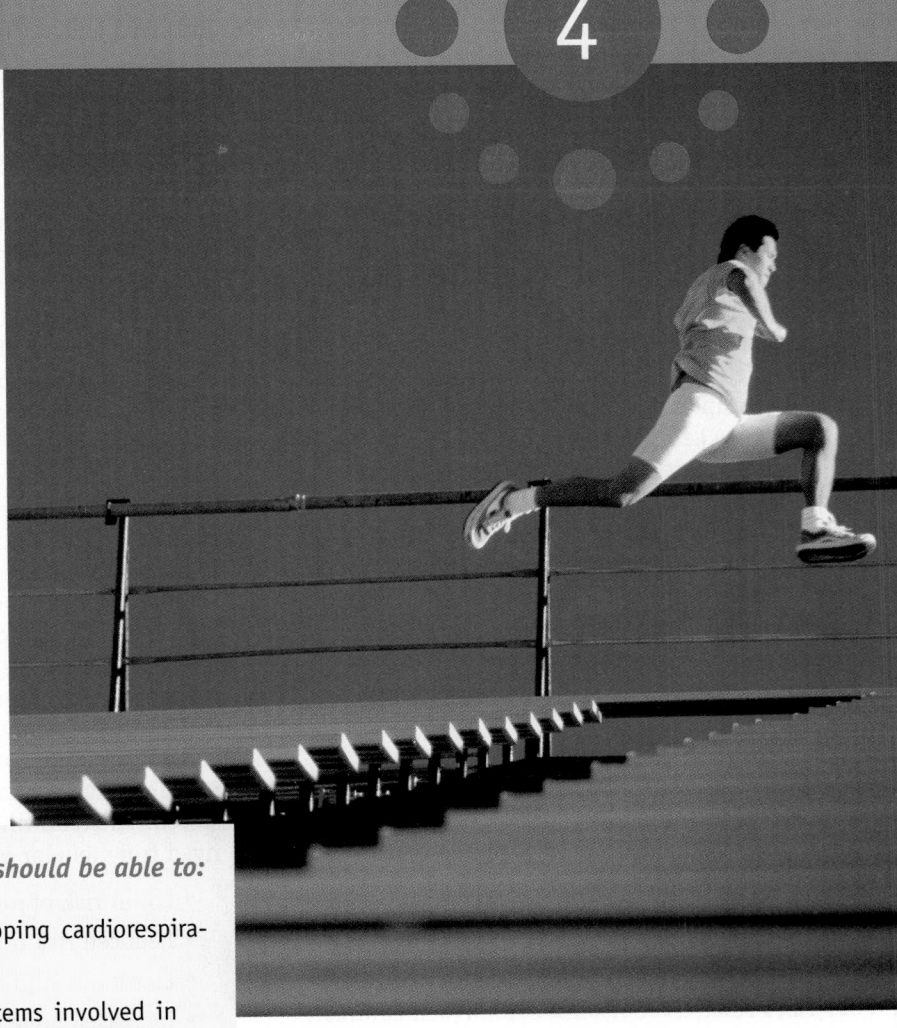

After studying this chapter, you should be able to:

1. Explain the benefits of developing cardiorespiratory fitness.

2. Identify the three energy systems involved in the production of adenosine triphosphate for muscular contraction.

3. Discuss the role of the circulatory and respiratory systems during exercise.

4. Define $\dot{V}O_{2max}$.

5. Identify the major changes that occur in skeletal muscles, the circulatory system, and the respiratory system in response to aerobic training.

6. List several modes of training used to improve cardiovascular fitness.

7. Outline the general components of an exercise prescription designed to improve cardiorespiratory fitness.

8. Design an exercise program for improving cardiorespiratory endurance.

Exercise Prescription Guidelines: Cardiorespiratory Fitness

Much of the current interest in cardiorespiratory training began in 1968 with the publication of Dr. Kenneth Cooper's best-selling fitness book, *Aerobics* (1). After the book's appearance, the term **aerobics** became commonly used to describe all forms of low-intensity exercise designed to improve cardiorespiratory fitness (such as jogging, walking, cycling, and swimming). Because aerobic exercise has proven effective in promoting weight loss (2) and reducing the risk of cardiovascular disease (3), many exercise scientists consider cardiorespiratory fitness to be one of the most important components of health-related physical fitness.

In the first three chapters of this book we discussed the health benefits of exercise, fitness assessment, and the general principles of exercise training. In the next three chapters we describe how to design a comprehensive, scientifically based exercise program to promote health-related physical fitness. This chapter describes techniques for promoting cardiorespiratory fitness. Before we discuss the exercise prescription for cardiovascular fitness, however, let's review the benefits of cardiorespiratory fitness and some basic concepts concerning how your body works during aerobic exercise.

☀ Benefits of Cardiorespiratory Fitness

Although most people consider health and fitness to be one and the same, there is now general agreement among experts that, although health and fitness certainly share many components, there are significant differences. Indeed, fitness is performance oriented and describes some level of work capacity. In contrast, health is disease oriented and is evaluated by various physiological and psychological measures. Health can be accomplished with much less exercise than what is needed to improve fitness.

Some are looking to maximize fitness gains while others are looking to improve health. If you are new to exercise, try focusing on health rather than fitness. Success breeds exercise adherence, and adherence is necessary for the success of good health and fitness.

The benefits of cardiorespiratory fitness are many. A key advantage is that people with high levels of cardiorespiratory fitness have a lower risk of heart disease and increased longevity. Other health benefits include a reduced risk of type II diabetes, lower blood pressure, and increased bone density in weight-bearing bones (4).

Another positive factor associated with developing cardiorespiratory fitness is that as fitness improves, energy for work and play increases. This translates into the ability to perform more work with less fatigue. Indeed, people with high levels of cardiorespiratory fitness often state that one of the reasons they exercise is because they feel better as a result.

Development of cardiorespiratory fitness through regular exercise has been shown to improve self-esteem (5). This improvement probably comes from several factors. First, starting and maintaining a regular exercise program provides a strong sense of accomplishment. Second, regular exercise improves muscle tone and assists in weight control. Combined, these factors result in an improved appearance and therefore improved self-esteem. Finally, studies have shown that people with high levels of cardiorespiratory fitness sleep better than less fit individuals (6). Fit individuals tend to sleep longer without interruptions (i.e., they enjoy more restful sleep) compared with less fit people. This exercise-related improved sleep results in a better night's rest and a more complete feeling of being mentally restored. The following list summarizes the benefits derived from regular exercise:

- Lower risk of heart disease
- Reduced risk of type II diabetes
- Lower blood pressure
- Increased bone density
- Increased energy for work and play
- Increased feeling of well-being
- Improved self-esteem
- Increased muscle tone and endurance
- Easier weight control
- Improved sleep

☀ Physiological Basis for Developing Cardiorespiratory Fitness

ENERGY TO PERFORM EXERCISE

The prolonged type of exercise that is necessary to develop cardiovascular fitness requires that an enormous amount of energy be supplied to the exercising

---

aerobics A common term to describe all forms of low-intensity exercise designed to improve cardiorespiratory fitness (e.g., jogging, walking, cycling, and swimming). Because aerobic exercise has proved effective in promoting weight loss and reducing the risk of cardiovascular disease, many exercise scientists consider cardiorespiratory fitness to be one of the most important components of health-related physical fitness.

muscles. Where do muscles get the energy to contract during exercise? The answer is: from the chemical energy released by the breakdown of food. However, food energy cannot be used directly for energy by the muscles. Instead, the energy released from the breakdown of food is used to manufacture another biochemical compound, called **adenosine triphosphate (ATP)**, a high-energy compound that is synthesized and stored in small quantities in muscle and other cells. The breakdown of ATP results in the release of energy that can be used to fuel muscular contraction. ATP is the only compound in the body that can provide this immediate source of energy. Therefore, for muscles to contract during exercise, a supply of ATP must be available.

Two "systems" in muscle cells can produce ATP. One system does not require oxygen and is called the **anaerobic** (without oxygen) system. The second system requires oxygen and is called the **aerobic** (with oxygen) system.

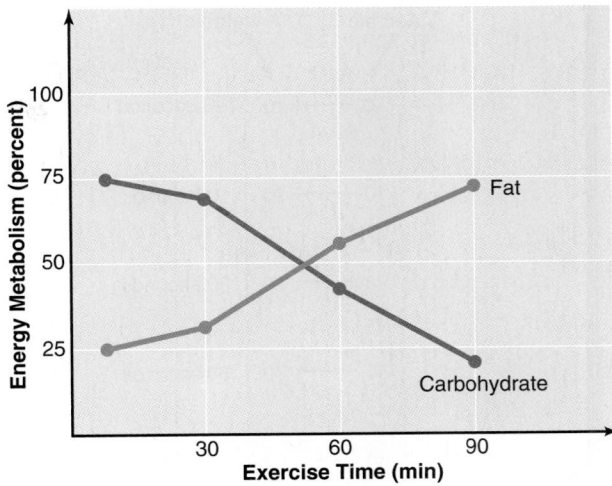

FIGURE 4.1
Changes in carbohydrate and fat use during 90 minutes of aerobic exercise.

ANAEROBIC ATP PRODUCTION

Most of the anaerobic ATP production in muscle occurs in a metabolic process called *glycolysis,* which breaks down carbohydrates (sugars) in cells. The end result of glycolysis is the anaerobic production of ATP and often the formation of lactic acid. Because lactic acid is often a by-product of glycolysis, this pathway for ATP production is often called the **lactic acid system**. The lactic acid system can use only carbohydrates as an energy source. Carbohydrates are supplied to muscles from blood sugar (*glucose*) and from muscle stores of glucose (a compound called *glycogen*).

Conceptually, it is convenient to think of the lactic acid system as the energy pathway that produces ATP at the beginning of exercise and during short-term (30–60 seconds) high-intensity exercise. For instance, most of the ATP required to sprint 400 meters (which may require 60–80 seconds) would be derived from the lactic acid system. During this type of intense exercise, muscles produce large amounts of lactic acid because the lactic acid system is operating at high speed. The accumulation of lactic acid in muscles results in fatigue and explains the decline in running speed of a 400-meter runner struggling toward the finish line.

AEROBIC ATP PRODUCTION

Exercise lasting longer than 60 seconds requires ATP production by the aerobic system. Therefore, activities of daily living and many types of exercise depend on aerobic ATP production.

Whereas the anaerobic lactic acid system uses only carbohydrate as a food source, aerobic metabolism can use all three foodstuffs (fats, carbohydrates, and protein) to produce ATP. In a healthy individual consuming a balanced diet, however, proteins play a limited role as an energy source during exercise; therefore, carbohydrates and fats are the primary sources. In general, at

the beginning of exercise, carbohydrate is the principal foodstuff broken down during aerobic ATP production. During prolonged exercise (i.e., longer than 20 minutes' duration), there is a gradual shift from carbohydrate to fat as an energy source. This process is illustrated in Figure 4.1.

THE ENERGY CONTINUUM

Although it is common to speak of aerobic versus anaerobic exercise, in reality the energy to perform many types of exercise comes from both sources. Figure 4.2(a) illustrates the anaerobic–aerobic energy continuum as a function of the exercise duration. Anaerobic energy production dominates

adenosine triphosphate (ATP)   A high-energy compound that is synthesized and stored in small quantities in muscle and other cells. The breakdown of ATP results in a release of energy that can be used to fuel muscular contraction. ATP is the only compound in the body that can provide this immediate source of energy.

anaerobic   Means "without oxygen"; in cells pertains to energy-producing biochemical pathways that do not require oxygen to produce energy.

aerobic   Means "with oxygen"; in cells pertains to energy-producing biochemical pathways that use oxygen to produce energy.

lactic acid   A by-product of glucose metabolism. Produced primarily during intense exercise (i.e., greater than 50–60% of maximal aerobic capacity). Results in inhibition of muscle contraction and, therefore, fatigue.

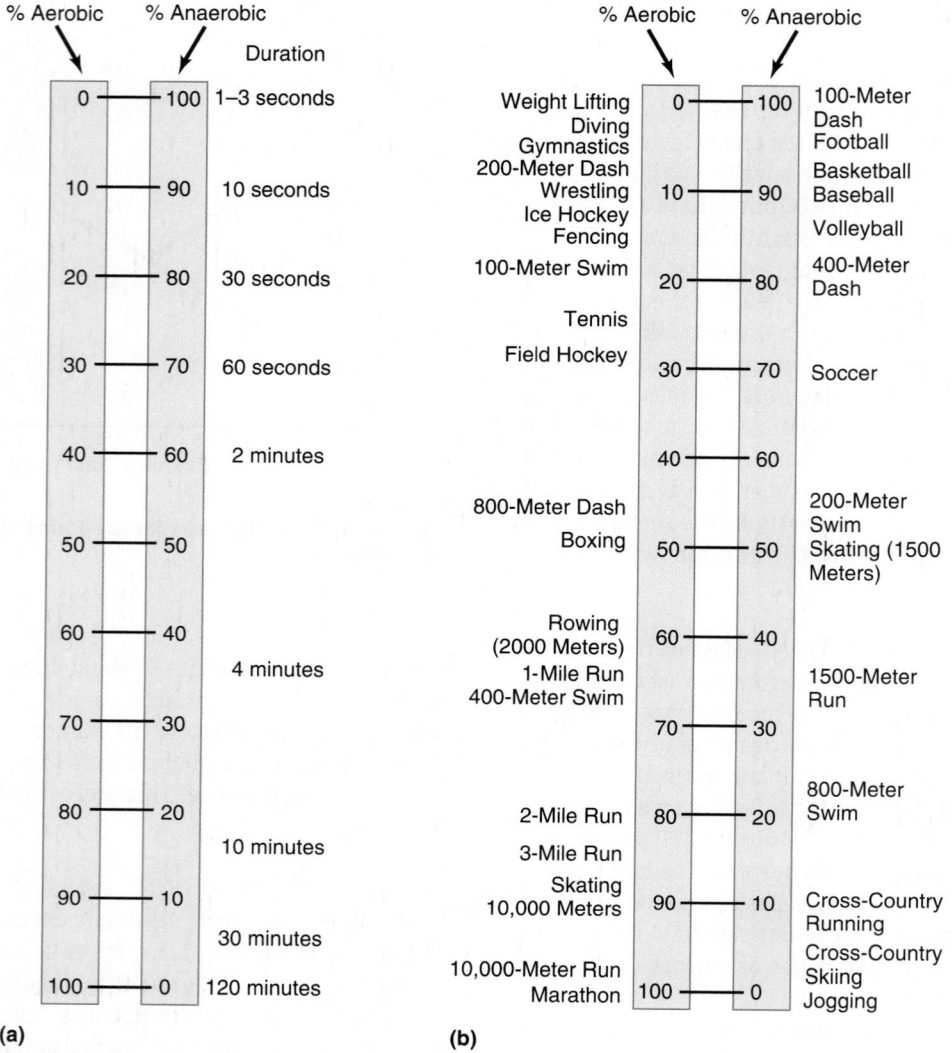

(a)

(b)

FIGURE 4.2
Contributions of aerobically and anaerobically produced ATP to energy metabolism during exercise. (a) Contributions as a function of exercise duration. (b) Contributions for various sport activities.

during short-term exercise, whereas aerobic energy production is greatest during long-term exercise. For example, maximal exercise of 10 seconds' duration uses anaerobic energy sources almost exclusively. On the other end of the energy spectrum, notice that aerobic energy production dominates during 2 hours of continuous exercise. Running a maximal-effort 800-meter race (exercise of 2–3 minutes' duration) is an example of an exercise duration that uses almost an equal amount of aerobic and anaerobic energy sources.

Figure 4.2(b) applies the anaerobic–aerobic energy continuum to various sports activities. Weight lifting, gymnastics, and football are examples of sports that use anaerobic energy production almost exclusively.

Boxing and skating (1500 meters) are examples of sports that require an equal contribution of anaerobic and aerobic energy production. Finally, cross-country skiing and jogging are examples of activities in which aerobic energy production dominates.

☀ IN SUMMARY

- ATP is required for muscular contraction and can be produced by two energy systems: the anaerobic (without oxygen) system and the aerobic (with oxygen) system.

- In general, anaerobic energy production dominates in short-term exercise, whereas aerobic energy production dominates during prolonged exercise.

Nutritional Links
TO HEALTH AND FITNESS

What Nutrients Are Most Important for Endurance Performance?

Whether you're an athlete or fitness enthusiast, nutrition is fundamental to your performance. A balanced eating plan that accounts for the type and level of activity is essential for cardiorespiratory endurance. Your diet should not vary considerably from a normal diet—that is, it should include plenty of fluids and low-fat, high-carbohydrate foods for energy. You should tailor the caloric content of your diet to reflect the amount of energy you expend during workouts. Carbohydrates should constitute at least 60% of the calories you consume, because they are the most critical supply of energy. Since muscles replenish stored carbohydrates most efficiently within the first 2 hours following exercise, you should consume 200–400 calories as soon as possible after exercise. Some good things to eat as a source of complex carbohydrates just after exercising include the following:

Two pieces of fruit

1 cup nonfat yogurt + 1 cup fruit topping

1 oz. cereal + 1/2 cup skim milk

1 low-fat muffin + 1/2 cup skim milk

12 oz. fruit juice

1 cup grapes + 1 bagel

1 cup vegetable soup + 1 slice bread

The intake of fluids is critical during exercise. Fluids are necessary to maintain blood volume and to replenish water lost through sweating. Because thirst is not a good regulator of fluid balance over the short run, fluids should be consumed before, during, and after your workout. Consume about 6 oz. of water 30 minutes before the workout, 3–6 oz. every 15 minutes during the workout, and 16 oz. for every pound lost during the workout.

☀ Exercise and the Cardiorespiratory System

The term *cardiorespiratory system* refers to the cooperative work of the circulatory and respiratory systems. Together they are responsible for the delivery of oxygen and nutrients as well as for the removal of waste products (e.g., carbon dioxide) from tissues. Exercise poses a major challenge to the cardiorespiratory system by increasing the muscular demand for oxygen and nutrients. The cardiorespiratory system must meet this demand to allow the individual to continue exercising. In the following sections we present a brief overview of cardiorespiratory function during exercise.

THE CIRCULATORY SYSTEM

The circulatory system is a closed loop composed of the heart and blood vessels. The pump in this system is the heart, which, by contracting, generates pressure to move blood through the system. Figure 4.3 illustrates that the heart can be considered two pumps in one. The right side pumps oxygen-depleted (deoxygenated) blood through the lungs through a pathway called the **pulmonary circuit**, while the left side pumps oxygen-rich (oxygenated) blood to tissues throughout the body through a pathway called the **systemic circuit**. Let's consider these two circuits in more detail.

In the systemic circuit, blood carrying oxygen leaves the heart in **arteries**, which branch to form microscopic vessels called *arterioles;* arterioles eventually branch into beds of smaller vessels called *capillaries*. **Capillaries** are thin-walled vessels that permit the exchange of gases (oxygen and carbon dioxide) and nutrients between the blood and tissues. After this exchange, blood passes from the capillaries into microscopic vessels called *venules*. As venules move back toward the heart, they increase in size and form **veins**, which carry oxygen-depleted blood back to the heart.

Venous blood (i.e., blood carried by veins) from all parts of the body returns to the right side of the heart and is pumped through the lungs. In the lungs, oxygen

---

pulmonary circuit   The blood vascular system that circulates blood from the right side of the heart, through the lungs, and back to the left side of the heart.

systemic circuit   The blood vascular system that circulates blood from the left side of the heart, throughout the body, and back to the right side of the heart.

arteries   The blood vessels that transport blood away from the heart.

capillaries   Thin-walled vessels that permit the exchange of gases (oxygen and carbon dioxide) and nutrients between the blood and tissues.

veins   Blood vessels that transport blood toward the heart.

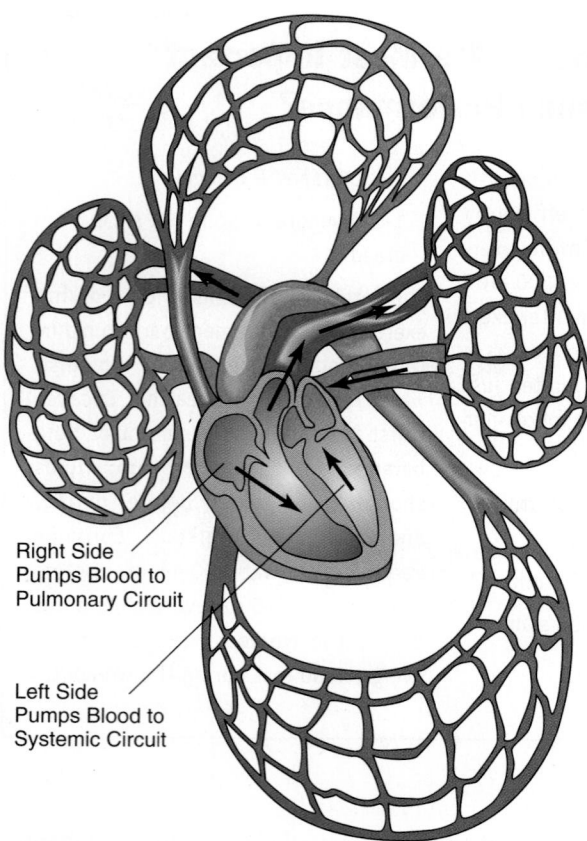

Right Side
Pumps Blood to
Pulmonary Circuit

Left Side
Pumps Blood to
Systemic Circuit

FIGURE 4.3
The concept of the heart as "two pumps in one."
Source: From Wilmore, J. H., and D. L. Costill, *Physiology of Sport and Exercise.*
Champaign, IL: Human Kinetics. Reprinted with permission.

is loaded into the blood, and carbon dioxide is removed from the blood into the lungs. The oxygen-rich blood is then returned to the left side of the heart and pumped to all body tissues by the systemic circuit.

The amount of blood the heart pumps per minute is called **cardiac output**. Cardiac output is the product

---

cardiac output   The amount of blood the heart pumps per minute.
heart rate   Number of heartbeats per minute.
stroke volume   The amount of blood pumped per heartbeat (generally expressed in milliliters).
systolic blood pressure   The pressure of the blood in the arteries at the level of the heart during the contraction phase of the heart (systole).
diastolic blood pressure   The pressure of the blood in the arteries at the level of the heart during the resting phase of the heart (diastole).
hypertension (high blood pressure)   Usually considered to be a blood pressure of greater than 140 for systolic or 90 for diastolic.

---

of the **heart rate** (number of heartbeats per minute) and the **stroke volume** (how much blood is pumped per heartbeat, generally expressed in milliliters). During exercise, cardiac output can be increased by increasing either heart rate or stroke volume or both. Stroke volume does not increase beyond light work rates (i.e., low-intensity exercise). Therefore, the increase in cardiac output needed for moderate work rates and above is achieved by increases in heart rate alone. (Changes in cardiac output in response to exercise are discussed later in this chapter.)

Maximal cardiac output declines in both men and women after approximately 20 years of age, primarily due to a decrease in maximal heart rate. The decrease in maximal heart rate (HR_{max}) with age can be estimated by the formula

$$HR_{max} = 220 - \text{age (in years)}$$

According to this formula, a 20-year-old individual would have a maximal HR of 200 beats per minute ($220 - 20 = 200$), whereas a 60-year-old would have a maximal HR of 160 beats per minute ($220 - 60 = 160$).

BLOOD PRESSURE   Blood is moved through the circulatory system by pressure generated by the pumping heart. The pressure that blood exerts against the walls of arteries is called *blood pressure.* Measurement of arterial blood pressure is generally attained by a device called a *sphygmomanometer* (Figure 4.4). During contraction of the heart (called *systole*), arterial blood pressure reaches its highest value. Blood pressure during systole is called **systolic blood pressure;** the normal resting systolic blood pressure for a young male adult is approximately 120 mm Hg (women may register 10–20 mm Hg lower). During the relaxation phase of the heart (called *diastole*), blood pressure declines and reaches its lowest value. Blood pressure during diastole is called **diastolic blood pressure;** normal diastolic blood pressure for a young male adult is approximately 80 mm Hg (again, women may register 10–20 mm Hg lower). It is important to measure both systolic and diastolic blood pressure because it is the combination of these two pressures that determines your mean (average) arterial pressure.

The walls of arteries are elastic, and they expand during the contraction of the heart. The increase in blood pressure during systole causes a pulsation in the arteries that can be felt by placing your finger (don't use the thumb) on the skin near a major artery. One pulse represents one heartbeat. This technique can be used to count your heart rate during or after exercise (discussed in Chapter 2).

Approximately 25% of all adults living in the United States (7) have abnormally high blood pressure, or **hypertension.** Systolic blood pressure of 140 mm Hg, and diastolic blood pressure of 90 mm Hg, are

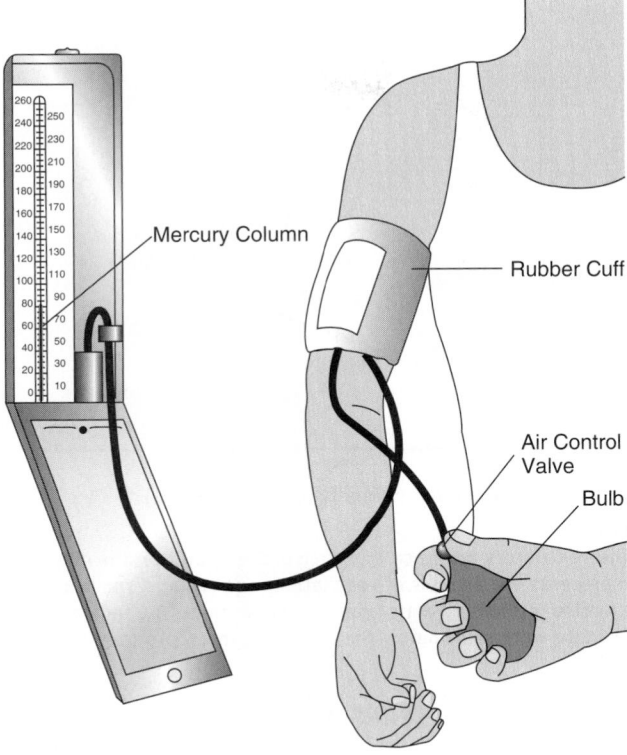

FIGURE 4.4
Measuring blood pressure using a sphygmomanometer.

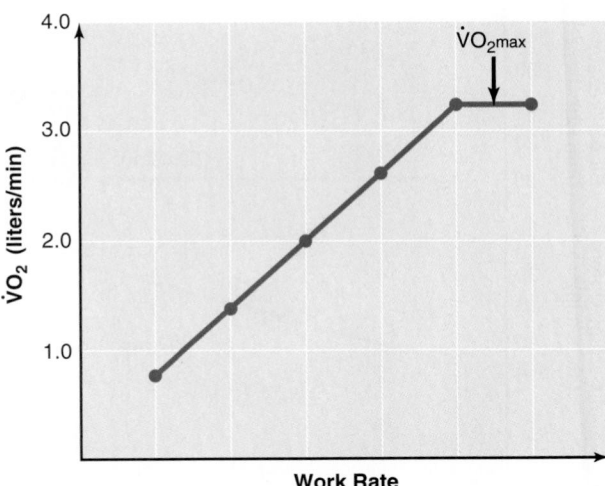

FIGURE 4.5
The relationship between exercise intensity (work rate) and $\dot{V}O_2$. $\dot{V}O_{2max}$ is the highest oxygen uptake that can be obtained during heavy exercise.

"threshold" blood pressure values; all higher values indicate hypertension. Hypertension is a serious health problem because it increases the risk of heart attack and stroke (8). As we saw in Chapter 1, regular exercise has been shown to reduce blood pressure in many individuals. Therefore, physicians often prescribe light exercise for hypertensive patients in an effort to lower their blood pressure.

THE RESPIRATORY SYSTEM

The primary purpose of the respiratory system (also called the *pulmonary system*) is to provide a means of supplying oxygen to the blood and removing carbon dioxide from the blood. This is achieved by bringing oxygen-rich air into the lungs, which we do by breathing. Oxygen then moves from the lungs into the blood, and carbon dioxide moves from the blood into the lungs and is then exhaled.

MAXIMAL CARDIORESPIRATORY FUNCTION: $\dot{V}O_{2max}$

The body's maximum ability to transport and use oxygen during exercise (called $\dot{V}O_{2max}$ or *maximal aerobic capacity*) was introduced in Chapter 2. $\dot{V}O_{2max}$ is considered by many exercise physiologists to be the most

valid measurement of cardiorespiratory fitness. Indeed, graded exercise tests designed to measure $\dot{V}O_{2max}$ are often conducted by fitness experts to determine an individual's cardiorespiratory fitness. These tests require expensive equipment to measure oxygen consumption and are usually conducted on a treadmill or stationary exercise cycle. This type of test is often called an incremental exercise test.

Figure 4.5 illustrates the change in oxygen consumption (called *oxygen uptake*) at every exercise intensity (work rate) during a typical incremental exercise test. Note that oxygen uptake increases in a straight line with respect to work rate until $\dot{V}O_{2max}$ is reached; thus, $\dot{V}O_{2max}$ represents a "physiological ceiling" for the ability of the cardiorespiratory system to transport oxygen and for the muscles to use it.

PHYSIOLOGICAL RESPONSES TO EXERCISE

Now that we have an idea how the cardiovascular, respiratory, and energy-producing systems function, let's discuss the specifics of how these systems respond to exercise.

CIRCULATORY RESPONSES Exercise increases the body's need for oxygen. To meet this need, blood flow (and therefore oxygen delivery) to working muscle must increase in proportion to the demand. Increased oxygen

$\dot{V}O_{2max}$ The highest oxygen consumption achievable during exercise. Practically speaking, $\dot{V}O_{2max}$ is a laboratory measure of the endurance capacity of both the cardiorespiratory system and exercising skeletal muscles.

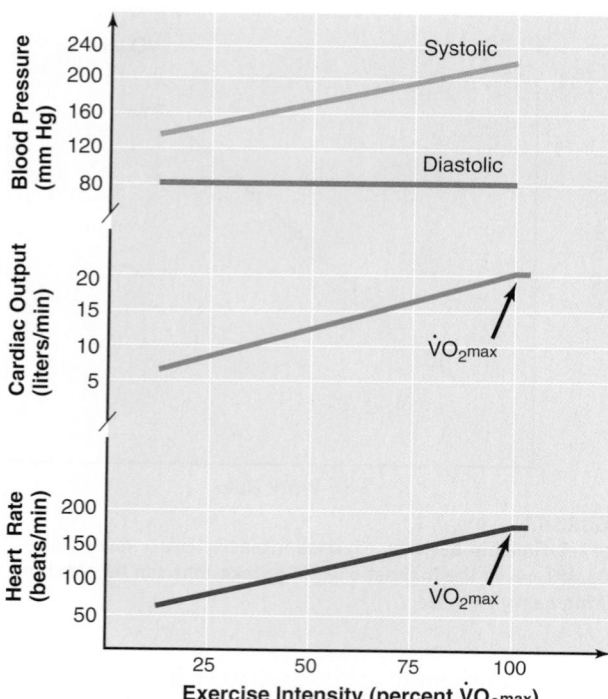

FIGURE 4.6
Changes in blood pressure, cardiac output, and heart rate as a function of exercise intensity.

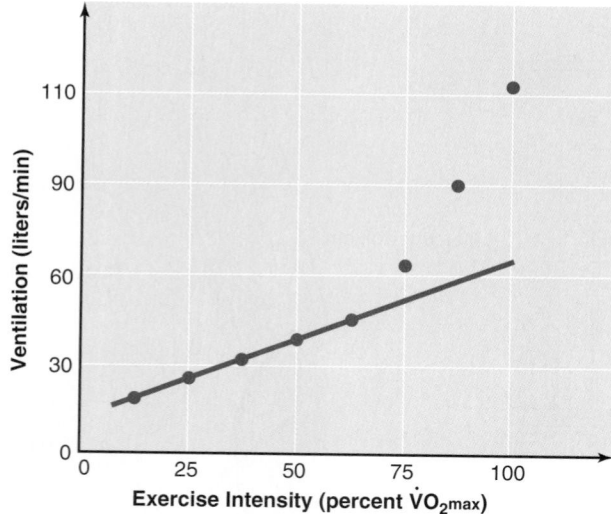

FIGURE 4.7
The ventilatory response to exercise. Each point on the graph represents the amount of ventilation required at a specific exercise intensity. Points lying on the straight line indicate exercise work rates below the anaerobic threshold (see A Closer Look).

transport to skeletal muscle is accomplished by increasing cardiac output and redistributing blood flow toward working muscle. The change in cardiac output, heart rate, and blood pressure in response to exercise of various intensities is illustrated in Figure 4.6. Note that both heart rate and cardiac output increase in a straight line as exercise intensity increases.

The fact that heart rate increases as a function of exercise intensity is useful for monitoring the intensity of exercise or the amount of physiological stress. For instance, a person riding a bicycle or running can stop exercising and quickly check heart rate (the pulse) to measure how hard he or she is working. Because it is easy to check heart rate during exercise, this has become the standard means of determining exercise intensity. Also, notice in Figure 4.6 that both heart rate and cardiac output reach a plateau when $\dot{V}O_{2max}$ is achieved. Again, $\dot{V}O_{2max}$ represents a physiological ceiling of the body's ability for delivery and utilization of oxygen in exercising muscles.

Finally, let's consider the changes in blood pressure in response to exercise of varying intensity (Figure 4.6). The key point in Figure 4.6 is that systolic blood pressure increases as the exercise intensity rises; in contrast, note that diastolic blood pressure remains relatively unchanged from the resting state. The rise in systolic blood pressure with higher exercise intensity provides the increased driving pressure to push blood toward the exercising muscles.

RESPIRATORY RESPONSES The responsibility of the respiratory system during exercise is to maintain constant arterial oxygen and carbon dioxide levels. Therefore, because exercise increases oxygen consumption and carbon dioxide production, the breathing rate must increase to bring more oxygen into the body and to remove carbon dioxide. Notice in Figure 4.7 that breathing (called *ventilation*) increases in proportion to exercise intensity up to approximately 65% of $\dot{V}O_{2max}$. At higher work rates, breathing increases rapidly, to enhance removal of carbon dioxide.

RESPONSES OF THE ENERGY-PRODUCING SYSTEMS
Recall that the energy needed to perform many types of exercise comes from both anaerobic and aerobic sources, and that anaerobic exercise dominates in high-intensity exercise, whereas aerobic energy production is greatest in low-intensity exercise. The relationship between exercise intensity and anaerobic energy production is discussed in detail in A Closer Look on p. 91.

☀ IN SUMMARY

- The term *cardiorespiratory system* refers to the cooperative work of the circulatory and respiratory systems.

- The primary function of the circulatory system is to transport blood carrying oxygen and nutrients to body tissues.

- The principal function of the respiratory system is to load oxygen into and remove carbon dioxide from the blood.

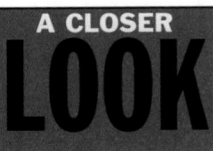

Exercise Intensity and Lactic Acid Production: Concept of the Anaerobic Threshold

High-intensity exercise results in an increased production of lactic acid. The relationship between exercise intensity and blood levels of lactic acid is illustrated in the figure in this box. Note that blood levels of lactic acid during exercise remain low until an exercise intensity of 50–60% of $\dot{V}O_{2max}$ is achieved. However, exercise above 50–60% of $\dot{V}O_{2max}$ results in a rapid accumulation of blood lactic acid. The exercise intensity that results in an increased rate of muscle lactic acid accumulation is called the **anaerobic threshold** (9).

During exercise above the anaerobic threshold, muscles begin to produce large amounts of lactic acid, resulting in muscular fatigue. This explains why exercise below the anaerobic threshold can be tolerated for a long period, whereas exercise above the anaerobic threshold results in rapid fatigue. Those of us who have experimented with finding the maximum speed that we can maintain while running or cycling have had ex-

perience with the anaerobic threshold. We learn that there is some maximal speed we can tolerate for the full duration of the exercise session, and that any attempt to pick up the pace results in muscle fatigue that forces us to slow our pace. This is so because the maximal speed we can

maintain represents an exercise intensity close to but below the anaerobic threshold. Accordingly, prolonged exercise sessions (i.e., 20–60 minutes' duration) aimed at improving cardiorespiratory fitness are generally performed at exercise intensities below the anaerobic threshold.

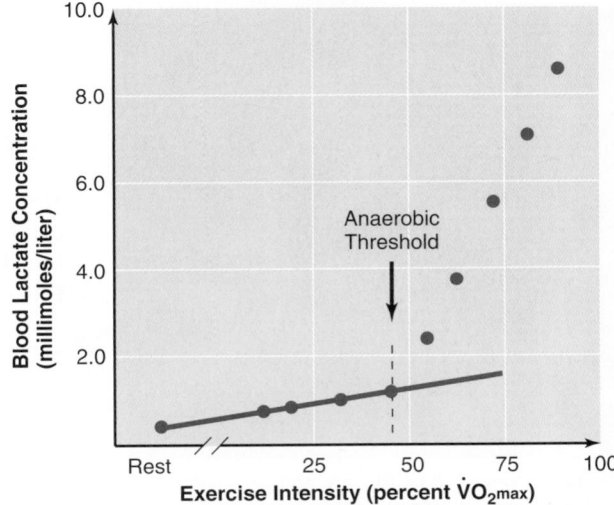

The relationship between blood lactic acid concentration and exercise intensity. Points lying on the straight line indicate exercise work rates below the anaerobic threshold.

- The maximum capacity to transport and utilize oxygen during exercise is called $\dot{V}O_{2max}$.
- $\dot{V}O_{2max}$ is considered by many exercise physiologists to be the most valid measure of cardiorespiratory fitness.
- During exercise, cardiac output, systolic blood pressure, heart rate, and breathing rate increase as a function of exercise intensity.

☀ Exercise Prescription for Cardiorespiratory Fitness

After assessing your health status and evaluating your current cardiorespiratory fitness level (Chapter 2), you are ready to develop your exercise prescription to

improve your cardiorespiratory fitness. As we have discussed, the exercise training session is composed of three primary elements: warm-up, workout (primary conditioning period), and cool-down.

WARM-UP

Every workout should begin with a warm-up. For an activity such as jogging, the warm-up might consist of the following steps:

anaerobic threshold The work intensity during graded, incremental exercise at which there is a rapid accumulation of blood lactic acid. This usually occurs at 50–60% of $\dot{V}O_{2max}$ and contributes to muscle fatigue.

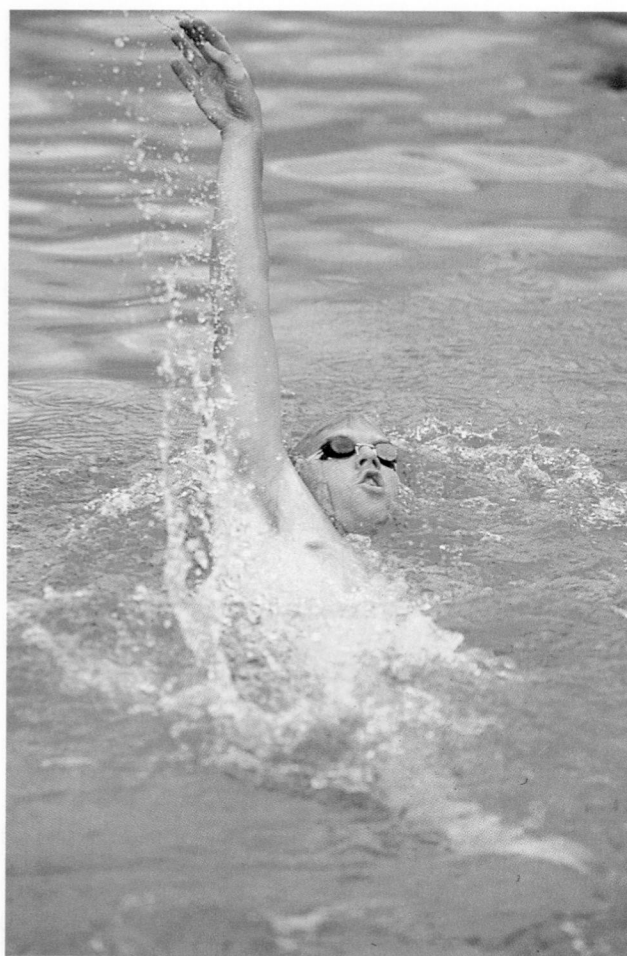

**TABLE 4.1
Popular Activities That Promote
Cardiorespiratory Fitness**

Aerobic dance
Bicycling
Calisthenics (heavy)
Cross-country skiing
Rope skipping
Rowing
Running
Skating (ice or roller)
Stair climber
Swimming
Walking

Swimming, walking, jogging, and cycling are popular modes of exercise that can be used to improve cardiorespiratory fitness.

WORKOUT: PRIMARY CONDITIONING PERIOD

The components of an exercise prescription to improve cardiovascular fitness include the mode, frequency, intensity, and duration of exercise. Let's discuss each of these factors briefly.

MODE   Several modes of exercise can be used to improve cardiorespiratory fitness. Some of the most common are walking, jogging, cycling, and swimming. In general, any activity that uses a large muscle mass (e.g., the legs) in a slow, rhythmical pattern can be used to improve cardiorespiratory fitness. Table 4.1 lists several activities that have been shown to improve cardiorespiratory fitness.

There are several key factors to consider when choosing an exercise mode. First, the activity must be fun! Choose an exercise mode that you enjoy. Your chances of sticking with an exercise program are much greater if you choose an activity that you like. A second consideration is that the type of exercise you choose must be convenient and accessible. For example, don't choose swimming if the nearest pool is 50 miles from your home. Similarly, don't choose cycling if you don't have use of a bicycle. A final factor is the risk of injury. High-impact activities such as running present a greater risk of injury than low-impact activities such as cycling and swimming. A commonsense rule when choosing an exercise mode is that if you tend to be injury prone, choose a low-impact activity. In contrast, if you rarely experience exercise-related injuries, feel free to choose either a high- or low-impact activity mode.

Historically, most exercise prescriptions for improving cardiorespiratory fitness have used only one activity mode. However, there is a current trend toward

1. 1 to 3 minutes of light calisthenics
2. 1 to 3 minutes of walking at a pace that elevates heart rate by 20 to 30 beats/min above rest
3. 2 to 4 minutes of stretching (optional; see Chapter 6 for details)
4. 2 to 5 minutes of jogging at a slow pace to gradually elevate the heart rate toward the desired target heart rate (discussed later in the section on intensity).

If the workout is to consist of exercise modes other than jogging, the same general warm-up routine could be followed by substituting other exercise modes, as in steps 2 and 4. For instance, if cycling is the primary mode of exercise, low-intensity cycling exercise would take the place of walking and jogging in steps 2 and 4.

TABLE 4.2
The Relationship of Target Heart Rate (THR) to Percent $\dot{V}O_{2max}$ and Percent HR_{max} for a 20-Year-Old Individual

THR (beats/minute*)	% $\dot{V}O_{2max}$	% HR_{max}
186	90	93
180	85	90
173	80	87
166	75	83
160	70	80
153	65	76
146	60	73
140	55	70
134	49	67

Heart rate based on a HR_{max} of 200 beats/min.

Source: Adapted from Fox, E., R. Bowers, and M. Foss. The Physiological Basis for Exercise and Sport. 1989. Reprinted by permission of McGraw Hill Companies.

---

using **cross training** (i.e., a variety of activity modes) for training the cardiorespiratory system. Many fitness experts feel that participating in only one mode of exercise is boring and leads to more exercise dropouts. Further, cross training may also reduce the frequency of injury. (Cross training is discussed in detail later in this chapter.)

FREQUENCY   Although cardiorespiratory fitness gains can be achieved with as few as two exercise sessions per week, the general recommendation for exercise frequency is three to five sessions per week to achieve near-optimal gains in cardiorespiratory fitness with minimal risk of injury (10). If you remain injury free while training, then if you desire you could increase exercise frequency to 5 days per week. It is, however, unlikely that even greater health or fitness benefits will accrue from exercising more than 5 days per week.

INTENSITY   Improvements in cardiorespiratory fitness occur when the training intensity is approximately 50% of $\dot{V}O_{2max}$ (this work rate is often called the **training threshold**). Although improvements in cardiorespiratory fitness can be achieved by exercising at $\dot{V}O_{2max}$, most people could only exercise for 1 to 2 minutes at that intensity. Thus, the recommended range of exercise intensity for improving health-related physical fitness is between 50% and 85% $\dot{V}O_{2max}$.

Recall that training intensity can be monitored indirectly by measurement of heart rate. The range of heart rates that corresponds to an exercise intensity sufficient to improve health-related physical fitness is called the **target heart rate (THR)**. The most popular method of determining THR is the percentage of maximal heart rate (HR_{max}) method. This method works on the principle that exercise intensity (i.e., % $\dot{V}O_{2max}$) can be estimated by measuring exercise heart rate. To compute your THR using this method, simply multiply your HR_{max} by both 90% and 70% to arrive at the high and low ends of your THR. For example, the maximal HR of a 20-year-old college student can be estimated by the formula

$$HR_{max} = 220 - 20 = 200 \text{ beats/min}$$

The THR is then computed as

$$200 \text{ beats/min} \times 0.70 = 140 \text{ beats/min}$$
$$200 \text{ beats/min} \times 0.90 = 180 \text{ beats/min}$$
$$THR = 140 \text{ to } 180 \text{ beats/min}$$

---

cross training   The use of a variety of activity modes for training the cardiorespiratory system.

training threshold   The training intensity above which there is an improvement in cardiorespiratory fitness. This intensity is approximately 50% of $\dot{V}O_{2max}$.

target heart rate (THR)   The range of heart rates that corresponds to an exercise intensity of approximately 50–85% $\dot{V}O_{2max}$. This is the range of training heart rates that results in improvements in aerobic capacity.

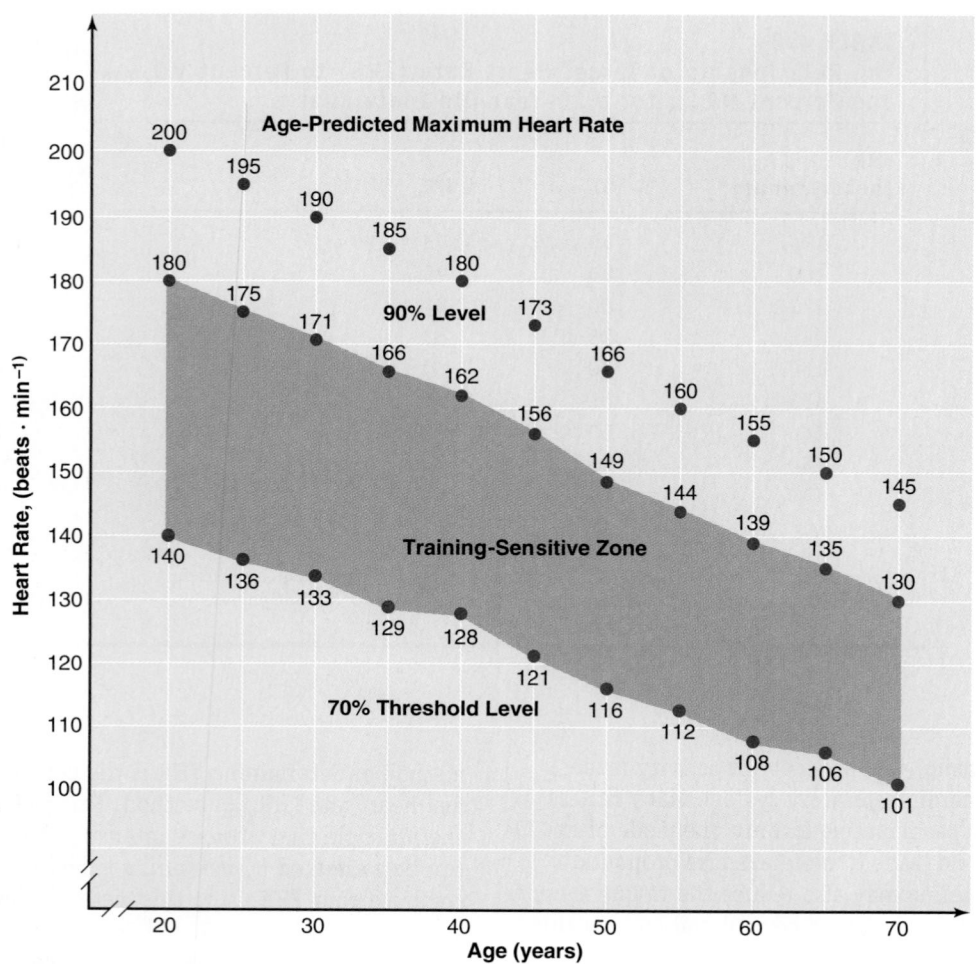

FIGURE 4.8
Target heart rate zones for individuals of ages 20 through 70. The zones cover 70–90% of maximum heart rate, which is indicated above the zones for selected ages.
Source: Donald Neiman, *Exercise Testing Prescription: A Health-Related Approach, 1995.* Reprinted by permission of McGraw Hill Companies.

In this example, the THR to be maintained during a workout to improve cardiorespiratory fitness is between 140 and 180 beats/min; this range of exercise intensities is sometimes called the *training sensitive zone.*

The reasoning behind using 70% and 90% of your maximal heart rate to compute your target rate is based on the relationship between percent HR_{max} and percent $\dot{V}O_{2max}$ (Table 4.2). Note that 70% of HR_{max} represents the heart rate associated with an exercise intensity that is close to 50% $\dot{V}O_{2max}$ (the lower end of the

training sensitive zone), and that 90% of the HR_{max} represents 85% $\dot{V}O_{2max}$ (the upper end of the recommended training sensitive zone).

Finally, it is important to remember that your THR will change as you get older due to the decrease in maximal heart rate. This point is illustrated in Figure 4.8. For instance, while the THR for a 20-year-old college student is between 140 and 180 beats per min, the THR for a 60-year-old is 108 to 139 beats per min.

Another way to estimate exercise intensity is to use the **Borg Rating of Perceived Exertion** (15). Perceived exertion is how hard you think your body is exercising. The collective efforts of breathing, sweating, and muscle exertion determine how hard the heart is working to circulate blood. Thus, it stands to reason that your subjective "rating" of these efforts would correlate to your heart rate. And it does!

Borg Rating of Perceived Exertion   A subjective way of estimating exercise intensity based on a numerical scale of 6–20.

Below is a table that shows the Rating of Perceived Exertion (RPE) scale and the corresponding exercise insensity estimate. The estimate is possible because of the linear relationship between heart rate and exercise intensity. (See Laboratory 4.3 on p. 113.)

INSTRUCTIONS FOR USING RATING OF PERCEIVED EXERTION (RPE) SCALE
During exercise, rate your perception of exertion. Combine all sensations and feelings of physical stress, effort, and fatigue. Do not focus on any one factor such as leg pain or shortness of breath.

Look at the rating scale while you are exercising. Find the best descriptor of your effort on the right and choose the associated number on the left. Your RPE multiplied by 10 will give you a rough estimate of the actual heart rate during the exercise. For example, if your RPE is 13, your heart rate could be estimated by multiplying 13 by 10 to get 130. This is a very rough estimate but will give you a reasonable idea of the intensity level of your activity, and you can use this information to speed up or slow down your movements to reach your desired range.

Try to appraise your feeling of exertion as honestly as possible, without thinking about the actual physical load. It is important to rate your own feeling of effort and exertion and not compare yours to that of someone else.

6	No exertion at all
7	Extremely light
8	
*9	Very light
10	
11	Light
12	
**13	Somewhat light
14	
15	Hard (heavy)
16	
***17	Very hard
18	
****19	Extremely hard
20	Maximal Exertion

*9—corresponds to "very light" exercise. For a healthy person, it is like walking slowly at his or her own pace for some minutes:

**13—on the scale is "somewhat hard" exercise, but it still feels OK to continue.

***17—"very hard" is very strenuous. A healthy person can still go on, but he or she really has to push him- or herself. It feels very heavy, and the person is very tired.

****19—on the scale is an extremely strenuous exercise level. For most people this is the most strenuous exercise they have ever experienced.

Source: Borg-RPE-scale ® from G. Borg, (1998), *Borg's Perceived Exertion and Pain Scales.* Champaign, IL: Human Kinetics. © Gunnar Borg, 1970, 1985, 1994, 1998. Used with permission of Dr. G. Borg. For correct usage of the scale the exact design and instructions given in Borg's folders must be followed.

Exercise Intensity

70–90% of HR $_{max}$

Exercise Duration

20–60 minutes per session

Exercise Frequency

| S | M | T | W | Th | F | S |

3–5 times per week

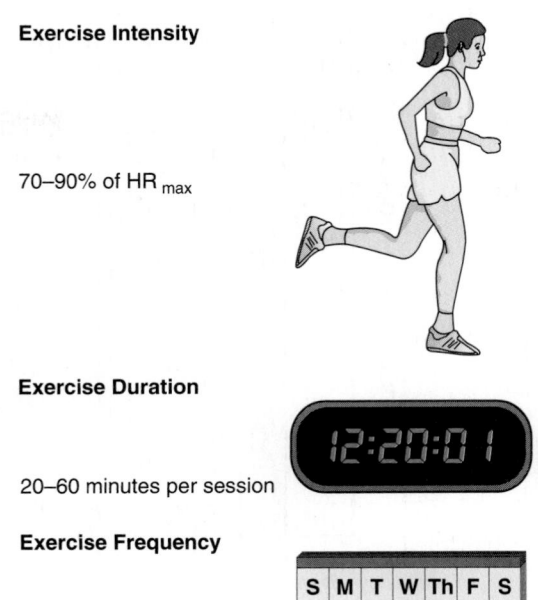

FIGURE 4.9
The suggested intensity, duration, and frequency of exercise necessary for improving cardiorespiratory fitness.

DURATION   Recall that the duration of exercise does not include the warm-up or cool-down. In general, exercise durations that have been shown to be most effective in improving cardiorespiratory fitness are between 20 and 60 minutes (10). The reason for this large "window" of duration is that the time required to obtain training benefits depends on both the individual's initial level of fitness and the training intensity. For example, a poorly conditioned individual may only require 20 to 30 minutes of daily exercise at his or her THR to improve cardiorespiratory fitness. In contrast, a highly trained person may require daily exercise sessions of 40 to 60 minutes' duration to improve cardiorespiratory fitness.

Another key point to understand is that improvement of cardiorespiratory fitness by engaging in low-intensity exercise requires a longer daily training duration than high-intensity exercise. For example, an individual training at 50% of $\dot{V}O_{2max}$ may require a daily exercise duration of 40 to 50 minutes to improve cardiorespiratory fitness. In contrast, the same person exercising at 70% of $\dot{V}O_{2max}$ may require only 20 to 30 minutes of daily exercise to achieve the same effect. A summary of the guidelines for improving cardiorespiratory fitness is illustrated in Figure 4.9.

SAFETY: IMPROVING CARDIORESPIRATORY FITNESS WITHOUT INJURY

What is the optimal combination of exercise intensity, duration, and frequency to promote cardiorespiratory fitness while minimizing risk of injury? The answer to

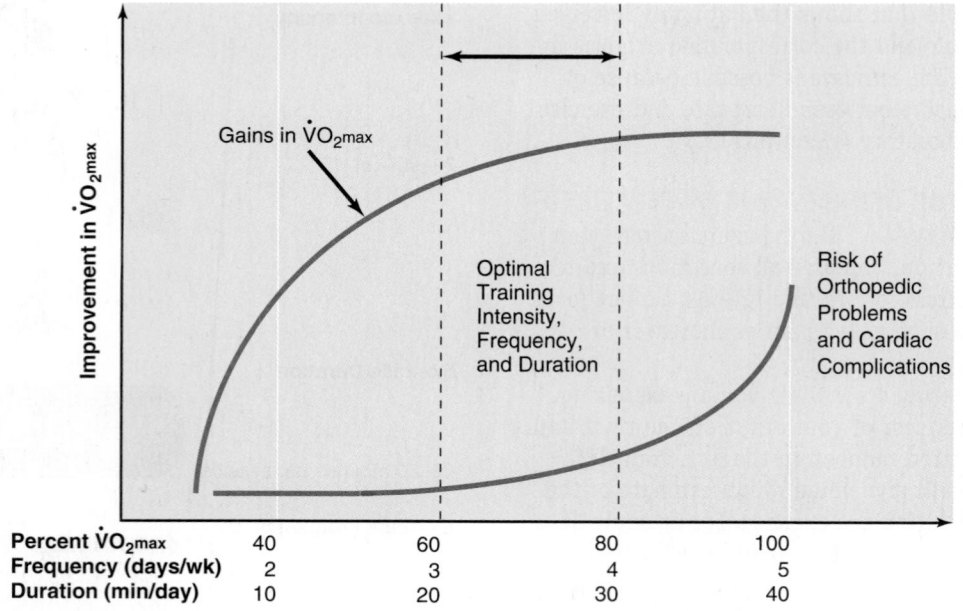

FIGURE 4.10
The effects of increasing intensity, frequency, and duration on the improvements in $\dot{V}O_2$max versus the increased risk of injury.

Source: From Scott Powers and Edward Howley, *Exercise Physiology: Theory and Application to Fitness and Performance.*
Copyright © 2004 The McGraw-Hill Companies. Reprinted by permission.

this question is illustrated in Figure 4.10. The optimal exercise intensity to improve cardiorespiratory fitness without increasing the risk of injury is between 60% and 80% of $\dot{V}O_2$max. Further, note that the optimal frequency and duration are 3 to 4 days per week and 20 to 30 minutes per day, respectively.

COOL-DOWN

Every training session should conclude with a cool-down (5–15 minutes of light exercises and stretching). A primary purpose of a cool-down is to promote blood return to the heart, thereby preventing blood from pooling in the arms and legs, which could result in dizziness and/or fainting. A cool-down may also decrease the muscle soreness and cardiac irregularities that sometimes appear after a vigorous workout. Although cardiac irregularities are rare in healthy individuals, it is prudent to cool down and reduce the risk.

A general cool-down of at least 5 minutes (of light exercise such as walking and calisthenics) should be followed by 5 to 30 minutes of flexibility exercises. In general, stretching exercises should focus on the muscles used during training. The type and duration of the stretching session depends on your flexibility goals (Chapter 6).

☀ IN SUMMARY

- A key factor in prescribing exercise to improve cardiorespiratory fitness is knowledge of the individual's initial fitness and health status.
- Three primary elements make up the exercise prescription: (1) warm-up; (2) workout, or primary conditioning period; and (3) cool-down.
- The purpose of a warm-up is to slowly elevate heart rate, muscle blood flow, and body temperature.
- The components of the workout are the mode, frequency, intensity, and duration of exercise.
- In general, the best mode of exercise is one that uses a large muscle mass in a slow, rhythmical pattern for 20 to 60 minutes.
- The intensity of the workout is gauged by the target heart rate, which should be in the range of exercise heart rates that correspond to 50–85% of $\dot{V}O_2$max.
- The recommended frequency of exercise to improve cardiorespiratory fitness is three to five times per week.
- The purpose of a cool-down is to slowly decrease the pulse rate and return blood to the heart. To accomplish this, the activity used during the training phase should be continued, but the intensity gradually decreased.

☀ Starting and Maintaining a Cardiorespiratory Fitness Program

Two key elements in any fitness program are the specific short-term and long-term goals. Without these, motivation to continue training is hard to maintain. Many fitness experts agree that the lack of goals is a major contributor to the high dropout rates seen in many organized fitness programs (11). It pays to establish both short-term and long-term fitness goals *before* you start your training program.

If your training plans include running, walking, aerobic dance, or other weight-bearing activities, it is important to exercise in good shoes. Unfortunately, good running, walking, or aerobics shoes are not cheap (costs range from $50–$150). However, investing in good shoes is important for both comfort and injury prevention. Look for a well-cushioned shoe with the following features: soft, comfortable upper material; adequate toe room (as indicated by comfort); well-padded heel and ankle collar; firm arch support; and a heel lift (a wedge that raises the heel about 1/2 inch higher than the sole). Many athletic shoe stores have well-trained sales personnel to assist you in the selection process.

DEVELOPING AN INDIVIDUALIZED EXERCISE PRESCRIPTION

Regardless of your initial fitness level or your choice of exercise mode, the exercise prescription for improving cardiovascular fitness usually has three stages: the starter phase, the slow progression phase, and the maintenance phase. Let's see how each of these training phases can be tailored to an individual's needs.

STARTER PHASE   The quickest way to extinguish enthusiasm for an exercise program is to try to accomplish too much too soon. Many people begin an exercise program with great excitement and anticipation of improved fitness levels and weight loss. Unfortunately, this early excitement can lead to exercising too hard during the first training session! This can promote sore muscles and undue fatigue. Therefore, start your fitness program slowly.

The objective of the starter phase is to permit the body to adapt gradually to exercise and to avoid soreness, injury, and personal discouragement. This phase usually lasts 2 to 6 weeks, depending on your initial fitness level. For example, if you are in a poor cardiorespiratory fitness category, you may spend 6 weeks in the starter phase. In contrast, if you have a relatively high initial cardiorespiratory fitness level, you may spend only 2 weeks in the starter phase.

The starter program should include a warm-up, a low-intensity training phase, and then a cool-down. In general, the intensity of exercise during the starter phase should be relatively low (up to 70% of HR_{max}). The following are key points to remember during the starter phase of an exercise program:

1. Start at an exercise intensity that is comfortable for you.
2. Don't increase your training duration or intensity if you are not comfortable.
3. Be aware of new aches or pains. Pain is a symptom of injury and indicates that rest is required to allow the body to repair itself. (See Chapter 11 for a discussion of injury prevention and treatment.)

SLOW PROGRESSION PHASE   The slow progression phase may last 12 to 20 weeks, with exercise progression being more rapid than during the starter phase. The intensity can be gradually elevated, and the frequency and duration of exercise increased, depending on fitness goals and the presence or absence of injuries. In general, this stage should involve an exercise frequency of 3 to 4 times per week and an exercise duration of at least 30 minutes per session. Exercise intensity should range between 70% and 90% HR_{max}, depending on your personal fitness goals.

MAINTENANCE PHASE   The average college-age student will generally reach the maintenance phase of the exercise prescription after 16 to 28 weeks of training. At this stage you should have achieved your fitness goal and are no longer interested in increasing your training load. The objective now is to maintain this level of fitness. As the old saying goes, "Fitness is not something you can put in the bank." To maintain cardiorespiratory fitness, you must continue to train on a regular basis. The key question now is, How much training is required during the maintenance phase to prevent a decline in cardiorespiratory fitness?

Several studies have shown that the primary factor in maintaining cardiorespiratory fitness is the intensity of exercise (12). If the exercise intensity and duration remain the same as during the final weeks of the slow progression phase, frequency can be reduced to as few as 2 days per week without a significant loss in fitness. In addition, if frequency and intensity remain the same as during the final weeks of the slow progression phase, duration can be reduced to as few as 20 to 25 minutes per day. In contrast, when frequency and duration are held constant, a one-third decrease in intensity results in a significant decline in cardiorespiratory fitness. To summarize, if exercise intensity is maintained, the exercise frequency and duration necessary to maintain a

TABLE 4.3
Sample Cardiorespiratory Exercise Program Designed for People in the Very Poor or Poor Fitness Category

General guidelines:
1. Begin each session with a warm-up.
2. Don't progress to the next level until you feel comfortable with your current level of exercise.
3. Monitor your heart rate during each training session.
4. End each session with a cool-down.
5. Be aware of aches and pains. If you are injury prone, choose a low-impact activity mode, and limit your exercise duration to 20 to 30 minutes per day.

Week No.	Phase	Duration (min/day)	Intensity (% of HR_{max})	Frequency (days/wk)
1	Starter	10	60	3
2	Starter	10	60	3
3	Starter	12	60	3
4	Starter	12	70	3
5	Starter	15	70	3
6	Starter	15	70	3
7	Slow progression	20	70	3
8	Slow progression	20	70	3
9	Slow progression	25	70	3
10	Slow progression	25	70	3
11	Slow progression	30	70	3
12	Slow progression	30	70	3
13	Slow progression	35	70	3
14	Slow progression	35	70	3
15	Slow progression	40	70	3
16	Slow progression	40	70	3
17	Slow progression	40	75	3
18	Slow progression	40	75	3
19	Slow progression	40	75	3
20	Slow progression	40	75	3–4
21	Slow progression	40	75	3–4
22	Slow progression	40	75	3–4
23	Maintenance	30	75	3–4
24	Maintenance	30	75	3–4
25	Maintenance	30	75	3–4
26	Maintenance	30	75	3–4

given level of cardiorespiratory fitness are substantially less than those required to improve fitness levels.

SAMPLE EXERCISE PRESCRIPTIONS As mentioned, the exercise prescription must be tailored to the individual. The key factor to consider when designing a personal training program is your current fitness level. Programs designed for people with good or excellent cardiorespiratory fitness levels start at a higher level and progress more rapidly, compared with programs designed for people in poor condition. Tables 4.3 through

4.5 illustrate three sample cardiorespiratory training programs designed for college-aged people who are beginning a fitness program. Table 4.3 contains an exercise prescription that might be appropriate for people in very poor or poor cardiorespiratory fitness. Table 4.4 illustrates a sample program designed for people in good or average cardiorespiratory fitness, while Table 4.5 on p. 100 contains a program aimed at people with a cardiorespiratory rating of excellent or above. Note that these programs are merely sample programs, and each can be modified to meet your

TABLE 4.4
Sample Cardiorespiratory Exercise Program Designed for People in the Average or Good Fitness Category

General guidelines:
1. Begin each session with a warm-up.
2. Don't progress to the next level until you feel comfortable with your current level of exercise.
3. Monitor your heart rate during each training session.
4. End each session with a cool-down.
5. Be aware of aches and pains. If you are injury prone, choose a low-impact activity mode, and limit your exercise duration to 20 to 30 minutes per day.

Week No.	Phase	Duration (min/day)	Intensity (% of HR_{max})	Frequency (days/wk)
1	Starter	10	70	3
2	Starter	15	70	3
3	Starter	15	70	3
4	Starter	20	70	3
5	Slow progression	25	70	3
6	Slow progression	25	75	3
7	Slow progression	25	75	3
8	Slow progression	30	75	3
9	Slow progression	30	75	3
10	Slow progression	35	75	3
11	Slow progression	35	75	3
12	Slow progression	40	75	3
13	Slow progression	40	75	3
14	Slow progression	40	75	3
15	Slow progression	40	80	3
16	Slow progression	40	80	3–4
17	Slow progression	40	80	3–4
18	Slow progression	40	80	3–4
19	Maintenance	30	80	3–4
20	Maintenance	30	80	3–4
21	Maintenance	30	80	3–4
22	Maintenance	30	80	3–4

individual fitness levels and goals. If you feel that none of these training programs meet your training needs, use Laboratory 4.1 on p. 109 to develop your personal exercise prescription. After designing your cardiorespiratory training program, use Laboratory 4.2 on p. 111 to keep a record of your exercise training habits. The following is an illustration of a typical training record:

Date	Activity	Duration	Exercise Heart Rate	Comments

☀ IN SUMMARY

- Establishing both short-term and long-term fitness goals is essential before beginning a fitness program.
- Regardless of your initial fitness level, an exercise prescription to improve cardiorespiratory fitness has three phases: (1) the starter phase, (2) the slow progression phase, and (3) the maintenance phase.

TABLE 4.5
Sample Cardiorespiratory Exercise Program Designed for People in the Excellent Fitness Category

General guidelines:
1. Begin each session with a warm-up.
2. Don't progress to the next level until you feel comfortable with your current level of exercise.
3. Monitor your heart rate during each training session.
4. End each session with a cool-down.
5. Be aware of aches and pains. If you are injury prone, choose a low-impact activity mode, and limit your exercise duration to 20 to 30 minutes per day.

Week No.	Phase	Duration (min/day)	Intensity (% of HR_{max})	Frequency (days/wk)
1	Starter	15	75	3
2	Starter	20	75	3
3	Slow progression	25	75	3
4	Slow progression	30	75	3
5	Slow progression	35	75	3
6	Slow progression	40	75	3
7	Slow progression	40	75	3–4
8	Slow progression	40	75	3–4
9	Slow progression	40	80	3–4
10	Slow progression	40	80	3–4
11	Slow progression	40	80	3–4
12	Slow progression	40	80–85	3–4
13	Slow progression	40	80–85	3–4
14	Slow progression	40	80–85	3–4
15	Maintenance	30	80–85	3–4
16	Maintenance	30	80–85	3–4
17	Maintenance	30	80–85	3–4
18	Maintenance	30	80–85	3–4

☀ Training Techniques

Endurance training is a generic term that refers to any mode of exercise aimed at improving cardiorespiratory fitness. Over the years, numerous endurance training techniques have evolved. In the next section we discuss several common ones.

CROSS TRAINING

As previously mentioned, cross training is a popular form of training that uses several different training modes. It may mean running on one day, swimming on another day, and cycling on another day. One advantage of cross training is that it reduces the boredom of performing the same kind of exercise day after day. Further, it may reduce the incidence of injuries by avoiding overuse of the same body parts. The disadvantage of cross training is the lack of training specificity. For example, jogging does not improve swimming endurance because the arm muscles are not trained during jogging. Similarly, swimming does not improve jogging endurance. In general, to improve endurance in a particular activity, training should consist of exercises similar to that activity.

LONG, SLOW DISTANCE TRAINING **Long, slow distance training**, or continuous training, requires a steady, submaximal exercise intensity (i.e., the intensity is generally around 70% HR_{max}). It is one of the most popular cardiorespiratory training techniques and can be applied to any mode of exercise. During the progression phase of the exercise program, an individual may find this type of training enjoyable because the exercise intensity does not increase. If injuries are not a problem, there is no reason why the duration of the training cannot be extended to 40 to 60 minutes per

---

long, slow distance training The term used to indicate continuous exercise that requires a steady, submaximal exercise intensity (i.e., the intensity is generally around 70% HR_{max}).

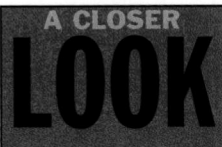

Frequently Asked Questions About Aerobic Workouts

What is a simple way to judge my workout intensity?

A very simple way to gauge intensity is the talk test. You should be able to talk without gasping for air while exercising. If you cannot, you should slow down. In contrast, if your intensity allows you to laugh and sing, then you need to work harder.

Is it better to exercise for several short sessions, or exercise for one longer period?

Either approach can be beneficial. You do need to warm-up for 5 to 10 minutes and cool-down for 5 to 10 minutes no matter the session length. So if you exercise for one 60-minute period, 40 to 50 minutes of that time should be for aerobic training, with the remainder for warm-up and cool-down. If you exercise for shorter periods, make sure to get at least 15 to 20 minutes of aerobic training.

Should I train my muscles in addition to doing aerobic activity?

Yes. Weight training is an important part of any aerobic program because strength will help protect you from injuries. Moreover, when you are strong it is easier to maintain proper form.

Can steam, the sauna, or a hot tub be helpful after a workout?

After an aerobic workout, blood vessels in the skin are open because blood is sent to the skin to aid in cooling the body. Any form of additional heat tends to open the blood vessels there even more, which diverts blood from critical areas such as the brain, the heart, and muscles. Therefore, heating up the body right after exercise is not the best thing to do. However, if you have thoroughly cooled down and have waited until your heart rate has returned to near its normal resting rate, you might use steam, the sauna, or a hot tub to help relax. If you feel any weakness or dizziness, however, get out immediately.

I am bored with aerobics. Is there something else I can do that will be just as effective?

Yes, try cardio boxing. Cardio boxing is an intensive, aerobic, full-body workout that combines boxing basics such as punching, kicking, and drills with aerobic exercise. You can work on strength, coordination, and endurance and, unlike boxing, you do not make physical contact with others. Jumping rope is part of the warm-up and many programs focus on developing strong abdominal muscles. Along with the total body workout that can burn as many as 750 calories an hour, many people report gaining an added bonus of increased self-confidence and a sense of empowerment. Other names for this type of workout include cardio kickboxing, aerobic boxing, kickboxing aerobics, and Tae Bo.

How good are exercise gadgets?

Trends and fads come and go in the fitness industry. Some gadgets are useful and will help you reach your fitness goals, but some are worthless. Before buying a new gadget, follow the guidelines in this text to determine if the equipment is useful. In general, the best piece of cardiovascular training equipment is the one that you will actually use. If you are simply concerned with which modality burns the most calories, the best piece is the one that you use for the *longest amount of time*.

Is the meal before a workout important, and what should it be?

Most of the energy expended during the workout will come from the meals you ate the previous day. That energy was stored in your muscles and liver. Thus, the pre-workout meal is important in that it (1) should be something easily digestible to keep from upsetting your stomach and thus preventing your workout, and (2) high in complex carbohydrates to replace the energy expended in the workout.

What is the best time of day to exercise?

The same principle that applies to choosing exercise equipment applies here: The best time of day to exercise is the time of day that you are most likely to maintain your workout routine. The best time of day to work out is when you want to exercise, so pick a time of day that works best for you.

Should I train if I'm sick?

Generally, if the sickness is above the neck (sinus, headache, sore throat, etc.), light exercise may not be a problem. Just take it easy, and be sure to respect others who aren't sick by wiping off any equipment that you use when you are finished with it and by washing your hands frequently.

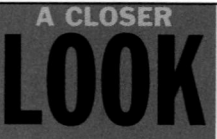

Spinning—Rev It Up?

Do you like to exercise with a group? Do you like biking but find it hard to do in your locale? Find a spinning class! Spinning is a type of aerobic exercise that is performed on specially designed stationary bikes via an indoor group ride led by an instructor.

Spinning is usually performed in a class with music playing to provide motivation while the instructor leads you through a 30–60-minute workout using visualization techniques, leading you to feel as if you are cycling over hills and through valleys.

Spinning was popularized in California by a man called Johnny G. He developed a stationary bike similar to the ones you see in gyms and fitness centers today. However, like the first stationary bikes, it has a flywheel that is turned by the pedals which allows you to quickly change the speed and resistance of pedaling. It is very

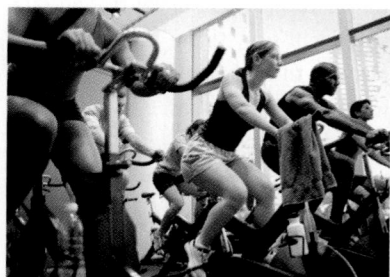

hard to get it started, but that is the uniqueness of the bike. Once you do get it started, the momentum of the flywheel lets you spin the pedals like you would on a ride through the countryside on a real bike.

Spinning bikes are designed to be much more comfortable than the typical stationary bike. The seats adjust forward, backward, up and down, while the handle bars also adjust to multiple positions.

Spinning is excellent for burning calories, consuming about 600 calories in an hour depending on the speed and resistance. It is one of the best exercises possible for improving cardiorespiratory fitness and increasing endurance of the quadriceps muscles.

session. An advantage of continuous training is that risk of injury is lower than in more intensive training.

INTERVAL TRAINING   **Interval training** means undertaking repeated sessions or intervals of relatively intense exercise. The duration of the intervals can be varied, but a 1- to 5-minute duration is common. Each interval is followed by a rest period, which should be equal to, or slightly longer than, the interval duration. For example, if you are running 400-meter intervals on a track, and it takes you approximately 90 seconds to complete each run, your rest period between efforts should be at least 90 seconds.

Interval training is a common training technique among athletes who have already established a base of endurance training and wish to attain much higher fitness levels in order to be more competitive in a particular sport. With correct spacing of exercise and rest periods, more work can be accomplished with interval training than with long, slow distance training. A major advantage of interval training is the variety of workouts it allows, which may reduce the tedium associated with other forms of training.

FARTLEK TRAINING

Fartlek is a Swedish word meaning "speed play," and it refers to a popular form of training for long-distance runners. **Fartlek training** is much like interval training, but it is not as rigid in its work-to-rest interval ratios. It consists of inserting sprints into long, slow running done on trails, roads, golf courses, and the like. An advantage of fartlek training is that these workouts provide variety and reduce the possibility of boredom. A modern type of Fartlek training is called "spinning." (See A Closer Look box above.)

interval training   Repeated sessions or intervals of relatively intense exercise. The duration of the intervals can be varied, but a 1- to 5-minute duration is common. Each interval is followed by a rest period, which should be equal to or slightly longer than the interval duration.

fartlek training   *Fartlek* is a Swedish word meaning "speed play," and it refers to a popular form of training for long-distance runners. It is much like interval training, but it is not as rigid in its work-to-rest interval ratios. It consists of inserting sprints into long, slow running done on trails, roads, golf courses, and so on.

☼ IN SUMMARY

- Common endurance training techniques to improve cardiorespiratory fitness include cross training; long, slow distance training; interval training; and fartlek training.

- Each of these techniques manipulates the frequency, intensity, and duration of training to improve endurance.

FITNESS AND WELLNESS FOR ALL

Wellness Issues Across the Population

DON'T LET A DISABILITY STOP YOU!

Although any type of temporary or permanent disability can certainly be a disincentive to exercise, you can take comfort in knowing that even with most disabilities you can obtain all of the benefits of cardiovascular exercise. Swimming and other water activities are popular ways to take away the burden of supporting your body weight and safely exercise capable muscle groups. Exercise in water is beneficial for several reasons:

- Exercising in water eliminates the dangers of falling.
- Flexibility exercises are much easier to do in water.
- Water provides resistance that allows capable muscle groups to work at an intensity that provides progressive overload to the cardiorespiratory system.
- A variety of water aids, including hand paddles, pull-buoys, flotation belts, and kick boards can be used to help maintain buoyancy and

balance as well as help you work in the water.

You must take responsibility for knowing about the medical complications associated with your disability, and for knowing how you can prevent and/or control those complications. Finally, remember that the potential for drowning always exists; never swim or work out in the water while alone.

☀ Aerobic Exercise Training: How the Body Adapts

How does the body adapt to aerobic exercise training? Endurance exercise training induces changes in the cardiovascular and respiratory systems, skeletal muscles and the energy-producing systems, $\dot{V}O_{2max}$, flexibility, and body composition, in response to regular aerobic training. A brief overview of each of these adaptations follows.

CARDIOVASCULAR SYSTEM

Several adaptations occur in the cardiovascular system as a result of endurance training (13). First, although endurance training does not alter maximal heart rate, this type of training results in a decrease in heart rate during submaximal exercise compared to before training. This reduction in heart rate results because the stroke volume at submaximal loads is increased with training. Further, endurance exercise results in an increase in maximal stroke volume (SV) and a corresponding increase in maximal cardiac output (because maximal cardiac output = maximal HR × maximal SV). An increased maximal cardiac output results in an increased oxygen delivery to the exercising muscles and improved exercise tolerance.

RESPIRATORY SYSTEM

Some fitness proponents report that exercise improves lung function by expanding the volume of the lungs

and increasing the efficiency of oxygen and carbon dioxide exchange. Unfortunately, there is no scientific evidence to support this belief. However, although endurance training does not alter the structure or function of the respiratory system, it does increase respiratory muscle endurance (14). That is, the diaphragm and other key muscles of respiration can work harder and longer without fatigue. This improvement in respiratory muscle endurance may reduce the sensation of breathlessness during exercise and eliminate the pain in the side (often called a *stitch*) that is sometimes associated with exercise.

SKELETAL MUSCLES AND ENERGY-PRODUCING SYSTEMS

Endurance training increases the muscles' capacity for aerobic energy production. The practical result of an improvement in muscle aerobic capacity is an improved ability to use fat as an energy source and an increase in muscular endurance (13). Note that these changes occur only in those muscles used during the training activity. For example, endurance training using a stationary exercise cycle results in an improvement in muscular endurance in leg muscles, but has little effect on arm muscles. Finally, although endurance training improves muscle tone, this type of exercise training does not result in large increases in muscle size or muscular strength.

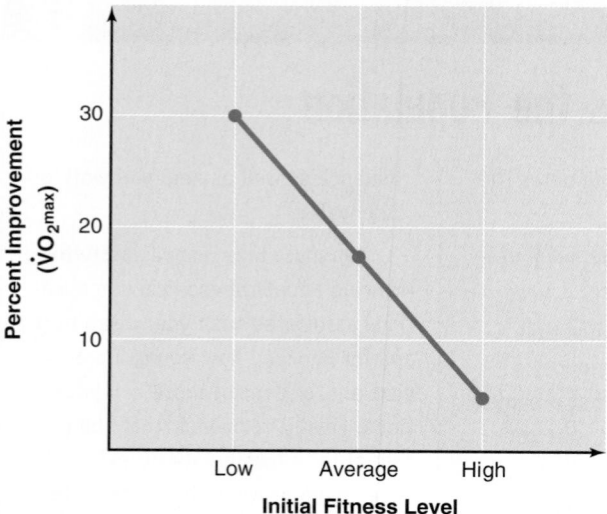

FIGURE 4.11
The relationship between initial fitness levels and improvements in $\dot{V}O_{2max}$ after a 12-week training period.

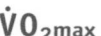

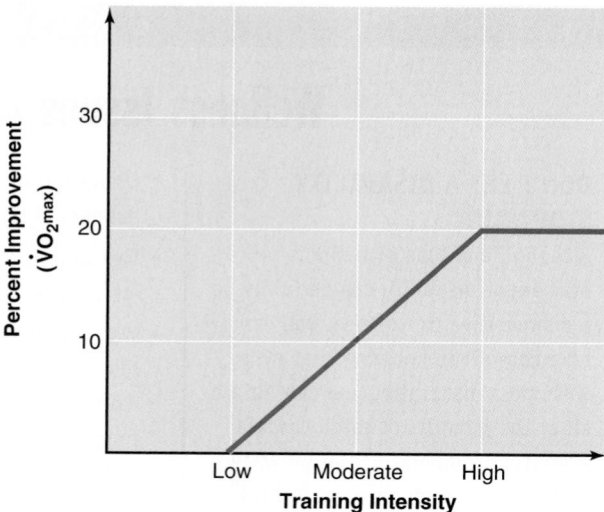

FIGURE 4.12
The relationship between training intensity and improvements in $\dot{V}O_{2max}$ following a 12-week training period.

$\dot{V}O_{2max}$

Recall that $\dot{V}O_{2max}$ is considered by many exercise physiologists to be the best single measure of cardiorespiratory fitness. Therefore, improvement in $\dot{V}O_{2max}$ is an important physiological adaptation that occurs in response to endurance training. In general, 12 to 15 weeks of endurance exercise results in a 10–30% improvement in $\dot{V}O_{2max}$ (13). This improvement is due to a combination of improved aerobic capacity in skeletal muscles and increased maximal cardiac output. The net result is increased oxygen delivery and use by skeletal muscles during exercise. Therefore, an increase in $\dot{V}O_{2max}$ translates to improved muscular endurance and less fatigue during routine daily activities.

How much $\dot{V}O_{2max}$ increases after an endurance training program is dependent on several factors: fitness status at the beginning of the training program, intensity of the training program, and nutritional status during the training program. In general, people who start exercise programs with high $\dot{V}O_{2max}$ values improve less than those with low initial $\dot{V}O_{2max}$ values. For example, a person entering an endurance training program with a high $\dot{V}O_{2max}$ may achieve only a 5% improvement over a 12-week period, whereas an individual with a low $\dot{V}O_{2max}$ may improve as much as 30% (Figure 4.11). The explanation for this is that a physiological ceiling or limit for improvement in $\dot{V}O_{2max}$ exists. Those people who enter fitness programs with relatively high $\dot{V}O_{2max}$ values are probably closer to their limits than are people who enter programs with low $\dot{V}O_{2max}$ values.

The magnitude of the exercise-induced increase in $\dot{V}O_{2max}$ is directly related to the intensity of the training program (12). High-intensity training programs result in greater $\dot{V}O_{2max}$ gains than low-intensity and short-duration programs (Figure 4.12). Notice that a plateau exists in the relationship between training intensity and improvement in $\dot{V}O_{2max}$. Therefore, once a high intensity of training is reached, increasing the intensity does not result in further improvement in fitness. In fact, training at extremely high intensities may increase the risk of injury and illness.

Finally, failure to maintain proper nutritional habits during an endurance training program will impair improvements in $\dot{V}O_{2max}$. Proper nutrition means a diet that provides all of the necessary nutrients for good health. In Chapter 7 we discuss how to construct the proper diet for health and fitness.

FLEXIBILITY

Most endurance training programs do not improve flexibility. In fact, several months of endurance training may reduce the range of motion at some joints due to muscle and tendon shortening. Therefore, to prevent a loss of flexibility, stretching exercises should always be a part of an endurance training program (Chapter 6).

BODY COMPOSITION

Endurance training generally results in a reduction in the percent of body fat (13). However, a loss of body fat in response to endurance training is not guaranteed. Whether or not an individual loses body fat due to exercise training is a result of many factors, including diet and the amount of exercise performed. More is said about this topic in Chapter 8.

☀ **IN SUMMARY**

- Endurance exercise training results in improvements in maximal cardiac output, endurance of muscles of respiration, skeletal muscle endurance, and $\dot{V}O_2max$.
- Endurance exercise can assist in the loss of body fat.
- Endurance training does not improve flexibility and may even reduce flexibility if regular stretching exercises are not performed.

☀ Motivation to Maintain Cardiorespiratory Fitness

Every year, millions of people make the decision to start an exercise routine. Unfortunately, over half those who begin a cardiorespiratory fitness program quit within the first 6 months (11). Although there are many reasons for this high dropout rate, a lack of time is commonly cited as a major one. Although finding time for exercise in a busy schedule is difficult, it is not impossible. The key is to schedule a regular time for exercise and to stick with it. A small investment in time to exercise can reap large improvements in fitness and health. Think about the time required to improve cardiorespiratory fitness in the following way. There are 168 hours in every week. All you need is three, 30-minute workouts per week to improve cardiorespiratory fitness. Including the associated warm-ups, cool-downs, and showers, this is about 3 hours per week, which is less than 2% of the total week. This leaves you with 165 hours per week to accomplish all of the other things you need to do. The bottom line is, with proper time management, anyone can find time to exercise.

In order for you to keep your commitment to develop cardiorespiratory fitness, exercise must be fun. Therefore, choose a training technique that you enjoy. Further, your chosen exercise mode should be convenient. Failure to meet either of these criteria increases your risk of becoming an exercise dropout.

One of the things that makes exercise enjoyable is the interaction with friends. Therefore, exercising with a partner is an excellent idea because it makes physical activity more fun and helps maintain your sense of commitment to a regular exercise routine. In choosing an exercise partner, choose someone that you enjoy interacting with and someone who is a good exercise role model.

Keeping a record of your training program is helpful in several ways. It assists you in keeping track of your training progress and serves as a motivating factor when you begin to notice improvements in your fitness level.

Finally, it is normal to experience some discomfort and soreness associated with your first several exercise sessions. Don't let this discourage you. In a short time the soreness will fade and the discomfort associated with exercise will begin to disappear. As your fitness level improves, you will start to feel better and look better. Although reaching and maintaining a reasonable level of cardiorespiratory fitness will always require time and effort, the rewards will be well worth the labor.

Summary

1. Benefits of cardiorespiratory fitness include a lower risk of disease, feeling better, increased capacity to perform everyday tasks, and improved self-esteem.

2. Adenosine triphosphate, which is required for muscular contraction, can be produced in muscles by two systems: anaerobic (without oxygen) and aerobic (with oxygen).

3. The energy to perform many types of exercise comes from both anaerobic and aerobic sources. In general, anaerobic energy production dominates in short-term exercise, whereas aerobic energy production dominates during prolonged exercise.

4. The term *cardiorespiratory system* refers to the cooperative work of the circulatory and respiratory systems. The primary function of the circulatory system is to transport blood carrying oxygen and nutrients to body tissues. The principal function of the respiratory system is to load oxygen into and remove carbon dioxide from the blood.

5. The maximum capacity to transport and utilize oxygen during exercise is called $\dot{V}O_2max$; many exercise physiologists consider $\dot{V}O_2max$ to be the most valid measurement of cardiorespiratory fitness.

6. Cardiac output, systolic blood pressure, and heart rate increase as a function of exercise intensity. Breathing (ventilation) also increases in proportion to exercise intensity.

7. A key factor in prescribing exercise to improve cardiorespiratory fitness is knowledge of the individual's initial fitness and health status.

8. Three primary elements make up the exercise prescription: warm-up, workout (primary conditioning period), and cool-down.

9. The components of the workout are the mode, frequency, intensity, and duration of exercise.

10. In general, the mode of exercise to be used to obtain increased cardiorespiratory endurance is one that uses a large muscle mass in a slow, rhythmical pattern for 20 to 60 minutes.

11. The target heart rate is the range of exercise heart rates that lie between 70% and 90% of maximal heart rate.

12. The recommended frequency of exercise to improve cardiorespiratory fitness is three to five times per week.

13. Establishing both short-term and long-term fitness goals is essential before beginning a fitness program.

14. Regardless of your initial fitness level, an exercise prescription for improving cardiorespiratory fitness has three phases: the starter phase, the slow progression phase, and the maintenance phase.

15. Common endurance training techniques to improve cardiorespiratory fitness include cross training; long, slow distance training; interval training; and fartlek training.

16. Aerobic exercise training results in an improvement in cardiorespiratory fitness ($\dot{V}O_{2max}$) and muscular endurance and can result in a reduction in percent body fat.

17. Maintaining a regular exercise routine requires proper time management and the choice of physical activities that you enjoy.

Study Questions

1. Discuss the two energy pathways used to produce muscle ATP during exercise.

2. Which energy pathway (aerobic or anaerobic) is predominantly responsible for production of ATP during the following activities: 100-meter dash, 800-meter run, 10,000-meter run, tennis, football, and weight lifting?

3. What is meant by the term *cardiorespiratory system*? List the major functions of the circulatory and respiratory systems.

4. Why is the heart considered "two pumps in one"?

5. Define the following terms:
   adenosine triphosphate (ATP)
   cross training
   hypertension
   target heart rate

6. Graph the changes in heart rate, blood pressure, cardiac output, and ventilation as a function of exercise intensity.

7. Define $\dot{V}O_{2max}$.

8. Discuss the relationship between exercise intensity and lactic acid production in muscles. Define the anaerobic threshold. What is the practical significance of the anaerobic threshold for exercise?

9. What physiological changes occur as a result of endurance training?

10. Will endurance training alone result in improvement in all of the components of health-related physical fitness? Why or why not?

11. What information is necessary to develop an individualized exercise prescription?

12. List the criteria that must be met to obtain improvement in aerobic capacity.

13. What effect does mode of training have on obtaining increased aerobic capacity?

14. What range in frequency of exercise is needed to improve aerobic capacity?

15. Define training threshold and give the range of intensities that are considered necessary to elicit an increase in $\dot{V}O_{2max}$.

16. What training techniques are generally used in exercise programs for improving cardiorespiratory fitness?

Suggested Reading

American College of Sports Medicine. American College of Sports Medicine position stand: The recommended quantity and quality of exercise for developing and maintaining cardiorespiratory and muscular fitness and flexibility in healthy adults. *Medicine and Science in Sports and Exercise* 30:975–991, 1998.

Blair, S. N., M. J. LaMonte, and M. Z. Nichaman. The evolution of physical activity recommendations: How much is enough? *American Journal of Clinical Nutrition* 79(5):913S–920S, 2004.

Brisswalter J., M. Collardeau, and A. Rene. Effects of acute physical exercise characteristics on cognitive performance. *Sports Medicine* 32(9):555–566, 2002.

Chobanian, A. V., G. L. Bakris, H. R. Black, W. C. Cushman, L. A. Green, J. L. Izzo Jr, D. W. Jones, B. J. Materson, S. Oparil, J. T. Wright Jr, and E. J. Roccella. National Heart, Lung, and Blood Institute Joint National Committee on Prevention, Detection, Evaluation, and Treatment of High Blood Pressure; National High Blood Pressure Education Program Coordinating Committee. The Seventh Report of the Joint National Committee on Prevention, Detection, Evaluation, and Treatment of High Blood Pressure: The JNC 7 report. *Journal of the American Medical Association* 21;289(19):2560–2572, 2003.

Neiman, D. C. *Fitness and Sports Medicine: A Health-Related Approach,* 3rd ed. Palo Alto, CA: Bull Publishing, 1995.

Pollock, M. L., and J. H. Wilmore. *Exercise in Health and Disease,* 3rd ed. Philadelphia: W. B. Saunders, 1998.

Powers, S., and E. Howley. *Exercise Physiology: Theory and Application to Fitness and Performance,* 4th ed. Dubuque, IA: McGraw-Hill, 2004.

Robertson, Robert. *Perceived Exertion for Practitioners: Rating Effort With the OMNI Picture System.* Champaign, IL: Human Kinetic Publishers, 2004.

Spriet, L. L., and M. J. Gibala. Nutritional strategies to influence adaptations to training. *Journal of Sports Science* 22(1):127–141, 2004.

Warburton, D. E., N. Gledhill, and A. Quinney. Musculoskeletal fitness and health. *Canadian Journal of Applied Physiology* 26(2):217–237, 2001.

For links to the web sites below visit The Total Fitness and Wellness Website at www.aw-bc.com/powers.

About.com

Provides information about many aspects of cardiovascular fitness, health benefits of exercise, and wellness.

WebMD.com

General information about exercise, fitness, and wellness. Great articles, instructional information, and updates.

ACSM.org

Comprehensive web site providing information, articles, equipment recommendations, how-to articles, books, and position statements about all aspects of health and fitness.

FitnessOnline

Provides information, tools, and support to achieve health and fitness goals. Online home of *Shape, Men's Fitness, Muscle & Fitness, Flex, Natural Health,* and *Fit Pregnancy* magazines.

Sympatico: Health

Includes numerous articles, book reviews, and links to nutrition, fitness, and wellness topics.

Gatorade Sports Science Institute

Presents many articles relating to fluid replacement during exercise. Enables registration to be on a mailing list to receive new articles.

The Running Page

Contains information about racing, running clubs, places to run, running-related products, magazines, and treating running injuries.

Meriter Fitness

Contains information on injury prevention and treatment, weight training, flexibility, exercise prescriptions, and more.

References

1. Cooper, K. H. *Aerobics.* New York: Bantam Books, 1968.

2. Ross, R., and I. Janssen. Physical activity, total and regional obesity: Dose-response considerations. *Medicine and Science in Sports and Exercise* 33(6):S345–S641, 2001.

3. Kohl, H. W. Physical activity and cardiovascular disease: Evidence for a dose response. *Medicine and Science in Sports and Exercise* 33(6):S472–S483, 2001.

4. Kesaniemi, Y. A., E. Danforth, M. D. Jensen, P. G. Kopelman, P. Lefebvre, and B. A. Reeder. Dose-response issues concerning physical activity and health: An evidence-based symposium. *Medicine and Science in Sports and Exercise* 33(6):S351–S358, 2001.

5. Dunn, A. L., M. H. Trivedi, and H. A. O'Neal. Physical activity dose-response effects on outcomes of depression and anxiety. *Medicine and Science in Sports and Exercise* 33(6):S587–S597, 2001.

6. Gambelunghe, C., R. Rossi, G. Mariucci, M. Tantucci, and M. V. Ambrosini. Effects of light physical exercise on sleep regulation in rats. *Medicine and Science in Sports and Exercise* 33(1):57–60, 2001.

7. American Heart Association. *Are You at Risk of Heart Attack or Stroke?* Dallas: American Heart Association, 1999.

8. American Heart Association. *2001 Heart and Stroke Statistical Update.* Dallas: American Heart Association, 2000.

9. Svedahl, K. and B. R. MacIntosh. Anaerobic threshold: The concept and methods of measurement. *Canadian Journal Applied Physiology* 28(2):299–323, 2003.

10. *ACSM's Resource Manual for Guidelines for Exercise Testing and Prescription,* 4th ed. Philadelphia: Lippincot Williams, & Wilkins 2001.

11. Mullineaux, D. R., C. A. Barnes, and E. F. Barnes. Factors affecting the likelihood to engage in adequate physical activity to promote health. *Journal of Sports Sciences* 19(4):279–288, 2001.

12. Laursen, P. B., and D. G. Jenkins. The scientific basis for high-intensity interval training: optimising training programmes and maximising performance in highly trained endurance athletes. *Sports Medicine* 32(1):53–73, 2002.

13. Powers, S., and E. Howley. *Exercise Physiology: Theory and Application to Fitness and Performance,* 4th ed. Dubuque, IA: McGraw-Hill, 2001.

14. Powers, S., S. Grinton, J. Lawler, D. Criswell, and S. Dodd. High intensity exercise training–induced metabolic alterations in respiratory muscles. *Respiration Physiology* 89:169–177, 1992.

15. Borg, G. *Borg's Perceived Exertion and Pain Scales.* Champaign, IL; Human Kinetics, 1998.

Developing Your Personal Exercise Prescription

NAME _____ DATE _____

Using Tables 4.3 through 4.5 as models, develop your personal exercise prescription based on your current fitness level and goals. Record the appropriate information in the spaces provided below. Monitor your fitness levels periodically and adjust your prescription accordingly.

Week No.	Phase	Duration (min/day)	Intensity (% of HR_{max})	Frequency (days/wk)	Exercise Mode	Comments
1						
2						
3						
4						
5						
6						
7						
8						
9						
10						
11						
12						
13						
14						
15						
16						

Cardiorespiratory Training Log

(Note: Make additional copies as needed)

NAME _____   DATE _____

In the spaces below keep a record of your exercise training program. Exercise heart rate can be recorded as the range of heart rates measured at various times during the training session. Use the comments section to record any useful information concerning your exercise session, such as weather conditions, time of day, how you felt, and so on.

Date	Activity	Warm-Up Duration	Exercise Duration	Cool-Down Duration	Exercise Heart Rate	Comments

Rate of Perceived Exertion

NAME_____ **DATE**_____

Ratings of perceived exertion were originally structured to correspond to heart rates. Adding a zero to the numerical rating produces the expected heart rate range for that rating. However, people perceive exertion differently, so ratings do not always match heart rate values. The important thing to learn is the RPE number that corresponds to your threshold of training heart rate and the RPE that represents the upper limit heart rate of your target heart rate (THR) zone. Typically, numerical RPE ratings for exercise in the THR zone will fall between 12 and 16. With practice, you can learn to make accurate ratings.

Use the following RPE scale to rate your exertion.

Scale	Verbal Rating
6	No exertion at all
7	Extremely light
8	
9	Very light
10	
11	Light
12	
13	Somewhat hard
14	
15	Hard (heavy)
16	
17	Very hard
18	
19	Extremely hard
20	Maximal exertion

Source: Borg-RPE-scale ® from G. Borg, (1998), *Borg's Perceived Exertion and Pain Scales.* Champaign, IL: Human Kinetics. © Gunnar Borg, 1970, 1985, 1994, 1998. Used with permission of Dr. G. Borg. For correct usage of the scale the exact design and instructions given in Borg's folders must be followed.

Perform the following exercises:

 a. Walk for 3 minutes at a brisk pace.

 b. Jog for 3 minutes at a slow pace.

 c. Jog for 3 minutes at a pace that will elevate your heart rate to your threshold level.

After each exercise bout, count your heart rate. Also, rate the intensity of the exercise at the end of the third minute using the RPE scale above. Record this in the table on the following page.

(continued on next page)

Next perform a more intense 3-minute run that elevates your heart rate to the upper one-third of your THR zone. When finished with this run, count your heart rate and give an RPE value.

Activity	Heart Rate (bpm)	Rating of Perceived Exertion
Walk	_____	_____
Slow	_____	_____
Threshold Jog	_____	_____
Intense Run	_____	_____

	Yes	No
1. Did the walk or slow jog elevate your heart rate to threshold level?	_____	_____
2. Was your RPE number less than 12 for the walk or slow jog?	_____	_____
3. Was your RPE number for the threshold jog in the range of 12 to 16?	_____	_____
4. Did your final intense run get your heart rate well into your target heart rate zone?	_____	_____
5. Was your RPE number in the intense run in the range of 12 to 16?	_____	_____

With practice, do you think you could learn to use the RPE scale to determine if you are exercising with enough intensity to build cardiovascular fitness? *Note:* If the last two runs do not elevate your heart rate into the target zone, learning to make accurate ratings of perceived exertion will be compromised.

Using the Rating of Perceived Exertion Scale

(Make additional copies as needed)

NAME _____ DATE _____

This lab requires students to divide into groups of three partners each. Partner #1 performs a graded, incremental exercise test as described in Chapter 3. Partner #2 records heart rate at the end of each increment while partner #3 records the exercise RPE using the RPE Scale from laboratory 4.3. While partner #2 records heart rate over the last 30 seconds of each exercise stage, partner #3 holds the RPE scale in front of partner #1 and asks him/her to rate the perceived exertion level. Record the results in the table below. (Note: It is not necessary to complete all stages of the test.)

	Heart Rate (HR)	RPE	DIFFERENCE HR − (RPE × 10)
Rest			
Stage 1			
Stage 2			
Stage 3			
Stage 4			
Stage 5			
Stage 6			
Stage 7			
Stage 8			
Stage 9			
Stage 10			
1' Post-test			
5' Post-test			
10' Post-test			

On a separate piece of paper, graph the response of RPE (y axis) to the change in heart rate (x axis). What can you conclude from this comparison?

Blood Pressure Response to Exercise

(Make additional copies as needed)

NAME _____ DATE _____

This lab can only be performed if the necessary equipment and individuals trained to take blood pressure are available. The lab requires one or more students to perform a graded, incremental exercise test as described in Chapter 3. At the end of each stage, someone trained to take blood pressure will determine blood pressure and record both systolic and diastolic pressure in the chart below. Another person will record heart rate. (Note: It is not necessary to complete all stages of the test.)

	Systolic BP	Diastolic BP	Heart Rate
Rest			
Stage 1			
Stage 2			
Stage 3			
Stage 4			
Stage 5			
Stage 6			
Stage 7			
Stage 8			
Stage 9			
Stage 10			
1' Post-test			
5' Post-test			
10' Post-test			

On a separate piece of paper, graph the response of systolic BP (*y* axis) to the change in heart rate (*x* axis). On a separate graph, plot the diastolic BP to heart rate. What can you conclude from these comparisons?

Determination of Target Heart Rate

NAME_____ **DATE**_____

Practice counting the number of pulses felt at both the carotid and radial locations. The carotid pulse is felt just lateral to the larynx, beneath the lower jaw. The radial pulse is located on the inside of the wrist, directly in line with the base of the thumb. Use a stopwatch to count for 15, 30, and 60 seconds. To determine your heart rate in beats per minute (bpm), multiply your 15-second count by four, and your 30-second count by two. Try locating and counting the pulse of another person at both the radial and carotid locations. Record your resting pulse counts in the spaces provided.

Carotid Pulse Count (Self)	Heart Rate (bpm)	Radial Pulse Count (Self)	Heart Rate (bpm)
_____ 15 seconds × 4	_____	_____ × 4	_____
_____ 30 seconds × 2	_____	_____ × 2	_____
_____ 60 seconds × 1	_____	_____ × 1	_____

Carotid Pulse Count (Partner)	Heart Rate (bpm)	Radial Pulse Count (Partner)	Heart Rate (bpm)
_____ 15 seconds × 4	_____	_____ × 4	_____
_____ 30 seconds × 2	_____	_____ × 2	_____
_____ 60 seconds × 1	_____	_____ × 1	_____

The target heart rate (THR) zone is calculated indirectly by subtracting your age (in years) from 220, and multiplying this number by 70% and 90%. Calculate your exercise THR:

$$220 - \underset{\text{age}}{\underline{\hspace{2cm}}} = \underset{\substack{\text{maximum} \\ \text{heart rate}}}{\underline{\hspace{3cm}}} \text{ bpm}$$

$$\underset{\substack{\text{max} \\ \text{heart rate}}}{\underline{\hspace{2cm}}} \times 0.70 = \underset{\substack{\textbf{lower end} \\ \textbf{of THR}}}{\underline{\hspace{2.5cm}}}$$

$$\underset{\substack{\text{max} \\ \text{heart rate}}}{\underline{\hspace{2cm}}} \times 0.90 = \underset{\substack{\textbf{upper end} \\ \textbf{of THR}}}{\underline{\hspace{2.5cm}}}$$

1. Which of the resting pulses did you find easiest to locate on yourself? Carotid or radial?

2. Which resting pulse was easiest to locate on your partner? Carotid or radial?

3. Which of the two locations would you prefer to use when counting exercise heart rate? Why?

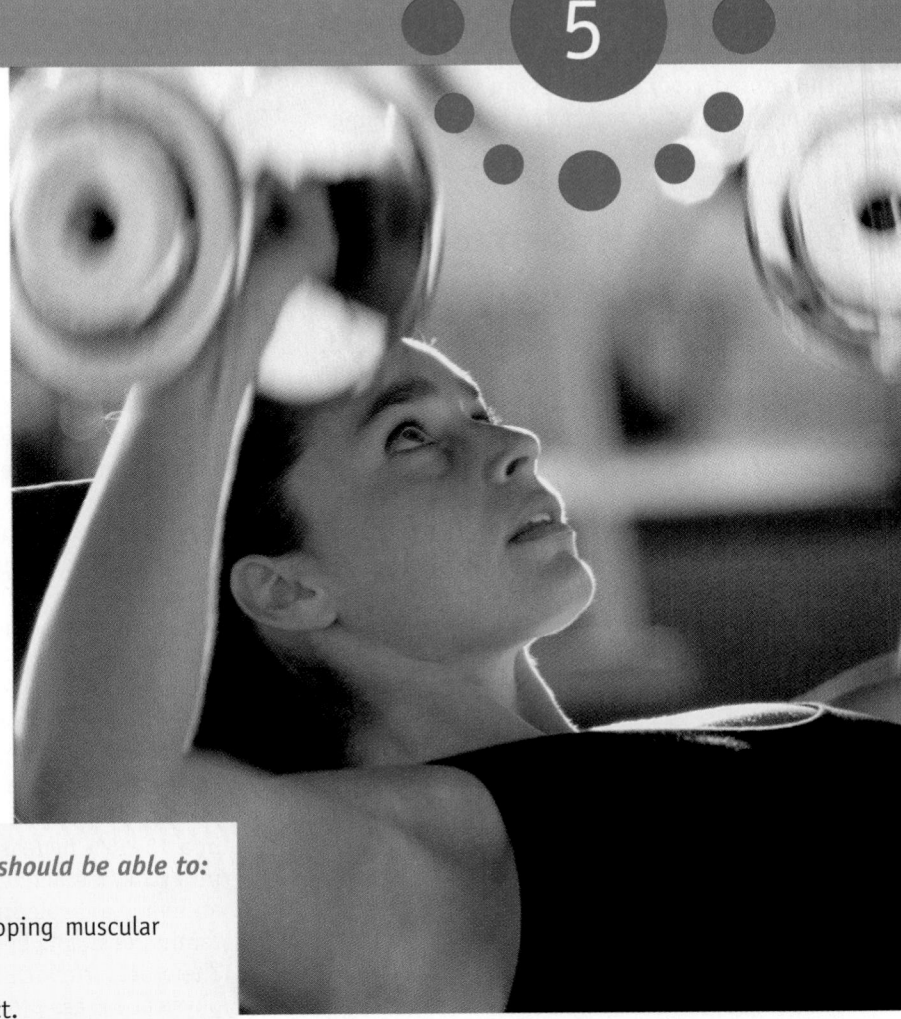

5

After studying this chapter, you should be able to:

1. Explain the benefits of developing muscular strength and endurance.

2. Describe how muscles contract.

3. Distinguish among the various types of muscle fibers.

4. Classify the types of muscular contractions.

5. Identify the major changes that occur in skeletal muscles in response to strength training.

6. List the factors that determine muscle strength and endurance.

7. Outline the general principles used in designing a strength and endurance program.

8. Distinguish among the various types of training programs for improving strength and endurance.

9. Design a program for improving strength and endurance.

Improving Muscular Strength and Endurance

Lifting weights or performing other types of resistance exercises to build muscular strength and endurance is commonly referred to as weight training or strength training. This chapter discusses the principles and techniques employed in strength training programs. We begin with a brief overview of the benefits associated with developing muscular strength and endurance.

❄ Benefits of Muscular Strength and Endurance

Regular strength training promotes numerous health benefits. For example, we know that the incidence of low back pain, a common problem in both men and women, can be reduced with the appropriate strengthening exercises for the lower back and abdominal muscles (1). Further, recent studies demonstrate that muscle-strengthening exercises may reduce the occurrence of joint and/or muscle injuries that may occur during physical activity (2). In addition, strength training can

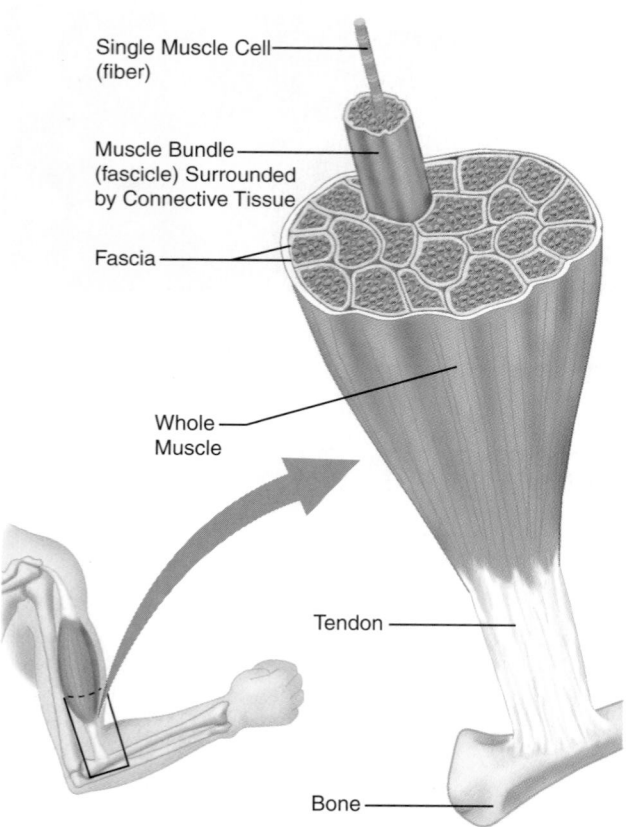

FIGURE 5.1
Muscle structure.
Source: Johnson, Michael, *Human Biology.* Benjamin Cummings, San Francisco, 2006.

delay the decreases in muscle strength experienced by sedentary older individuals (4), as well as contribute to the prevention of the bone-wasting disease called osteoporosis (4).

Another positive aspect of strength training is the improvement in personal appearance and self-esteem associated with increased muscular tone and strength (5). Also, increased muscular strength has many practical benefits in daily activities, such as an improved ability to carry heavy boxes, perform routine yard work, or do housework.

One of the most important benefits of strength training is that increasing muscle size results in an elevation in resting energy expenditure (14). Resting energy expenditure (called *resting metabolic rate*) is the total amount of energy that the body requires to perform all of the necessary functions associated with maintaining life. Resting metabolic rate includes the energy required to drive the heart and respiratory muscles and to build and maintain body tissues.

How does strength training influence resting metabolic rate? One of the primary results of strength training is an increase in muscle mass. Because muscle tissue requires energy even at rest, muscular enlargement promotes an increase in resting energy expenditure. An increase of 1 pound of muscle elevates resting metabolism by approximately 2–3%. Further, this increase can be magnified with larger gains in muscle. For instance, a 5-pound increase in muscle mass would result in a 10–15% increase in resting metabolic rate. Changes in resting metabolic rate of this magnitude can play an important role in assisting in weight loss or maintaining desirable body composition throughout life. Therefore, strength training is a key component of any physical fitness program.

❄ Physiological Basis for Developing Strength and Endurance

The human body contains approximately 600 skeletal muscles, the primary function of which is to provide force for bodily movement. The body and its parts move when the appropriate muscles shorten and apply force to the bones. Skeletal muscles also assist in maintaining posture and regulating body temperature during cold exposure by causing heat production through the mechanism of shivering in cold weather. Because all fitness activities require the use of skeletal muscles, some appreciation of their structure and function is essential for anyone entering a physical fitness program.

Before we discuss how muscles work, let's revisit the definitions of muscular strength and endurance. Muscular strength and endurance are related, but they

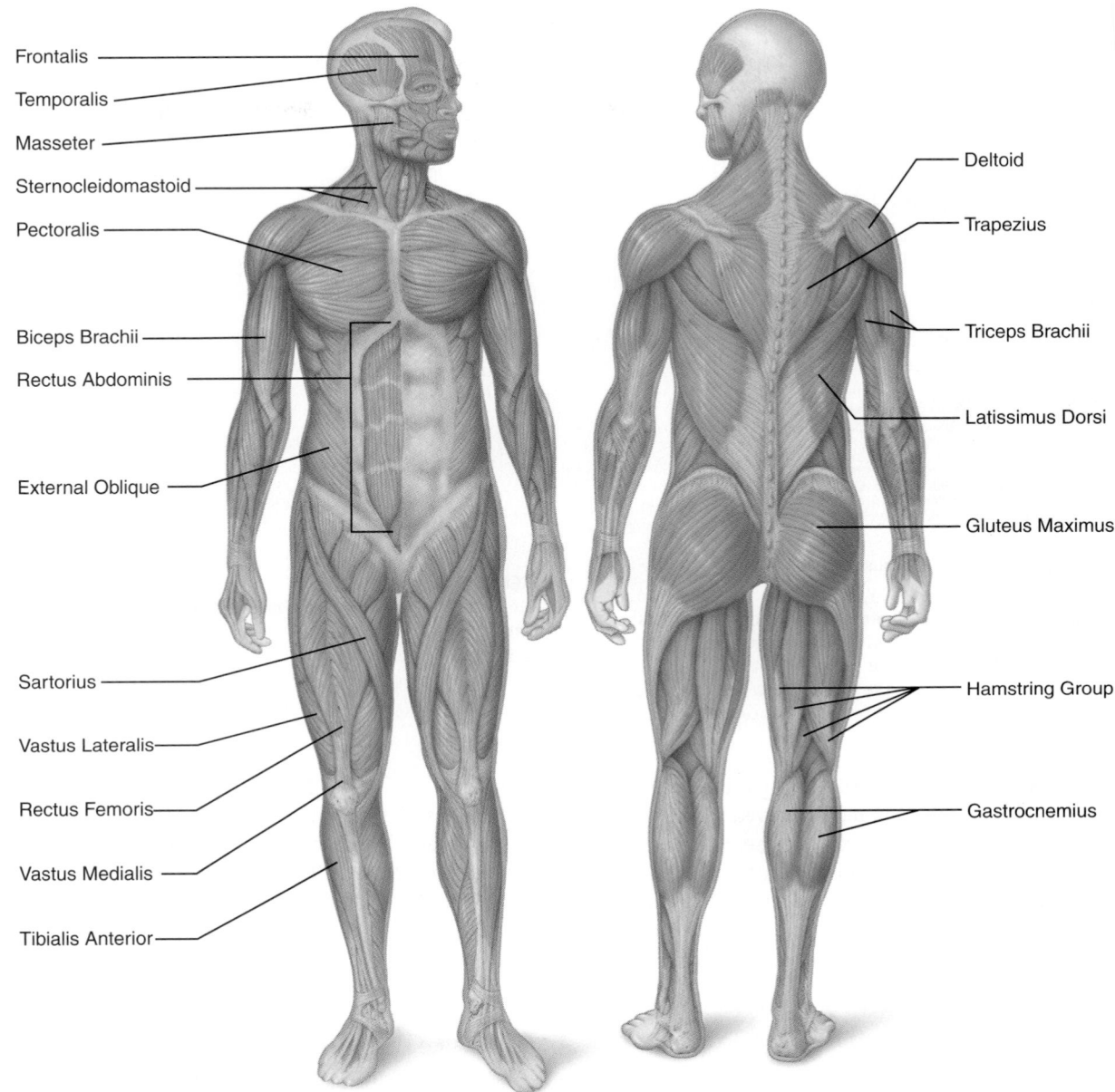

FIGURE 5.2
Major muscles of the human body.
Source: Johnson, Michael, *Human Biology*. Benjamin Cummings, San Francisco, 2006.

are not the same thing. Recall that muscular strength is defined as the ability of a muscle to generate maximal force (Chapter 1). In simple terms, muscular strength is the amount of weight that an individual can lift during one maximal effort. In contrast, muscular endurance is defined as the ability to generate force over and over again. In general, increasing muscular strength by exercise training will increase muscular endurance as well. However, training aimed at improving muscular endurance does not always result in significant improvements in muscular strength. Techniques to improve both muscular strength and muscular endurance are discussed later in this chapter.

MUSCLE STRUCTURE AND CONTRACTION

MUSCLE STRUCTURE Skeletal muscle is a collection of long thin cells called *fibers*. These fibers are surrounded by a dense layer of connective tissue called *fascia* that holds the individual fibers together and separates muscle from surrounding tissues (Figure 5.1).

Muscles are attached to bone by connective tissues known as *tendons*. Muscular contraction causes the tendons to pull on the bones, thereby causing movement. Many of the muscles involved in movement are illustrated in Figure 5.2.

CNS Spinal Cord

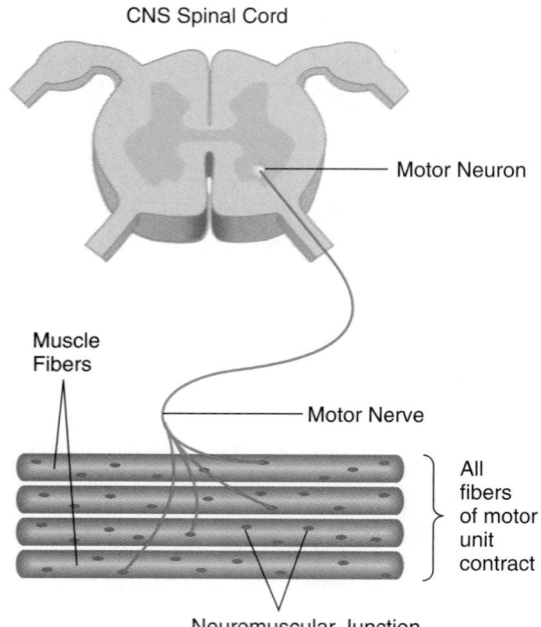

Motor Neuron

Muscle Fibers

Motor Nerve

All fibers of motor unit contract

Neuromuscular Junction

FIGURE 5.3
The concept of a motor unit. A motor nerve from the central nervous system is shown innervating several muscle fibers. With one impulse from the motor nerve, all fibers contract.
Source: Fox, E., R. Bowers, and M. Foss, *The Physiological Basis of Physical Education and Athletics.* Reprinted by permission of McGraw Hill Companies.

Isometric vs. Isotonic Contraction

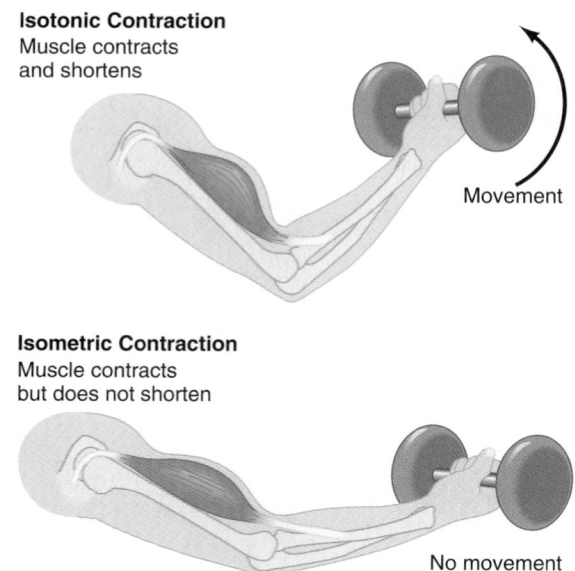

Isotonic Contraction
Muscle contracts and shortens

Movement

Isometric Contraction
Muscle contracts but does not shorten

No movement

FIGURE 5.4
Illustration of isotonic (also called dynamic) and isometric contractions.
Source: Powers, S., and E. Howley, *Exercise Physiology: Theory and Application to Fitness and Performance.* Dubuque, IA: McGraw-Hill, 2003.

MUSCLE CONTRACTION Muscle contraction is regulated by signals coming from motor nerves. Motor nerves originate in the spinal cord and send messages to individual muscles throughout the body. A motor nerve and an individual muscle fiber meet and make contact at a neuromuscular junction. The relationship between a motor nerve and skeletal muscle fibers is

illustrated in Figure 5.3. Note that each motor nerve branches and then connects with numerous individual muscle fibers. The motor nerve and all of the muscle fibers it controls is called a **motor unit.**

A muscle contraction begins when a message to contract (called a *nerve impulse*) reaches the neuromuscular junction (Figure 5.3). The arrival of the nerve impulse triggers the contraction process by permitting the interaction of contractile proteins in muscle.

Because the nerve impulse initiates the contractile process, it is logical that the removal of the nerve signal from the muscle would "turn off" the contractile process. Indeed, when a motor nerve ceases to send signals to a muscle, the contraction stops. Occasionally, however, an uncontrolled muscular contraction occurs, which is referred to as a muscle cramp.

TYPES OF MUSCLE CONTRACTIONS

Muscle contractions are classified into two major categories: isotonic and isometric. **Isotonic** (also called **dynamic**) contractions are those that result in movement of a body part. Most exercise or sports skills utilize isotonic contractions. For example, lifting a dumbbell (Figure 5.4, top) involves movement of a body part and is therefore classified as an isotonic contraction. An **isometric** (also called **static**) contraction requires

---

motor unit A motor nerve and each of the muscle fibers it innervates.

isotonic Refers to muscle contractions in which there is movement of a body part. Most exercise or sports skills use isotonic contractions.

dynamic Means "movement"; in reference to muscle contractions, dynamic contraction is synonymous with isotonic contraction.

isometric Refers to muscle contractions in which muscular tension is developed but no movement of body parts takes place.

static Stationary; in reference to muscle contractions, static contraction is synonymous with isometric contraction.

the development of muscular tension but results in no movement of body parts (Figure 5.4, bottom). A classic example of isometric contraction involves an individual exerting force against an iron bar mounted on the wall of a building; the muscle is developing tension but the wall is not moving, and therefore neither is the body part. Isometric contractions occur commonly in the postural muscles of the body during sitting or standing; for instance, isometric contractions are responsible for holding the head upright.

Note that isotonic contractions can be further subdivided into concentric, eccentric, and isokinetic contractions. **Concentric contractions** are isotonic muscle contractions that result in muscle shortening. The upward movement of the arm in Figure 5.5 is an example of a concentric contraction. In contrast, **eccentric contractions** (also called *negative contractions*) are defined as contractions in which the muscle exerts force while it lengthens. An eccentric contraction occurs when, for example, an individual resists the pull of a weight during the lowering phase of weight lifting (Figure 5.5). Here, the muscle is developing tension, but the force developed is not great enough to prevent the weight from being lowered.

Isokinetic contractions are concentric or eccentric contractions performed at a constant speed. That is, the speed of muscle shortening or lengthening is regulated at a fixed, controlled rate. This is generally accomplished by a weight-lifting machine that controls the rate of muscle shortening.

MUSCLE FIBER TYPES

There are three types of skeletal muscle fibers: slow twitch, fast twitch, and intermediate. These fiber types differ in their speeds of contraction and in fatigue resistance (6). Because most human muscles contain a mixture of all three fiber types, it is helpful to have an understanding of each before beginning the strength-training process.

SLOW-TWITCH FIBERS   As the name implies, **slow-twitch fibers** contract slowly and produce small amounts of force; however, these fibers are highly resistant to fatigue. Slow-twitch fibers, which are red in appearance, have the capacity to produce large quantities of ATP aerobically, making them ideally suited for a low-intensity prolonged exercise like walking or slow jogging. Further, because of their resistance to fatigue, most postural muscles are composed primarily of slow-twitch fibers.

FAST-TWITCH FIBERS   **Fast-twitch fibers** contract rapidly and generate great amounts of force but fatigue quickly. These fibers are white and have a low aerobic capacity, but they are well equipped to produce ATP

Concentric Contraction

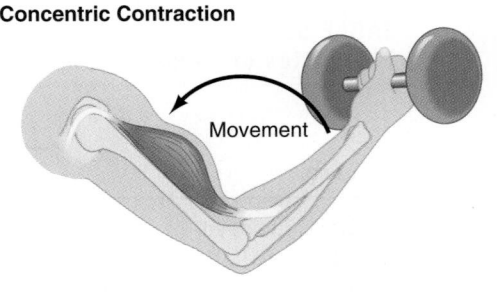

Eccentric Contraction

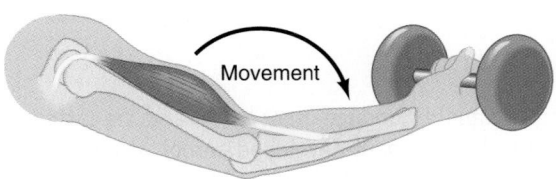

FIGURE 5.5
Illustration of concentric and eccentric contractions.
Source: Adapted from Powers, S., and E. Howley, *Exercise Physiology: Theory and Application to Fitness and Performance,* copyright 1994. Reprinted by permission of McGraw Hill Companies.

anaerobically. With their ability to shorten rapidly and produce large amounts of force, fast-twitch fibers are used during activities requiring rapid or forceful movement, such as jumping, sprinting, and weight lifting.

INTERMEDIATE FIBERS   **Intermediate fibers,** although more red in color, possess a combination of the characteristics of fast- and slow-twitch fibers. They

---

concentric contractions   Isotonic muscle contractions that result in muscle shortening.
eccentric contractions   Isotonic contractions in which the muscle exerts force while the muscle lengthens (also called *negative contractions*).
isokinetic contractions   Concentric or eccentric isotonic contractions performed at a constant speed.
slow-twitch fibers   Muscle fibers that contract slowly and are highly resistant to fatigue. Red in appearance, they have the capacity to produce large quantities of ATP aerobically, making them ideally suited for low-intensity, prolonged exercise like walking or slow jogging.
fast-twitch fibers   Muscle fibers that contract rapidly but fatigue quickly. These fibers are white and have a low aerobic capacity, but they are well equipped to produce ATP anaerobically.
intermediate fibers   Muscle fibers that possess a combination of the characteristics of fast- and slow-twitch fibers. They contract rapidly and are fatigue resistant due to a well-developed aerobic capacity.

TABLE 5.1
Properties of Human Skeletal Muscle Fiber Types

Property	Fiber Type		
	Slow-twitch	Intermediate	Fast-twitch
Contraction speed	Slow	Intermediate	Fast
Resistance to fatigue	High	Intermediate	Low
Predominant energy system	Aerobic	Combination aerobic and anaerobic	Anaerobic
Force generation	Low	Intermediate	High

contract rapidly, produce great force, and are fatigue resistant due to a well-developed aerobic capacity. Intermediate fibers contract more quickly and produce more force than slow-twitch fibers but contract more slowly and produce less force than fast-twitch fibers. They are more fatigue resistant than fast-twitch fibers but less fatigue resistant than slow-twitch fibers. Table 5.1 summarizes the properties of all three fiber types.

RECRUITMENT OF MUSCLE FIBERS DURING EXERCISE

Many types of exercise use only a small fraction of the muscle fibers available in a muscle group. For example, walking at a slow speed may use fewer than 30% of the muscle fibers in the legs. More intense types of exercise, however, require more force. In order for a muscle group to generate more force, a greater number of muscle fibers must be called into play. The process of involving more muscle fibers to produce increased muscular force is called fiber **recruitment.** Figure 5.6 illustrates the order of recruitment of muscle fibers as the intensity of exercise increases. Note that during low-intensity exercise, only slow-twitch fibers are used. As the exercise intensity increases, progressive recruitment of fibers occurs, from slow-twitch to intermediate fibers and finally to fast-twitch fibers. High-intensity activities like weight training recruit large numbers of fast-twitch fibers.

GENETICS AND FIBER TYPE

People vary in the percentage of slow-twitch, intermediate, and fast-twitch fibers their muscles contain. Research by exercise scientists has shown that a relationship exists between muscle fiber type and success in athletics. For example, champion endurance athletes, such as marathon runners, have a predominance of slow-twitch fibers. This is logical, because endurance sports require muscles with high fatigue resistance. In contrast, elite sprinters, such as 100-meter dash runners, possess a predominance of fast-twitch fibers. The average non-athlete generally has equal numbers of all three fiber types.

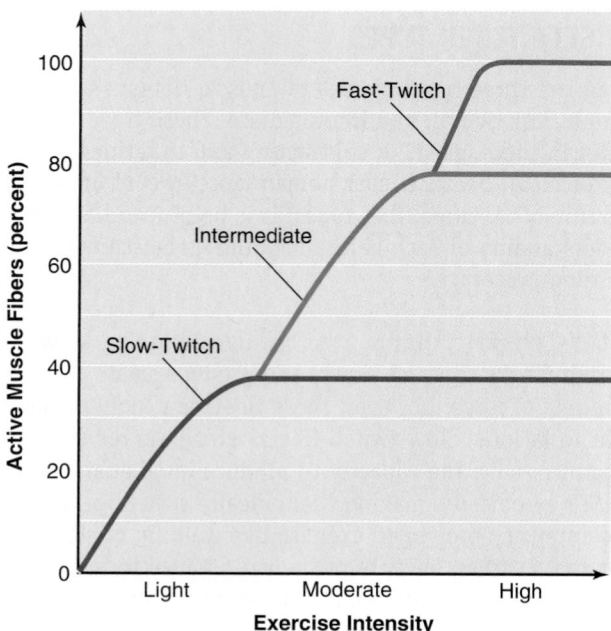

FIGURE 5.6
The relationship between exercise intensity and recruitment of muscle-fiber type.
Source: Adapted from Powers, S., and E. Howley, *Exercise Physiology: Theory and Application to Fitness and Performance,* copyright 1994. Reprinted by permission of McGraw Hill Companies.

recruitment   The process of involving more muscle fibers to increase muscular force.

Nutritional Links

TO HEALTH AND FITNESS

Do Weight Lifters Need Large Amounts of Protein in Their Diets?

Although many nutritional supplement companies claim that weight lifters require large quantities of protein in their diets, organizations such as the American College of Sports Medicine (ACSM), American Dietetic Association (ADA), and Dietitians of Canada (DC) have concluded that athletes have only slightly higher protein require-

ments than non-athletes. They have also found that most athletes consume protein in their normal diets far in excess of any increased protein requirement. Provided that sound nutrition principles are followed and energy intake is sufficient to maintain body weight, athletes require about 10–15% of their total caloric intake

from protein and do not need to fortify their diets with expensive protein powders or amino acid supplements. The table below illustrates the daily energy and protein requirements for the average endurance or strength athlete.

Protein requirements for active individuals.[*]

Type of athlete	Energy (calories/day)	Daily Requirement for a 154 lb Individual		
		Protein		
		Grams protein per lb body weight per day	Grams/day	% of daily calories
Endurance	3800	0.55–0.64	84–98	9–10%
Strength	3200	0.73–0.77	112–119	14–15%

[*]Values are based on ACSM/ADA/DC Joint Position Statement (16) and assume a resting energy expenditure equivalent to 40 Kcals per kilogram (18 Kcals/lb) of body weight per day; a male runner who runs 10 miles per day at a pace of 6 minutes per mile with an energy expenditure of running of 0.11 Kcals per minute per pound of body weight; and an additional cost of 2.7 Kcals per pound body weight per day for heavy resistance training.

Although endurance exercise training has been shown to cause some fiber type conversion (6), the number and percentage of skeletal muscle fiber types is primarily determined by genetics. Because of the interrelationship among genetics, fiber type, and athletic success, some researchers have jokingly suggested that if you want to be a champion athlete, you must pick your parents wisely!

FACTORS THAT DETERMINE MUSCULAR STRENGTH

Two primary physiological factors determine the amount of force that a muscle can generate: the size of the muscle and the number of fibers recruited during the contraction.

MUSCLE SIZE The primary determinant of how much force a muscle can generate is its size. The larger the muscle, the greater the force it can produce. Although

there is no difference in the chemical makeup of muscle in men and women, men are generally stronger than women because men have more muscle mass (i.e., larger muscles). The larger muscle mass in men is due to hormonal differences between the sexes; men have higher levels of the male sex hormone testosterone. The fact that testosterone promotes an increase in muscle size has led some athletes to attempt to improve muscular strength with drugs (see A Closer Look on p. 128).

MUSCLE FIBER RECRUITMENT We have seen that muscle fiber recruitment influences the production of muscle force. The more muscle fibers that are stimulated to shorten, the greater the muscle force generation, because the force generated by individual fibers is additive (Figure 5.7).

Muscle fiber recruitment is regulated voluntarily through the nervous system. That is, we determine how many muscle fibers to recruit by voluntarily making a decision about how much effort to put into a particular

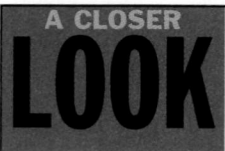

Anabolic Steroid Use Increases Muscle Size but Has Serious Side Effects

The abuse of **anabolic steroids** (synthetic forms of the hormone testosterone, which is important in muscle growth) and their precursors have mushroomed over the past several decades. The fierce competition in body building and sports in which strength and power are necessary for success has driven both men and women to risk serious health consequences in order to develop large muscles.

The large doses of steroids needed to increase muscle mass produce several health risks. A partial list of the side effects caused by abusing steroids and their precursors includes liver cancer, increased blood pressure, increased levels of "bad" cholesterol, severe depression, and prostate cancer. Prolonged use and high doses of steroids can be lethal.

In recent years, chemical precursors to the formation of testosterone in the body have come into favor with athletes and bodybuilders. One of the most popular, androstenedione, is used to increase blood testosterone with the intent to increase strength, lean body mass, and sexual performance. However, the most reliable research indicates that androstene-dione does not significantly increase strength and/or lean body mass. Another presuror to testosterone production in the body, dehydroepiandrosterone (DHEA), has also been used to increase testosterone in the body. DHEA is also advertised as an antiobesity and antiaging supplement capable of improving libido, vitality, and immunity levels. However, the best evidence demonstrates that DHEA supplementation does not increase testosterone concentrations or increase strength in men, and it may have masculinizing effects in women.

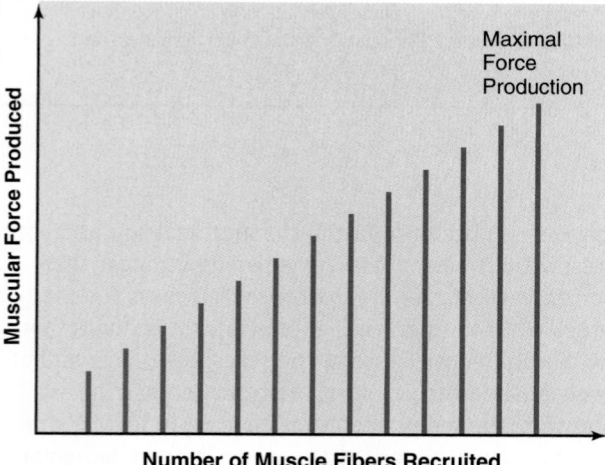

FIGURE 5.7
The relationship between motor unit recruitment and muscular force production.

anabolic steroids   Hormones produced by the body that enhance muscle growth. Usually refers to the synthetic form of the hormone testosterone.

movement. For instance, when we choose to make a minimal effort in lifting an object, we recruit only a few motor units, and the muscle develops limited force. However, if we make a decision to exert our maximal effort in lifting a heavy object, many muscle fibers are recruited and great force is generated (Figure 5.7).

☀ IN SUMMARY

- Strength training can reduce low back pain, reduce the incidence of exercise-related injuries, decrease the incidence of osteoporosis, and aid in maintenance of functional capacity that normally decreases with age.

- Muscular strength is the ability to generate maximal force, whereas muscular endurance is the ability to generate force over and over again.

- Skeletal muscle is composed of various types of fibers that are attached to bone by tendons. These fibers range from those generating high force with low endurance, to those generating less force with high endurance.

- Muscle contraction is regulated by signals coming from motor nerves. A motor unit comprises a motor nerve and all the muscle fibers it controls.

- Isotonic, or dynamic, muscle contractions result in movement of a body part, whereas isometric contractions result in no movement.
- Slow-twitch muscle fibers shorten slowly but are fatigue resistant. Fast-twitch fibers shorten rapidly but fatigue rapidly. Intermediate fibers shorten quickly but fatigue slowly.
- The process of involving more muscle fibers to produce increased muscular force is called *fiber recruitment.*
- The percentages of slow-twitch, intermediate, and fast-twitch fibers vary among individuals and play a major role in determining success in athletics.
- Two factors that determine muscle force are the size of the muscle and the number of fibers recruited.

Guiding Principles for Designing a Strength and Endurance Program

In Chapter 3 we discussed the general principles for developing training programs to improve physical fitness. Before we discuss the specifics of how to develop a strength training program, let's discuss several principles that should be considered in developing a muscular strength and endurance training program.

Progressive Resistance Exercise

The concept of **progressive resistance exercise (PRE)** is an application of the overload principle applied to strength and endurance exercise programs. Even though the two terms can be used interchangeably, PRE is preferred when discussing weight training. Progressive resistance exercise means that as strength and endurance are increased, the load against which the muscle works must be periodically elevated if strength and endurance gains are to be realized.

PRINCIPLE OF SPECIFICITY OF TRAINING

The principle of **specificity of training** means that development of muscular strength and endurance is specific to both the muscle group that is exercised and the training intensity. First, only those muscles that are trained will improve in strength and endurance. For example, if an individual has low back pain and wishes to improve the strength of the supporting musculature of the lower back, it would be of no benefit to strengthen the arm muscles. The specific muscles involved with movement of the lower back should be the ones trained. Second, the training intensity determines whether the muscular adaptation is primarily an increase in strength or endurance. High-intensity training (i.e., lifting heavy weights four to six times) results in an increase in both muscular strength and size with only limited improvements in muscular endurance. Conversely, high-repetition, low-intensity training (i.e., lifting light weights 20–25 times or more) promotes an increase in muscular endurance, with only limited improvements in muscular size and strength.

Designing a Training Program for Increasing Muscle Strength

There are numerous approaches to the design of weight-training programs. Any program that adheres to the basic principles described earlier will result in an improvement in strength and endurance. However, the type of weight-training program that you develop for yourself depends on your goals and the types of equipment available to you. Next, we discuss several other considerations in the development of a weight-training program.

SAFETY CONCERNS

Before we discuss the specifics of how to develop a weight-training program, the need for safety should be emphasized. Although weight training can be performed safely, some important guidelines should be followed:

1. When using free weights (like barbells), have spotters (helpers) assist you in the performance of exercises. They can help you if you are unable to complete a lift. Many weight machines reduce the need for spotters.

---

progressive resistance exercise (PRE) The application of the overload principle applied to strength and endurance exercise programs. Even though the overload principle and PRE can be used interchangeably, PRE is preferred when discussing weight training.

specificity of training The concept that the development of muscular strength and endurance, as well as cardiorespiratory endurance, is specific to both the muscle group exercised and the training intensity.

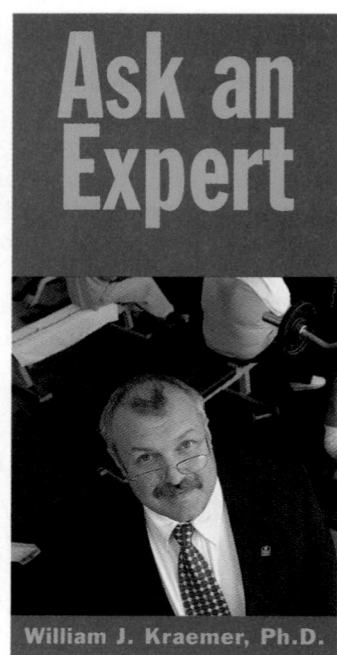

Ask an Expert

William J. Kraemer, Ph.D.

Resistance Training

Dr. Kraemer is Director of Research in the Human Performance Lab at the University of Connecticut. He is an internationally known expert on the adaptation of muscle to resistance training programs. He has published many scientific papers, books, and book chapters related to the acute and chronic adaptations to resistance exercise. In the following interview, Dr. Kraemer addresses several questions related to resistance training.

Q: I am beginning to work out with weights and want to improve my strength and understand that there is controversy over how many sets are best—one set or three sets. What is your advice?

A: When starting a program you should use the principle of "progressive resistance training" in your program. How many sets you should do depends on your training goals. Start out with one set to allow your body to develop toleration to the stress of resistance exercise. If your goal is to see continued improvement beyond a base level of fitness, progress to a multiple set program. Understand that not all exercises in a program need to be performed with the same number of sets. The number of sets are part of a volume of exercise equation (sets × reps × resistance = exercise volume). The volume of exercise can also be manipulated over time with the concept of periodization, where you may have training days or training cycles with very low, low-moderate, high, or very high training volumes for the entire body or a particular body part. Most advanced programs utilize multiple sets to expose the body to more total work, and such programs have been found to be significantly better than single set programs in producing strength, power, local muscular endurance, and muscle size gains.

Q: After starting a weight training program several months ago, my strength gains have plateaued.

What can I do to further my strength gains?

A: Studies overwhelmingly show that gains in strength are highest early in training and that the rate of improvement decreases as higher levels of strength are achieved. To surpass a plateau, adhere to three basic principles of progression: 1) progressive overload; 2) specificity; and 3) variation (periodization).

Progressive overload entails that the program gradually become more difficult. Overload may be introduced for improved strength, hypertrophy, endurance, and power in several ways:
1) increase load;
2) add repetitions;
3) alter repetition speed with submaximal loads;
4) shortened rest periods for endurance improvements or lengthened for strength and power;
5) increase volume within reasonable limits; and/or
6) any combination of the above.

Specificity refers to training that targets one particular (specific) group of muscles. The adaptation of this group of muscles will be specific to the particular muscle action, speed of movement, range of motion, muscle group, energy system, and intensity and volume of training.

Variation (or periodization) refers to systematic alteration in the volume and intensity of work. The technique of variation optimizes the development of strength by increasing the intensity while decreasing volume.

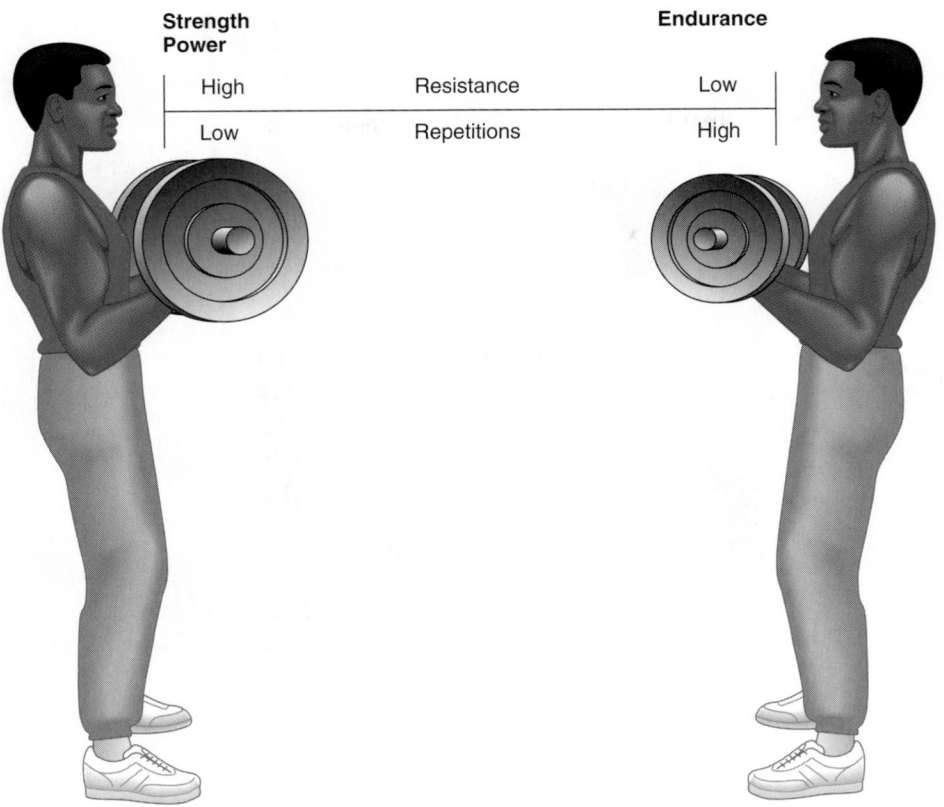

Strength Power		Endurance
High	Resistance	Low
Low	Repetitions	High

FIGURE 5.8
The strength-endurance continuum. Strength is achieved by using low repetitions/high weight, and endurance is achieved by using high repetitions/low weight.

2. Be sure that the collars on the end of the bars of free weights are tightly secured to prevent the weights from falling off. Dropping weight plates on toes and feet can result in serious injuries. Again, many weight machines reduce the potential risk of dropping weights.

3. Warm up properly before doing any weight-lifting exercise. Stretching the intended muscles and lifting very light weight is a good way to start.

4. Do not hold your breath during weight lifting. A recommended breathing pattern to prevent breath holding during weight lifting is to exhale while lifting the weight and inhale while lowering. Also, breathe through both your nose and mouth.

5. Although debate continues as to whether high-speed weight lifting is superior to slow-speed lifting in terms of strength gains, slow movements may reduce the risk of injury. Therefore, because slow movement during weight lifting certainly results in an increase in both muscle size and strength, it would be wise to take this approach.

6. Use light weights in the beginning so that the proper maneuver can be achieved in each exercise. This is particularly true when lifting free weights.

TRAINING TO IMPROVE STRENGTH VERSUS TRAINING TO IMPROVE ENDURANCE

Weight-training programs specifically designed to improve strength and programs designed to improve muscular endurance differ mainly in the number of repetitions (i.e., the number of lifts performed) and the amount of resistance (8). Note in Figure 5.8 that a weight-training program using low repetitions and high resistance results in the greatest strength gains, whereas a weight-training program using high repetitions and low resistance results in the greatest improvement in muscular endurance. However, it is important to appreciate that while low-repetition/high-resistance training appears to be the optimal training method to increase strength, this type of training improves muscular endurance as well. In contrast, although weight training using high repetition and low resistance improves endurance, this training method results in only small strength increases, particularly in less fit individuals.

TYPES OF WEIGHT-TRAINING PROGRAMS

Weight-training programs can be divided into three general categories classified by the type of muscle contraction involved: isotonic, isometric, and isokinetic.

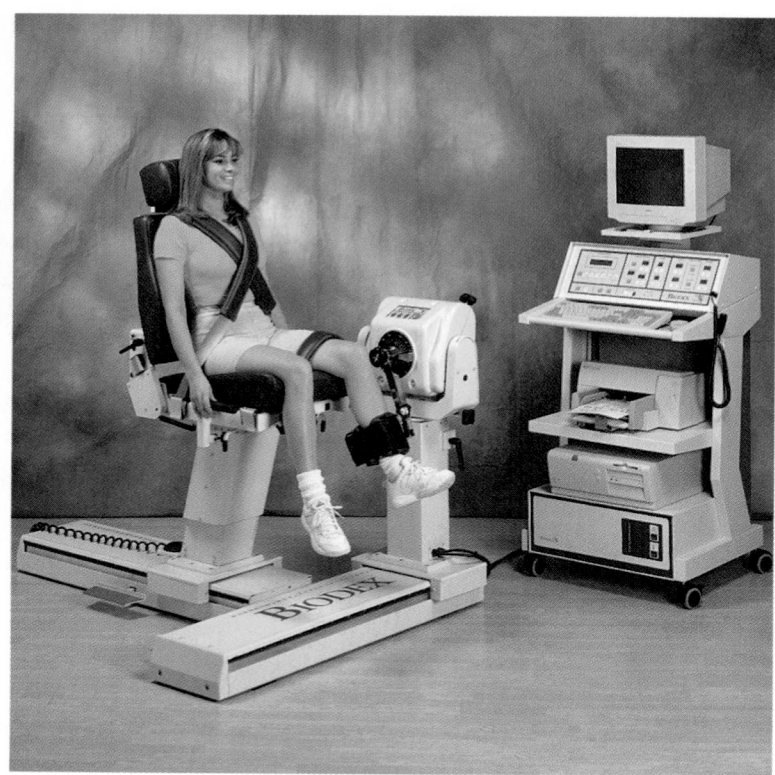

A commercially available isokinetic weight-training device.

ISOTONIC PROGRAMS Isotonic programs, like isotonic contractions, involve the concept of contracting a muscle against a movable load (usually a free weight or weights mounted by cables or chains to form a weight machine). Isotonic programs are very popular and are the most common type of weight-training program in use today.

ISOMETRIC PROGRAMS An isometric strength-training program is based on the concept of contracting a muscle at a fixed angle against an immovable object, using an isometric or static contraction. Interest in strength training increased dramatically during the 1950s with the finding that maximal strength could be increased by contracting a muscle for 6 seconds at two-thirds of maximal tension once per day for 5 days per week! Although subsequent studies suggested that these claims were exaggerated (7), it is generally agreed that isometric training can increase muscular strength and endurance.

valsalva maneuver   Breath holding during an intense muscle contraction; can reduce blood flow to the brain and cause dizziness and fainting.

Two important aspects of isometric training make it different from isotonic training. First, in isometric training, the development of strength and endurance is specific to the joint angle at which the muscle group is trained (9). Therefore, if isometric techniques are used, isometric contractions at several different joint angles are needed to gain strength and endurance throughout a full range of motion. In contrast, because isotonic contractions generally involve the full range of joint motion, strength is developed over the full movement pattern. Second, the static nature of isometric muscle contractions can lead to breath holding (called a **valsalva maneuver**), which can reduce blood flow to the brain and cause dizziness and fainting. In an individual at high risk for coronary disease, the maneuver could be extremely dangerous and should always be avoided. Remember: Continue to breathe during any type of isometric or isotonic contraction!

ISOKINETIC PROGRAMS Recall that isokinetic contractions are isotonic contractions performed at a constant speed (*isokinetic* refers to constant speed of movement). Isokinetic training is a relatively underutilized strength training method, so limited research exists to describe its strength benefits compared with those of isometric and isotonic programs. Isokinetic exercises require the use of machines that govern the speed of movement during muscle contraction. The first

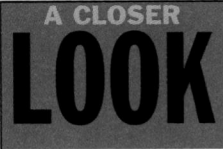

Plyometric Training Is Not for Everyone

You may have heard the term *plyometrics* used in reference to training for athletes. Athletes use this technique to develop explosive power. Plyometric training is performed by quickly stretching a muscle prior to initiating a maximal contraction. A common example is a simple vertical jump. You may have noticed that when you attempt to jump as high as possible, you almost always bend your knees quickly and "rebound" in order to maximize your jump height. You can certainly jump higher by using this "rebound" than by starting the jump with your knees already bent.

Plyometric training is based on the principle that stretching a muscle prior to contraction enables a greater force to be generated by the muscle. The most common method of plyometric training is called "drop jump-

ing"—dropping from a height and rebounding. (See the figure below.) This exercise requires the athlete to drop (not jump) to the ground from a platform or box, and then immediately jump. The drop prestretches the muscles, and the jump overloads the muscles with the ensuing concentric contraction. The exercise is more effective the shorter the time the feet are in contact with the ground. The amount of load placed on the muscles is determined in part by the height of the drop, which should be in the

range of 12–30 in. Drop jumping is a relatively high-impact form of training and should not be introduced until after an athlete has used lower-impact alternatives, such as two-footed jumping on the ground.

Because of the dynamic nature of plyometric training, there is great potential for injury to both muscles and joints. For a basic fitness program, there is no need to include a high-risk type of training when a low-risk activity will accomplish the same goal. This training technique is best reserved for athletes looking for a competitive edge and for rehabilitation programs that are closely supervised.

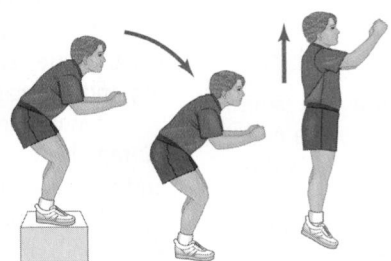

A drop jump.

isokinetic machines available were very expensive and were used primarily in clinical settings for injury rehabilitation. Recently, less expensive machines use a piston device (much like a shock absorber on a car) to limit the speed of movement throughout the range of the exercise. Today, these machines are found in fitness centers across the United States.

IN SUMMARY

- The overload principle states that a muscle will adapt only when it works against a workload that is greater than normal. The application of the overload principle to weight training is called progressive resistance exercise (PRE).
- The greatest strength gains are made with a training program using low repetitions and high resistance, whereas the greatest improvement in endurance is made using high repetitions and low resistance.
- Isotonic programs include exercises with moveable loads. Isometric training includes exercises in

which a muscle contracts at a fixed angle against an immovable object. Isokinetic exercises involve machines that govern speed of movement during muscle contraction.

Exercise Prescription for Weight Training: An Overview

We introduced the general concepts of the intensity, duration, and frequency of exercise required to improve physical fitness in Chapter 3. Although these same concepts apply to improving muscular strength and endurance via weight training, the terminology used to monitor the intensity and duration of weight training is unique. For example, the intensity of weight training is measured not by heart rate but by the number of "repetition maximums." Similarly, the duration of weight training is monitored not by time but by the number of sets performed. Let's discuss these two concepts briefly.

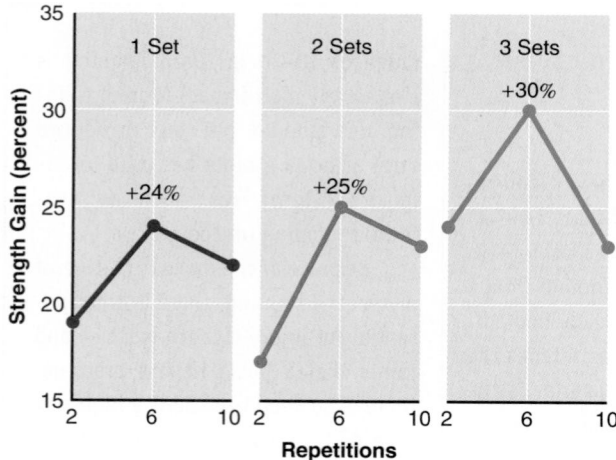

FIGURE 5.9
Strength gains from a resistance training program consisting of various sets and repetitions. All programs were performed 3 days a week for 12 weeks. Note that the greatest strength gains (+30% improvement) were obtained using 3 sets of 6 reps per set.

Source: Adapted from Fox, E., R. Bowers, and M. Foss, *Fox's Physiological Basis of Exercise and Sports.* Copyright 1998, McGraw-Hill.

The intensity of exercise in both isotonic and isokinetic weight-training programs is measured by the concept of the **repetition maximum (RM).** The RM is the maximal load that a muscle group can lift a specified number of times before tiring. For example, 6 RM is the maximal load that can be lifted six times. Therefore, the amount of weight lifted is greater when performing a low number of RMs than a high number of RMs; that is, the weight lifted while performing 4 RMs is greater than the weight lifted while performing 15 RMs.

The number of repetitions (reps) performed consecutively without resting is called a **set.** In the example of 6 RM, 1 set = 6 reps. Because the amount of rest required between sets will vary among individuals depending on how fit they are, the duration of weight training is measured by the number of sets performed, not by time.

Although disagreement exists as to the optimum number of reps and sets required to improve strength and endurance, some general guidelines can be provided. To improve strength, 3–5 sets of 6 RMs for each exercise are generally recommended. The concept of progressive resistance applied to a strength-training program involves increasing the amount of weight to be lifted a specific number of reps. For example, suppose that 3 sets of 6 RMs were selected as your exercise prescription for increasing strength. As the training progresses and you become stronger, the amount of weight lifted must be increased. A good rule of thumb is that once 8 reps can be performed, the load should be increased to a level at which 6 reps are again maximal. Figure 5.9 illustrates the relationship between strength improvement and various combinations of reps and sets. Note that in each strength-training program, 6 reps result in the greatest strength improvement. A key point in Figure 5.9 is that programs involving 3 sets result in the greatest strength gains. This is because the third set requires the greatest effort and thus is the greatest overload for the muscle. Although it may seem that adding a fourth set would elicit even greater gains, most studies suggest 4 or more sets results in overtraining and decreased benefits.

To improve muscular endurance, 4 to 6 sets of 18 to 20 reps for each exercise are recommended. Note that endurance could be improved by either increasing the number of reps progressively while maintaining the same load, or increasing the amount of weight while maintaining the same number of reps. The advantage of the latter program is that it would also improve muscular strength.

What role does training frequency play in the development of strength? Most research suggests that 2 to 3 days of exercise per week is optimal for strength gains (10). However, studies have shown that once the desired level of strength has been achieved, one high-intensity training session per week is sufficient to maintain the new level of strength. Finally, although limited research exists regarding the optimal frequency of training to improve muscular endurance, 3 to 5 days per week seem adequate (12).

☀ Starting and Maintaining a Weight-Training Program

You should begin your weight-training program with both short- and long-term goals. Identifying goals is an important means of maintaining interest and enthusiasm for weight training. A key point is to establish realistic short-term goals that can be reached in the first several weeks of training. Reaching these goals provides the motivation needed to continue training.

---

repetition maximum (RM) The measure of the intensity of exercise in both isotonic and isokinetic weight-training programs. The RM is the maximal load that a muscle group can lift a specified number of times before tiring. For example, 6 RM is the maximal load that can be lifted six times.
set The number of repetitions performed consecutively without resting.

TABLE 5.2
Guidelines and Precautions to Follow Prior to Beginning a Strength-Training Program

- Warm up before beginning a workout. This involves 5 to 10 minutes of movement (calisthenics) using all major muscle groups.
- Start slowly. The first several training sessions should involve limited exercises and light weight!
- Use the proper lifting technique, as shown in the Isotonic Strength-Training Exercises in this chapter. Improper technique can lead to injury.
- Follow all safety rules (see the section on safety concerns on p. 129).
- Always lift through the full range of motion. This not only develops strength throughout the full range of motion but also assists in maintaining flexibility.

DEVELOPING AN INDIVIDUALIZED EXERCISE PRESCRIPTION

An exercise prescription for strength training has three stages: the starter phase, the slow progression phase, and the maintenance phase.

STARTER PHASE   The primary objective of the starter phase is to build strength gradually without developing undue muscular soreness or injury. This can be accomplished by starting your weight-training program slowly—beginning with light weights, a high number of repetitions, and only 2 sets per exercise. The recommended frequency of training during this phase is twice per week. The duration of this phase varies from 1 to 3 weeks, depending on your initial strength fitness level. A sedentary person might spend 3 weeks in the starter phase, whereas a relatively well-trained person may only spend 1 to 2 weeks.

SLOW PROGRESSION PHASE   This phase may last 4 to 20 weeks depending on your initial strength level and your long-term strength goal. The transition from the starter phase to the slow progression phase involves three changes in the exercise prescription: increasing the frequency of training from 2 to 3 days per week; increasing the amount of weight lifted and decreasing the number of repetitions; and increasing the number of sets performed from 2 to 3 sets.

The objective of the slow progression phase is to gradually increase muscular strength until you reach your desired level. After reaching your strength goal, your long-term objective becomes to maintain this level of strength by entering the maintenance phase of the strength-training exercise prescription.

MAINTENANCE PHASE   After reaching your strength goals, the problem now becomes, How do I maintain this strength level? The bad news is that maintaining strength will require a lifelong weight-training effort. Strength is lost if you do not continue to exercise. The good news is that the effort required to maintain muscular strength is less than the initial effort needed to gain strength. Research has shown that as little as one workout per week is required to maintain strength. A sample exercise prescription incorporating all three training phases follows.

SAMPLE EXERCISE PRESCRIPTION FOR WEIGHT TRAINING

GETTING STARTED   Similar to training to improve cardiorespiratory fitness, the exercise prescription for improving muscular strength must be tailored to the individual. Before starting a program, keep in mind the guidelines and precautions presented in Table 5.2.

DETAILS OF THE PRESCRIPTION   Table 5.3 illustrates the stages of a suggested strength-training exercise prescription. As mentioned earlier, the durations of both the starter and slow progression phases will vary depending on your initial strength fitness level. When the strength goals of the program are reached, the maintenance phase begins. This period utilizes the same routine as used during the progression phase but may be done only once per week.

SAMPLE STRENGTH-TRAINING EXERCISES   The isotonic strength-training program contains 12 exercises that are designed to provide a whole body workout. Although specific machines are used in the following examples, barbells may be used for performing similar exercises. However, it is important to remember that safety and proper lifting technique are especially important when using barbells. Before beginning a program using barbells, it is a good idea to get advice from someone experienced with their use.

Follow the exercise routines described and illustrated in Exercises 5.1 through 5.12, and develop your program using the guidelines provided in Table 5.3. This selection of exercises is designed to provide a

TABLE 5.3
Suggested Isotonic Strength-Training Routine to Be Included in a Basic Fitness Program
The durations of the starter and slow progression phases will depend on your initial strength level.

Week No.	Phase	Frequency	Sets	Reps	Weight
1–3	Starter	2/week	2	15	15 RM
4–20	Slow progression	2–3/week	3	6	6 RM
20+	Maintenance	1–2/week	3	6	6 RM

TABLE 5.4
Priorities for Selection of Resistance Exercises to Economize Time

Selection Priority	Muscle Group	Exercises
Highest priority	Hips/Thighs	5.3-5.8-Lunges
	Chest	5.4-5.12-Push up
	Upper Back	5.7-Pull up, seated rowing
	Lower Back	5.6
	Biceps	5.1
	Abdominals	5.2-Curl-Ups
Moderate priority	Lower legs	Toe Raises
	Triceps	5.11
	Lateral Abdominals	5.10-5.9
	Hamstrings	5.5
	Shoulders	5.9

comprehensive strength-training program that focuses on the major muscle groups. Although many more exercises exist, some of them use the same muscle groups as those covered here. Be aware of which muscle groups are involved in an exercise in order to avoid overtraining any one muscle group (Figure 5.2). Note that it is not necessary to perform all 12 exercises in one workout session; you can perform half of the exercises on one day and the remaining exercises on an alternate day.

In order to help economize your time in the weight room, Table 5.4 gives you an idea of how you might prioritize exercises. Use Laboratory 5.1 on p. 149 to keep a record of your training progress. Remember: Maintenance and review of your training progress will help motivate you to continue your strength-training program!

☀ IN SUMMARY

- In developing a strength-training program, divide it into three phases: a starter phase, a slow progression phase, and a maintenance phase.

☀ Strength Training: How the Body Adapts

What physiological changes occur as a result of strength training? How quickly can muscular strength be gained? Do men and women differ in their responses to weight-training programs? Let's address each of these questions separately.

PHYSIOLOGICAL CHANGES DUE TO WEIGHT TRAINING

It should now be clear that programs designed to improve muscular strength can do so only by increasing muscular size and/or by increasing the number of muscle fibers recruited. In fact, both these factors are altered by strength training (8). Research has shown that strength-training programs increase muscular strength by first altering fiber recruitment patterns due to changes in the nervous system and then by increasing muscle size (Figure 5.10).

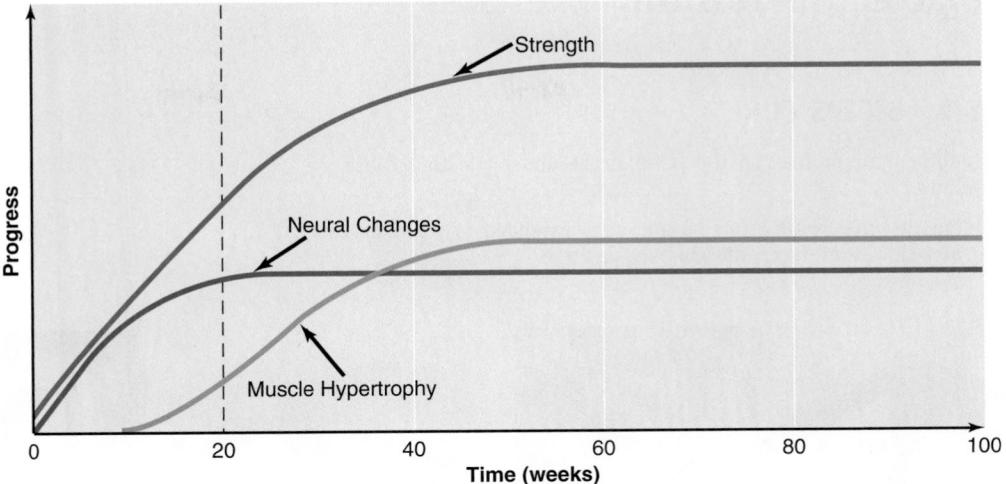

FIGURE 5.10
The relative roles of the nervous system and muscular adaptation in strength development. Strength training increases muscular strength first through changes in the nervous system and then by increasing muscle size.

Source: Whitmore, J. H., and D. L. Costill, *Physiology of Sport and Exercise,* Champaign, IL: Human Kinetics, 2004.

How do muscles increase in size? Muscle size is increased primarily through an increase in fiber size, called **hypertrophy** (8). Most research has shown that strength training has little effect on the formation of new muscle fibers, a process called **hyperplasia.** To date, the role that hyperplasia plays in the increase in muscle size due to strength training remains controversial. Regardless, the increase in muscle size due to strength training depends on diet, the muscle fiber type (fast fibers may hypertrophy more than slow fibers), blood levels of testosterone, and the type of training program.

Although strength training does not result in significant improvements in cardiorespiratory fitness (11), a regular weight-training program can provide positive changes in both body composition and flexibility. For most men and women, rigorous weight training results in an increase in muscle mass and a loss of body fat, the end result being a decrease in the percent of body fat.

If weight-training exercises are performed over the full range of motion possible at a joint, flexibility can be improved (7). In fact, many diligent weight lifters have excellent flexibility. Therefore, the notion of weight lifters becoming muscle-bound and losing flexibility is generally incorrect.

RATE OF STRENGTH IMPROVEMENT WITH WEIGHT TRAINING

How rapidly does strength improvement occur? The answer depends on your initial strength level. Strength gains occur rapidly in untrained people, whereas gains are more gradual in individuals with relatively higher strength levels (Figure 5.11 on p. 144). Indeed, an exciting point about weight training for a novice lifter is that strength gains occur very quickly (12). These rapid strength gains provide motivation to continue a regular weight-training program.

GENDER DIFFERENCES IN RESPONSE TO WEIGHT TRAINING

In terms of absolute strength, men tend to be stronger than women because men generally have a greater muscle mass. The difference is greater in the upper body, where men are approximately 50% stronger than women; men are only 30% stronger than women in the lower body.

Do men and women differ in their responses to weight-training programs? The answer is "no" (13). On a percentage basis, women gain strength as rapidly as men during the first 12 weeks of a strength-training

Text continues on p. 144

hypertrophy   An increase in muscle fiber size.
hyperplasia   An increase in the number of muscle fibers.

Isotonic Strength-Training Exercises

EXERCISE 5.1   BICEPS CURL

Purpose: To strengthen the muscles in the front of the upper arm that cause flexion at the elbow.

Movement: Holding the grips with palms up and arms extended (a), curl up as far as possible (b) and slowly return to the starting position.

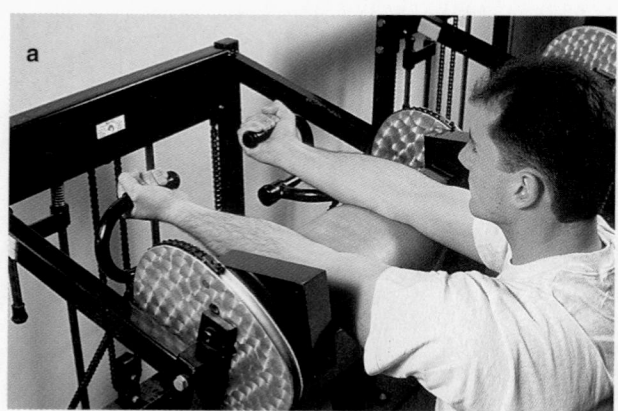 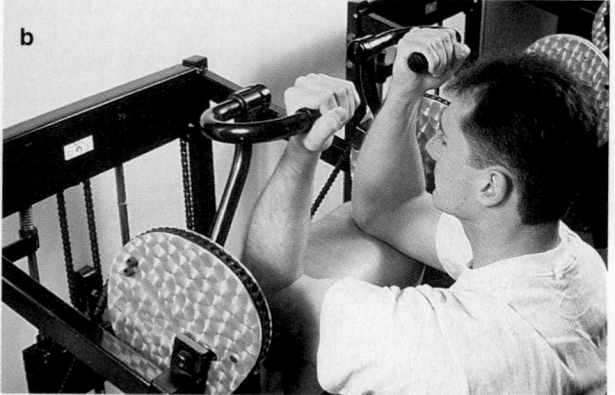

EXERCISE 5.2   ABDOMINAL CURL

Purpose: To strengthen the abdominal muscles.

Movement: Place hands on the abdomen (a) and curl forward, bringing the chest toward the knees (b). Slowly return to the upright position.

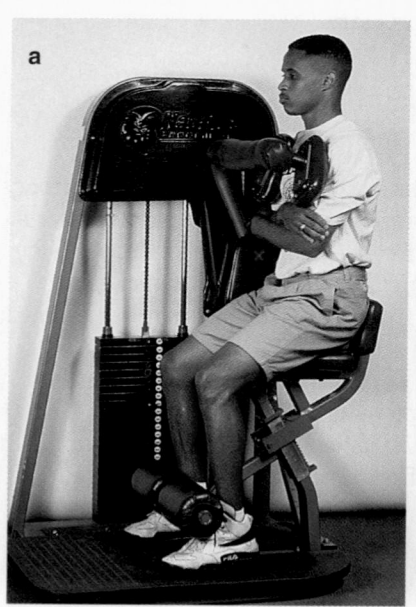 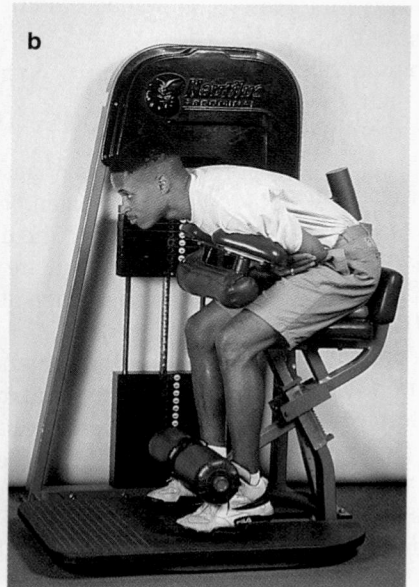

Isotonic Strength-Training Exercises

EXERCISE 5.3   LEG EXTENSION

Purpose: To strengthen the muscles in the front of the upper leg.

Movement: Sitting in a nearly upright position, grasp the handles on the side of the machine (a). Extend the legs until they are completely straight (b) and then slowly return to the starting position.

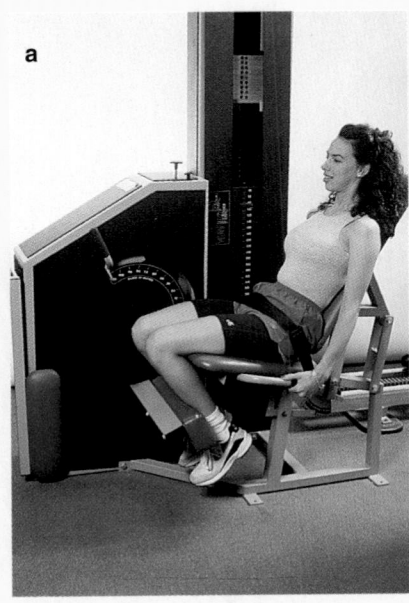
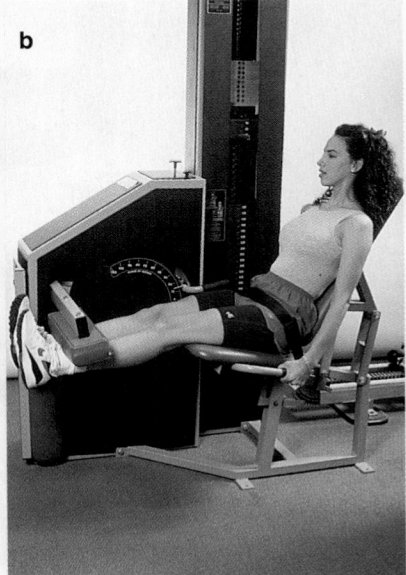

EXERCISE 5.4   BENCH PRESS

Purpose: To strengthen the muscles in the chest, the front of the shoulders, and the back of the upper arm.

Movement: Lie on the bench with the bench press bar above the chest and the feet flat on the foot rest (a). Grasp the bar handles and press upward until the arms are completely extended (b). Return slowly to the original position. **Caution:** Do not arch the back while performing this exercise.

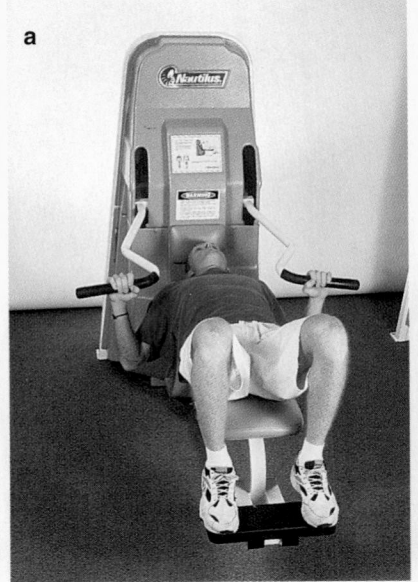
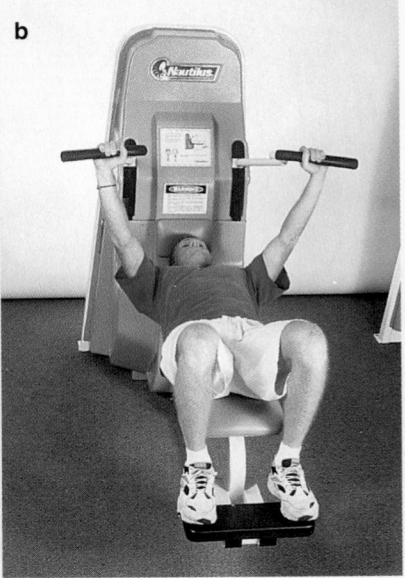

Isotonic Strength-Training Exercises

EXERCISE 5.5   LEG CURL

Purpose: To strengthen the muscles on the back of the upper leg and buttocks.

Movement: Lying on the left side, place the back of the feet over the padded bar (a). Curl the legs to at least a 90° angle (b) and then slowly return to the original position.

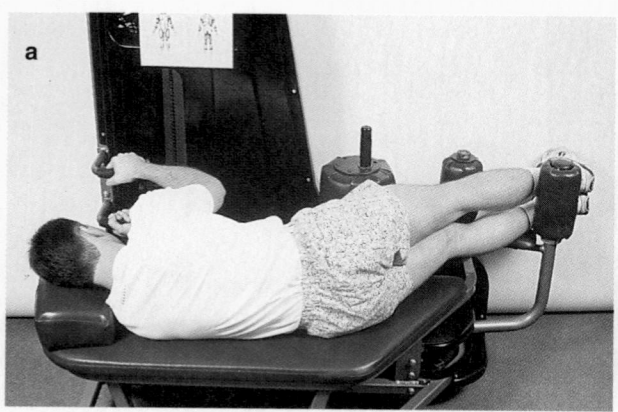
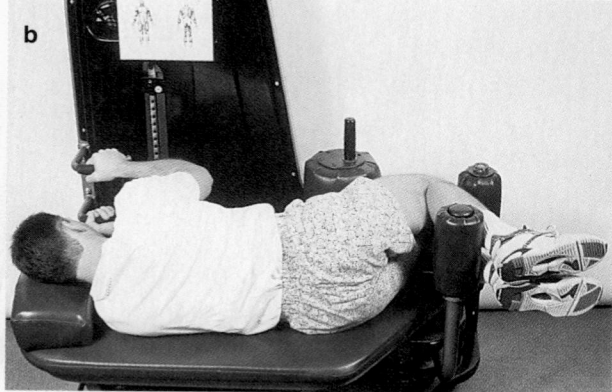

EXERCISE 5.6   LOWER BACK EXTENSION

Purpose: To strengthen the muscles of the lower back and buttocks.

Movement: Position the thighs and upper back against the padded bars (a). Buckle the strap around the thighs. Slowly press backward against the padded bar until the back is fully extended (b). Slowly return to the original position.

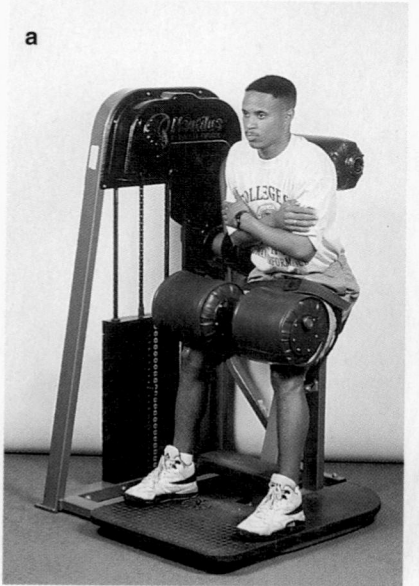
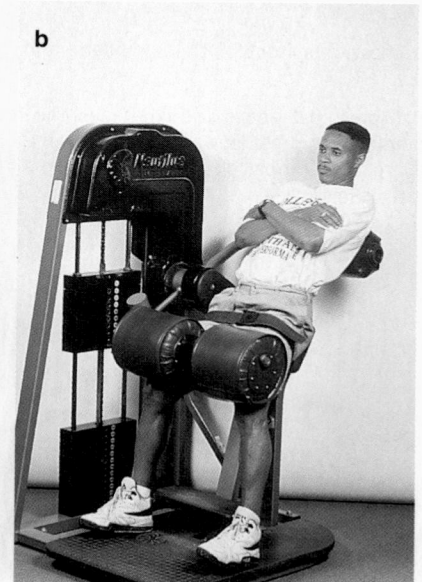

Isotonic Strength-Training Exercises

EXERCISE 5.7   UPPER BACK

Purpose: To strengthen the muscles of the upper back.

Movement: Sit in the machine with elbows bent and the backs of the arms resting against the padded bars (a). Press the arms back as far as possible, drawing the shoulder blades together (b). Slowly return to the original position.

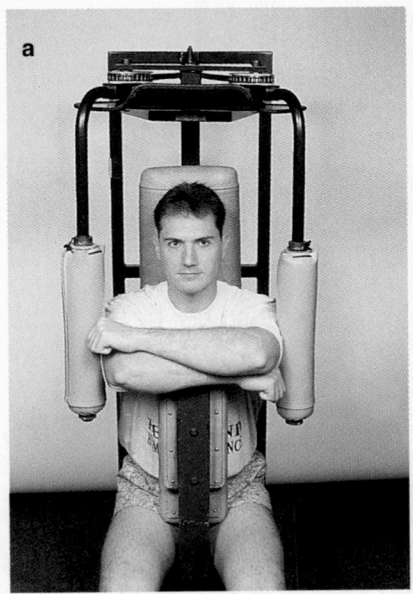
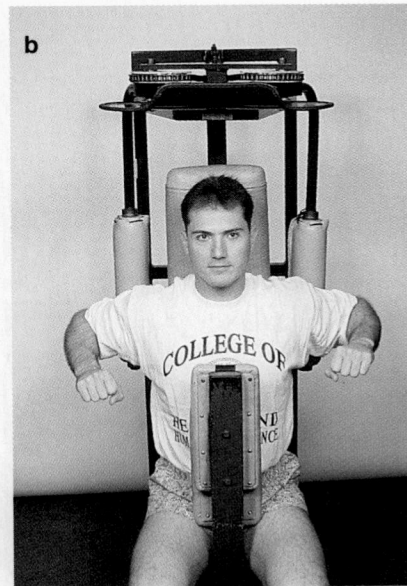

EXERCISE 5.8   HIP AND BACK

Purpose: To strengthen the muscles of the hip and lower back.

Movement: Lying on the left side, grasp the handles at both sides for stability. Place the back of the knees against the padded bars (a). Press the legs back until fully extended (b). Slowly return to the original position.

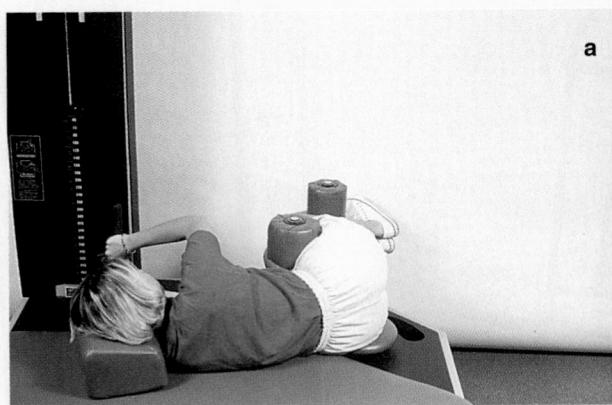
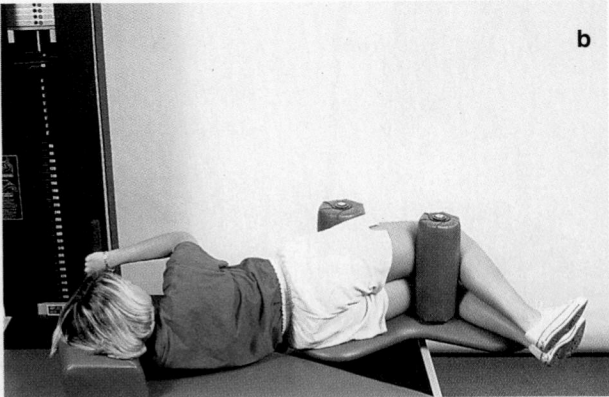

Isotonic Strength Training Exercises

EXERCISE 5.9 PULLOVER

Purpose: To strengthen the muscles of the chest, shoulder, and side of the trunk.

Movement: Sit with elbows against the padded end of the movement arm and grasp the bar behind your head (a). Press forward and down with the arms, pulling the bar overhead and down to the abdomen (b). Slowly return to the original position.

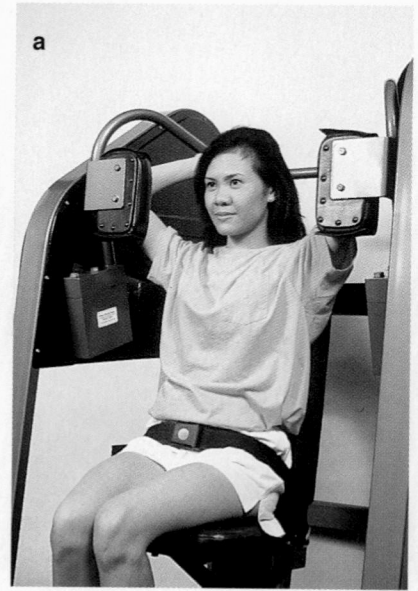
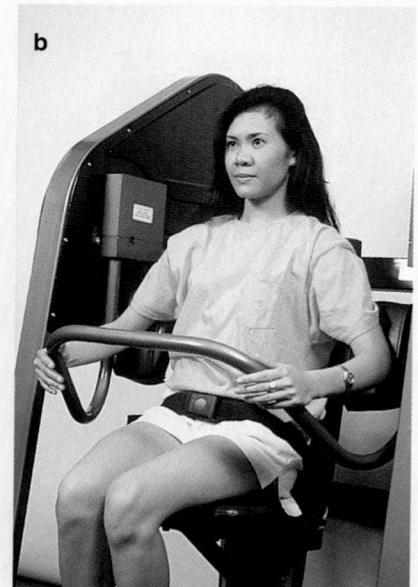

EXERCISE 5.10 TORSO TWIST

Purpose: To strengthen the muscles on the sides of the abdomen.

Movement: Sitting upright with the elbows behind the padded bars, twist the torso as far as possible to one side (a). Slowly return to the original position and repeat to the other side (b).

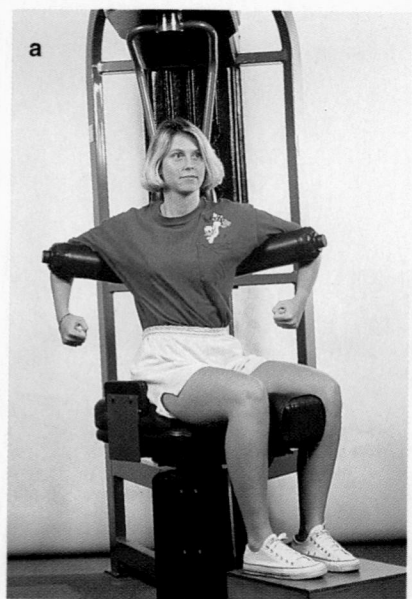
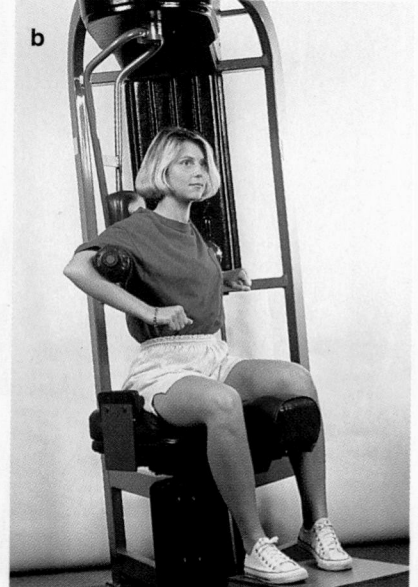

Isotonic Strength Training Exercises

EXERCISE 5.11 TRICEPS EXTENSION

Purpose: To strengthen the muscles on the back of the upper arm.

Movement: Sit upright with elbows bent (a). With the little-finger side of the hand against the pad, fully extend the arms (b) and then slowly return to the original position.

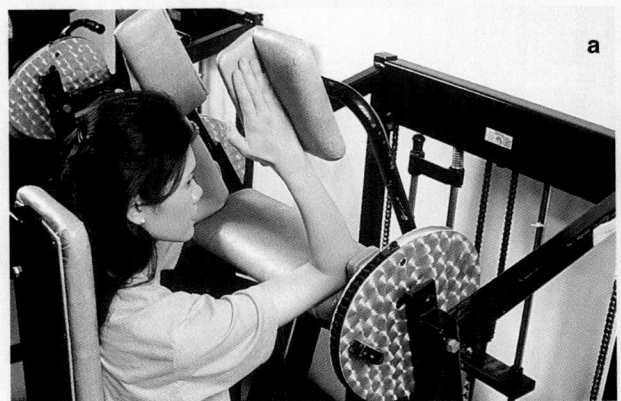
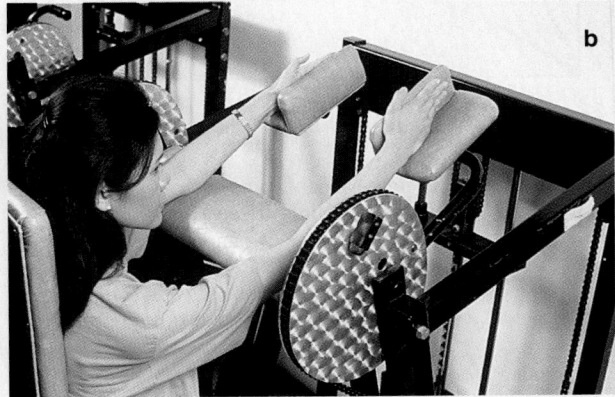

EXERCISE 5.12 CHEST PRESS

Purpose: To strengthen the muscles of the chest and shoulder.

Movement: With the elbows bent at a 90° angle and the forearms against the pads (a), press the arms forward as far as possible, leading with the elbows (b). Slowly return to the original position.

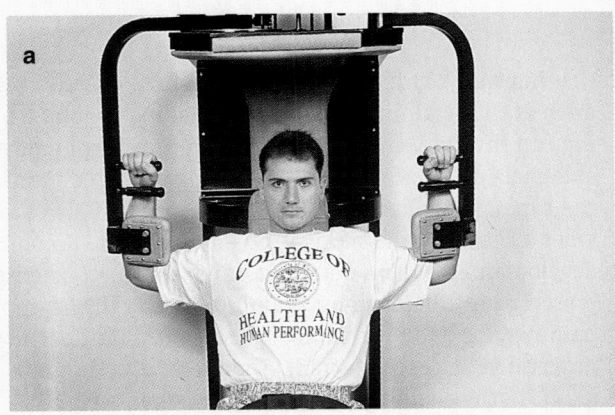
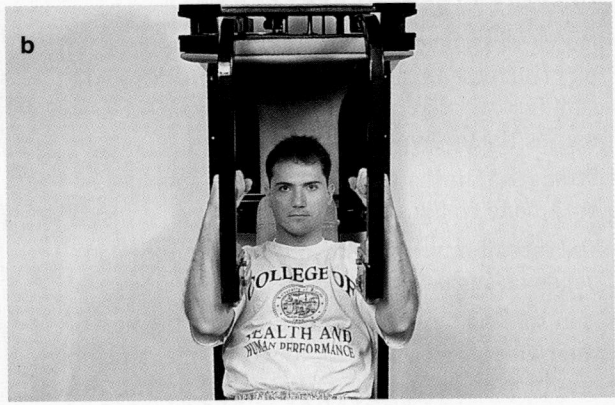

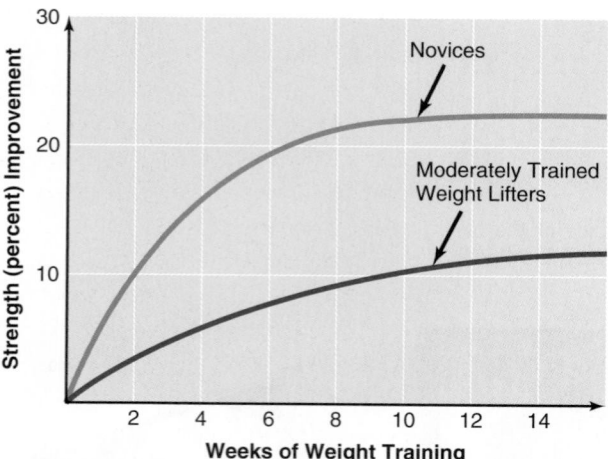

FIGURE 5.11
Time course of strength improvement in novice weight lifters versus moderately well-trained weight lifters. The rate of improvement and the total percent strength improvement is greater in novices compared with moderately trained weight lifters. This occurs because moderately trained weight lifters began the weight-training program with higher initial strength levels.

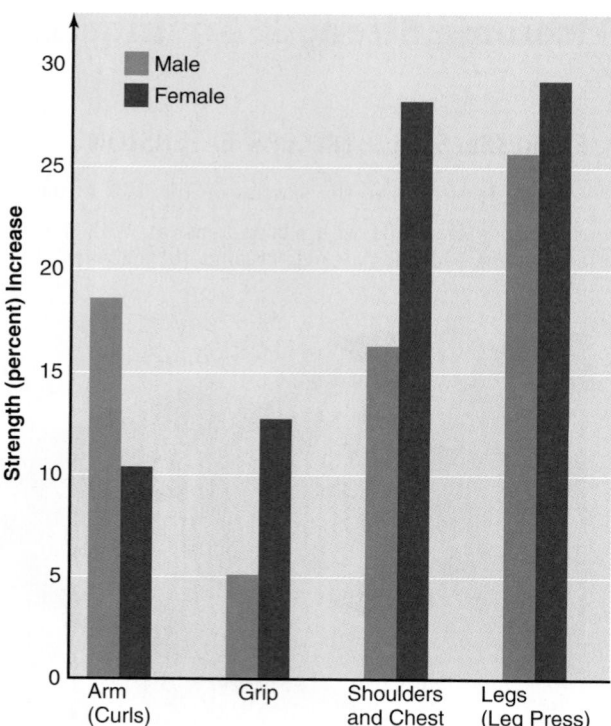

FIGURE 5.12
A comparison of strength gains for men and women. In relation to beginning strength levels, the increase in strength for women over the first 12 weeks of training is equal to or greater than that seen in men for most muscle groups.
Source: Adapted from Whitmore, J. Body composition and strength development, *Journal of Physical Education Research* 46(1):38–40, 1975. Reprinted by permission of author.

program (Figure 5.12). However, as a result of long-term weight training, men generally exhibit a greater increase in muscle size than do women. This occurs because men have 20 to 30 times more testosterone (a male sex hormone that builds muscles) than do women.

☀ IN SUMMARY

- Muscle size increases primarily because of hypertrophy (increase in size) of muscle fibers. Strength training can also promote the formation of new muscle fibers (hyperplasia).
- Strength training promotes positive changes in both body composition and flexibility.
- The rate of improvement in weight training depends on initial strength level.
- Men tend to be stronger than women because of their greater muscle mass. Testosterone, a predominantly male hormone, is responsible for this difference.
- Women gain strength as fast as men early in a weight-training program.

☀ Motivation to Maintain Strength Fitness

The problems associated with starting and maintaining a weight-training program are similar to those associated with cardiorespiratory training. You must find time to train regularly, so good time management is critical.

Another key feature of any successful exercise program is that training must be fun. Making weight training fun involves several elements. First, find an enjoyable place to work out. Locate a facility that contains the type of weights that you want to use and also provides a pleasant and motivating environment. Second, develop an enjoyable weight-training routine (exercise prescription). Designing a training routine that is too hard may be good for improving strength but does not increase your desire to train. Therefore, design a program that is challenging, but fun. Further, weight training is more enjoyable if you have a regular training partner. Select a friend who is highly motivated to exercise and has strength abilities similar to yours.

Although the benefits of weight training are numerous, recent studies have shown that improved appearance, elevated self-esteem, and the overall feeling of well-being that result from regular weight training are the most important factors in motivating people to continue to train regularly. Looking your best and feeling good about yourself are excellent reasons to maintain a regular weight-training program.

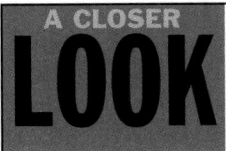

Frequently Asked Questions About Weight Training

How much rest is necessary between training sessions?

Getting the correct amount of rest is as important as doing the proper exercises! Weight training depletes energy stores and damages muscle fibers. With the proper rest, water intake, and nutrition, the muscles grow stronger by replenishing and repairing themselves. If you do not get the proper rest, your muscles will not reach their potential. Depending on the muscle groups used and the intensity and volume of training, you may need 24 to 72 hours to recover and allow muscles to repair themselves. Also, you should try to get 6 to 8 hours of sleep per night.

What is the best kind of equipment for weight training?

No particular kind of resistance-training equipment is "better" than any other. All exercise accessories have their advantages and disadvantages. As discussed in this chapter, equipment should be safe and provide the ability to overload the muscle groups you want to train. Remember, the best piece of equipment is the one that you use regularly!

Should I train a muscle if it's sore?

No. If your legs are sore from squatting and you want to work an upper-body muscle group, that's okay. But if your legs are still sore from the last leg workout, take at least another day off before working the same muscle group again.

Will doing aerobics retard muscle growth?

If you're training for maximum muscle mass, aerobics will slow down muscle growth. However, if you are developing an all-purpose fitness program, both aerobics and resistance training are necessary.

Should I use a lifting belt?

Most people don't need to use a lifting belt. Using a belt all the time actually weakens the abdominals and the lower back by making them work less. Weight belts are recommended for max squats or heavy lifting above the head.

I have reached a plateau in strength gains. What can I do?

First, you could be overtraining. Try taking a week off, and when you come back take it easy for a few weeks while reevaluating your workout. Second, make sure your caloric intake is adequate and rich in nutrients. Don't overeat—doing so will not build muscle. Third, if you have been using the same routine/exercise for every workout, change your routine and use different muscle groups. Remember, the muscles will only respond if overloaded. Finally, you may be hitting your genetic limits. Taking a break, eating more, and changing your workout should help when you hit a strength plateau.

Should I use free weights or machines?

This argument has been ongoing for years. Free weights indirectly work more muscles (those needed for stability and balance), and they allow a larger range of motion. Machines isolate muscles better and are safer since you don't need a spotter. Most people who train use both, and many others use whatever type is available. But realize that a lot can be accomplished by doing exercises with neither, such as push-ups, pull-ups, one-legged squats, lunges, and so on. Each exercise or piece of equipment works the muscles at a slightly different angle. Experiment to find what works for you. For most people, ensuring that the workout is safe should be the prime concern.

What exercises should I avoid?

Any exercise can cause an injury when done improperly. Again, safety is a primary concern, so go slow, don't bounce, and don't cheat. If you feel any pain during any exercise, STOP!

I have heard that creatine supplementation is safe and effective in building muscle. Is this true?

Creatine phosphate is a molecule used in the body for quick conversion of chemical energy to energy for muscle contraction. Some athletes have used creatine supplementation to replenish energy for the muscle when they do repetitive bouts of high-intensity exercise. Bodybuilders have used creatine under the assumption that it will build muscle. The best evidence suggests that creatine, itself, does not build muscle. It is likely, however, that creatine does prolong intense workouts and this may allow additional overloading of muscle and the subsequent strength gains that many research studies have reported. The evidence for this remains controversial (15). What is not known about creatine is the long-term health effects. In addition, there have been many reports of unintended chemicals in some brands. For these reasons and the fact that there is no benefit for the normal fitness enthusiast, do not take supplements such as creatine because the risks are too great.

Will unexercised muscle turn into fat?

No! Muscle and fat are different types of tissue. In any given area of the body, both muscle mass and fat stores can get either smaller or larger. However, neither one is converted to the other. Fat is gained with increases in caloric intake and/or a reduction in caloric expenditure. Muscle mass can be increased with resistance training.

I don't want to look like a bodybuilder. Should I still lift weights?

YES! For most people, adding muscle is very difficult. Hard work, eating right, and having the right genetics are all needed to get the bodybuilder look. It also takes years, and most often a lot of steroids, to put on the kind of mass that you see in magazines. If you find yourself getting larger muscles than you'd like, you can stop training and they will shrink due to lack of work.

Summary

1. The importance of training to improve strength and endurance is evident from the fact that strength training can reduce low back pain, reduce the incidence of exercise-related injuries, decrease the incidence of osteoporosis, and aid in maintenance of functional capacity, which normally decreases with age.

2. Muscular strength is defined as the ability of a muscle to generate maximal force (Chapter 1). In simple terms, this refers to the amount of weight that an individual can lift during one maximal effort. In contrast, muscular endurance is defined as the ability of a muscle to generate force over and over again. In general, increasing muscular strength by exercise training will increase muscular endurance as well. In contrast, training aimed at improving muscular endurance does not always result in significant improvements in muscular strength.

3. Skeletal muscle is composed of a collection of long thin cells (fibers). Muscles are attached to bone by thick connective tissue (tendons). Therefore, muscle contraction results in the tendons pulling on bone, thereby causing movement.

4. Muscle contraction is regulated by signals coming from motor nerves. Motor nerves originate in the spinal cord and send nerve fibers to individual muscles throughout the body. The motor nerve and all of the muscle fibers it controls is called a *motor unit.*

5. Isotonic or dynamic contractions are contractions that result in movement of a body part. Isometric contractions involve the development of force but result in no movement of body parts. Concentric contractions are isotonic muscle contractions involving muscle shortening. In contrast, eccentric contractions (negative contractions) are defined as isotonic contractions in which the muscle exerts force while the muscle lengthens.

6. Human skeletal muscle can be classified into three major fiber types: slow-twitch, fast-twitch, and intermediate fibers. Slow-twitch fibers shorten slowly but are highly fatigue resistant. Fast-twitch fibers shorten rapidly but fatigue rapidly. Intermediate fibers possess a combination of the characteristics of fast- and slow-twitch fibers.

7. The process of involving more muscle fibers to produce increased muscular force is called fiber recruitment.

8. The percentages of slow-, intermediate, and fast-twitch fibers vary among individuals. Research by sports scientists has shown that a relationship exists between muscle fiber type and success in athletics. For example, champion endurance athletes (e.g., marathon runners) have a high percentage of slow-twitch fibers.

9. Two primary physiological factors determine the amount of force that can be generated by a muscle: the size of the muscle and the neural influences (i.e., number of fibers recruited).

10. Muscle size is increased primarily because of an increase in fiber size (hypertrophy). Further, recent research has shown that strength training can also promote the formation of new muscle fibers (hyperplasia).

11. The overload principle states that a muscle will increase in strength and/or endurance only when it works against a workload that is greater than normal.

12. The concept of progressive resistance exercise (PRE) is the application of the overload principle to strength and endurance exercise programs.

13. A weight-training program using low repetitions/high resistance results in the greatest strength gains, whereas a weight-training program using high repetitions/low resistance results in the greatest improvement in muscular endurance.

14. Isotonic programs, like an isotonic contraction, involve the concept of contracting a muscle against a movable load (usually a free weight or weights mounted by cables or chains to form a weight machine). An isometric strength-training program is based on the concept of contracting a muscle(s) at a fixed angle against an immovable object (isometric or static contraction). Isokinetic exercises require the use of machines that govern the speed of movement during muscle contraction throughout the range of motion.

15. To begin a strength-training program, divide the program into three phases: starter phase—2 to 3 weeks with 2 workouts per week using 2 sets at 15 RM; slow progression phase—20 weeks with 2 to 3 workouts per week using 3 sets at 6 RM; and maintenance phase—continues for life with 1 workout per week using 3 sets at 6 RM.

Study Questions

1. Define the following terms:
   anabolic steroid
   hyperplasia
   hypertrophy
   motor unit
   progressive resistance exercise
   static contraction
   valsalva maneuver

2. List at least three reasons why training for strength and endurance is important.

3. List and discuss the characteristics of slow-twitch, fast-twitch, and intermediate skeletal muscle fibers.

4. Discuss the pattern of muscle fiber recruitment with increasing intensities of contraction.

5. Discuss the relationship of muscle fiber type to success in various types of athletic events.

6. What factors determine muscle strength?

7. What are some of the consequences of steroid abuse?

8. What physiological changes occur as a result of strength training?

9. Compare and contrast the overload principle and progressive resistance exercise.

10. Discuss the concept of specificity of training.

11. Compare and contrast the differences in training to increase strength versus training to increase endurance.

12. Define the concept of repetition maximum.

13. List the phases of a strength and endurance training program and discuss how they differ.

14. Distinguish between *concentric* and *eccentric* contractions.

15. Describe each of the following types of muscle contraction: isokinetic, isometric, and isotonic.

Suggested Reading

American College of Sports Medicine, American Dietetic Association, and Dietitians of Canada. Joint Position Statement: Nutrition and athletic performance. *Medicine and Science in Sports and Exercise* 32:2130–2145, 2000.

American College of Sports Medicine. The recommended quantity and quality of exercise for developing and maintaining cardiorespiratory and muscular fitness, and flexibility in healthy adults. *Medicine and Science in Sports and Exercise* 30:975–991, 1998.

Blair, S. N., M. J. LaMonte, M. Z. Nichaman. The evolution of physical activity recommendations: How much is enough? *American Journal of Clinical Nutrition* 79(5):913S–920S, 2004.

Fleck, S. J., and W. J. Kraemer. *Designing Resistance Training Programs*. Champaign, IL: Human Kinetics, 1997.

Howley, E. Type of activity: Resistance, aerobic and leisure versus occupational physical activity. *Medicine and Science in Sports and Exercise* 33(6):S364–S369, 2001.

Komi, P. *Strength and Power in Sport*. Oxford: Blackwell Publishers, 2002.

Kraemer, W. J., N. A. Ratamess, and D. N. French. Resistance training for health and performance. *Current Sports Medicine Report* 1(3):165–171, 2002.

Lemon, P. W., J. M. Berardi, and E. E. Noreen. The role of protein and amino acid supplements in the athlete's diet: Does type or timing of ingestion matter? *Current Sports Medicine Report* 1(4):214–121, 2002.

Phillips, S. M. (2002). Assessment of protein status in athletes. In: J. A. Driskell and I. Wolinsky (eds.) *Nutritional Assessment of Athletes*. Boca Raton, FL: CRC Press, pp. 283–316.

Powers, S., and E. Howley. *Exercise Physiology: Theory and Application to Fitness and Performance*, 4th ed. Dubuque, IA: McGraw-Hill, 2003.

Sandler, D. *Weight Training Fundamentals*. Champaign, IL: Human Kinetics, 2003.

Spriet, L. L., and M. J. Gibala. Nutritional strategies to influence adaptations to training. *Journal of Sports Science* 22(1):127–141, 2004.

For links to the web sites below visit The Total Fitness and Wellness Website at www.aw-bc.com/powers.

ACSM.org

Comprehensive Web site providing information, articles, equipment recommendations, how-to articles, books and position statements about all aspects of health and fitness.

About.com

Provides information about many aspects of fitness, and health benefits of exercise, and wellness.

Women Fitness

Provides basic information and programs, current articles, and exercises for beginner level strength training.

HealthAtoZ

Shows you techniques, tips, and news to make the most out of your strength training.

WebMD.com

General information about exercise, fitness, wellness. Great articles, instructional information, and updates.

Meriter Fitness

Discusses injury prevention and treatment, weight training, flexibility, exercise prescriptions, and more.

Muscle Physiology

Includes in-depth discussions of how muscle works as well as recent research articles from a world-renowned muscle physiology lab.

References

1. Mannion, A. F., A. Junge, S. Taimela, M. Muntener, K. Lorenzo, and J. Dvorak. Active therapy for chronic low back pain, Part 3. Factors influencing self-rated disability and its change following therapy. *Spine* 26(8):920–929, 2001.

2. Buckwalter J. A. Sports, joint injury, and posttraumatic osteoarthritis. *Journal of Orthopedics Sport and Physical Therapy* 33(10):578–588, 2003.

3. Spirduso, W. W., and D. L. Cronin. Exercise dose-response effects on quality of life and independent living in older adults. *Medicine and Science in Sports and Exercise* 33(6): S598–S608, 2001.

4. Seguin, R., and M. E. Nelson. The benefits of strength training for older adults. *American Journal of Preventive Medicine* 25(3 Suppl 2):141–149, 2003.

5. Dunn, A. L., M. H. Trivedi, and H. A. O'Neal. Physical activity dose-response effects on outcomes of depression and anxiety. *Medicine and Science in Sports and Exercise* 33(6):S587–S597, 2001.

6. Pette, D. Perspectives: Plasticity of mammalian skeletal muscle. *Journal of Applied Physiology* 90(3):1119–1124, 2001.

7. Kraemer, W. L., N. D. Duncan, and J. S. Volek. Resistance training and elite athletes: Adaptations and program considerations. *Journal of Orthopedic Sports and Physical Therapy* 28(2):110–119, 1998.

8. Fleck, S. J., and W. J. Kraemer. *Designing Resistance Training Programs.* Champaign, IL: Human Kinetics, 2004.

9. Kitai, T. A. Specificity of joint angle in isometric training. *European Journal of Applied Physiology* 58:744, 1989.

10. Powers, S., and E. Howley. *Exercise Physiology: Theory and Application to Fitness and Performance,* 4th ed. Dubuque, IA: McGraw-Hill, 2003.

11. Hakkinen, K., M. Alen, W. J. Kraemer, E. Gorostiaga, M. Izquierdo, H. Rusko, J. Mikkola, A. Hakkinen, H., Valkeinen, E. Kaarakainen, S. Romu, V. Erola, J. Ahtiainen, and L. Paavolainen. Neuromuscular adaptations during concurrent strength and endurance training versus strength training. *European Journal of Applied Physiology* 89(1):42–52, 2003.

12. Duchateau, J., and R. M. Enoka. Neural adaptations with chronic activity patterns in able-bodied humans. *American Journal of Physical Medicine Rehabilitation.* 81(11 Suppl):S17–27, 2002.

13. Shephard, R. J. Exercise and training in women, Part 1: Influence of gender on exercise and training responses. *Canadian Journal of Applied Physiology* 25(1):19–34, 2000.

14. Winett, R. A., and R. N. Carpinelli. Potential health-related benefits of resistance training. *Preventive Medicine* 33(5):503–513, 2001.

15. Spriet, L. L., and M. J. Gibala. Nutritional strategies to influence adaptations to training. *Journal of Sports Science* 22(1):127–141, 2004.

16. American College of Sports Medicine, American Dietetic Association, and Dietitians of Canada. Joint Position Statement: Nutrition and athletic performance. *Medicine and Science in Sports Exercise* 32:2130–2145, 2000.

Strength-Training Log

NAME _____ DATE _____

The purpose of this log is to provide a record of progress in building strength in the upper and lower body.

DIRECTIONS

Record the date, number of sets, reps, and the weight for each of the exercises listed in the left column.

St/RP/Wt = Sets/Reps/Weights
Example: 2/6/80 = 2 sets of 6 reps each with 80 lbs.

Date							
Exercise	St/Rp/Wt	St/Rp/Wt	St/Rp/Wt	St/Rp/Wt	St/Rp/Wt	St/Rp/Wt	St/Rp/Wt
Biceps curl							
Abdominal curl							
Leg extension							
Bench press							
Leg curl							
Lower back extension							
Upper back							
Hip and back							
Pullover							
Torso twist							
Triceps extension							
Chest press							

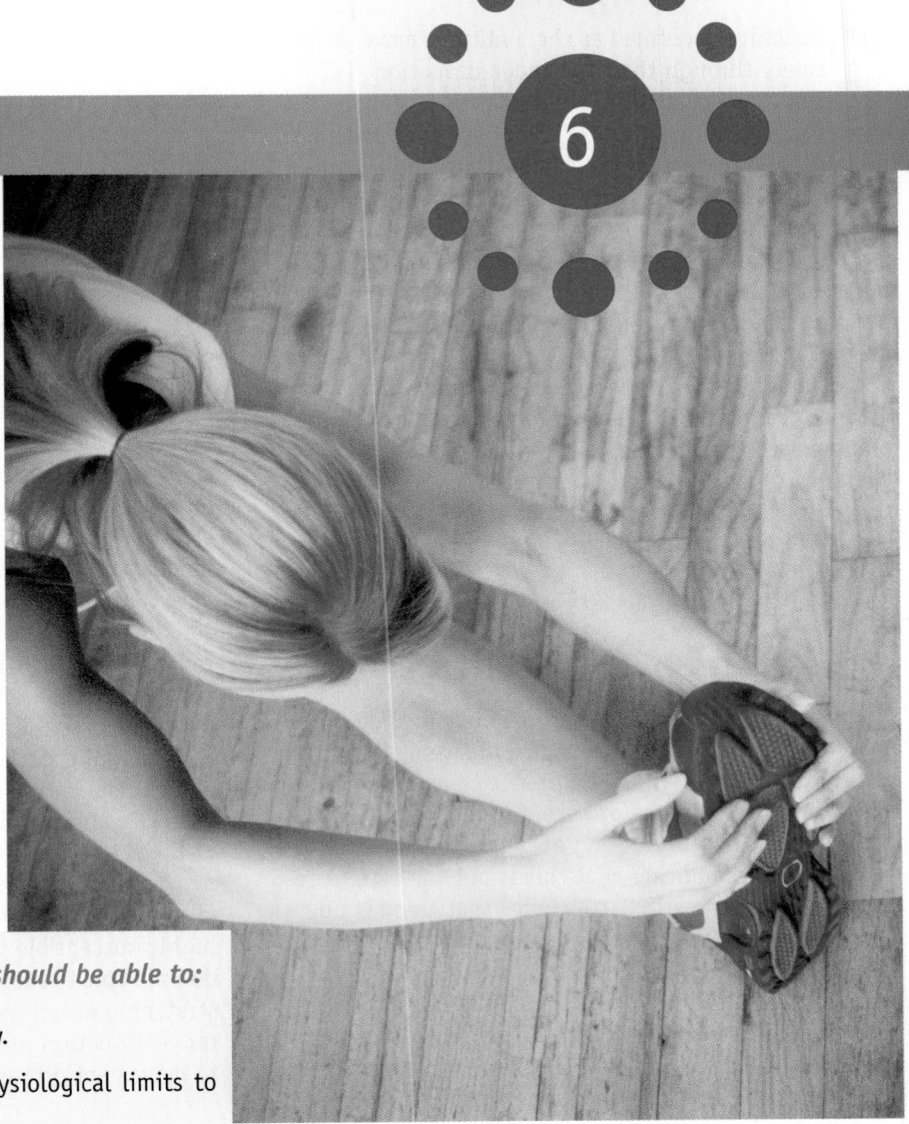

After studying this chapter, you should be able to:

1. Discuss the value of flexibility.

2. Identify the structural and physiological limits to flexibility.

3. Discuss the stretch reflex.

4. Describe the three categories of stretching techniques.

5. Design a flexibility exercise program.

Improving Flexibility

Flexibility is defined as the ability to move joints freely through their full range of motion. The full range of motion is determined in part by the shapes and positions of the bones that make up the joint, and in part by the composition and arrangement of muscles and tendons around the joint. For example, movement of the elbow (a hinge-type joint) is not limited solely by the arrangement of the bones themselves, because the soft connective tissues surrounding the joint also impose major limitations on the range of movement (1, 2).

Although flexibility varies among individuals because of differences in body structure, it is important to appreciate that flexibility is not a fixed property. The range of motion of most joints can be increased with proper training techniques or can decline with disuse. This chapter introduces exercises designed to improve flexibility.

⁂ Benefits of Flexibility

The many benefits of increased flexibility include increased joint mobility, efficient body movement, and good posture (1, 3, 4). Although it is commonly believed that stretching before exercise reduces the incidence of muscle injury during exercise, data from most research studies indicate that this is not the case. A recent critical review article concludes that there is no good evidence that stretching reduces muscle injury and, in fact, cites evidence suggesting that stretching may contribute to injury (5). The only studies suggesting that stretching offers protection from muscle injury combined the stretching with a general warm-up.

While all of these flexibility benefits are important, a key reason to improve flexibility is its role in the prevention of low back problems. For example, most low back pain is due to misalignment of the vertebral column and pelvic girdle caused by a lack of flexibility and/or weak muscles. This topic is discussed in a later section.

⁂ Physiological Basis for Developing Flexibility

We have already noted that the limits to flexibility are determined by the way the joint is constructed as well as by the associated muscles and tendons. Let's discuss these factors in more detail.

STRUCTURAL LIMITATIONS TO MOVEMENT

Five primary factors contribute to the limits of movement: bone; muscle; connective tissue within the joint capsule (the joint capsule is composed of **ligaments**, which hold bones together, and **cartilage**, which cushions the ends of bones); **tendons**, which connect muscle to bones and to connective tissue surrounding joints; and skin. Exercise aimed at improving flexibility does not change the structure of bone, but it alters the soft tissues (i.e., muscle, joint connective tissue, and tendons) that contribute to flexibility. Table 6.1 lists the contribution of the various soft tissues to total joint flexibility. Note that the structures associated with the joint capsule, muscles, and tendons provide most of the body's resistance to movement. Therefore, exercises aimed at improving flexibility must alter one of these three factors in order to increase the range of motion around a joint. Stretching the ligaments in the joint capsule may lead to a loose joint that would be highly susceptible to injury. However, muscle and tendon are soft tissues that can lengthen over time with stretching exercises. Stretching exercises increase the range of motion in the joint by reducing the resistance to movement offered by tight muscles and tendons.

STRETCHING AND THE STRETCH REFLEX

Before we examine specific exercises for improving flexibility, it is useful to discuss a key physiological response to stretching exercises. Muscles contain special receptors, called *muscle spindles*, that are sensitive to stretch. When a doctor taps you on the knee with a

---

ligaments   Connective tissue within the joint capsule that holds bones together.
cartilage   A tough, connective tissue that forms a pad on the end of bones in certain joints, such as the elbow, knee, and ankle. Cartilage acts as a shock absorber to cushion the weight of one bone on another and to provide protection from the friction due to joint movement.
tendons   Connective tissue that connects muscles to bones.

TABLE 6.1
Contribution of Soft-Tissue Structures to Limiting Joint Movement

Structure	Resistance to Flexibility (% of total)
Joint capsule	47
Muscle	41
Tendon	10
Skin	2

Nutritional Links

Can Diet Supplements Improve Joint Health?

The ends of the bones in joints are covered by a firm, resilient type of connective tissue called *cartilage,* which absorbs shock and provides smooth surfaces that aid joint movement. Cartilage mostly consists of a gel-like matrix of water, collagen fibers, and chains of sugar-based molecules (glycans) produced by cartilage cells. Joint injury, arthritis, and the natural process of aging can cause deterioration of cartilage in joints, which can lead to pain and reduced flexibility. As a result, preventing joint deterioration and stimulating the re-

generation of cartilage is important to joint health.

Several recent studies have investigated the effects of dietary supplements containing two key substances the body uses to produce cartilage. One substance, chondroitin, is thought to be important in reducing joint wear by combining with other molecules to increase the strength and resiliency of cartilage. The other substance, glucosamine, promotes regeneration of damaged cartilage matrix. Several of these studies have shown that individuals with cartilage deterio-

ration who take glucosamine and chondroitin have thicker joint cartilage compared to controls (6).

Although these results and the apparent lack of side effects of taking these supplements are encouraging, it is not yet known whether taking chondroitin and glucosamine provides long-term improvements in joint health. If you have joint pain or other joint problems, consult your physician to determine whether supplementation with these products might be beneficial for you.

---

rubber hammer, for example, the rapid stretching of muscle spindles results in a "reflex" contraction of the muscle to prevent it from stretching too far too fast. This reflex contraction, called **stretch reflex,** is counterproductive to stretching exercises because the muscle is shortening instead of lengthening. Fortunately, the stretch reflex can be avoided when muscles and tendons are stretched very slowly. In fact, if a muscle stretch is held for several seconds, the muscle spindles allow the muscle being stretched to further relax and permit an even greater stretch (2, 3). Therefore, stretching exercises are most effective when they avoid promoting a stretch reflex.

☀ IN SUMMARY

- Flexibility is defined as the range of motion of a joint.
- Improved flexibility results in the following benefits: increased joint mobility, resistance to muscle injury, prevention of low back problems, efficient body movement, and improved posture and personal appearance.
- The structural and physiological limits to flexibility are (1) bone, (2) muscle, (3) structures within the joint capsule, (4) the tendons which connect muscle to bones and to connective tissue surrounding joints, and (5) skin.
- If muscle spindles are stretched suddenly, they respond by initiating a stretch reflex that causes the

muscle to contract and shorten. However, if the muscles and tendons are stretched slowly, the stretch reflex can be avoided.

☀ Designing a Flexibility Training Program

Three kinds of stretching techniques are commonly used to increase flexibility: ballistic stretching, static stretching, and proprioceptive neuromuscular facilitation (2, 7). Ballistic, also called dynamic, stretching can be useful for athletes who perform ballistic movements in their sport. With this type of stretching, the athlete can cause the nervous system to adapt to the quick, jerking-type movements that they routinely perform. However, for the average fitness enthusiast seeking to increase flexibility, these ballistic movements may activate the stretch reflex (discussed earlier) causing injury to muscles and tendons. For this reason, we do not discuss ballistic stretching techniques. A brief discussion of static and proprioceptive neuromuscular facilitation techniques follows.

---

stretch reflex   Involuntary contraction of a muscle that occurs due to rapid stretching of that muscle.

STATIC STRETCHING

Static stretching is extremely effective for improving flexibility and has gained popularity over the last decade (2, 4). Static stretching slowly lengthens a muscle to a point at which further movement is limited (slight discomfort is felt) and requires holding this position for a fixed period of time. The optimal amount of time to hold the stretch for maximal improvement in flexibility is unknown. However, it is generally agreed that holding the stretch position for 20 to 30 seconds (repeated three to four times) results in an improvement in flexibility (4). Compared with ballistic stretching, the risk of injury associated with static stretching is minimal. Another benefit of static stretching is that, when performed during the cool-down period, it may reduce the muscle stiffness associated with some exercise routines (2, 4).

PROPRIOCEPTIVE NEUROMUSCULAR FACILITATION

A relatively new technique for improving flexibility, **proprioceptive neuromuscular facilitation (PNF)**, combines stretching with alternating contraction and relaxation of muscles. There are two common types of PNF stretching: contract-relax (CR) stretching and contract-relax/antagonist contract (CRAC) stretching. The CR stretch technique calls for first contracting the muscle to be stretched. Then, after relaxing the muscle, the muscle is slowly stretched. The CRAC method calls for the same contract-relax routine but adds to this the contraction of the **antagonist** muscle, the muscle on the opposite side of the joint. The purpose of contracting the antagonist muscle is to promote a reflex relaxation of the muscle to be stretched.

How do PNF techniques compare with ballistic and static stretching? First, PNF has been shown to be safer and more effective in promoting flexibility than ballistic stretching (7). Further, studies have shown PNF programs to be equal to, or in some cases superior to,

static stretching for improving flexibility (8). However, one disadvantage of PNF stretching is that some stretches require a partner.

The following steps illustrate how a CRAC procedure can be done with a partner (Figure 6.1):

1. After the assistant moves the limb in the direction necessary to stretch the desired muscles to the point of tightness (mild discomfort is felt), the subject isometrically contracts the muscle being stretched for 3 to 5 seconds and then relaxes them.

2. The subject then moves the limb in the opposite direction of the stretch by isometrically contracting the antagonist muscles. The subject holds this isometric contraction for approximately 5 seconds, during which time the muscles to be stretched relax. While the desired muscles are relaxed, the assistant may increase the stretch of the desired muscles.

3. The subject then isometrically contracts the antagonist muscles for another 5 seconds, which relaxes the desired muscles, and then the assistant again stretches the desired muscles to the point of mild discomfort.

This cycle of three steps is repeated three to five times. Figure 6.1 illustrates a partner-assisted CRAC procedure for stretching the calf muscles.

Figure 6.2 shows how some PNF stretches can be done without a partner.

☀ Lower Back Health

Approximately 15% of Americans will be disabled by low back pain (LBP) in their lifetime. However, up to 8 out of 10 people will experience LBP (10). Why is this problem so widespread? There are several reasons. LBP has often been labeled as a hypokinetic disease, that is, a disease associated with a lack of exercise. Here is a list of the top potential contributors to the problem.

- low back lumbar flexibility
- hamstring flexibility
- hip flexor flexibility
- strength and endurance of the forward and lateral abdominals
- strength and endurance of the back extensor muscles

Males and females are affected equally by back pain and it is usually experienced between the ages of 25 and 60. Most pain in the lower back goes away in a few days or weeks. If you continue to have low back pain for six months, it is considered chronic.

---

static stretching   Stretching that slowly lengthens a muscle to a point where further movement is limited.
proprioceptive neuromuscular facilitation (PNF) A technique that combines stretching with alternating contraction and relaxation of muscles to improve flexibility. There are two common types of PNF stretching: contract-relax (CR) stretching and contract-relax/antagonist contract (CRAC) stretching.
antagonist   The muscle on the opposite side of the joint.

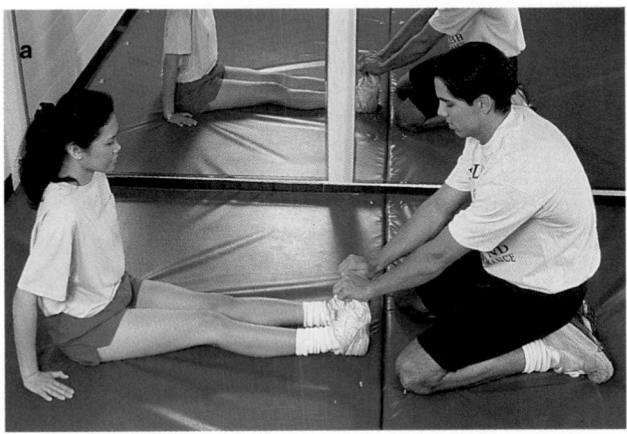

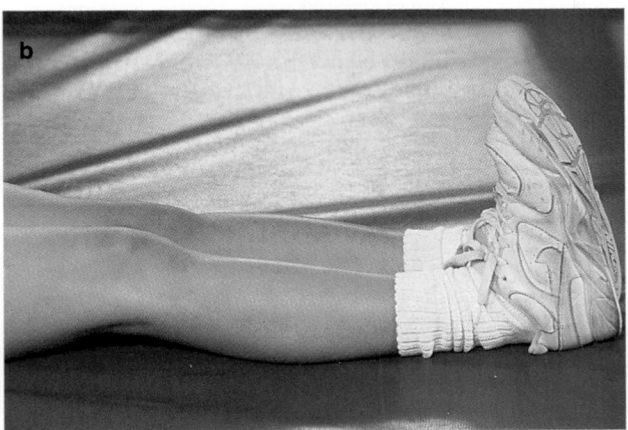

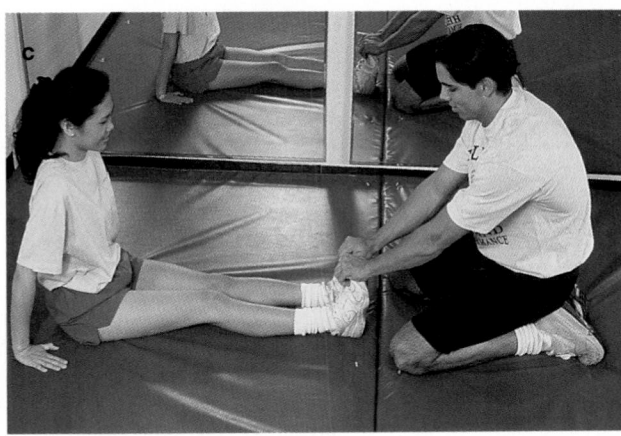

FIGURE 6.1
An example of a partner-assisted CRAC procedure for stretching the calf muscles. The subject contracts the calf muscles against resistance provided by the assistant (a). Unassisted, the subject contracts the shin (antagonist) muscles, which relaxes the calf muscles (b). While the subject continues the contraction of the shin muscles, the assistant stretches the calf muscles (c).

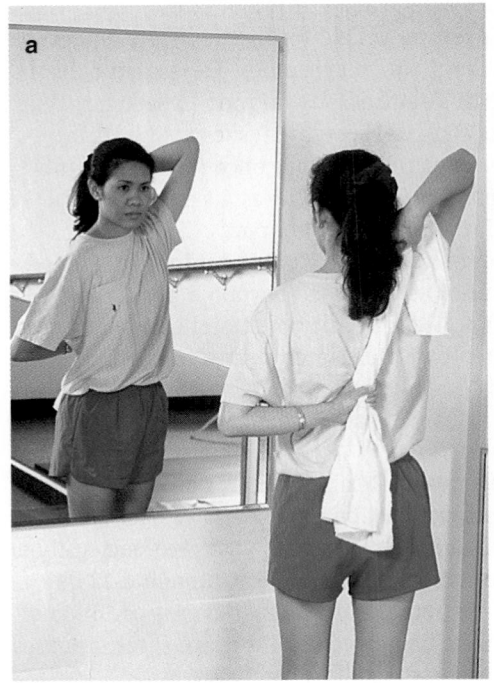

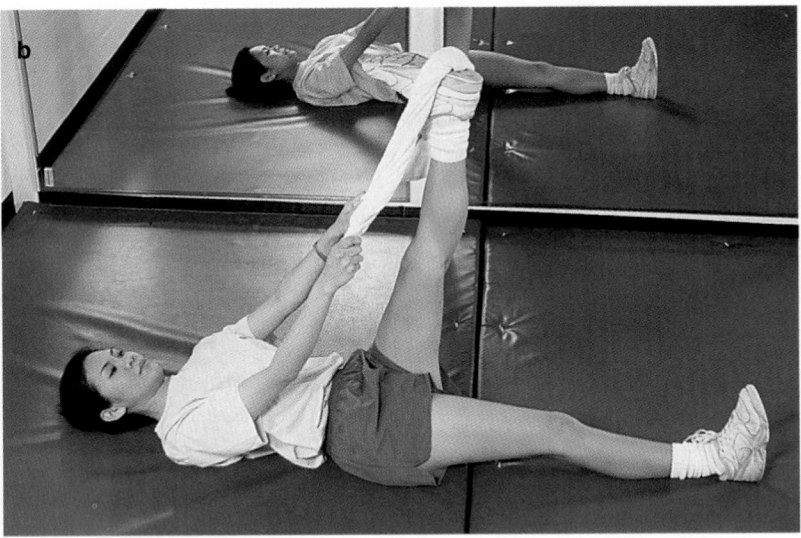

FIGURE 6.2
Examples of how PNF stretches may be done without a partner. What other creative ways to self-assist with PNF stretches can you devise?

TABLE 6.2
Sample Flexibility Program with Considerations for Duration of Stretch Hold, Number of Repetitions, and Frequency of Training

Week No.	Phase	Duration of Stretch Hold	Repetitions	Frequency (times/wk)
1	Starter	15 sec	1	1
2	Slow progression	20 sec	2	2
3	Slow progression	25 sec	3	3
4	Slow progression	30 sec	4	3
5	Slow progression	30 sec	4	3–4
6	Slow progression	30 sec	4	4–5
7 +	Maintenance	30 sec	4	4–5

Chronic use of backpacks has recently come under scrutiny because of the potential to cause problems in the lower back while trying to maintain stability. Indeed, in a recent study (11), curvature of the spine was significantly increased as subjects wearing backpacks fatigued. Interestingly, after the subjects rested for several minutes, both trunk and head angles were not significantly different from the fatigued condition. Although this study did not examine resulting back problems from the chronic wearing of a backpack, the findings certainly suggest that long-term backpack use can result in misalignment in the lower back.

Although many studies have tried to calculate the costs, the psychological, social, and physical costs cannot begin to be calculated. The medical, insurance, and business/industry costs are generally considered to be in the billions of dollars per year. The development and maintenance of healthy low back function requires a balance of flexibility, strength, and endurance.

The stretching exercises presented in this chapter should help you maintain a healthy back. Focus on the following stretches: One-leg stretch (6.3), Lower back stretch (6.4), Thigh stretch (6.7), Spine twister (6.8), Leg stretch (6.11), Trunk twister (6.12), Leg pull, Sitting hamstring stretch, Curl up, and the Knee-to-toe touch.

☀ IN SUMMARY

- Static stretches involve stretching a muscle to the limit of movement and holding the stretch for an extended period of time.
- Proprioceptive neuromuscular facilitation (PNF) combines stretching with alternating contraction and relaxation of muscles to improve flexibility.
- Flexibility of the hamstrings and lower back and strong abdominal muscles are important for a healthy back.

☀ Exercise Prescription for Improving Flexibility

For safety reasons, all flexibility programs should consist of either PNF or static stretching exercises. The frequency and duration of a stretching exercise prescription should be 2 to 5 days per week for 10 to 30 minutes each day. The first week of a stretching regimen is considered the starter phase. The first week should consist of one stretching session, and one session should be added per week during the first 4 weeks of the slow progression phase of the program. Initially, the duration of each training session should be approximately 5 minutes and should increase gradually to 20 to 30 minutes following 6 to 12 weeks of stretching during the slow progression phase. The physiological rationale for increasing the duration of stretching is that each stretch position is held for progressively longer durations as the program continues. For example, begin by holding each stretched position for 15 seconds, then add 5 seconds each week up to 30 seconds. Start by performing each of the exercises once (1 rep) and progress to 4 reps. Table 6.2 illustrates a sample exercise prescription for a flexibility program.

What about the intensity of stretching? In general, a limb should not be stretched beyond a position of mild discomfort. The intensity of stretching is increased simply by extending the stretch nearer to the limits of your range of motion. Your range of motion will gradually increase as your flexibility improves during the training program.

To improve overall flexibility, all major muscle groups should be stretched. Just because you have good flexibility in the shoulders does not mean your flexibility will be good in the hamstrings. Exercises 6.1 through 6.12 on pp. 158–165 illustrate the proper methods of performing 12 different stretching exercises. Integrate these exercises into the program outlined in Table 6.2.

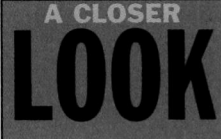

Pilates—More Than Stretching?

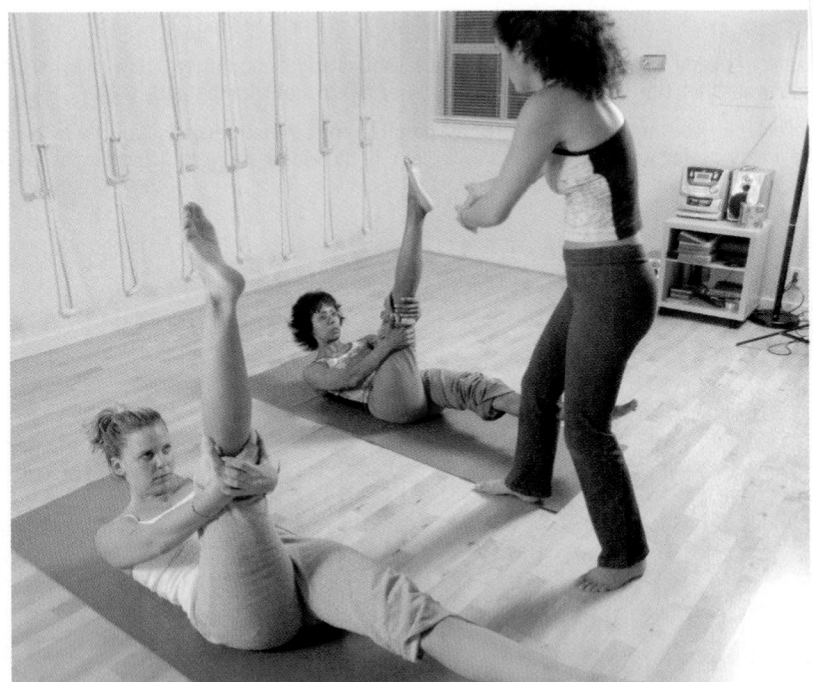

In the mid 1990s, the Pilates method of exercise (named after the German-born Joseph Pilates) came into vogue in rehabilitation hospitals and clinics across the United States. This form of exercise stressed the gentle, subtle stretching and contraction of muscles that produce very fluid, controlled movements that stress a mind–body interaction. The basic Pilates program consists of a variety of exercises that utilize two pieces of equipment (although many more specialized pieces exist today). *Mat Work* consists of a series of exercises performed on a padded mat. It is considered best for a general workout and, when done correctly, the most difficult. *The Reformer* is a moving carriage on a horizontal frame with straps and springs. There are a series of up to 100 exercises performed on it without stopping. Most forms of Pilates emphasize the following basic principles and claims of benefits:

- Concentration—The mind–body connection. This stresses that conscious control of movement enhances body awareness.
- Control/Precision—It's not about intensity or multiple "reps," it's more about proper form.
- Centering—This declares that a mental focus within the body calms the spirit and a particular focus on the torso develops a strong core and enables the rest of the body to function efficiently. All action initiates from the trunk and flows outward to the extremities.
- Stabilizing—Before you move you have to be still. Makes for a safe starting place for mobility.
- Breathing—Deep, coordinated, conscious diaphragmatic patterns of inhalation and exhalation initiate movement, help activate deep muscles, and keep you focused.
- Alignment—Proper alignment is key to good posture. You'll be aware of the position of your head and neck on the spine and pelvis, right down through the legs and toes.
- Fluidity—Smooth, continuous motion rather than jarring repetitions.
- Integration—Several different muscle groups are engaged simultaneously to control and support movement. All principles come together, making for a holistic mind–body workout.

To date, no data-based research has validated the health and fitness benefits that have been claimed by the various Pilates instructional schools (12).

These exercises are designed to be used in a regular program of stretching to increase flexibility. The exercises presented involve the joints and major muscle groups for which range of motion tends to decrease with age and disuse. The exercises include both static and PNF movements and may require a partner.

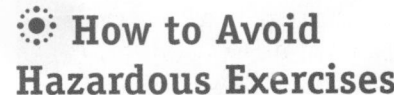

How to Avoid Hazardous Exercises

Many exercises are potentially harmful to the musculoskeletal system. Which exercises actually cause injury

Text continues on p. 166

Sample Flexibility Exercises

EXERCISE 6.1   LOWER LEG STRETCH

Purpose: To stretch the calf muscles and the Achilles' tendon.

Position: Stand on the edge of a surface that is high enough to allow the heel to be lower than the toes. Have a support nearby to hold for balance.

Movement: Rise on the toes as far as possible for several seconds (a), then lower the heels as far as possible (b). Shift your body weight from one leg to the other for added stretch of the muscles.

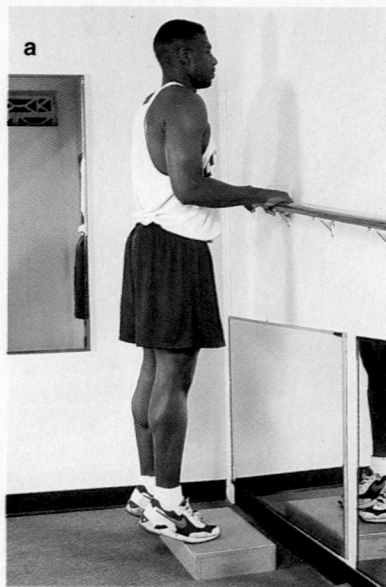 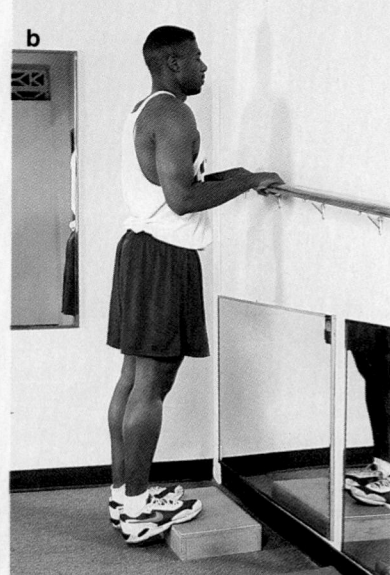

Lower leg stretch

EXERCISE 6.2   INSIDE LEG STRETCH

Purpose: To stretch the muscle on the inside of the thighs.

Position: Sit with bottoms of the feet together and the hands placed just below the knees.

Movement: Using the hands and forearms to resist an effort to raise the knees. Then relax and, using your hands, press the knees toward the floor and hold for several seconds.

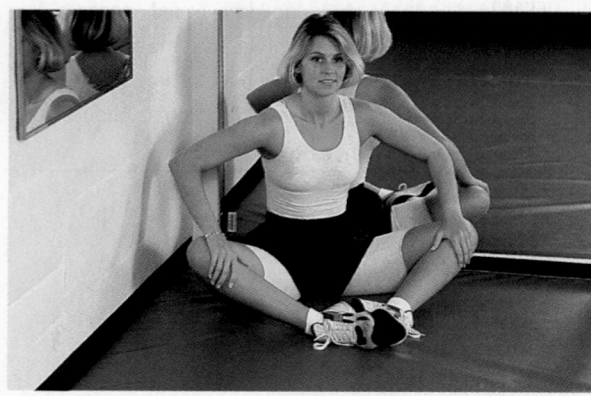

Inside leg stretch

Sample Flexibility Exercises

EXERCISE 6.3 ONE-LEG STRETCH

Purpose: To stretch the lower back muscles and muscles in the back of the thigh.

Position: Stand with the heel of one foot on a support approximately knee-to-waist high. Keep both legs straight.

Movement: Press the heel down on the support for several seconds (a); then relax and bend forward at the waist and attempt to touch your head to your knee, and hold for several seconds (b). Return to the upright position and alternate legs.

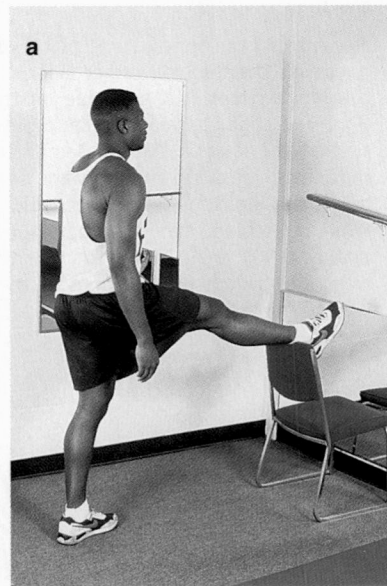 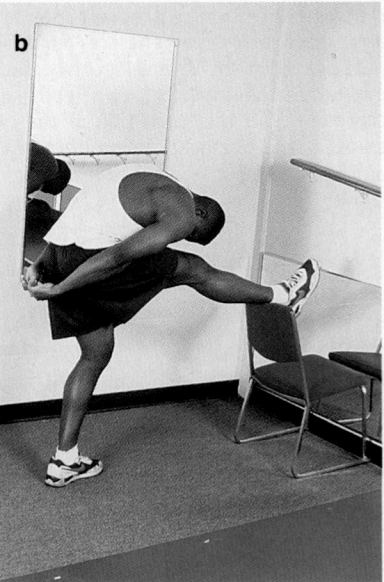

One-leg stretch

EXERCISE 6.4 LOWER BACK STRETCH

Purpose: To stretch the lower back and buttocks muscles.

Position: Lying on your back with the feet flat on the floor.

Movement: First, arch your back and lift the hips off the floor, and hold for several seconds (a). Relax and place your hands behind the knees. Pull the knees to the chest and hold for several seconds (b). Repeat the sequence for the desired number of repetitions.

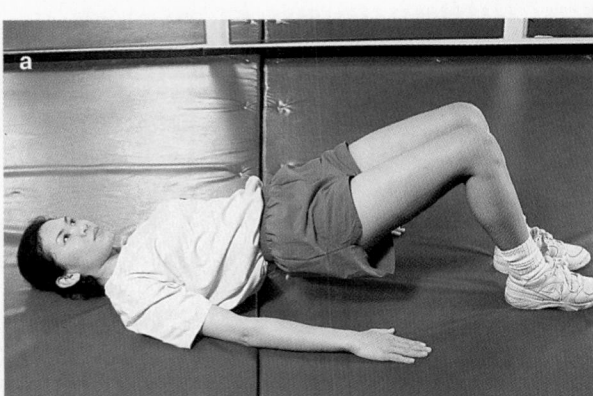 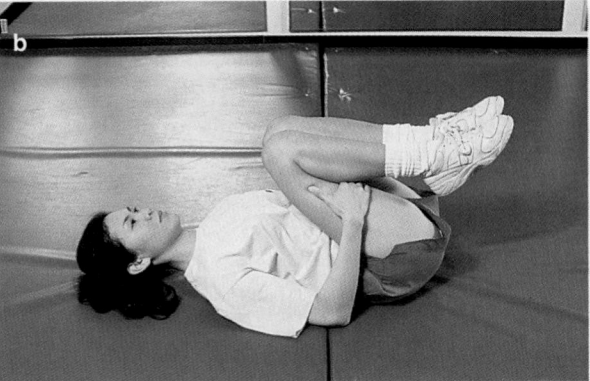

Lower back stretch

Sample Flexibility Exercises

EXERCISE 6.5
CHEST STRETCH

Purpose: To stretch the muscles across the chest.

Position: Stand in a doorway and grasp the frame of the doorway at shoulder height.

Movement: Press forward on the frame for ~5 seconds. Then, relax and shift your weight forward until you feel the stretch of muscles across the chest, and hold for several seconds.

EXERCISE 6.6
SIDE STRETCH

Purpose: To stretch the muscles of the upper arm and side of the trunk.

Position: Sitting on the floor with legs crossed.

Movement: Stretch one arm over the head while bending at the waist in the same direction. With the opposite arm, reach across the chest as far as possible. Hold for several seconds. Do not rotate the trunk; try to stretch the muscle on the same side of the trunk as the overhead arm. Alternate arms to stretch the other side of the trunk.

EXERCISE 6.7
THIGH STRETCH

Purpose: To stretch the muscles in the front of the thigh of the extended (rear) leg.

Position: Kneel on one knee, resting the rear foot on the ball of the foot and placing the forward foot flat on the floor.

Movement: Lean forward and place your hands on the floor on either side of the forward foot. Lift the knee off the floor and slide the rear leg backward so that the knee is slightly behind the hips; then press the hips forward and down, and hold for several seconds. While stretching, maintain approximately a 90° angle at the knee of the front leg. Switch the positions of the legs to stretch the other thigh.

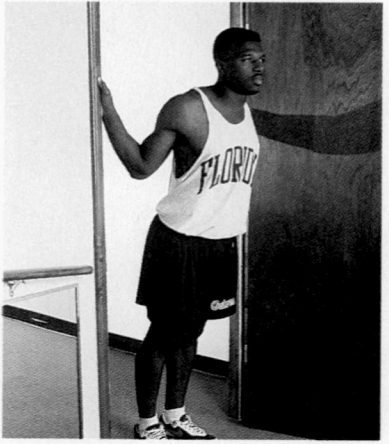

Chest stretch

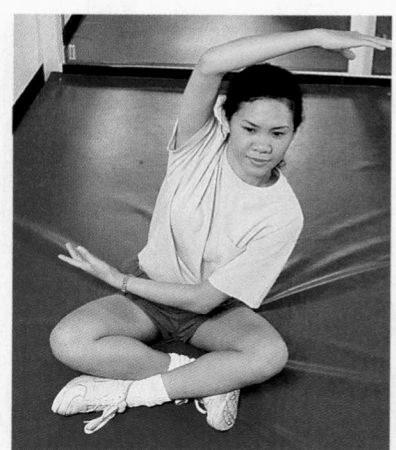

Side stretch

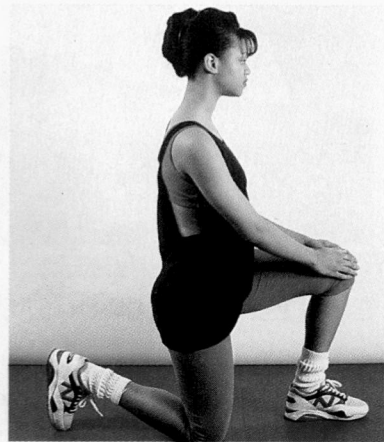

Thigh stretch

EXERCISE 6.8   SPINE TWISTER

Purpose: To stretch the muscles that rotate the trunk and thighs.

Position: Lie on your back, with one leg crossed over the other and both shoulders and both arms on the floor (a).

Movement: Rotate the trunk such that the crossed-over leg stays on top and both knees approach or touch the floor (b); hold for several seconds. The shoulders and arms should remain on the floor all during the stretch. Reverse the positions of the legs and repeat the stretch.

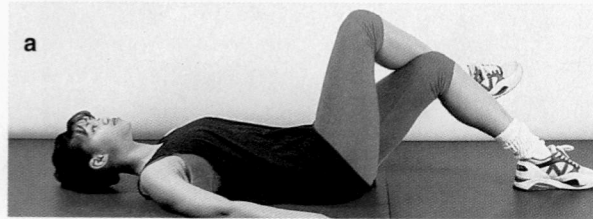

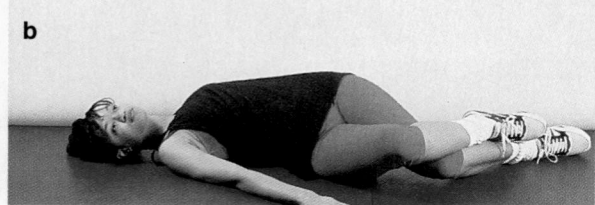

Spine twister

Sample Flexibility Exercises

EXERCISE 6.9   NECK STRETCH

Purpose: To stretch the muscles that rotate the neck.

Position: After turning the head to one side, place the hand against the cheek with fingers toward the ear and elbow forward.

Movement: Try to turn the head and neck against the resistance of the hand; hold for a few seconds. Remove the hand and relax, and then turn the head as far as possible in the same direction as before. Hold this position for several seconds. Then repeat the stretch, this time turning in the other direction.

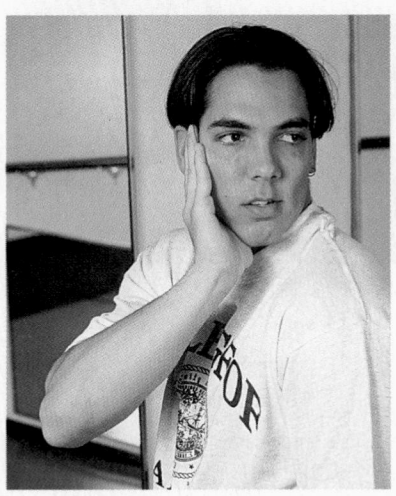

Neck stretch

EXERCISE 6.10   SHIN STRETCH

Purpose: To stretch the muscles of the shin.

Position: Kneel on both knees, with the trunk rotated to one side and the hand on that side pressing down on the ankle.

Movement: While pressing down on the ankle, move the pelvis forward; hold for several seconds. Repeat on the other side.

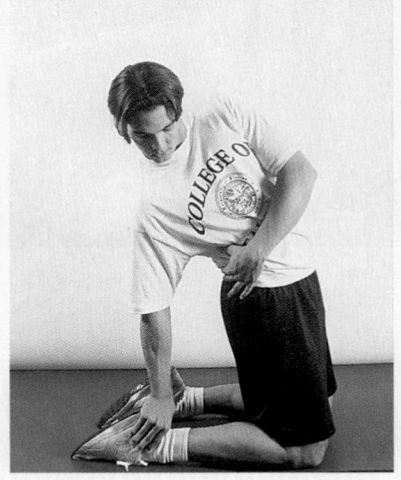

Shin stretch

EXERCISE 6.11   LEG STRETCH

Purpose: To stretch the muscles on the back of the hip, the back of the thigh, and the calf.

Position: Lying on your back, bring one knee toward the chest and grasp the toes with the hand on the same side. Place the opposite hand on the back of the leg just below the knee.

Movement: Pull the knee toward the chest while pushing the heel toward the ceiling and pulling the toes toward the shin. Straighten the knee until you feel sufficient stretch in the muscles of the back of the leg, and hold for several seconds. Repeat for the other leg.

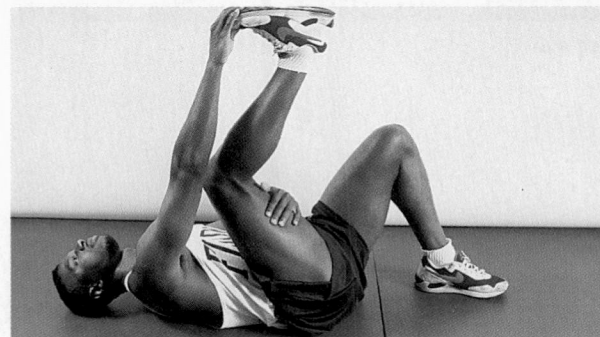

Leg stretch

EXERCISE 6.12   TRUNK TWISTER

Purpose: To stretch the trunk muscles and the muscles of the hip.

Position: Sit with the left leg extended, the right leg bent and crossed over the left knee, and the right foot on the floor. Place the right hand on the floor behind the buttocks.

Movement: Placing the left arm on the right side of the right thigh and the left hand on the floor, use the left arm to push against the right leg while twisting the trunk to the right. Hold for several seconds. Then assume the starting position with the right leg extended and so forth, and stretch the opposite side of the body.

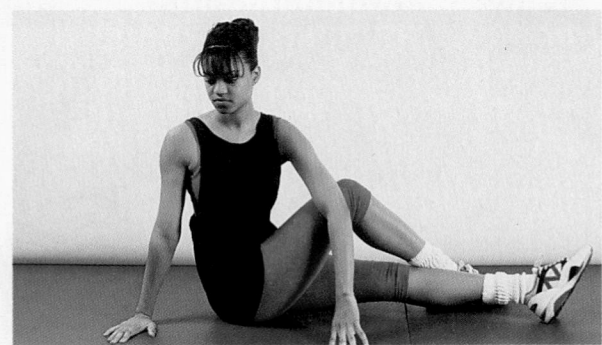

Trunk twister

Contraindicated Exercise

ARM CIRCLES (PALMS DOWN)

Purpose: To strengthen the muscles of the shoulder and upper back.

Problem: May result in irritation of the shoulder joint and, if circled forward and down, results in the use of the chest muscles instead of back muscles.

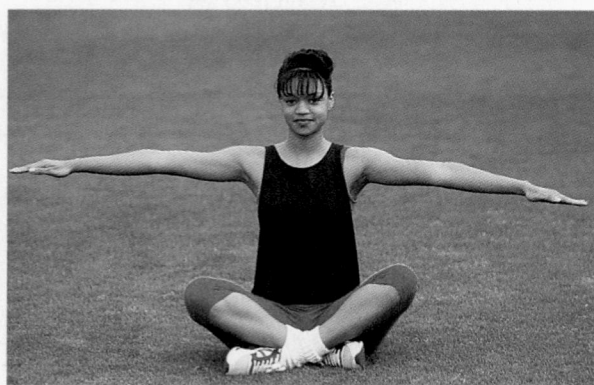

Arm circles (palms down)

KNEE PULL

Purpose: To stretch the lower back and buttocks.

Problem: Places undue stress on the knee joint.

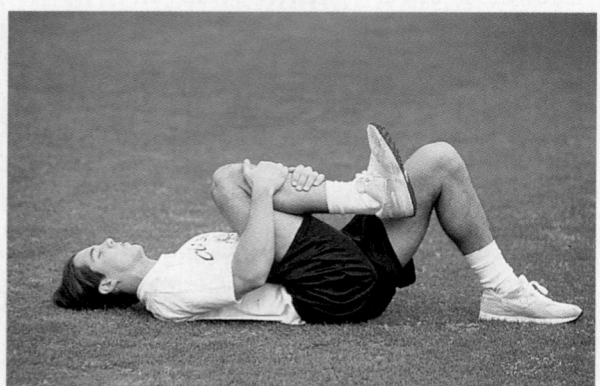

Knee pull

Substitute Exercise

ARM CIRCLES (PALMS UP)

In a sitting position, turn the palms up and circle the arms backward and up.

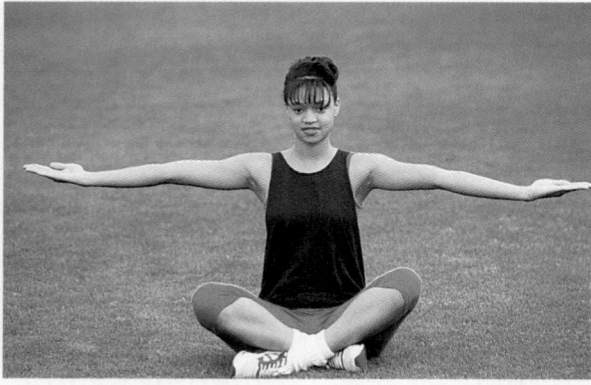

Arm circles (palms up)

LEG PULL

Lying on your back, pull the knee toward the chest by pulling on the back of the leg just below the knee. Then, extend the knee joint and point the sole of the foot straight up. Continue to pull the leg toward your chest. Repeat several times with each leg.

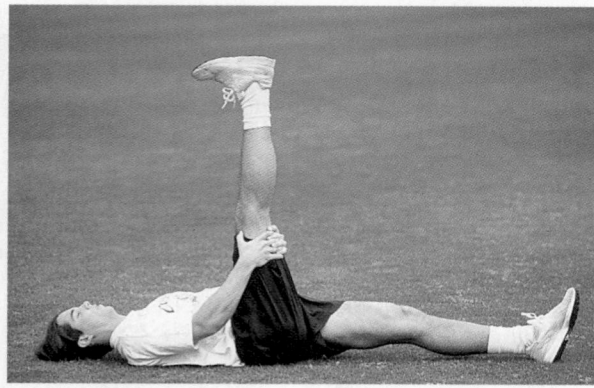

Leg pull

Contraindicated Exercise

DEEP KNEE BENDS

Purpose: To strengthen the upper leg and stretch the lower leg.

Problem: This movement hyperflexes the knee and "opens" the joint while stretching the ligaments.

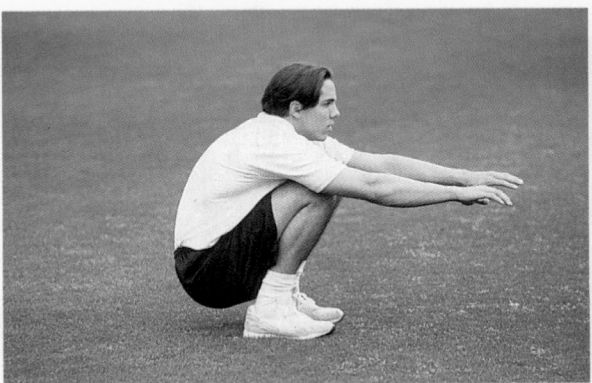

Deep knee bends

LEG LIFTS

Purpose: To strengthen the abdominal muscles.

Problem: This exercise primarily recruits the hip flexor muscles and thus does not accomplish the intended purpose. These muscles are likely strong enough and do not need strengthening. In addition, this exercise produces excess compression on the vertebral disks.

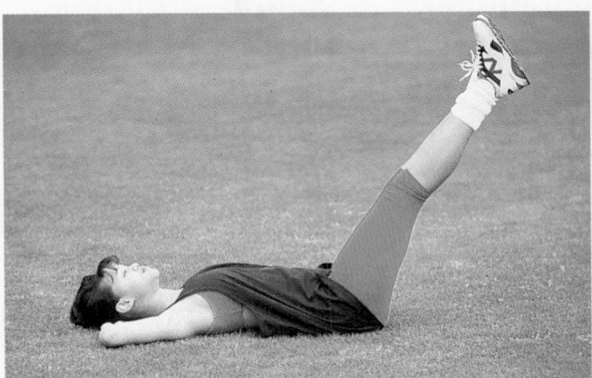

Leg lifts

Substitute Exercise

LUNGES

While standing, step forward with either foot and touch the opposite knee to the ground. Repeat with the opposite leg.

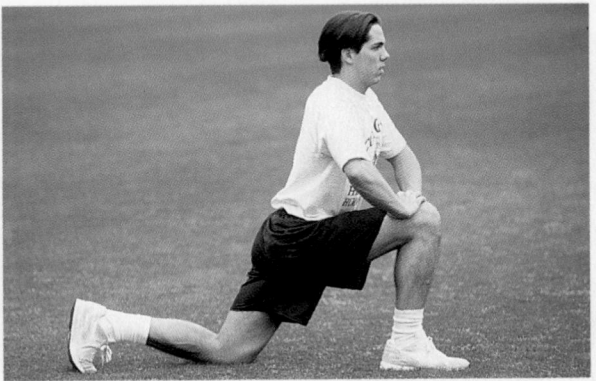

Lunges

REVERSE CURL

Lie on your back with the knees bent and the arms and feet flat on the ground. Maintaining about the same degree of bend at the knee joint, pull the knees up toward the chest so that the hips leave the ground. Do not allow the knees to go past the shoulders. Lower the legs back to the ground and repeat.

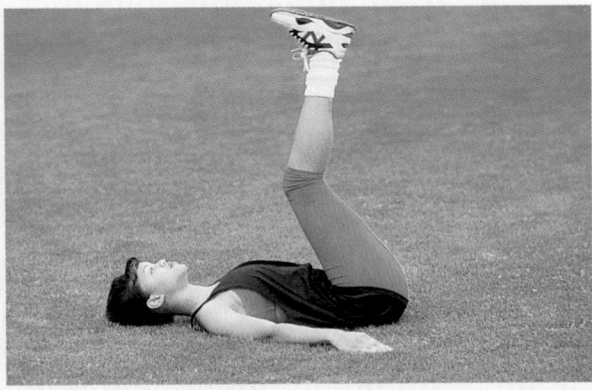

Reverse curl

Contraindicated Exercise

STANDING TOE TOUCH

Purpose: To stretch the lower back, buttocks, and hamstrings.

Problems: First, hyperflexion of the knee could cause damage to ligaments and, second, if performed with the back flat, damage could occur to the lower back.

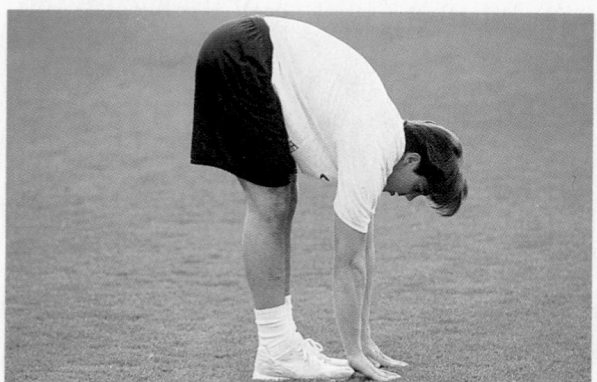

Standing toe touch

SIT-UP (HANDS BEHIND HEAD)

Purpose: To strengthen the abdominal muscles.

Problem: With hands behind the head, there is a tendency to jerk on the head and neck to "throw" yourself up. This could cause hyperflexion of the neck. In addition, sitting up with the back straight places undue strain on the lower back.

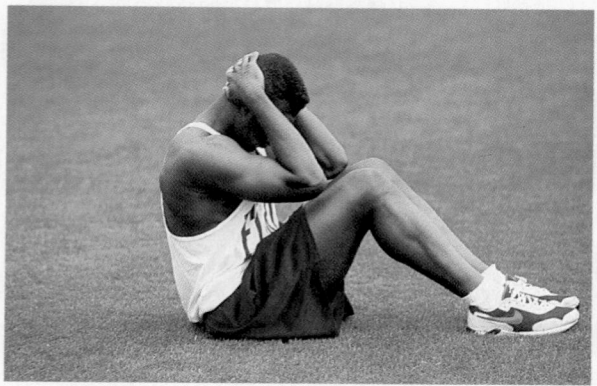

Sit-up (hands behind head)

Substitute Exercise

SITTING HAMSTRING STRETCH

Sit at leg-length from a wall. With your foot on the wall and the other knee bent with the foot between the wall and buttocks, bend forward keeping the lower back straight. The bent knee can fall to the side.

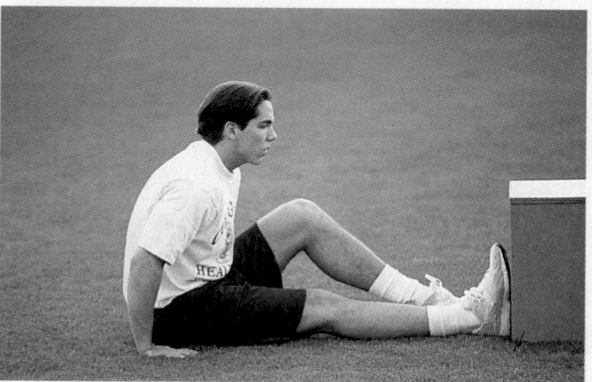

Sitting hamstring stretch

CURL UP

Keeping the knees bent while lying on your back, cross your arms over your chest so that your fingers rest on your shoulders. Using the abdominal muscles, curl up until the upper half of the back is off the floor and then return to the starting position.

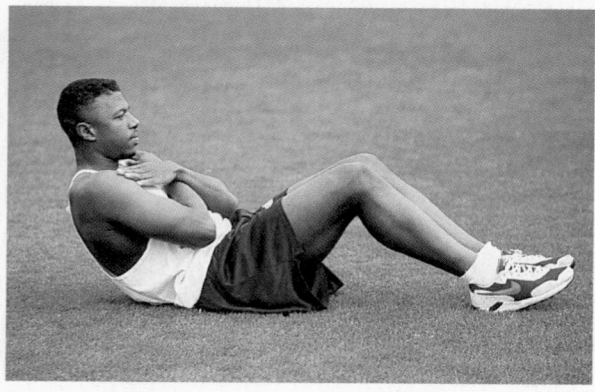

Curl up

Contraindicated Exercise

NECK CIRCLES

Purpose: To stretch the neck muscles.

Problem: Hyperextension of the neck should always be avoided. This can pinch arteries and nerves, as well as damage disks in the spine.

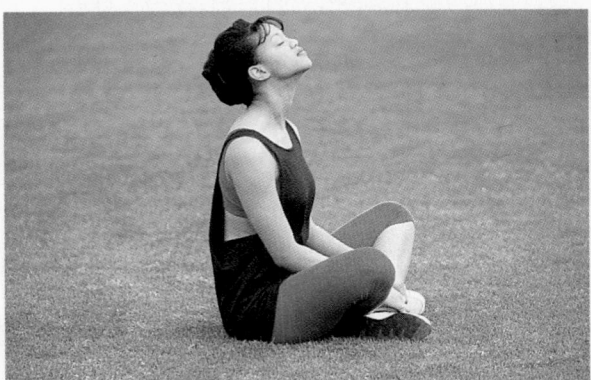

Neck circles

DONKEY KICK

Purpose: To stretch and strengthen the buttocks.

Problem: When kicking the leg back, most people hyperextend the neck and/or back.

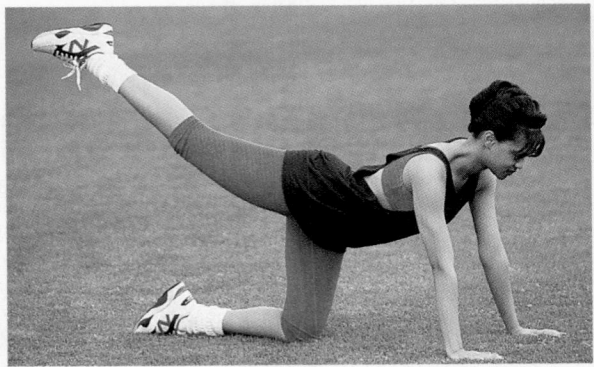

Donkey kick

Substitute Exercise

NECK STRETCHES

In a sitting position, with your head and neck straight, move your head down to flex the neck, and return the head upright. Then, slowly turn your head from side to side as far as possible; attempt to point your chin at each shoulder.

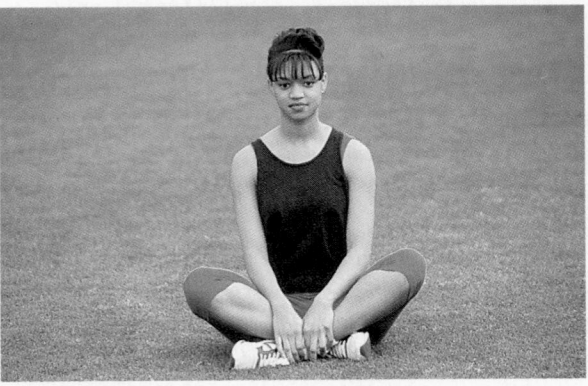

Neck stretches

KNEE-TO-NOSE TOUCH

While on your hands and knees, lift one knee toward your nose and then extend that leg to horizontal. Alternate legs. Remember: Your leg should not go higher than your hips, and your neck should remain in line with your back.

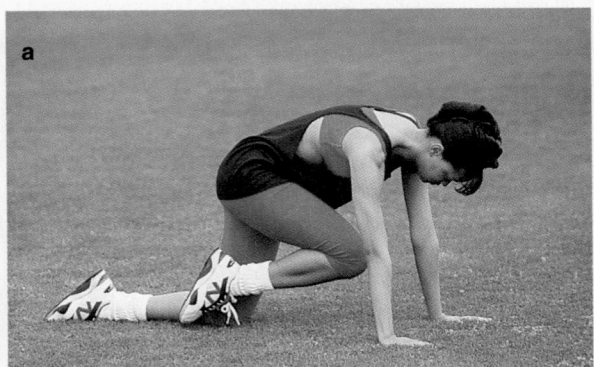

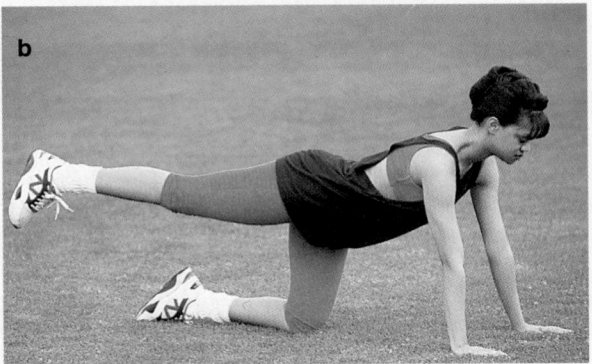

Knee-to-nose touch

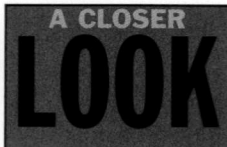

When Muscles Cramp

Muscle cramps are one of the most common problems encountered in sports and exercise. For many years the primary causes of muscle cramps were thought to be dehydration and/or electrolyte imbalances. Accordingly, drinking enough fluids and ensuring that the diet contains sufficient amounts of sodium (from table salt, for example) and potassium (from bananas, for example) have long been encouraged as preventive measures. Whenever muscles cramp, stretching and/or massage have been used to relieve the cramping until electrolyte balance can be restored.

More recent research, however, suggests that cramping may be due to abnormal spinal control of motor neuron activity, especially when a muscle contracts while shortened (9). Thus, for example, the cramping that often occurs in the calf muscles of recreational swimmers when their toes are pointed may occur because those calf muscles are contracting while they are shortened.

The most prevalent risk factors for cramps during exercise are muscle fatigue and poor stretching habits (failure to stretch regularly and long enough during each session). Other risk factors include older age, higher body mass index, and a family history of muscle cramps.

If cramping occurs, you should:

- Passively stretch the muscle. Such stretching induces receptors that sense the stretch to initiate nerve impulses that inhibit muscle stimulation.

- Drink plenty of water to avoid dehydration or electrolyte imbalances. Sports drinks can help replenish glucose and electrolytes, but do *not* use salt tablets.

- Seek medical attention if multiple muscle groups are involved, because this could be a sign of more serious problems.

Although no strategies for preventing muscle cramping during exercise have been proven effective, regular stretching using PNF techniques, correction of muscle balance and posture, and proper training for the exercise activity involved may be beneficial.

---

depends on how they are performed. Remember the following key points during an exercise session to help prevent injury:

- Avoid breathholding. Try to breathe as normally as possible during the exercise.
- Avoid full flexion of the knee or neck.
- Avoid full extension of the knee, neck, or back.
- Do not stretch muscles that are already stretched, such as the abdominal muscles.
- Do not stretch to the point that joint pain occurs.
- Use extreme caution when using an assistant to help with passive stretches.
- Avoid forceful extension and flexion of the spine.

Many commonly practiced exercises may cause injuries and are therefore contraindicated. The illustrations starting on p. 162 show some of these exercises (contraindicated exercises) and provide alternatives (substitute exercises) to accomplish the same goals.

☀ IN SUMMARY

- Stretching exercises should be performed 2 to 5 days per week for 10 to 30 minutes each day.

- Week one, the "starter" phase, consists of one stretching session lasting approximately 5 minutes.
- Weeks 2 through 4 are "progression" weeks during which one session should be added each week.
- The duration of stretching exercise sessions should be increased gradually up to 20–30 minutes over 10 to 12 weeks.
- The intensity of a stretch is considered to be maximal where "mild discomfort" is felt.

☀ Motivation to Maintain Flexibility

Maintaining flexibility requires a lifetime commitment to performing regular stretching. Just as in other types of fitness training, good time management is critical if you are going to succeed. Set aside time for 3 to 5 stretching periods per week, and stick to your schedule. A key point to remember is that stretching can be performed almost anywhere because it does not require special equipment. So take advantage of "windows" of free time in your day and plan stretching workouts.

You are not likely to maintain a lifetime stretching program if you do not enjoy your workouts. One suggestion for making stretching more fun is to perform stretching workouts while listening to music or during a television program you enjoy. This will allow time to pass more rapidly and will make your stretching workout more pleasant.

As in other aspects of physical fitness, establishing short-term and long-term flexibility goals is important in maintaining the motivation to stretch. Further, keeping a record of your workouts and improvements allows you to follow your flexibility progress and plan your future training schedule (Laboratory 6.1, p. 169). So, establish your stretching goals today and get started toward a lifetime of flexibility.

Summary

1. *Flexibility* is defined as the range of motion of a joint.
2. Improved flexibility results in the following benefits: increased joint mobility, prevention of low back problems, efficient body movement, and improved posture and personal appearance.
3. The five structural and physiological limits to flexibility are bone, muscle, structures within the joint capsule, the tendons that connect muscle to bones and connective tissue that surrounds joints, and skin.
4. If muscle spindles are suddenly stretched, they respond by initiating a stretch reflex that causes the muscle to contract. However, if the muscles and tendons are stretched slowly, the stretch reflex can be avoided.
5. Static stretches involve stretching a muscle to the limit of movement and holding the stretch for an extended period of time.
6. Proprioceptive neuromuscular facilitation combines stretching with alternating contraction and relaxation of muscles to improve flexibility.

Study Questions

1. Define the following terms:
   antagonist
   cartilage
   flexibility
   proprioceptive neuromuscular facilitation
2. Describe the difference in function between ligaments and tendons.
3. Compare static and ballistic stretching.
4. List three primary reasons why maintaining flexibility is important.
5. List all of the factors that limit flexibility. Which factors place the greatest limitations on flexibility?
6. Compare and contrast the two recommended methods of stretching.
7. Briefly outline the exercise prescription for improvement of flexibility.
8. Describe why the stretch reflex is counterproductive to stretching, and explain how this reflex can be avoided.

Suggested Reading

American College of Sports Medicine. The recommended quantity and quality of exercise for developing and maintaining cardiorespiratory and muscular fitness, and flexibility in healthy adults. *Medicine and Science in Sports and Exercise* 30:975–991, 1998.

Bishop, D. Warm up II: performance changes following active warm up and how to structure the warm up. *Sports Medicine* 33(7):483–498, 2003.

Blair, S. N., M. J. LaMonte, and M. Z. Nichaman. The evolution of physical activity recommendations: how much is enough? *American Journal of Clinical Nutrition* 79(5):913S–920S, 2004.

Guissard, N., and J. Duchateau. Effect of static stretch training on neural and mechanical properties of the human plantar-flexor muscles. *Muscle Nerve* 29(2):248–255, 2004.

Weldon, S. M., and R. H. Hill. The efficacy of stretching for prevention of exercise-related injury: A systematic review of the literature. *Manual Therapy* 8(3):141–150, 2003.

Wilmore, J., and D. Costill. *Physiology of Sport and Exercise.* 3rd Ed. Champaign, IL: Human Kinetics, 2004.

For links to the web sites below visit The Total Fitness and Wellness Website at www.aw-bc.com/powers.

About.com

Provides information about many aspects of fitness, health benefits of exercise, and wellness.

WebMD.com

General information about exercise, fitness, wellness. Great articles, instructional information, and updates.

ACSM.org

Comprehensive Web site providing information, articles, equipment recommendations, how-to articles, books, and position statements about all aspects of health and fitness.

References

1. Kubo, K., H. Kanehisa, Y. Kawakami, and T. Fukunaga. Influence of static stretching on viscoelastic properties of human tendon structures in vivo. *Journal of Applied Physiology* 90(2):520–526, 2001.

2. Guissard, N., and J. Duchateau. Effect of static stretch training on neural and mechanical properties of the human plantar-flexor muscles. *Muscle Nerve* 29(2):248–255, 2004.

3. McGill, S. M. Low back stability: From formal description to issues for performance and rehabilitation. *Exercise and Sport Sciences Review* 29(1):26–31, 2001.

4. American College of Sports Medicine. The recommended quantity and quality of exercise for developing and maintaining cardiorespiratory and muscular fitness, and flexibility in healthy adults. *Medicine and Science in Sports and Exercise* 30(6):975–991, 1998.

5. Thacker, S. B., J. Gilchrist, D. F. Stroup, and C. D. Kimsey. The impact of stretching on sports injury risk: A systematic review of the literature. *Medicine and Science in Sports Exercise* 36(3):371–378, 2004.

6. Reginster, J. Y., O. Bruyere, M. P. Lecart, and Y. Henrotin. Naturocetic (glucosamine and chondroitin sulfate) compounds as structure-modifying drugs in the treatment of osteoarthritis. *Current Opinion in Rheumatology* 15(5):651–655, 2003.

7. McAtee, Robert. *Facilitated Stretching,* 2nd ed. Champaign, IL: Human Kinetics, 1999.

8. Chalmers, G. Re-examination of the possible role of Golgi tendon organ and muscle spindle reflexes in proprioceptive neuromuscular facilitation muscle stretching. *Sports Biomechanics* 3(1):159–183, 2004.

9. Bentley, S. Exercise-induced muscle cramp. Proposed mechanisms and management. *Sports Medicine* 21(6): 409–420, 1996.

10. Plowman, S. A. Physical fitness and healthy low back function. *Research Digest*. The Presidents Council on Physical Fitness, 1(3); 2004.

11. Orloff, H. A., and C. M. Rapp. The effects of load carriage on spinal curvature and posture. *Spine* 29(12):1325–1329, 2004.

12. Anderson, B. D., and A. Spector. Introduction to Pilates-based rehabilitation. *Orthopedic and Physical Therapy Clinics of North America* 9(3); 396–410, 2000.

Flexibility Progression Log

NAME _____ **DATE** _____

The purpose of this log is to provide a record of progress in increasing flexibility in selected joints.

DIRECTIONS

Record the date, sets, and hold time for each of the exercises listed in the left column.

St/Hold = Sets and hold time

Example: 2/30 = 2 sets held for 30 seconds each.

DATE _____

Exercise	St/Hold	St/Hold	St/Hold	St/Hold	St/Hold	St/Hold	St/Hold
Lower leg stretch							
Inside leg stretch							
One-leg stretch							
Lower back stretch							
Chest stretch							
Side stretch							
Thigh stretch							
Spine twister							
Neck stretch							
Shin stretch							
Leg stretch							
Trunk twister							

Avoiding Harmful Stretches

NAME _____ DATE _____

There are some stretches once thought to improve flexibility that are now known to be potentially damaging to the musculoskeletal system. The common contraindicated exercises are listed here, along with alternative stretches that accomplish the same goal. Perform each of the substitute stretches instead of the contraindicated stretches. Hold stretches for 20-30 seconds, and repeat each exercise three times.

CONTRAINDICATED STRETCH

1. Arm circles (Palms down)

Purpose: To strengthen the muscles of the shoulder and upper back.

Problem: May result in irritation of the shoulder joint and, if circled forward and down, results in the use of the chest muscles instead of the back.

2. Knee Pull

Purpose: To stretch the buttocks and lower back.

Problem: Places unnecessary stress on the knee.

3. Deep Knee Bends

Purpose: To strengthen the knee extensors and stretch the hip flexors.

Problem: This exercise hyperflexes the knee.

4. Standing Toe Touch

Purpose: To stretch the lower back, hamstrings, and buttocks.

Problem: Hyperflexion of the knee can lead to ligament damage. If performed with the back flat, damage to the lower back can occur.

5. Neck Circle

Purpose: To stretch the neck muscles.

Problem: Hyperextension of the neck should be avoided. This can pinch arteries and nerves, as well as damage disks in the spine.

ALTERNATIVE STRETCH

Arm Circles (Palms up)

In a sitting position, turn the palms up and circle the arms backward.

Leg Pull

Lying on your back, pull one knee to your chest by pulling on the back of your leg just below the knee joint. Extend the knee and point your foot to the sky. Repeat on the other leg.

Lunges

While standing, step forward with one foot and touch the opposite knee to the floor. Bend the front knee to a 90° angle. Repeat with the opposite leg.

Sitting Hamstring Stretch

Sit at leg-length from a wall. With one foot against the wall and the other foot close to your buttock with a bent knee, bend forward keeping your lower back straight. Repeat on the other side.

Neck Stretches

In a sitting position, with your head and neck straight, move your head down to flex the neck, and return the head upright. Then, slowly turn your head from side to side as far as possible, attempting to point your chin to each shoulder.

(continued on next page)

1. Did each substitute stretch accomplish the same goal as the more harmful, contraindicated stretch?

2. Can you think of any other stretches that may cause damage to the musculoskeletal system? If so, is there an alternative stretch that is not harmful?

3. Adequate flexibility may help prevent or alleviate backaches associated with short, tight muscles. What stretching exercises would you recommend to a person suffering from backaches? How long should each stretch be held, and how often should they perform the stretching routine?

4. As you have learned in the text, flexibility is joint-specific. For the athletes/athletic maneuvers listed below, think of a sport- and joint-specific stretch that would be beneficial for each person or activity.

   Golfer: _____

   Baseball Pitcher: _____

   Football Quarterback: _____

   Tennis Serve: _____

   Track Sprinter: _____

   Distance cycling: _____

Here are some other tips to keep in mind as you improve your flexibility:

1. Avoid holding your breath as you stretch. Try to breathe as normally as possible.

2. Avoid full flexion of the knee or neck.

3. Avoid full extension of the knee, neck, or back.

4. Do not stretch any joint to the point that ligaments and joint capsules are stressed.

5. Practice extreme caution when using a partner to help with passive stretches.

6. Avoid forceful flexion and extension of the spine.

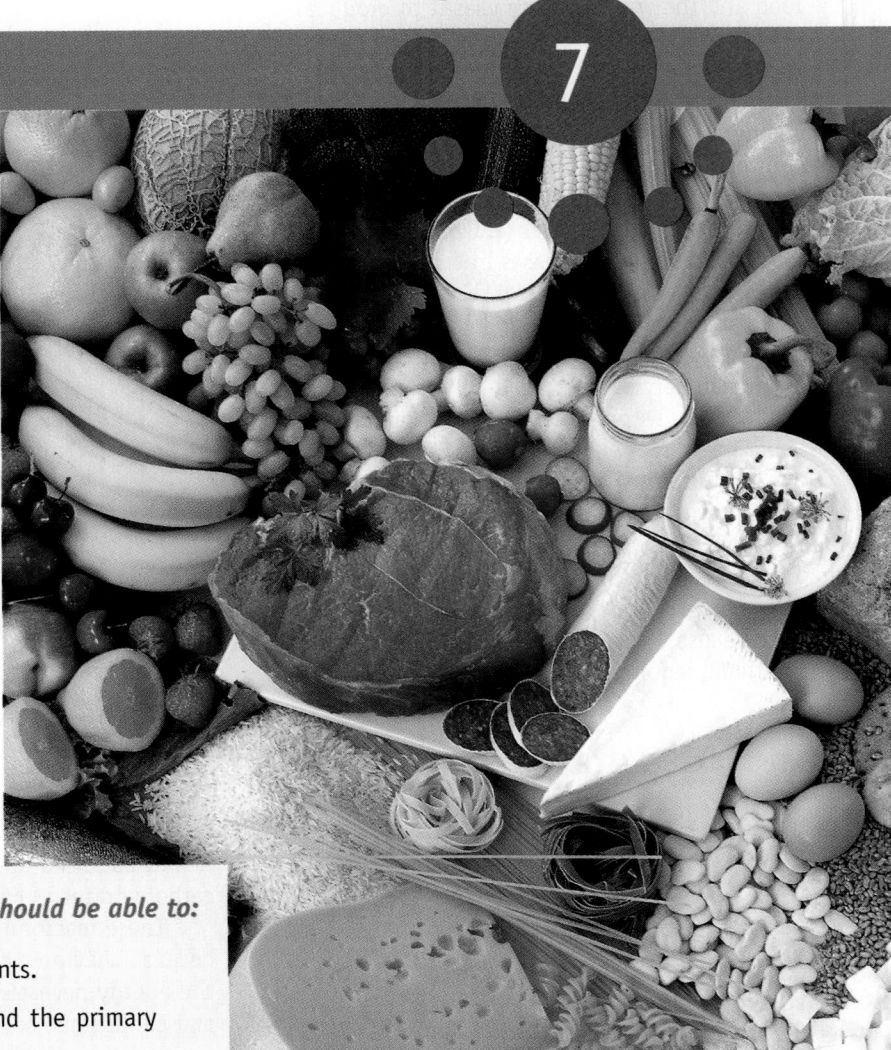

7

After studying this chapter, you should be able to:

1. Define macro- and micronutrients.

2. Describe the macronutrients and the primary functions of each.

3. Discuss the energy content of fats, carbohydrates, and proteins in the body.

4. Describe the micronutrients and the primary functions of each.

5. Discuss the value of water in the diet.

6. List the dietary guidelines for a well-balanced diet.

7. Define the term *calorie*.

8. Describe the need for protein, carbohydrate, and vitamins for physically active individuals.

9. Define the term *dietary supplement,* and discuss governmental regulations for marketing such supplements.

10. Discuss the benefits of irradiation of foods.

Nutrition, Health, and Fitness

Nutrition can be broadly defined as the study of food and the way the body uses it to produce energy and build or repair body tissues. Good nutrition means that an individual's diet supplies all of the essential foodstuffs required to maintain a healthy body. Although dietary deficiencies were once a problem in many industrialized countries, a primary danger associated with nutrition today is overeating.

Many diets are high in calories (A Closer Look), sugar, fats, and sodium, and diseases linked to these dietary excesses, such as cardiovascular disease, cancer, obesity, and diabetes, are the leading killers in the United States today (1). According to the U.S. Department of Health and Human Services, over one-half of all deaths in the United States are associated with health problems linked to poor nutrition (2). Nevertheless, through diet analysis and modification, it is possible to prevent many of these nutrition-related diseases. An elementary understanding of nutrition is therefore important for everyone. This chapter outlines the fundamental concepts of good nutrition and provides guidelines for developing a healthy diet. We also discuss how exercise training can modify nutritional requirements.

☀ Basic Nutrition

Substances in food that are necessary for good health are called **nutrients.** They can be divided into two categories: macronutrients and micronutrients. **Macronutrients,** which consist of carbohydrates, fats, and proteins, are necessary for building and maintaining body tissues and providing energy for daily activities. **Micronutrients** include all other substances in food, such as vitamins and minerals, that regulate the functions of the cells.

---

nutrients Substances in food that are necessary for good health.
macronutrients Carbohydrates, fats, and proteins, which are necessary for building and maintaining body tissues and providing energy for daily activities.
micronutrients Nutrients in food, such as vitamins and minerals, that regulate the functions of the cells.
carbohydrates One of the macronutrients; they are especially important during many types of physical activity because they are a key energy source for muscular contraction. Dietary sources of carbohydrates are breads, grains, fruits, and vegetables.
glucose The most noteworthy of the simple sugars because it is the only sugar molecule that can be used by the body in its natural form. All other carbohydrates must first be converted to glucose to be used for fuel.

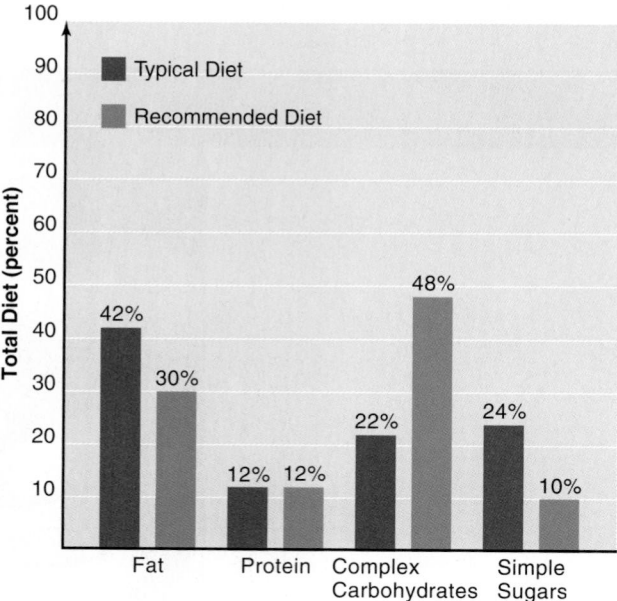

FIGURE 7.1
The recommended nutritionally balanced diet compared with the typical U.S. diet.
Source: Block, G. Junk foods account for 30% of caloric intake. *Journal of Food Composition and Analysis* 17:439-47, 2004.

MACRONUTRIENTS

A well-balanced diet is composed of approximately 58% carbohydrates, 30% fat, and 12% protein (Figure 7.1).

These macronutrients are called "fuel nutrients" because they are the only substances that can provide the energy necessary for bodily functions. Under normal conditions, carbohydrates and fats are the primary fuels used by the body to produce energy. The primary function of protein is to serve as the body's "building blocks" to repair tissues. However, when carbohydrate is in short supply or the body is under stress, protein can be used as a fuel.

Table 7.1 lists the major food sources and the energy contents of carbohydrates, proteins, and fats. Given the importance of dietary carbohydrates, proteins, and fats to health and fitness, we discuss these macronutrients in more detail.

CARBOHYDRATES **Carbohydrates** are especially important during many types of physical activity because they are a key energy source for muscular contraction. Dietary sources of carbohydrates are breads, grains, fruits, and vegetables. Carbohydrates can be divided into two major classes and several subclasses. (See Table 7.2.)

Simple Carbohydrates. Simple carbohydrates consist of one or two of the simple sugars shown in Table 7.2. **Glucose** is the most noteworthy of the simple sugars because it is the only sugar molecule that can be

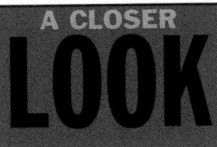

A CLOSER LOOK

What Is a Calorie?

A **calorie** is the unit of measure used to quantify the energy in foods or the energy expended by the body. Technically, a calorie is the amount of energy necessary to raise the temperature of 1 gram of water 1°C. The amount of energy contained in one serving of a particular food or the amount used during exercise is typically *several hundred thousand calories!* To simplify discussing such large numbers, we measure and report calories contained in foods and energy expended during exercise in thousands of calories, or kilocalories (kcals). For example, one serving of a particular food may contain 100,000 calories, or 100 kcals. Thus, when you read "100 calories" on a food label, this actually refers to 100 kcals. This textbook uses "calorie" and "kcal" interchangeably.

TABLE 7.1
Food Sources and Energy Content of the Macronutrients

Carbohydrate (4 calories/ gram)	Protein (4 calories/ gram)	Fat (9 calories/ gram)
Grains	Meats	Butter
Fruits	Fish	Margarine
Vegetables	Poultry	Oils
Concentrated sweets	Eggs	Shortening
Breads	Milk	Cream
Beans/peas	Beans	
	Rice	

TABLE 7.2
A Classification of Carbohydrates and the Sources of Each

Major Classifications of Carbohydrates	Subclasses of Carbohydrates	Food Sources
Simple carbohydrates (simple sugars)	Fructose	Fruits and honey
	Galactose	Breast milk
	Glucose	All sugars
	Lactose	Milk sugar
	Maltose	Malt sugar
	Sucrose	Table sugar
Complex carbohydrates	Starches	Potatoes, rice bread
		Fiber
		Fruits, vegetables, bread

---

used by the body in its natural form. To be used for fuel, all other carbohydrates must first be converted to glucose. After a meal, glucose is stored by skeletal muscles and the liver as **glycogen,** a molecule composed of a chain of glucose molecules. The glucose remaining in the blood thereafter is often converted to fat and stored in fat cells as a future source of energy.

The body requires glucose to function normally. Indeed, the central nervous system uses glucose almost exclusively for its energy needs. If dietary intake of carbohydrates is inadequate, the body must make glucose from protein. This is undesirable because it results in the breakdown of body protein for use as fuel. Dietary carbohydrate is not only important as a direct fuel source, but also important for its protein-sparing effect.

Other types of simple sugars include fructose, galactose, lactose, maltose, and sucrose. **Fructose,** or fruit sugar, is a naturally occurring sugar found in fruits and in honey. **Galactose** is a sugar found in the breast milk of humans and other mammals. **Lactose** (composed of galactose and glucose) and **maltose** (composed of two glucose molecules linked together)

---

calorie The unit of measure used to quantify food energy or the energy expended by the body. Technically, a calorie is the amount of energy necessary to raise the temperature of 1 gram of water 1°C.

glycogen The storage form of glucose in the liver and skeletal muscles.

fructose Also called *fruit sugar;* a naturally occurring sugar found in fruits and in honey.

galactose A simple sugar found in the breast milk of humans and other mammals.

lactose Also called *milk sugar;* a simple sugar found in milk products; it is composed of galactose and glucose.

maltose Also called *malt sugar;* a simple sugar found in grain products; it is composed of two glucose molecules linked together.

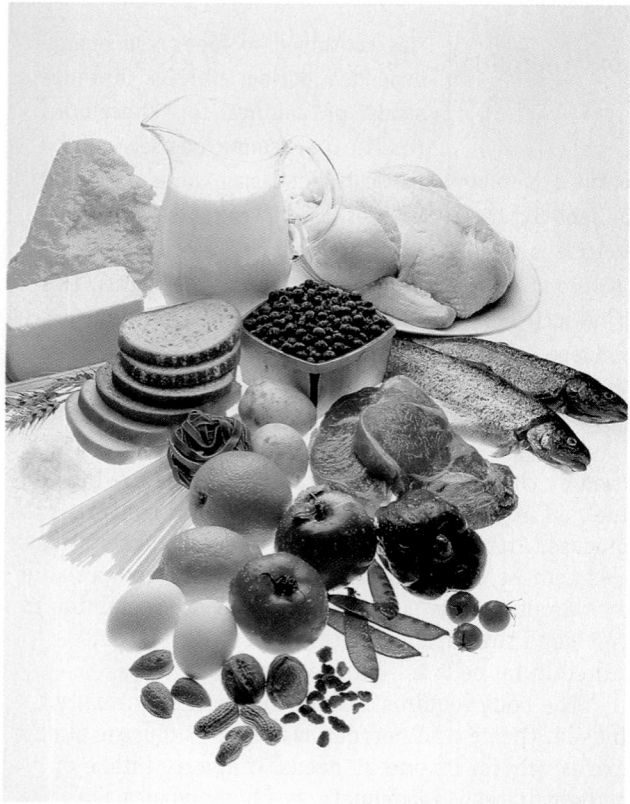

One of the main ingredients of a healthy lifestyle is a well balanced diet.

TABLE 7.3
Major Classes of Fats and
Common Examples of Each

Classes of Fat	Example
Simple fats	Triglyceride (one glycerol + three fatty acids)
Compound fats	Lipoprotein
Derived fats	Cholesterol

are best known as milk sugar and malt sugar, respectively. **Sucrose** (table sugar) is composed of glucose and fructose. A key point to remember about these simple sugars is that each must be converted to glucose before it can be used by the body.

Complex Carbohydrates. Complex carbohydrates provide both micronutrients and the glucose necessary

for producing energy. They are contained in starches and fiber. **Starches** are long chains of sugars commonly found in foods such as corn, grains, potatoes, peas, and beans. Starch is stored in the body as glycogen and, as previously discussed, is used for that sudden burst of energy we often need during physical activity. **Fiber** is a stringy, nondigestible carbohydrate found in whole grains, vegetables, and fruits in its primary form, cellulose. Because fiber is nondigestible, it is not a fuel source; nor does it provide micronutrients. It is, however, a key ingredient in a healthy diet.

In recent years, nutrition researchers have shown that dietary fiber provides bulk in the intestinal tract. This bulk aids in the formation and elimination of food waste products, thus reducing the time necessary for wastes to move through the digestive system and lowering the risk of colon cancer. Dietary fiber is also thought to be a factor in reducing the risk for coronary heart disease and breast cancer, and in controlling blood sugar in diabetics (3). Some types of fiber bind with cholesterol in the digestive tract and prevent its absorption into the blood, thereby reducing blood cholesterol levels.

Although a minimum of 25 grams of fiber are recommended on a daily basis, excessive amounts of fiber in the diet can cause intestinal discomfort and decreased absorption of calcium and iron into the blood (3). To increase the fiber in your diet, it is recommended that you:

- Eat a variety of foods.
- Eat at least five servings of fruits and vegetables and three to six servings of whole-grain breads, cereals, and legumes per day.
- Eat less processed food.
- Eat the skins of fruits and vegetables.
- Get your fiber from foods rather than pills or powders.
- Drink plenty of liquids.

sucrose Also called *table sugar;* a molecule composed of glucose and fructose.

complex carbohydrates Carbohydrates that provide both micronutrients and the glucose necessary for producing energy. They are contained in starches and fiber.

starches Long chains of sugars commonly found in foods such as corn, grains, potatoes, peas, and beans. Starch is stored in the body as glycogen and is used for that sudden burst of energy often needed during physical activity.

fiber A stringy, nondigestible carbohydrate found in whole grains, vegetables, and fruits in its primary form, cellulose.

TABLE 7.4
Classification of Fats According to Fatty Acid Type, and Their Dietary Sources and Effects on Cholesterol Levels

Type of Fatty Acid	Primary Sources	State at Room Temperature	Effect on Cholesterol
Monounsaturated	Canola* and olive oils; foods made from and prepared in them	Liquid	Lowers LDL; no effect on HDL
Polyunsaturated**	Soybean, safflower, corn, and cottonseed oils; foods made from and prepared in them	Liquid	Lowers both LDL and HDL
Saturated	Animal fat from red meat, whole milk, and butter; also, coconut and palm oils	Solid	Raises LDL and total cholesterol
Trans	Partially hydrogenated vegetable oils used in cooking, margarine, shortening, baked and fried foods, and snack foods	Semisolid	Raises LDL and total cholesterol

Many nutritionists consider canola oil the most healthful vegetable oil because it's low in saturated fat, high in monounsaturated fat, and has a moderate level of omega-3 polyunsaturated fat.

**Contains the omega-3 and omega-6 essential fatty acids that the human body can't make on its own.*

Source: Fats: The good, the bad, the trans. Health News, July 25, 1999, pp 1–2. Massachusetts Medical Society. Published by Englander Communications, LLC, an affiliate of Behavior Publications, Inc.

FAT   Fat is an efficient storage form for energy, because each gram of fat holds more than twice the energy content of either carbohydrate or protein (Table 7.1). Excess fat in the diet is stored in fat cells (called *adipose tissue*) located under the skin and around internal organs. Fat not only is derived from dietary sources, but also can be formed in the body from excess carbohydrate and protein in the diet. Although fat can be synthesized in the body, fat in the diet should not be totally eliminated. Indeed, dietary fat is the only source of linoleic and linolenic acids, fatty acids that are essential for normal growth and healthy skin.

Fat also gives protection to internal organs and assists in absorbing, transporting, and storing the fat-soluble vitamins A, D, E, and K. Fats are classified as simple, compound, or derived (Table 7.3). Let's discuss each of these subcategories of fat.

Simple Fats. The most common of the simple fats are **triglycerides**. Triglycerides constitute approximately 95% of the fats in the diet and are the storage form of body fat. This is the form of fat that is broken down and used to produce energy to power muscle contractions during exercise.

Fatty acids are the basic structural unit of triglycerides. Though important nutritionally because of their energy content, fatty acids contribute to cardiovascular disease through their effects on cholesterol. Based on structure, fatty acids are classified as monounsaturated, polyunsaturated, saturated, or trans. Table 7.4 lists the dietary sources and effects on cholesterol levels of the various types of fatty acids.

Monounsaturated and polyunsaturated fatty acids are both **unsaturated fatty acids,** which are found in plants (in peas, beans, grains, and vegetable oils) and are liquid at room temperature. Because monounsaturated fatty acids seem to lower bad cholesterol levels, they are thought to be the least harmful fatty acids to the cardiovascular system. Although polyunsaturated fatty acids were favored by nutritional researchers in the early 1980s, recent evidence suggests that polyunsaturated fatty acids may decrease levels of good cholesterol as well as bad cholesterol.

fat An efficient storage form for energy, because each gram of fat holds over twice the energy content of either carbohydrate or protein. Excess fat in the diet is stored in fat cells (called *adipose tissue*) located under the skin and around internal organs.

triglycerides The form of fat that is broken down and used to produce energy to power muscle contractions during exercise. Triglycerides constitute approximately 95% of the fats in the diet and are the storage form of body fat.

fatty acids The basic structural unit of triglycerides that are important nutritionally, not only because of their energy content, but also because they play a role in cardiovascular disease.

unsaturated fatty acid A type of fatty acid that comes primarily from plant sources and is liquid at room temperature.

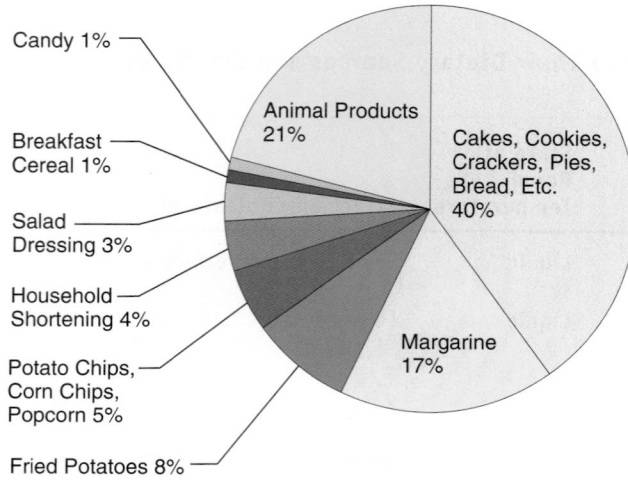

Candy 1%

Breakfast Cereal 1%

Salad Dressing 3%

Household Shortening 4%

Potato Chips, Corn Chips, Popcorn 5%

Fried Potatoes 8%

Animal Products 21%

Cakes, Cookies, Crackers, Pies, Bread, Etc. 40%

Margarine 17%

FIGURE 7.2
Major sources of trans fat in the diet.

One type of polyunsaturated fatty acid, called **omega-3 fatty acid,** has recently gained widespread attention. This fatty acid, which is found primarily in fresh or frozen mackerel, herring, tuna, and salmon, is reported to lower both blood cholesterol and triglycerides. However, omega-3 fatty acids are not present in canned fish because the canning process destroys the structure of these molecules. Some researchers have argued that one or two servings per week of fish containing omega-3 fatty acids reduces the risk of heart disease (4). Although this is an exciting possibility, more research is needed to confirm the claim.

omega-3 fatty acid A type of unsaturated fatty acid that lowers both blood cholesterol and triglycerides and is found primarily in fresh or frozen mackerel, herring, tuna, and salmon.

saturated fatty acid A type of fatty acid that comes primarily from animal sources (meat and dairy products) and is solid at room temperature.

trans fatty acid A type of fatty acid that increases cholesterol in the blood and is a major contributor to heart disease.

lipoproteins Combinations of protein, triglycerides, and cholesterol in the blood that are important because of their role in promoting heart disease.

derived fats A class of fats that do not contain fatty acids but are classified as fats because they are not soluble in water.

cholesterol A type of derived fat in the body which is necessary for cell and hormone synthesis. Can be acquired through the diet or can be made by the body.

Saturated fatty acids, which generally come from animal sources (meat and dairy products), are solid at room temperature. However, some saturated fatty acids, including coconut oil, come from plant sources. It is well accepted that saturated fatty acids increase blood levels of cholesterol. High cholesterol levels, in turn, promote the buildup in the coronary arteries of fatty plaque, which can eventually lead to heart disease (Chapter 9).

Trans fatty acids, which tend to have more complex structures than the other classes of fatty acids, tend to raise total cholesterol in the blood. Trans fatty acids are found in baked and fried foods.

In 2003, the FDA began requiring manufacturers to list trans fat on the Nutrition Facts panel of foods and some dietary supplements by 2006. With this rule, consumers have additional information to make healthier food choices that could lower their intake of trans fat as part of a heart-healthy diet. The FDA estimates that by three years from the effective date, trans fat labeling could prevent from 600 to 1,200 cases of chronic heart disease (CHD) and 250 to 500 deaths each year (17). Figure 7.2 shows major sources of trans fat in the diet.

Compound Fats. For health considerations, the most important compound fats are the **lipoproteins.** These molecules are combinations of protein, triglycerides, and cholesterol. Although lipoproteins exist in several forms, the two primary types are low-density lipoproteins (LDL cholesterol) and high-density lipoproteins (HDL cholesterol). LDL cholesterol consists of a limited amount of protein and triglycerides but contains large amounts of cholesterol. It is thus associated with promoting the fatty plaque buildup in the arteries of the heart that is the primary cause of heart disease. In contrast, HDLs are primarily composed of protein, have limited amounts of cholesterol, and are associated with a low risk of heart disease. We discuss HDL and LDL cholesterol again in Chapter 9.

Derived Fats. Even though they do not contain fatty acids, **derived fats** are classified as fats because they are not water soluble. The best example of a derived fat is **cholesterol,** which is present in many foods from animal sources, including meats, shellfish, and dairy products. Although a diet high in cholesterol increases your risk of heart disease, some cholesterol is essential for normal body function. Indeed, cholesterol is a constituent of cells and is used to manufacture certain types of hormones (e.g., male and female sex hormones).

Protein. The primary role of dietary protein is to serve as the structural unit to build and repair body tissues. Proteins are also important for numerous other bodily functions, including the synthesis of enzymes, hormones, and antibodies. These compounds regulate body metabolism and provide protection from disease.

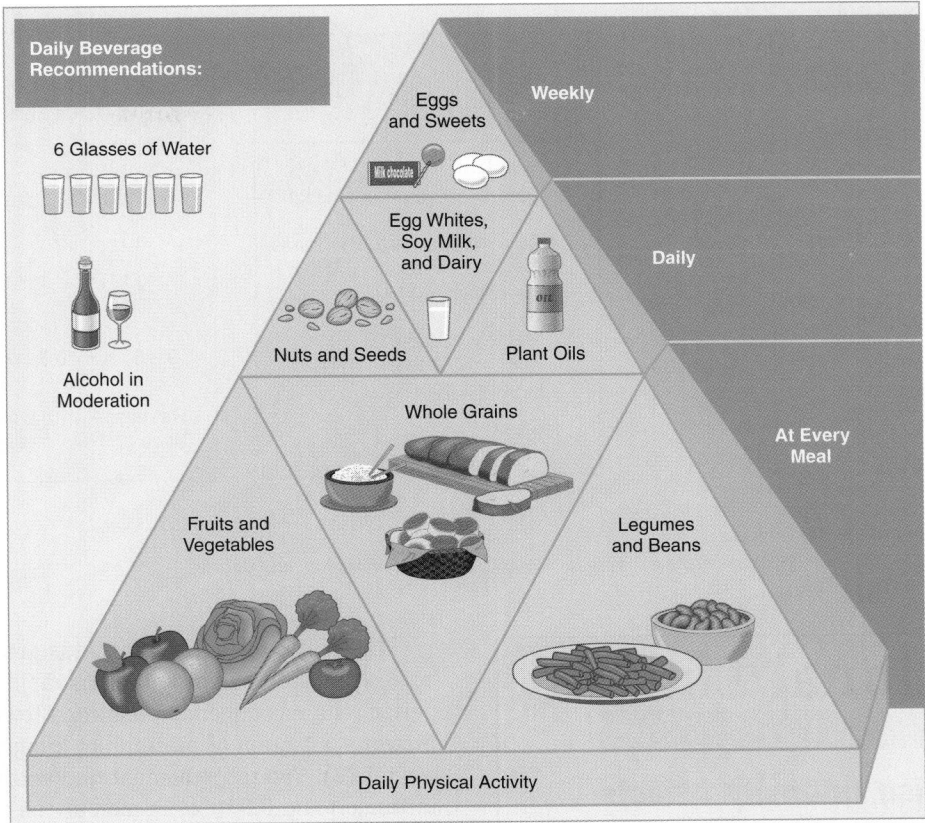

Daily Beverage Recommendations:

6 Glasses of Water

Alcohol in Moderation

Weekly

Eggs and Sweets

Egg Whites, Soy Milk, and Dairy

Daily

Nuts and Seeds

Plant Oils

Whole Grains

At Every Meal

Fruits and Vegetables

Legumes and Beans

Daily Physical Activity

FIGURE 7.3
The food guide pyramid for vegetarian meal planning. Eating a healthful diet requires that certain combinations of foods are consumed daily in order to consume all of the essential amino acids. Planning meals to conform to the proportions shown in the pyramid will result in combinations of foods that enable vegetarians to avoid protein deficiencies.

As mentioned earlier, proteins are not usually a major fuel source. Nevertheless, under conditions of low carbohydrate intake (e.g., dieting), proteins can be converted to glucose and used as fuel. During periods of adequate dietary carbohydrate intake, excess proteins consumed in the diet are converted to fats and stored in adipose tissue as an energy reserve.

The basic structural units of proteins are called **amino acids.** Twenty different amino acids exist and can be linked end-to-end in various combinations to create different proteins with unique functions. The body can make 11 of these amino acids; because they are not needed in the diet, they are referred to as **nonessential amino acids.** The remaining nine amino acids cannot be manufactured by the body; because they must be obtained in the diet, they are called **essential amino acids.**

Complete proteins contain all of the essential amino acids and are present only in foods of animal origin (meats and dairy products). **Incomplete proteins** are missing one or more of the essential amino acids and are present in numerous vegetable sources. There-

fore, vegetarians must be careful to combine a variety of foods in their diet in order to get all of the essential amino acids. (See Figure 7.3 above.)

amino acids The basic structural unit of proteins. Twenty different amino acids exist and can be linked end-to-end in various combinations to create different proteins with unique functions.
nonessential amino acids Eleven amino acids that the body can make and are therefore not necessary in the diet.
essential amino acids Amino acids that cannot be manufactured by the body and must therefore be consumed in the diet.
complete proteins Contain all the essential amino acids and are found only in foods of animal origin (meats and dairy products).
incomplete proteins Proteins that are missing one or more of the essential amino acids; can be found in numerous vegetable sources.

	RDA (g/kg)*
Adult Males	= 0.9
Adult Females	= 0.8
*The RDA is 10 g/day higher during pregnancy, 15 g/day higher during the first six months of lactation, and 12 g/day higher during the remainder of lactation	

Calculating Your Protein RDA
1. Determine your body weight
2. Convert pounds to kilograms (pounds divided by 2.2 lb/kg equals kilograms)
3. Multiply by 0.8 or 0.9 g/kg (adult RDA) to get an RDA in grams per day

40 Grams

Example (Adult Female)
1. Weight = 110 lbs
2. 110 ÷ 2.2 lb/kg = 50 kg
3. 50 Kg × 0.8 g/kg = 40g
Results: A 110-lb female would have an RDA of 40g of protein

FIGURE 7.4
Estimated daily protein needs for adults.
Source: An Invitation to Health: The Power of Prevention, 6th ed., by D. R. Hales 0805354808. Reprinted with permission of Brooks/Cole, a division of Thomson Learning.

Nutritional Links
TO HEALTH AND FITNESS

How Exercise Intensity Affects Fuel Use by the Muscle

The intensity of exercise is the prime determinant of whether fat or carbohydrate is the primary fuel used during exercise. Of course, the intensity of exercise also determines the length of time that you can exercise continuously. Thus, both intensity and duration of exercise will govern the predominant fuel used during an exercise session. The following table illustrates how intensity affects fuel use during endurance-type exercises.

Exercise Intensity	Fuel Used by Muscle
Less than 30% $\dot{V}O_{2max}$	Mainly muscle fat stores
40–60% $\dot{V}O_{2max}$	Fat and carbohydrate equally
75% $\dot{V}O_{2max}$	Mainly carbohydrate
Greater than 80% $\dot{V}O_{2max}$	Nearly 100% carbohydrate

vitamins Small molecules that play a key role in many bodily functions, including the regulation of growth and metabolism. They are classified according to whether they are soluble in water or fat.

The dietary need for protein is greatest during the adolescent years, when growth is rapid. During this period, the recommended dietary allowance (RDA) for proteins is 1 gram of protein per kilogram of body weight (3). The recommendation decreases to 0.8 g/kg in women and 0.9 g/kg in men at the end of adolescence (Figure 7.4). Because the average person in industrialized countries consumes more than enough protein in the diet, the nutritional problem associated with protein intake is one of excess. Protein foods from animal sources are often high in fat (and high in calories), which can lead to an increased risk of heart disease, cancer, and obesity.

MICRONUTRIENTS

The category of nutrients referred to as micronutrients consists of vitamins and minerals. Functionally, micronutrients are as important as macronutrients and are required for sustaining life. Although they do not supply energy, they are essential to the breakdown of the macronutrients.

VITAMINS **Vitamins** are small molecules that play a key role in many bodily functions, including the regulation of growth and metabolism. They are classified according to whether they are soluble in water or fat. The class of vitamins called *water-soluble vitamins* consists of several B complex vitamins and vitamin C. Because they are soluble in water, these vitamins can be eliminated from the body by the kidneys. The *fat-soluble vitamins* are soluble in fat only and consist of vitamins A, D, E, and K. Because they are stored in body fat, it is possible for these vitamins to accumulate in the body to toxic levels. Table 7.5 on p. 182 lists the dietary sources of both water-soluble and fat-soluble vitamins.

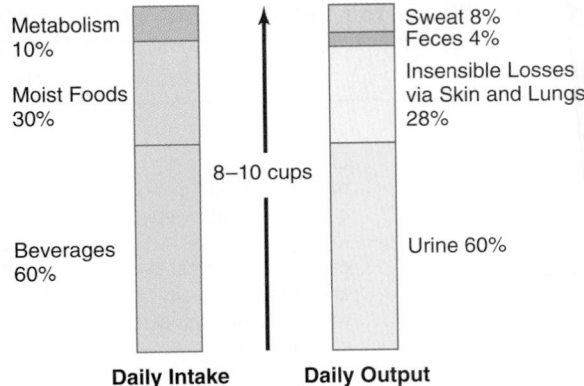

Daily Water Balance in the Body

Metabolism 10%

Moist Foods 30%

Beverages 60%

Daily Intake

8–10 cups

Sweat 8%
Feces 4%

Insensible Losses via Skin and Lungs 28%

Urine 60%

Daily Output

FIGURE 7.5
Daily water intake and output by the body.

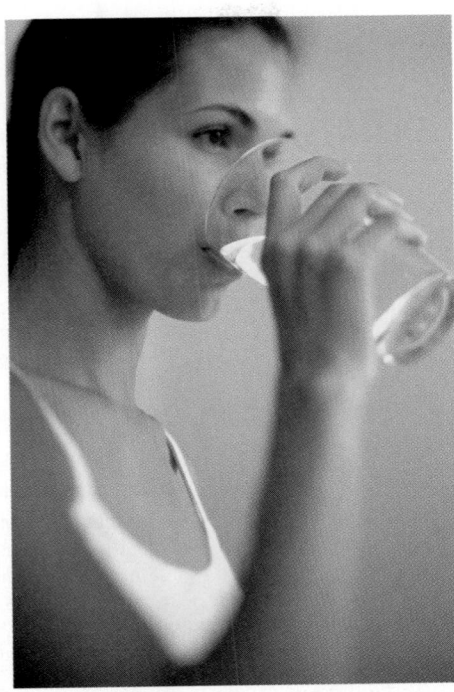

Although often overlooked nutritionally, water should be a key ingredient in any diet.

Most vitamins cannot be manufactured in the body and must therefore be consumed in the diet. The exceptions to this rule are vitamins A, D, and K, which can be produced by the body in small quantities. Vitamins in food can be destroyed in the process of cooking, so eating vegetables raw or lightly steamed is best for retaining their maximum nutritional value. Vitamins exist in almost all foods, and a balanced diet supplies all of the vitamins essential to body function.

Recent research indicates a new function for some vitamins and minerals as protectors against tissue damage (3, 5). This has important implications for individuals engaged in an exercise program. This potential new role for micronutrients is discussed later in this chapter.

MINERALS   **Minerals** are chemical elements such as sodium and calcium that are required by the body for normal function. Like vitamins, minerals are contained in many foods and play important roles in regulating key body functions, such as the conduction of nerve impulses, muscular contraction, enzyme function, and maintenance of water balance. Minerals serve a structural function as well; calcium, phosphorus, and fluoride all are important constituents of bones and teeth.

Table 7.6 on p. 184 illustrates the nutritionally important minerals and their functions. Three of the most widely recognized minerals are calcium, iron, and sodium. Calcium is important in its role in bone formation. A deficiency of calcium contributes to the devel-

opment of the bone disease called osteoporosis. A deficiency of dietary iron may lead to iron-deficiency anemia, which results in chronic fatigue. High sodium intake has been associated with hypertension, a major risk factor for heart disease.

WATER

Approximately 60–70% of the body is water. Because water is involved in all vital processes in the body, it is considered the nutrient of greatest concern to the physically active individual. An individual performing heavy exercise in a hot, humid environment can lose 1 to 3 liters of water per hour through sweating (6). A loss of 5% of body water causes fatigue, weakness, and the inability to concentrate; a loss of 15% can be fatal. Water is important for temperature control of the body, absorption and digestion of foods, formation of blood, and elimination of wastes. Chapter 11 provides guidelines for maintaining proper hydration during exercise training.

Water is contained in almost all foods, especially fruits and vegetables. Combining the water contained in foods and that consumed as beverages, you should consume the equivalent of 8–10 cups of water per day. This does not account for conditions that cause excess fluid loss such as excess sweating, donating blood, diarrhea, or vomiting. Figure 7.5 illustrates the balance between the body's sources of water intake and routes of water output.

minerals Chemical elements (e.g., sodium and calcium) that are required by the body for normal functioning.

TABLE 7.5
Vitamins: Where You Get Them and What They Do

Vitamin	Best Sources	Main Roles	Deficiency Symptoms	Risks of Megadoses
Fat Soluble				
A	Liver; eggs; cheese; butter; fortified margarine and milk; yellow, orange, and dark-green vegetables and fruits (e.g., carrots, broccoli, spinach, cantaloupe)	Assists in the formation and maintenance of healthy skin, hair, and mucous membranes; aids in the ability to see in dim light (night vision); needed for proper bone growth, teeth development, and reproduction.	Night blindness; rough skin and mucous membranes; infection of mucous membranes; drying of the eyes; impaired growth of bones and tooth enamel	Blurred vision, loss of appetite, headaches, skin rashes, nausea, diarrhea, hair loss, menstrual irregularities, extreme fatigue, joint pain, liver damage, insomnia, abnormal bone growth, injury to brain and nervous system
D	Fortified milk; egg yolk; liver; tuna: salmon; cod-liver oil. Made in skin in sunlight.	Aids in the formation and maintenance of bones and teeth; assists in the absorption and use of calcium and phosphorus.	In children, rickets; stunted bone growth, bowed legs, malformed teeth, protruding abdomen; in adults, osteomalacia, softening of the bones leading to shortening and fractures, muscle spasms, and twitching	In infants, calcium deposits in kidneys and excessive calcium in blood; in adults, calcium deposits throughout body, deafness, nausea, loss of appetite, kidney stones, fragile bones, high blood pressure, high blood cholesterol
E	Vegetable oils; margarine; wheat germ; whole-grain cereals and bread; liver; dried beans; green leafy vegetables	Aids in the formation of red blood cells, muscles, and other tissues; protects vitamin A and essential fatty acids from oxidation.	Prolonged impairment of fat absorption; lysis of red blood cells; nerve destruction	None definitely known. Reports of headache, blurred vision, extreme fatigue, muscle weakness; can destroy some vitamin K made in the gut.
K	Green leafy vegetables; cabbage; cauliflower; peas; potatoes; liver; cereals. Except in newborns, made by bacteria in human intestine.	Aids in the synthesis of substances needed for blood clotting; helps maintain normal bone metabolism.	Hemorrhage, especially in newborn infants	Jaundice in babies; anemia in laboratory animals
Water Soluble				
Thiamin (B_1)	Pork (especially ham); liver; oysters; whole-grain and enriched cereals, pasta, and bread; wheat germ; oatmeal; peas; lima beans	Helps release energy from carbohydrates; aids in the synthesis of an important nervous system chemical.	Beriberi: mental confusion, muscular weakness, swelling of the heart, leg cramps	None known. However, because B vitamins are interdependent, excess of one may produce deficiency of others.
Riboflavin (B_2)	Liver; milk; meat; dark-green vegetables; eggs; whole-grain and enriched cereals, pasta, and bread; dried beans and peas	Helps release energy from carbohydrates, proteins, and fats; aids in the maintenance of mucous membranes.	Skin disorders, especially around nose and lips; cracks at corners of mouth; sensitivity of eyes to light	None known. See Thiamin.
Niacin (B_3, nicotinamide, nicotinic acid)	Liver; poultry; meat; fish; eggs; whole-grain and enriched cereals, pasta, and bread; nuts; dried peas and beans	Participates with thiamin and riboflavin in facilitating energy production in cells	Pellagra, skin disorders, diarrhea, mental confusion, irritability, mouth swelling, smooth tongue	Duodenal ulcer, abnormal liver function, elevated blood sugar, excessive uric acid in blood, possibly leading to gout, skin flushing at >100 mg

TABLE 7.5
Vitamins: Where You Get Them and What They Do (continued)

Vitamin	Best Sources	Main Roles	Deficiency Symptoms	Risks of Megadoses
Pantothenic acid	Mushrooms; liver; broccoli; eggs	Molecule involved in energy metabolism and fat storage and breakdown	Tingling in hands, fatigue, headache, nausea	None
Biotin	Cheese; egg yolks; cauliflower; peanut butter; liver	Molecule involved in glucose production; fat storage	Dermatitis, tongue soreness, anemia, depression	Unknown
Choline	Lettuce; peanuts; liver, cauliflower	Regeneration of amino acids; nerve function	Liver malfunction	Nausea, diarrhea, vomiting
B_6 (pyridoxine)	Whole-grain (but not enriched) cereals and bread; liver; avocados; spinach; green beans; bananas; fish; poultry meats; nuts; potatoes; green leafy vegetables	Aids in the absorption and metabolism of proteins; helps the body use fats; assists in the formation of red blood cells.	Skin disorders, cracks at corners of mouth, smooth tongue, convulsions, dizziness, nausea, anemia, kidney stones	Dependency on high dose, leading to deficiency symptoms when one returns to normal amounts
B_{12} (cobalamin)	Only in animal foods; liver; kidneys; meat; fish; eggs; milk; oysters; nutritional yeast	Aids in the formation of red blood cells; assists in the building of genetic material; helps the functioning of the nervous system.	Pernicious anemia, anemia, pale skin and mucous membranes, numbness and tingling in fingers and toes that may progress to loss of balance and weakness and pain in arms and legs	None known
Folacin (folic acid)	Liver; kidneys; dark-green leafy vegetables; wheat germ; dried beans and peas. Stored in the body, so daily consumption is not crucial.	Acts with B_{12} in synthesis of genetic material; aids in the formation of hemoglobin in red blood cells.	Megaloblastic anemia; enlarged red blood cells, smooth tongue, diarrhea; during pregnancy, deficiency may cause loss of the fetus or fetal abnormalities. Women on oral contraceptives may need extra folacin.	Body stores it, so it is potentially hazardous. Can mask a B_2 deficiency. Diarrhea; insomnia
C (ascorbic acid)	Citrus fruits; tomatoes; strawberries, melon; green peppers; potatoes; dark-green vegetables	Aids in the formation of collagen; helps maintain capillaries, bones, and teeth; helps protect other vitamins from oxidation; may block formation of cancer-causing nitrosamines.	Scurvy; bleeding gums; degenerating muscles; wounds that don't heal; loose teeth; brown, dry, rough skin. Early symptoms include loss of appetite, irritability, weight loss.	Dependency on high doses, possibly precipitating symptoms of scurvy when withdrawn (especially in infants if megadoses taken during pregnancy); kidney and bladder stones; diarrhea; urinary tract irritation; increased tendency for blood to clot; breakdown of red blood cells in persons with certain common genetic disorders

Source: Reprinted from Jane Brody's Nutrition Book, *with permission of W. W. Norton & Company, Inc. Copyright © 1981 by Jane E. Brody.*

TABLE 7.6
Minerals: Where You Get Them and What They Do

Best Sources	Main Roles	Deficiency Symptoms	Risks of Megadoses
Macrominerals			
Calcium			
Milk and milk products; sardines; canned salmon eaten with bones; dark-green, leafy vegetables; citrus fruits; dried beans and peas	Building bones and teeth and maintaining bone strength; muscle contraction; maintaining cell membranes; blood clotting; absorption of B_2; activation of enzymes	In children: distorted bone growth (rickets); in adults: loss of bone (osteoporosis) and increased susceptibility to fractures	Drowsiness; extreme lethargy; impaired absorption of iron, zinc, and manganese; calcium deposits in tissues throughout body, mimicking cancer on X-ray
Phosphorus			
Meat; poultry; fish; eggs, dried beans and peas; milk and milk products; phosphates in processed foods, especially soft drinks	Building bones and teeth; release of energy from carbohydrates, proteins, and fats; formation of genetic material, cell membranes, and many enzymes	Weakness; loss of appetite; malaise; bone pain. Dietary shortages uncommon, but prolonged use of antacids can cause deficiency	Distortion of calcium-to-phosphorus ratio, creating relative deficiency of calcium
Magnesium			
Green, leafy, vegetables (eaten raw); nuts (especially almonds and cashews); soybeans; seeds; whole grains	Building bones; manufacture of proteins; release of energy from muscle glycogen; conduction of nerve impulse to muscles; adjustment to cold	Muscular twitching and tremors; irregular heartbeat; insomnia; muscle weakness; leg and foot cramps; shaky hands	Disturbed nervous system function because the calcium-to-magnesium ratio is unbalanced; catharsis: hazard to persons with poor kidney function
Potassium			
Orange juice; bananas; dried fruits; meats; bran; peanut butter; dried beans and peas; potatoes; coffee; tea; cocoa	Muscle contraction; maintenance of fluid and electrolyte balance in cells; transmission of nerve impulses; release of energy from carbohydrates, proteins, and fats	Abnormal heart rhythm; muscular weakness; lethargy; kidney and lung failure	Excessive potassium in blood, causing muscular paralysis and abnormal heart rhythms
Sulfur			
Beef; wheat germ; dried beans and peas; peanuts; clams	In every cell as part of sulfur-containing amino acids; forms bridges between molecules to create firm proteins of hair, nails, and skin	None known in humans	Unknown
Chlorine			
Table salt and other naturally occurring salts	Regulation of balance of body fluids and acids and bases; activation of enzyme in saliva; part of stomach acid	Disturbed acid-base balance in body fluids (very rare)	Disturbed acid-base balance

TABLE 7.6
Minerals: Where You Get Them and What They Do (continued)

Best Sources	Main Roles	Deficiency Symptoms	Risks of Megadoses
Trace Minerals			
Iron			
Liver; kidneys; red meats; egg yolk; green, leafy vegetables; dried fruits; dried beans and peas; potatoes; blackstrap molasses; enriched and whole-grain cereals	Formation of hemoglobin in blood and myoglobin in muscles, which supply oxygen to cells; part of several enzymes and proteins	Anemia, with fatigue, weakness, pallor, and shortness of breath	Toxic buildup in liver, pancreas, and heart
Copper			
Oysters; nuts; cocoa powder; beef and pork liver; kidneys; dried beans; corn-oil margarine	Formation of red blood cells; part of several respiratory enzymes	In animals: anemia; faulty development of bone and nervous tissue; loss of elasticity in tendons and major arteries; abnormal lung development; abnormal structure and pigmentation of hair	Violent vomiting and diarrhea. Cooking acid foods in unlined copper pots can lead to toxic accumulation of copper.
Zinc			
Meat; liver; eggs; poultry; seafood; milk; whole grains	Constituent of about 100 enzymes	Delayed wound healing; diminished taste sensation; loss of appetite; in children: failure to grow and mature sexually; prenatally: abnormal brain development	Nausea, vomiting; anemia; bleeding in stomach; premature birth and stillbirth; abdominal pain; fever. Can aggravate marginal copper deficiency. May produce atherosclerosis.
Iodine			
Seafood; seaweed; iodized salt; sea salt	Part of thyroid hormones; essential for normal reproduction	Goiter (enlarged thyroid with low hormone production); newborns: cretinism, retarded growth, protruding abdomen, swollen features	Not known to be a problem, but could cause iodine poisoning or sensitivity reaction.
Fluorine			
Fish; tea; most meats; fluoridated water; foods grown with or cooked in fluoridated water	Formation of strong, decay-resistant teeth; maintenance of bone strength	Excessive dental decay; possibly osteoporosis	Mottling of teeth and bones; in larger doses, a deadly poison
Manganese			
Nuts; whole grains; vegetables and fruits; tea; instant coffee; cocoa powder	Functioning of central nervous system; normal bone structure; reproduction; part of important enzymes	None known in human beings; in animals: poor reproduction; retarded growth; birth defects; abnormal bone development	Masklike facial expression; blurred speech; involuntary laughing; spastic gait; hand tremors

Source: Adapted from Jane Brody's Nutrition Book, *with the permission of W. W. Norton & Company, Inc. Copyright © 1981 by Jane E. Brody.*

☼ IN SUMMARY

- Nutrition is the study of food and its relationship to health and disease.

- A well-balanced diet is composed of approximately 58% complex carbohydrates, 30% fat, and 12% protein; collectively these three components of the diet are called macronutrients.

- The calorie is a unit of measure for quantifying the energy in food or the energy expended by the body.

- Carbohydrates constitute a primary source of fuel for the body. Simple carbohydrates consist of both simple sugars and sugars composed of two simple sugars. Complex carbohydrates include starches (long energy-yielding chains of sugars) and fiber (long nondigestible but essential chains of sugars).

- Fat is an efficient storage form for energy that can either come directly from the diet or be produced from excess carbohydrate and protein in the diet. Fats are either simple fats (e.g., triglycerides), compound fats (e.g., lipoproteins), or derived fats (e.g., cholesterol).

- Protein consumed in the diet serves as the structural unit for building and repairing cells in the body. Proteins are composed of amino acids, which are either made by the body (nonessential amino acids) or must be consumed in the diet (essential amino acids).

- Vitamins serve many important functions in the body. The water-soluble vitamins include several B complex vitamins and vitamin C. The fat-soluble vitamins are vitamins A, D, E, and K.

- Minerals are chemical elements in foods that, like vitamins, play important roles in many body functions.

- Water is the nutrient of greatest concern to physically active individuals because approximately 60% of body weight is water. It is recommended that people consume 8–10 cups of fluids each day.

☼ Guidelines for a Healthy Diet

Several national health agencies have suggested guidelines for healthy diets. Although they don't agree on all points, in essence, they do agree on the following, as suggested by the U.S. Department of Agriculture's "Dietary Guidelines for Americans, 2000":

Aim for fitness . . .

- Aim for a healthy weight.
- Be physically active each day.

Build a healthy base . . .

- Let the Pyramid guide your food choices.
- Choose a variety of grains daily, especially whole grains.
- Choose a variety of fruits and vegetables daily.
- Keep food safe to eat.

Choose sensibly . . .

- Choose a diet that is low in saturated fat and cholesterol and moderate in total fat.
- Choose beverages and foods to moderate your intake of sugars.
- Choose and prepare foods with less salt.
- If you choose to drink alcoholic beverages, do so in moderation.

The following sections provide general rules for selection of the macro- and micronutrients to meet the goals of a healthy diet. In addition, we discuss how to critically analyze your diet using a dietary record.

NUTRIENTS

The general rule for meeting the body's need for macronutrients is that an individual should consume approximately 58% of needed calories from carbohydrates (48% complex carbohydrates and 10% simple sugars), 30% or less in fats (approximately 10% saturated and 20% unsaturated fats), and 12% in proteins (3). Again, the daily protein requirement for adults is approximately 0.8 gram of protein per kilogram (2.2 lbs) of body weight.

To meet the need for micronutrients, the National Academy of Science (7) has established guidelines concerning the quantities of each micronutrient required to meet the minimum needs of most individuals. These Recommended Dietary Allowances (RDAs) are contained in Table 7.7 on p. 188.

Once you know the recommended daily requirements for nutrients, the key question is, "How do I choose foods to meet these goals?" Previous dietary guidelines suggested choosing foods from four basic food groups: fruits and vegetables; poultry, fish, meat, and eggs; beans, grains, and nuts; and dairy products. Although these guidelines are still generally acceptable, they do not represent the most desirable proportions of different foods. Government health agencies responsible for setting nutritional guidelines (7) have altered their recommendations about how we should choose foods from these groups. Figure 7.6 on p. 190 illustrates these latest recommendations for a healthy diet using the "eating-right pyramid."

The use of the eating-right pyramid in forming a diet accomplishes two important goals. First, the relative proportions of foods known to promote disease are minimized. Second, "nutrient-dense" foods—that is,

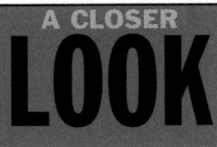

A CLOSER LOOK

Recommended Dietary Allowances of Nutrients

Recommended Dietary Allowances (also known as RDAs) are the daily amounts of the different food nutrients the National Academy of Sciences deems adequate for healthy individuals. Great effort has been made over the last few years to define these amounts more precisely, and an updated list of nutrients has now been published (7).

Over the past decade our increased knowledge about nutritional needs and the boom in the use of supplements have prompted the Academy to revise the way in which the values are reported. People now ask, "What are the minimal amounts of nutrients I need?" and "What are the maximal amounts that are safe?"

Even today, RDAs for some nutrients are not known. Thus, the Academy has changed the way in which recommendations are reported. In 1997 they issued several indices to guide people in monitoring their diets. They refer to these indices as Dietary Reference Intakes (DRIs). The new DRIs are divided into four categories, each of which addresses a different nutritional issue. (See the figure below.) The new DRIs are:

- **Recommended Dietary Allowance (RDA):** Unlike their predecessors, these RDAs are the amount of nutrient that will meet the needs of almost every healthy person in a specific age and gender group. Also, these RDAs are meant to reduce disease risk, not just prevent deficiency.

- **Adequate Intake (AI):** This value is used when the RDA is not known because the scientific data aren't strong enough to produce a specific recommendation, yet there is enough evidence to give a general guideline. Thus, it is an "educated guess" at what the RDA would be if it were known.

- **Estimated Average Requirement (EAR):** This is a value that is estimated to provide one-half of the RDA for that nutrient. It is primarily used to establish the RDA. In addition, it is used for evaluating and planning the diets of large groups of people (such as the army), not individuals.

- **Tolerable Upper Intake Level (UL):** This is the maximal amount that a person can take without risking "adverse health effects." Anything above this amount might result in toxicity. In most cases this number refers to the **total** intake of the nutrient—from food, fortified foods, and nutritional supplements.

The new guidelines have changed the categorization of nutrients to more closely group them according to the functional properties of each. The following list shows the groups, the year of the latest update, and the nutrients in each.

- **Micronutrients (2001):** Vitamin A, vitamin K, arsenic, boron, chromium, copper, iodine, iron, manganese, molybdenum, nickel, silicon, vanadium, and zinc

- **The B Vitamins and Choline (2000):** Thiamin (B_1), riboflavin (B_2), niacin (B_3), vitamin B_6, folate, vitamin B_{12}, pantothenic acid, biotin, and choline

- **Antioxidants (2000):** Vitamin C, vitamin E, selenium, and carotenoids

- **Calcium and Related Nutrients (1999);** Calcium, phosphorus, magnesium, vitamin D, and fluoride

Source: National Academy of Sciences. *Dietary Reference Intakes: Applications in Dietary Assessment.* Washington, DC: National Academy Press, 2001.

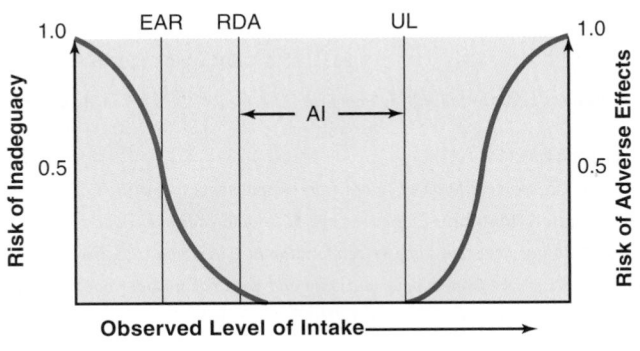

TABLE 7.7
Recommended Dietary Allowances of Selected Micronutrients (with upper limits in parentheses) Revised 2001

Life Stage and Gender	Vit A µg^e	Thiamin (B₁) mg	Riboflavin (B₂) mg	Niacin (B₃) mg	Pantothenic Acid mg	Biotin µg	Vit B₁₂ µg	Folate µg	Vit B₆ mg	Vit C# mg	Vit D µg^e	Vit E^c µg^e
Infants												
0–6 mos	400 (600)	0.2*	0.3*	2*	1.7*	5*	0.1*	65*	0.4*	40	5* (25)	4
7–12 mos	500 (600)	0.3*	0.4*	4*	1.8*	6*	0.3*	80*	0.5*	50	5* (25)	5
Children												
1–3 yr	300 (600)	0.5	0.5	6 (10)	2*	8*	0.5 (30)	150 (300)	0.9 (400)	15 (50)	5*	6 (200)
4–8 yr	400 (900)	0.6	0.6	8 (15)	3*	12*	0.6 (40)	200 (400)	1.2	25 (650)	5* (50)	7 (300)
Males												
9–13 yr	600 (1700)	0.9	0.9	12 (20)	4*	20*	1.0 (60)	300 (600)	1.8	45 (1200)	5* (50)	11 (600)
14–18 yr	900 (2800)	1.2	1.3	16 (30)	5*	25*	1.3 (80)	400 (800)	2.4	75 (1800)	5* (50)	15 (800)
19–30 yr	900 (3000)	1.2	1.3	16 (35)	5*	30*	1.3 (100)	400 (1000)	2.4	90 (2000)	5* (50)	15 (1000)
31–50 yr	900 (3000)	1.2	1.3	16 (35)	5*	30*	1.3 (100)	400 (1000)	2.4	90 (2000)	5* (50)	15 (1000)
51–70 yr	900 (3000)	1.2	1.3 (35)	16	5*	30*	1.7 (100)	400 (1000)	2.4*	90 (2000)	10* (50)	15 (1000)
>70 yr	900 (3000)	1.2	1.3 (35)	16	5*	30*	1.7 (100)	400 (1000)	2.4*	90 (2000)	15* (50)	15 (1000)
Females												
9–13 yr	600 (1700)	0.9	0.9	12 (20)	4*	20*	1.0 (60)	300 (600)	1.8	45 (1200)	5* (50)	11 (600)
14–18 yr	700	1	1	14 (30)	5*	25*	1.2 (80)	400^a (800)	2.4	65 (1800)	5* (50)	15 (800)
19–30 yr	700	1.1	1.1	14 (30)	5*	30*	1.3 (100)	400^a (1000)	2.4	75 (2000)	5* (50)	15 (1000)
31–50 yr	700	1.1	1.1	14 (30)	5*	30*	1.3 (100)	400^a (1000)	2.4	75 (2000)	5* (50)	15 (1000)
51–70 yr	700 (3000)	1.1	1.1	14 (30)	5*	30*	1.5 (100)	400^a (1000)	2.4^b	75 (2000)	10* (50)	15 (1000)
>70 yr	700 (3000)	1.1	1.1	14 (30)	5*	30*	1.5 (100)	400^a (1000)	2.4^b	75 (2000)	15* (50)	15 (1000)
Pregnant												
≤18 yr	750	1.4	1.4	18 (30)	6*	30*	1.9 (80)	600 (800)	2.6	80	5* (50)	15 (800)
≥19 yr	770	1.4	1.4	18 (35)	6*	30*	1.9 (100)	600 (1000)	2.6	85	5* (50)	15 (1000)
Lactating												
≤18 yr	1200	1.4	1.6	17 (30)	7*	35*	2.0 (80)	500 (800)	2.8	115	5* (50)	19 (800)
≥19 yr	1300	1.4	1.6	17 (35)	7*	35*	2.0 (100)	500 (1000)	2.8	120	5* (50)	19 (1000)

* Asterisk indicates Adequate Intake (AI) values because the RDA is unknown. RDA meets ~98% of needs and AI is at or above that value. See A Closer Look on p. 187 for further explanation.

Smokers should consume an additional 35 mg/day.

[a] Women capable of becoming pregnant should consume 400 ug of folate from supplements or fortified foods in addition to intake from a varied diet.

[b] Food-bound B₁₂ may have inadequate absorption. Therefore, those over age 50 should consume foods fortified with B₁₂ or a supplement.

[c] Alpha-tocopherol (other forms of vitamin E do not have the same effects); Vitamin E as alpha-tocopherol (1 mg = 1.5 IU).

[d] The upper limit (UL) for magnesium represents intake from supplement only and does not include food or water.

[e] Vitamin A: 1 µg = 1 retinol equivalent (RE) = 3.3 international units (IU).

Source: Reprinted with permission from Recommended Dietary Allowances, 11th edtion. Copyright © 2001 by National Academy of Sciences. Courtesy of the National Academy Press, Washington, D.C.

Minerals

Vit K μg	Choline mg (g)	Calcium mg (g)	Iodine μg	Iron mg	Magnesium[d] mg	Phosphorus mg (g)	Selenium μg	Zinc mg	Chromium mg	Fluoride mg
2.0*	125*	210*	110*	0.27* (40)	30*	100*	15 (450)	2.0*	0.2*	0.01* (0.7)
2.5*	150*	270*	130*	11 (40)	75*	275*	20 (60)	3	5.5*	0.5* (0.9)
30* (1g)	200*	500* (2.5g)	90 (200)	7 (40)	80 (65)	460 (3g)	20 (90)	3	11*	0.7* (1.3)
55*	250* (1g)	800* (2.5g)	90 (300)	10 (40)	130 (110)	500 (3g)	30 (150)	5	15*	1.0* (2.2)
60*	375* (2g)	1300* (2.5)	120 (600)	8 (40)	240 (350	1250 (4g)	40 (280)	8	25*	2* (10)
75*	550* (3g)	1300* (2.5)	150 (900)	11 (45)	410 (350)	1250 (4g)	55 (400)	11	35*	3* (10)
120*	550* (3.5g)	1000* (2.5)	150 (1100)	8 (45)	400 (350)	700 (4g)	55 (400)	11	35*	4* (10)
120*	550* (3.5g)	1000* (2.5)	150 (1100)	8 (45)	420 (350)	700 (4g)	55 (400)	11	35*	4* (10)
120*	550* (3.5g)	1200* (2.5)	150 (1100)	8 (45)	420 (350)	700 (4g)	55 (400)	11	30*	4* (10)
120*	550* (3.5g)	1200* (2.5)	150 (1100)	8 (45)	420 (350)	700 (4g)	55 (400)	11	30*	4* (10)
60*	375* (2g)	1300* (2.5g)	120 (600)	8 (40)	240 (350)	1250 (4g)	40 (280)	8	21*	2* (10)
75*	400* (3g)	1300* (2.5g)	150 (900)	15 (45)	360 (350)	1250 (4g)	55 (400)	9	24*	3* (10)
90*	425* (3.5g)	1000* (2.5g)	150 (1000)	18 (45)	310 (350)	700 (4g)	55(400)	8	25*	3* (10)
90*	425* (3.5g)	1000* (2.5g)	150 (1100)	18 (45)	320 (350)	700 (4g)	55 (400)	8	25*	3* (10)
90*	425* (3.5g)	1200* (2.5g)	150 (1100)	8 (45)	320 (350)	700 (4g)	55 (400)	8	20*	3* (10)
90*	425* (3.5g)	1200* (2.5g)	150 (1100)	8 (45)	320 (350)	700 (4g)	55 (400)	8	20*	3* (10)
75*	450* (3g)	1300* (2.5g)	220 (900)	27 (45)	400 (350)	1250 (3.5g)	60 (400)	12	29*	3* (10)
90*	450* (3.5g)	1000* (2.5g)	220 (1100)	27 (45)	360 (350)	700 (3.5g)	60 (400)	11	30*	3* (10)
75*	550* (3g)	1300* (2.5g)	290 (900)	10 (45)	360 (350)	1250 (3.5g)	70 (400)	13	44*	3* (10)
90*	550* (3.5g)	1000* (2.5g)	290 (1100)	9 (45)	320 (350)	700 (4g)	70 (400)	12	45*	3* (10)

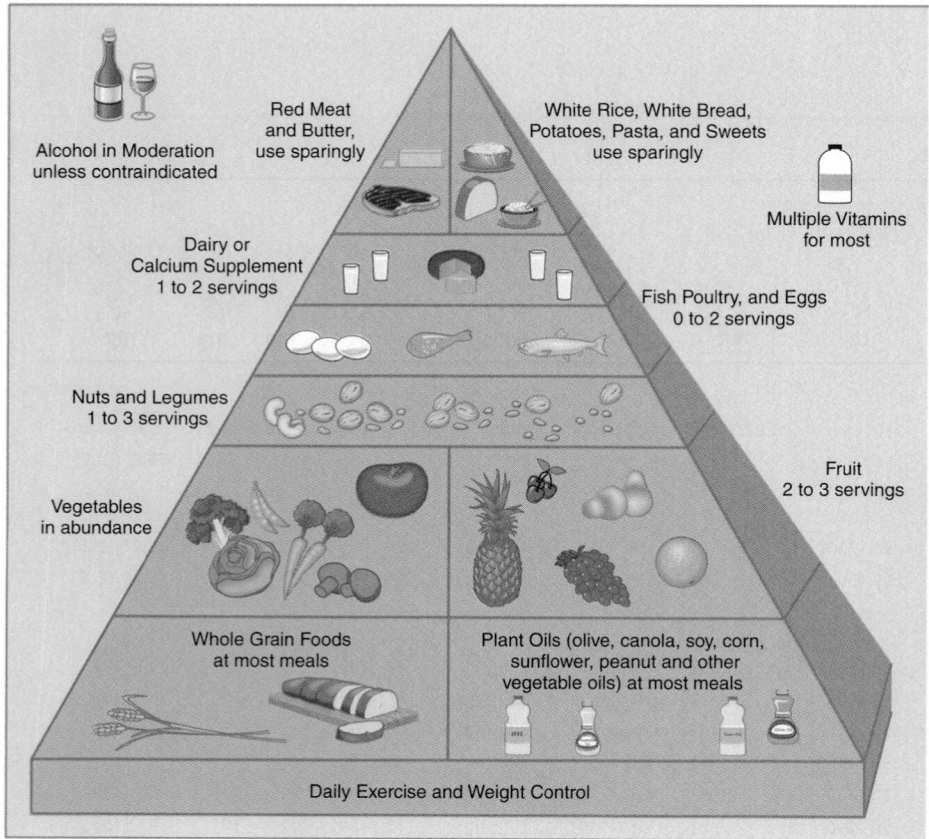

FIGURE 7.6

The "eating right pyramid". The basic diet should consist primarily of those foods on the lower two tiers of the pyramid, with decreasing amounts of foods from the top. This recent modification of the pyramid illustrates the latest research into the make-up of a healthy diet. Note in particular that 'healthy' fats found in some oils have moved to the bottom while, processed grains such white bread and white rice, have moved to the top.

foods high in micronutrients per calorie—are maximized. Thus, by following the pyramid approach, you are assured of getting the proper balance of macro- and micronutrients.

Until recently, nutrition labeling provided little help in choosing the right foods. Labels were required on only 60% of packaged foods, making it difficult to follow the RDA guidelines. Further, the terms used on labels were often undefined, poorly organized, and misleading. In 1994, consumer groups and major health organizations prompted the U.S. Food and Drug Administration to adopt a new set of requirements for food labeling. As illustrated in Figure 7.7 on p. 192, the labeling system now enables consumers to choose foods based on current, accurate, and easy-to-understand information.

CALORIES

The number of calories in the diet is a key consideration for developing good eating habits. As mentioned, the problem with most U.S. diets is not the lack of nutrients, but excess caloric content. Therefore, monitor your total caloric intake to prevent overconsumption of food energy.

When monitoring your dietary calories, remember these two important points. First, most people consume too many calories from simple sugars. The primary simple sugar in most diets is sucrose (i.e., table sugar). The principal nutritional problem related to simple sugars is that they contain many calories but few micronutrients. A second concern when determining caloric intake is the amount of fat in the diet. Fat is high in calories, often rich in cholesterol, and contains over twice as many calories as a gram of carbohydrate or protein (1 gram of fat = 9 calories; 1 gram of carbohydrate = 4 calories; and 1 gram of protein = 4 calories). Limiting fat in the diet both reduces the risk of heart disease and helps avoid excess caloric intake. We discuss how to determine the optimal caloric intake for a healthy body weight in much greater detail in Chapter 8.

DIETARY ANALYSIS

From the preceding discussions, it is clear that eating a balanced diet is the key to good nutrition. Now the critical question is, "How do I know if I'm eating a well-balanced diet?" The answer is to perform a dietary analysis by keeping a 3-day record of everything you eat. It is a good idea to include both weekdays and weekends in your record (two weekdays and one weekend day are generally recommended). At the end of each day, look up the nutrient content of each food (Appendices B and C) and

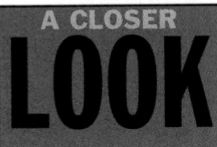

The Mediterranean Diet Can Help You with Dietary Planning

It is now well known that the dietary habits of some cultures around the world provide for a longer life, lower blood cholesterol, and less risk of heart disease and cancer. Researchers have discovered that people in the countries that border the Mediterranean Sea exhibit very low rates of heart disease compared to Americans and others. Over the past several years, extensive research has isolated key dietary habits as a vital part of this region's lower rates of chronic disease (18). This Mediterranean Diet consists mostly of grains, fruits, beans, and vegetables. In addition, the diet is closely tied to areas of olive oil cultivation in the Medi_terranean region. Another item that is prominent in Mediterranean dishes is garlic. Garlic may help prevent blood clots, lower your cholesterol level, and protect you against cancer.

This Mediterranean Diet Pyramid, shown below, does not use either the weight or the calories of foods in the diet, but is meant to give relative proportions and a general sense of frequency of servings, as well as an indication of which foods to favor in a healthy Mediterranean-style diet. The pyramid describes a diet for most healthy adults. Still in need of further research is the effect of this diet on children, women in their reproductive years, and other special population groups. For Americans and others who want to improve their diets though, this model provides a framework for change.

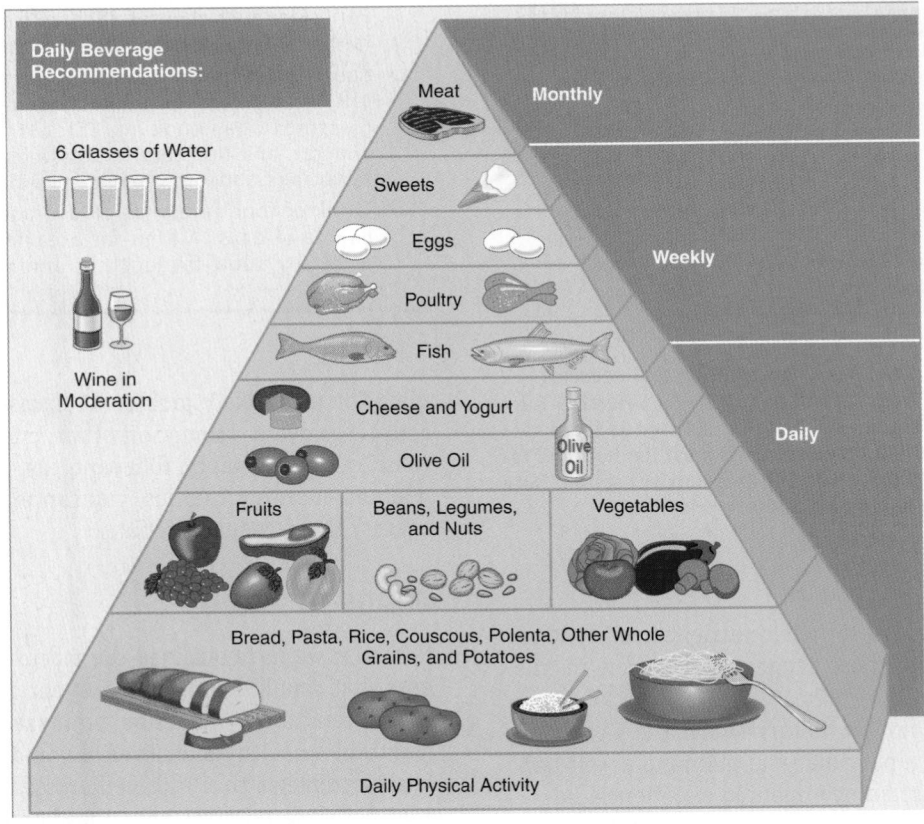

record this information in the tables provided in Laboratory 7.1. The process of analyzing your diet in this way is often time-consuming and can be simplified by using computerized dietary analysis software.

When you have recorded the nutritive values for each day of your 3-day record, compare your average nutrient intake with the recommended dietary allowances for your age and gender (Laboratory 7.1). These results will provide you with a good index of your dietary strengths and limitations. If you find your diet to be deficient in any macro- or micronutrient (compared with RDA values), you should modify your diet to include foods that will provide adequate amounts of that nutrient. In contrast, if you find your diet to be

Sample Label for
Macaroni and Cheese

Start Here

Nutrition Facts

Serving Size 1 cup (228g)
Servings Per Container 2

Amount Per Serving

Calories 250   Calories from Fat 110

% **Daily Value***

Total Fat 12g	**18%**
Saturated fat 3g	**15%**
Cholesterol 30mg	**10%**
Trans fat 1.5g	
Sodium 470mg	**20%**
Total Carbohydrate 31g	**10%**
Dietary Fiber 0g	**0%**
Sugars 5g	**0%**
Protein 5g	**10%**

Vitamin A	4%
Vitamin C	2%
Calcium	20%
Iron	4%

*Percent Daily Values are based on a 2,000 calorie diet.
Your Daily Values may be higher or lower depending on
your calorie needs:

	Calories:	2,000	2,500
Total Fat	Less than	65g	80g
Sat. Fat	Less than	20g	25g
Cholesterol	Less than	300mg	300mg
Sodium	Less than	2,400mg	2,400mg
Total Carbohydrate	Less than	300g	375g
Dietary Fiber		25g	30g

**Limit These
Nutrients**

**Quick Guide
to % Daily
Value**

5% or less is low
20% or more
is high

**Get Enough
of These
Nutrients**

Footnote

FIGURE 7.7
The 'Nutrition Facts' label has a new addition that becomes
mandatory in 2006. Trans fat will be just below Saturated Fat
on the label. It will not have % Daily Value listed as that has
not been established. All other nutrients must list both the total amount and the % Daily Value of each nutrient shown. Note
that daily values are based on a 2000-calorie diet.

excessive in any macro- or micronutrient, modify it to
reduce the values to those suggested elsewhere in this
chapter.

A careful and honest dietary analysis is a critical
step in modifying a poor diet and planning a well-balanced one. It is also an eye-opening experience, because most of us are not aware of the nutrient contents
of common foods. After performing a 3-day dietary
analysis, many people are surprised by their high fat
intake. The average U.S. diet contains approximately
42% fat (% of total calories), which is well above the
recommended 30% (Figure 7.1). As mentioned earlier,
a high fat intake results in an increased risk of disease
and obesity.

Thus, the most likely deficiency you will encounter
in dietary analysis is too few micronutrients in your

> **TABLE 7.8**
> **Guidelines for Cutting Fat from the Diet**
>
> - Read food labels. Keep in mind that 30% or less
>   of total calories should come from fat, and that
>   no more than 10% should be saturated fat.
> - Many foods are now fat free or low in fat and
>   should be chosen over high-fat foods.
> - For baking and sautéing, choose vegetable oils,
>   such as olive oil, that do not raise cholesterol
>   levels.
> - Choose only lean meats, fish, and poultry.
>   Always remove the skin before eating, and bake
>   or broil meats whenever possible. Meats that are
>   the most well-done have fewer calories and are
>   less likely to cause food poisoning. Drain off all
>   oils from meats after cooking.
> - Eliminate most cold cuts from your diet (e.g.,
>   bacon, sausage, hot dogs). Beware of meat
>   products that claim to be "95% fat-free,"
>   because they may still have a high fat content.
> - Select nonfat dairy products whenever possible.
>   Part skim milk cheeses such as mozzarella,
>   farmer's, lappi, and ricotta are the best choices.
> - Substitute other products for butter, margarine,
>   oils, sour cream, mayonnaise, and salad
>   dressings when cooking. Chicken broths, wine,
>   vinegar, and low-calorie dressings make good
>   flavorings and/or cooking ingredients.
> - Think of food intake as an average over a day or
>   couple of days. A high-fat breakfast can be
>   offset by a low-fat lunch or dinner.

diet. The most likely problem of excess you may encounter is overconsumption of fat, simple sugars, and
calories. Remember, by following the eating-right pyramid and counting calories, you can protect your diet
against these common pitfalls.

FOODS TO AVOID

Now that we have outlined the macro- and micronutrients that should be included in your diet, remember
that several foods should be minimized in order to
maintain a healthy diet. Even if you do not have the
health problems that will be discussed next, determine
whether close relatives have these problems. If they
do, you may be a prime candidate for developing the
problem later in life if you do not change your eating
habits now.

First and foremost on the list of foods to avoid are
those with a high fat content. Both saturated and unsaturated fats are linked to heart disease, obesity, and
certain cancers. In addition, it is often overlooked that
dietary fat contributes more to body fat than does protein or carbohydrate (3). Table 7.8 provides guidelines
to help you cut fat intake from your diet.

TABLE 7.9
The Cholesterol/Saturated Fat Index: Which Foods Promote Cardiovascular Disease?

The cholesterol/saturated fat index (CSI) compares the saturated fat in foods with the amount of cholesterol. The CSI value listed for each food indicates the relative contribution of that food to promoting cardiovascular disease. The lower the saturated fat and cholesterol, the lower the CSI. However, because saturated fat poses a greater risk than cholesterol in the diet, it is given a heavier weight in calculating CSI. For example, fruits and vegetables have a CSI of zero (the best). A food that is high in cholesterol but low in saturated fat would have an intermediate CSI value. Shrimp, for example, with 182 mg of cholesterol but virtually no saturated fat, has a CSI of 6. In contrast, lean hamburger, with approximately 95 mg of cholesterol and 6.3 grams of fat, has a CSI of 10 and carries a greater risk for promoting cardiovascular disease. For a healthy diet, the total daily CSI should range from 22 to 50, depending on the caloric content of your diet (22 for a 1200-calorie diet; 50 for a 2800-calorie diet).

	Cholesterol (mg)	Saturated Fat (g)	CSI
Fish, shellfish, cooked (3.5 oz)			
Sole	50	3	4
Salmon	74	1.5	5
Shrimp, crab, lobster	182	0.2	6
Poultry, no skin (3.5 oz.)	84.7	1	6
Beef, pork, lamb (3.5 oz.)			
15% fat (ground round)	94.6	6.3	10
30% fat (ground beef)	88.6	11.4	18
Cheeses (3.5 oz)			
1–2% fat (low-fat, cottage cheese)	7.9	1.2	1
5–10% fat (cottage cheese)	15.1	2.8	6
32–38% fat (cheddar, cream cheese)	104.7	20.9	26
Eggs			
Whites (3)	0	0	0
Whole (1)	246	2.41	15
Fats (1/4 cup, 4 tablespoons, or 55 g)			
Most vegetable oils	0	7	8
Soft vegetable margarines	0	7.8	10
Stick margarines	0	8.5	15
Butter	124	28.7	37
Frozen desserts (1 serving)			
Frozen low-fat yogurt	*	*	2
Ice milk	13.6	2.4	6
Ice cream (10% fat)	60.6	9	13
Specialty ice cream (22% fat)	*	*	34

Varies according to brand.

Source: Adapted with permission of Simon & Schuster Inc. from The New American Diet by Sonja L. Connor, M.S., R.D. and William E. Connor, M.D. Copyright © 1986 by Sonja L. Connor, M.S., R.D., and William E. Connor, M.D.

Although cholesterol is a substance that the body needs to function properly, too much contributes to heart disease. Lowering blood cholesterol by dietary modifications can lower your risk of heart disease. Improvement in one's coronary heart disease risk is closely related to a decrease in dietary cholesterol, and a 1% reduction in cholesterol results in a 2% reduction in risk (Chapter 9). The new food labeling system will help identify foods high in cholesterol; however, the cholesterol content of some unlabeled foods may surprise you. Many foods that are high in cholesterol are also high in fat. Table 7.9 will help you determine your cholesterol/saturated fat index in order to rate the cardiovascular risks of certain foods.

Although salt (sodium chloride) is a necessary micronutrient, the body's daily requirement is small (less than 1/4 of a teaspoon). For very active people who perspire a great deal, this need may increase to over 1 1/2 teaspoons/day. To put this into perspective, the average diet in the United States ranges from 3 to 10 teaspoons/day! Most people are totally unaware of the amount of salt in some foods. Figure 7.8 illustrates the "hidden" salt in an average pizza.

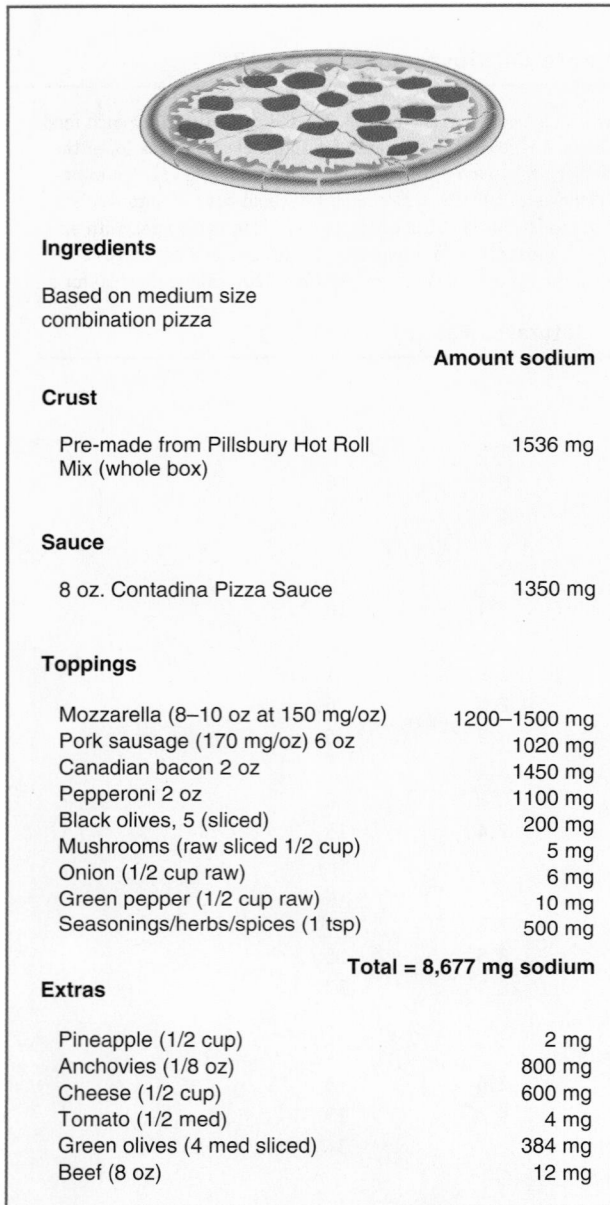

Ingredients

Based on medium size
combination pizza

                                                    Amount sodium

Crust

  Pre-made from Pillsbury Hot Roll   1536 mg
  Mix (whole box)

Sauce

  8 oz. Contadina Pizza Sauce   1350 mg

Toppings

  Mozzarella (8–10 oz at 150 mg/oz)   1200–1500 mg
  Pork sausage (170 mg/oz) 6 oz   1020 mg
  Canadian bacon 2 oz   1450 mg
  Pepperoni 2 oz   1100 mg
  Black olives, 5 (sliced)   200 mg
  Mushrooms (raw sliced 1/2 cup)   5 mg
  Onion (1/2 cup raw)   6 mg
  Green pepper (1/2 cup raw)   10 mg
  Seasonings/herbs/spices (1 tsp)   500 mg

                            Total = 8,677 mg sodium

Extras

  Pineapple (1/2 cup)   2 mg
  Anchovies (1/8 oz)   800 mg
  Cheese (1/2 cup)   600 mg
  Tomato (1/2 med)   4 mg
  Green olives (4 med sliced)   384 mg
  Beef (8 oz)   12 mg

FIGURE 7.8
The "hidden" salt in a typical medium pizza.

An excess of salt should be avoided because it is a complicating factor in people with high blood pressure. In countries where salt is not added to foods, either during cooking or at the table, high blood pressure is virtually unknown. Thus, even if you don't already have high blood pressure, you should limit salt in your diet to only the minimal daily requirements.

It has been estimated that half of the dietary carbohydrate intake of the average U.S. citizen is in the form of simple sugars as sucrose (table sugar) and corn syrup (commercial sweetener)(3). This represents more than 80 pounds of table sugar and 45 pounds of corn syrup per person each year! Sucrose and corn syrup are used to make cakes, candies, and ice cream, as well as to sweeten beverages, cereals, and other foods. Although overconsumption of these simple sugars has been linked to health problems—from hyperactivity in children to diabetes—there is little evidence to support these claims. However, several effects from overconsumption of these simple sugars should be avoided. First, the amount of sugar in sweets adds a tremendous amount of calories to the diet. This leads to obesity, which contributes to many health problems (e.g., diabetes). In addition, calories from sweets are considered "empty" calories because they provide little of the micronutrients the body needs to metabolize the macronutrients. Thus, complex carbohydrates are preferred because they are "loaded" with micronutrients. Second, sugar in sweets also leads to tooth decay. Although brushing your teeth after eating sweets can prevent this problem, it will not solve the other problems of overconsumption of sugar. One way of avoiding sucrose in the diet is to use fructose as a sweetener. Fructose is twice as sweet as sucrose, so you get equal sweetness for fewer calories.

Like table sugar, alcohol provides empty calories. In addition, chronic alcohol consumption tends to deplete the body's stores of some vitamins, which could lead to severe deficiencies. Thus, if for no other reason, alcohol consumption should be limited because it adds empty calories to your diet.

YOUR NEW DIET

Now that we have presented the guidelines for a healthy diet, let's put these principles into practice and illustrate how to construct a new diet. As we discuss the steps for choosing the right foods, refer to Table 7.10, which presents a sample healthful 1-day diet for a college-age woman weighing 110 pounds. Assuming light daily activities, her projected daily caloric need is approximately 1690 calories. For your use of this diet plan, adjust the quantities accordingly.

Because the diet should consist of mainly complex carbohydrates, let's start each meal with a selection of food from the lower two levels of the eating-right pyramid. This will provide mainly carbohydrates, which should be greater than 58% of the total caloric intake, or 980 calories. These calories may be spread out over the day in any proportion you choose. We will use foods from the upper two levels of the pyramid to "fill in" where certain nutrients are needed.

Breakfast. Our subject first chooses grapefruit, raisin bran cereal, a waffle, low-fat milk, and a banana. This gives her 2 fruits, 2 bread/cereals, and 1 dairy product to start the day. The breakfast is low in fat, cholesterol, and sodium. A large part of the protein need is met, as well as over 40% of the

TABLE 7.10
Sample Diet for a College-Age Female Weighing 110 Pounds, Assuming Light Daily Activities

	kcal	Fat (g)	Sat. Fat (g)	Chol. (mg)	Sod (mg)	CHO (g)	Pro (g)	Vit A (RE)	Vit C (mg)	Ca (mg)	Iron (mg)
Breakfast											
1/2 grapefruit	38	0.1	0.02	0	0	10.7	0.8	2	41.3	14	0.1
Raisin bran (1 cup)	127	0	0	0	244	33	3	0	0	16	5.5
1 Waffle (4 in. diam)	100	3	0.2	9	292	15	2	500	0	86	1.7
Lowfat milk (1 cup)	225	2.6	1.7	10	121	42	9	20	1.4	314	0.1
1 banana	105	1	0	0	1	27	1	93	10	7	0.4
Snack											
Low fat yogurt (1 cup)	130	2.6	1.7	10	121	44	9	20	1.4	314	0.1
Lunch											
Turkey sandwich											
Whole wheat w/mustard	191	3.7	0.7	9	784	25	9.4	0	0	78	2.2
Baby carrots (10)	36	1	0.1	0	35	8	1	1972	8	23	0.8
Whole wheat spaghetti (1 cup)	165	1	0.2	0	4	39	8	0	0	22	1.6
w/tomato sauce (1/2 cup)	39	0	0	0	182	9	2	1265	8	168	1
Snack											
1 slice pizza w/parmesan cheese	145	3	1.2	8	336	21	8	382	1	117	0.6
Dinner											
Broiled Salmon (1/2 fillet)	180	5	2	83	107	0	32	169	0	21	1.8
w/mushrooms (1/2 cup)	20	0	0	0	2	4	2	0	3	5	1.4
2 whole wheat dinner rolls	150	2	0.3	0	272	27	4	0	0	60	1.4
3 spears broccoli	26	0	0	0	25	5	3	1434	87	45	0.8
Lima beans (1/2 cup)	90	0	0	0	15	21	6	332	9	29	2.2
1 Peach	37	0	0	0	0	10	1	465	6	4	0.1
TOTALS	1669	25	8.02	129	2543	310.4	100.2	6672	177.1	1159	22.8
RDA	1690	<30%	<10%	<300	<3000	>58%	40	700	75	1000	18
% of RDA	99	45	43	43	85	128	251	953	236	116	127

Abbreviations: Sat. Fat, saturated fat; Chol., cholesterol; Sod., sodium; CHO, carbohydrate; Pro., protein; RE, retinol equivalents; Ca, calcium.

calcium and iron needs. The fruits alone provide almost all of the recommended vitamin A and C needs for the day!

Snack. A morning snack adds some energy and helps to suppress the appetite before lunch. Here our subject chooses a 2nd dairy product for the day (low-fat yogurt) that provides 130 kcals of energy and lots of calcium.

Lunch. For lunch, she chooses 1 meat, 4 more servings of breads/cereals, and 2 vegetables. This lunch

provides a low-calorie meal with lots of protein, vitamin A, and iron. The tomato sauce chosen was low in sodium. Be careful in choosing canned tomato sauce as it is extremely high in sodium. The lunch also includes a turkey sandwich, which can add considerable amount to the sodium intake, but also has the benefit of the protein and other nutrients.

Snack. Our subject chooses a piece of cheese pizza for afternoon snack to add her 3rd dairy and 7th

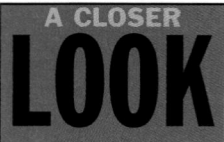

How Low Carb Foods Fit in Your Diet!

Beginning with the book *Dr. Atkins Diet Revolution*, low carbohydrate (CHO) diets have garnered increasing popularity over the last several years. These diets are based on the notion that some CHO foods cause a dramatic increase in blood insulin levels that results in increased storage of fat. While their effectiveness as tools for weight loss is controversial, there is mounting evidence that these diets are effective in controlling hunger, lowering high levels of blood fats, and lowering the risk of heart disease, cancer, and diabetes (19).

The diets are based on the glycemic index (GI) of foods that gives a measure of the speed at which CHO is broken down, and the rate of increase in blood glucose. The list here gives you an idea about the relative glycemic values of foods.

GLYCEMIC INDEX RANGE

Low GI	0–55
Medium GI	56–69
High GI	70–100

Equally important is the glycemic load (GL), which is the product of the glycemic index times the content of CHO [GI (%) x grams of carbohydrate per serving]. The GL allows you to determine the total glycemic load for the quantity of food that you eat. For example, one unit of GL would be equivalent to approximately the glycemic effect of 1 gram of glucose. The following list gives you an idea about the relative glycemic load of a particular serving.

GLYCEMIC LOAD RANGE

Low GL	10 or less
Medium GL	11–19
High GL	20 or more

Then you can sum the GL over the course of a meal or a day to determine the total glycemic effect of your diet. A typical diet has ~100 GL units over a day (80–120).

GLYCEMIC LOAD PER DAY

Low GL	< 80
High GL	> 120

The guidelines below show you how to lower the glycemic load in your diet. Notice that the suggestions offer healthy alternatives to the high-carb foods.

HOW TO SWITCH TO A LOWER GLYCEMIC INDEX DIET

- Use breakfast cereals based on oats, barley, and bran.
- Use dense, chewy breads made with whole seeds, not white bread.
- Eat fewer potatoes, but more al dente pasta.
- Choose basmati rather than white rice.
- Enjoy all types of vegetables.
- Eat plenty of salad vegetables with vinaigrette dressing.
- Balance a meal containing high glycemic index foods (GI) with extra low-GI foods.
- Adding food acids (like citrus fruits) helps slow stomach emptying and reduces the glycemic response.
- Eat fewer sugary foods like cookies, cakes, candy, and soft-drinks.

bread/cereal servings. Be careful in ordering pizza since some toppings (meats and additional cheese) can add lots of fat, sodium, and calories to your diet. In contrast, vegetable toppings can be added to get valuable nutrients without the fat, sodium, and calories.

Dinner. Our subject finishes the day by adding her 2nd serving of meat and 2 more vegetables, to make a total of 5. She also adds a peach for desert that provides lots of vitamin A. The salmon contains lots of protein and plenty of omega-3 fatty acids (heart healthy). The broccoli adds lots of vitamins A and C, and calcium, which is an important component of our subject's diet. The lima beans add lots of vitamin A and iron.

SPECIAL DIETARY CONSIDERATIONS

Several conditions require special dietary considerations, especially as they pertain to people who lead an active lifestyle. Following is a list of nutrients that may need to be supplemented, depending on your individual needs. Use these concepts to help complete Laboratory 7.2 on p. 217.

VITAMINS As mentioned previously, healthy people who eat a balanced diet generally do not need vitamin supplements. Some individuals, however, may not be getting proper nutrition because of poor diet or disease. Therefore, the following people may find a multivitamin supplement helpful:

Nutritional Links
TO HEALTH AND FITNESS

Choosing Your Fast Food More Wisely

As our lifestyles become faster, fast food has become a way of life. In 2003, we reached a significant milestone in the U.S. Now, over 50% of our total food dollars are spent on ready-prepared, ready-to-eat foods (20). The typical fast-food meal is high in fat and calories, factors that are major contributors to heart disease and obesity, so it is important to know how to choose foods during your next stop at the drive-through window. Keep the following guidelines in mind the next time you decide to grab a quick meal out:

- **Order small.** Don't "supersize" your meal. Consider these numbers: Depending on the restaurant, a double cheeseburger may contain 600–700 calories, 30–40 grams fat,

120–140 mg cholesterol, and 1000–1200 mg sodium.

- **Ask for sauce on the side.** Typically, tartar sauce contains about 20 grams of fat and about 220 mg sodium per tablespoon. Ketchup or pickle relish make a healthier sauce.

- **Order grilled meat instead of fried.** Breaded chicken typically contains double the amount of fat than if that same piece is broiled.

- **Try an Adult Health Meal** Several of the fast-food chains now offer "healthy meals" for nutrition conscious consumers. Generally, these offerings are salads, fruit bowls, or yogurt. Some even offer pedometers to motivate you to exercise.

- **Order salads without the dressing.** Most fast-food restaurants are adding more and more salad options. A side salad is an excellent way to include vegetables in your drive-through meal. Opting for a salad entree will provide a meal with less fat and sodium if you choose a nonfat salad dressing. However, you must choose wisely: At one fast-food restaurant, one serving of reduced calorie light Italian dressing contains 170 calories and 18 grams of fat!

On your next "drive-through," ask for the nutrition information sheet that most restaurants offer. Then you'll be able to choose fast food that is appealing to you *and* meets your dietary goals.

- strict vegetarians
- people with chronic illnesses that depress appetite or the absorption of nutrients
- people on medications that affect appetite or digestion
- athletes engaged in a rigorous training program
- pregnant women or women who are breast-feeding infants
- individuals on prolonged low-calorie diets
- the elderly

- Eat legumes, fresh fruits, whole-grain cereals, and broccoli, all of which are high in iron.
- Also eat foods high in vitamin C, which helps iron absorption.
- Eat lean red meats high in iron at least two or three times per week.
- Eat iron-rich organ meats, such as liver, once or twice per month.
- Don't drink tea with your meals; it interferes with iron absorption.

IRON   Iron is an essential component of red blood cells, which carry oxygen to all our tissues for energy production. A deficiency of iron can result in decreased oxygen transport to tissues and thus an energy crisis. Getting enough iron is a major problem for women who are menstruating, pregnant, or nursing. Indeed, only one-half of all women of child-bearing age get the necessary 15 mg of iron per day (3). Five percent suffer from iron-deficiency anemia! Although these individuals should not take iron supplements unless their physician prescribes them, they can modify their diets to assure getting the RDA of iron. To meet this requirement, the following dietary modifications should be undertaken:

CALCIUM   Calcium, the most abundant mineral in the body, is essential for building bones and teeth, as well as for normal nerve and muscle function. Adequate calcium is especially important for pregnant or nursing women. There is some evidence that calcium may help in the prevention of colon cancer (3).

The most recent RDAs call for a significant increase in calcium intake for both sexes beginning at age 9. Whereas the previous RDA for calcium for adults was 800 mg, now 1300 mg of calcium are recommended each day for individuals between 9 and 18 years of age. Adequate calcium intake during those years may be a crucial factor in preventing osteoporosis in later years, which strikes one of every four women over the age of

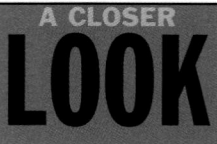

Choosing Fruits and Vegetables for High Nutrient Content

As the "eating-right pyramid" suggests, a good diet is based on at least two servings of fruit and at least three servings of vegetables each day, whether they are fresh, frozen canned, or dried. Often, the brighter the fruit or vegetable, the higher the content of vitamins and minerals. So, to eat a healthful diet, choose fruits and vegetables of a variety of colors and kinds, especially dark-green leafy vegetables, bright orange fruits and vegetables, and cooked dried peas and beans.

The following list can serve as a guide for choosing the best sources of four important nutrients:

- **Sources of vitamin A (carotenoids)**

  Bright orange vegetables (carrots, sweet potatoes, pumpkins)

  Dark-green leafy vegetables (spinach, collards, turnip greens)

  Bright orange fruits (mangoes, cantaloupes, apricots)

- **Sources of vitamin C**

  Citrus fruits and juices, kiwis, strawberries, and cantaloupes

Broccoli, peppers, tomatoes, cabbage, and potatoes

Leafy greens (romaine lettuce, turnip greens, spinach)

- **Sources of folate**

  Cooked dried beans and peas

  Oranges, orange juice

  Dark-green leafy vegetables (spinach, mustard greens)

- **Sources of potassium**

  Potatoes, sweet potatoes, spinach, winter (orange) squash

  Bananas, plantains, many dried fruits, orange juice

Source: National Academy of Sciences. *Dietary Reference Intakes: Applications in Dietary Assessment.* Washington, DC: National Academy Press, 2001.

---

60 (8). The following recommendations can help you get the calcium you need:

- Add dairy products to your diet, but remember, choose those low in fat.
- Choose other calcium-rich alternatives, such as canned fish (packed in water), turnip and mustard greens, and broccoli.
- Eat foods rich in vitamin C to boost absorption of calcium.
- Use an acidic dressing, made with citrus juices or vinegar, to enhance calcium absorption from salad greens.
- Add a supplement if you can't get enough calcium in the foods you like. However, beware of supplements made with dolomite or bone meal, as they may be contaminated with lead.

⚙ IN SUMMARY

- The basic goals of developing good nutritional habits are to maintain ideal body weight; eat a variety of foods following the "eating-right pyramid" model; avoid consuming too much fat, saturated fat, and cholesterol; eat foods with adequate starch and fiber; avoid consuming too much simple sugar; avoid consuming too much sodium; and if you drink alcohol, do so in moderation.

- The general rule for meeting the body's need for macronutrients is that an individual should consume approximately 58% of needed calories in carbohydrates (about 48% complex carbohydrates and 10% simple sugars), 30% or less in fats (approximately 10% saturated and 20% unsaturated fats), and 12% in proteins.

- The calorie is a unit of measure of the energy value of food or the energy required for physical activity.

⚙ Nutritional Aspects of Physical Fitness

The number of myths about physical fitness and nutrition increases every year. Radio, T.V., newspaper, and magazine advertisements create a never-ending source of fallacies. Successful athletes are often viewed as experts by the public, and their endorsements of various nutritional products are attempts to convince the public that a particular food or beverage is responsible for their success. Even though most of the claims made in commercial endorsements are not supported by research, the claims are so highly publicized that they often become accepted as fact. The truth is, there are no miracle foods to improve physical fitness or exercise performance. In the paragraphs that follow we discuss the specific needs of individuals engaging in a regular exercise program.

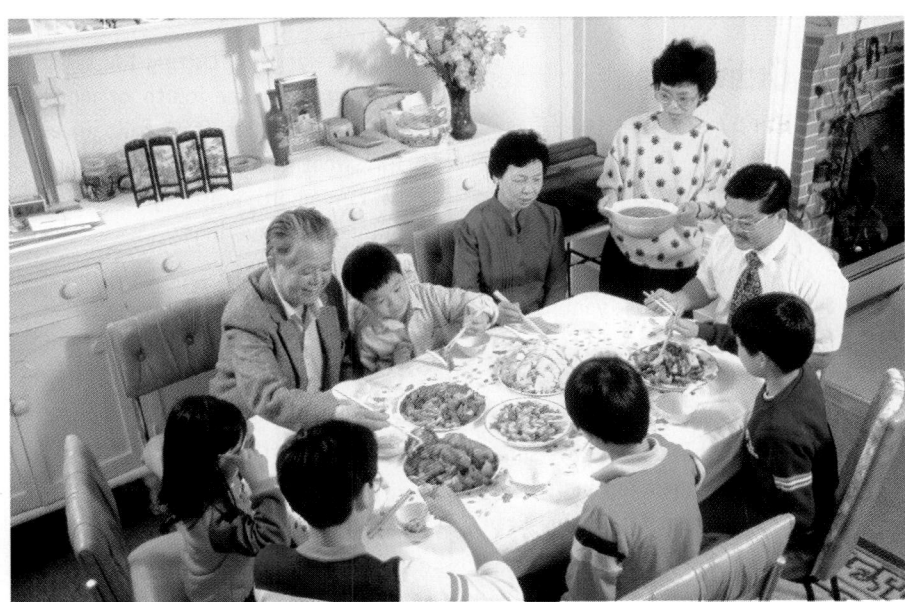

Family and cultural influences often dictate the foods we choose.

CARBOHYDRATES

The increased energy expenditure during exercise creates a greater demand for fuel. Recall that the primary fuels used to provide energy for exercise are carbohydrates and fat. Because even very lean people have a large amount of energy stored as fat, lack of fat for fuel is not a problem during exercise. In contrast, the carbohydrate stores in the liver and muscles can reach critically low levels during intense or prolonged exercise (6) (Figure 7.9).

Because carbohydrates play a critical role in providing energy during exercise, some exercise scientists have suggested that people participating in daily exercise programs should increase the complex carbohydrates in their diet from 58–70% of the total calories consumed (fat intake is then reduced to 18% of total caloric intake) (6). If exercise is intense, carbohydrates can be depleted from the liver and muscles, and the result is fatigue. The intensity of the exercise dictates whether carbohydrates or fat is the predominant source of energy production (6, 9).

Manufacturers of sweets have perpetrated the notion that candy can give you a quick burst of energy when needed. Does a candy bar consumed prior to exercise provide a quick burst of energy? The answer is "no." In fact, there are at least two potential problems with this type of carbohydrate consumption. First, simple sugar in the form of sweets contains only minimal amounts of the micronutrients necessary for energy production. Second, consumption of candy results in a rapid rise in blood glucose, which promotes hormonal changes that reduce blood glucose levels below normal and can create a feeling of fatigue. In this case, the

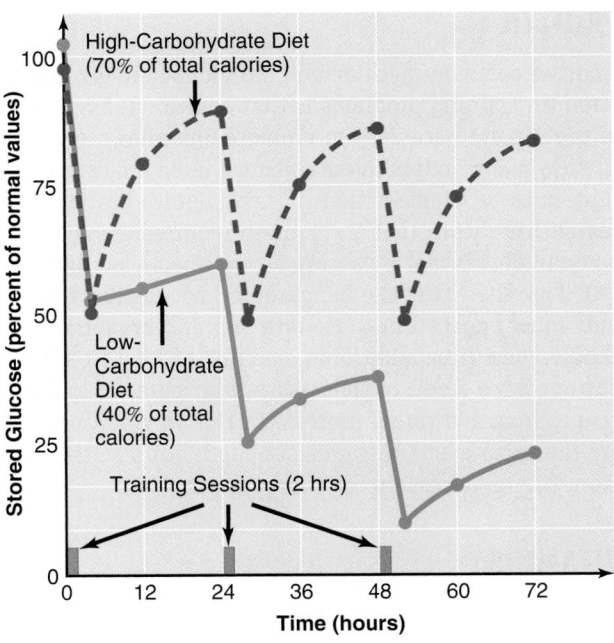

FIGURE 7.9
The importance of a high-carbohydrate diet during exercise training. With a low-carbohydrate diet (solid line), glucose stored in muscles as glycogen is depleted by daily training sessions. If a high-carbohydrate diet is consumed (dashed line), muscle glycogen levels are maintained at near normal levels.
Source: David C. Nieman, *Exercise Testing and Prescription: A Health Related Approach.*
Copyright © 2003. Reprinted by permission of the McGraw-Hill Companies.

effect is opposite of the one intended. Increasing the percentage of complex carbohydrates in the diet and maintaining sufficient caloric intake can ensure that an adequate supply of energy from carbohydrates is stored in the muscles and the liver to meet the needs of a rigorous exercise training program.

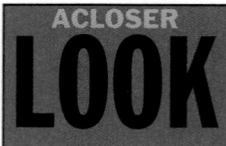 **How to Control Cravings for Sweets**

The following guidelines can help in your quest to control your sweet tooth.

- Know how to spot sugar. When you see terms such as *sucrose, glucose, maltose, dextrose, fructose,* or *corn syrup* on food labels, beware. These are all forms of sugar.

- If sugar or its "pseudos" are in the first three ingredients on a label, avoid the product. It has a high sugar content by weight.

- Cut back on all sugars, including honey, brown sugar, and white sugar.

- Eat graham crackers, yogurt, fresh fruits, popcorn, and other healthy substitutes for high-sugar sweets when you have the munchies.

- Buy cereals that do not have sugars listed among their top ingredients. Shredded Wheat®, Raisin Bran, and oatmeal are among the best choices.

- When baking, try cutting the sugar in recipes by one-fourth or more; you can also substitute fruit juices for sweetness or use spices such as cinnamon, anise, ginger, and nutmeg for flavorings.

- If you can't resist sweets, at least eat foods that give you some nutritional value. For example, put bananas on your oatmeal rather than brown sugar, or make oatmeal cookies rather than sugar cookies.

Source: Boyle, M., and G. Zyla. *Personal Nutrition.* St. Paul, MN: West Publishers, 1991.

PROTEIN

Another common myth among individuals involved in strength training programs is that additional amounts of protein are necessary to promote muscular growth. In fact, many bodybuilders consume large quantities of protein to supplement their normal dietary protein. Research has shown that the protein requirements of most bodybuilders is met by a normal, well-balanced diet (10, 11). Therefore, the increased caloric needs of an individual engaged in a strength training program should come from additional amounts of food from the bottom three levels of the eating-right pyramid and not simply from additional protein. In this way, not only are the extra macronutrients supplied, but also the micronutrients necessary for energy production.

VITAMINS

Some vitamin manufacturers have argued that megadoses of vitamins can improve exercise performance. This belief is based on the notion that exercise increases the need for energy and, because vitamins are necessary for the breakdown of foods for energy, an extra load of vitamins should be helpful. There is no evidence to support this claim (14). The energy supplied for muscle contraction is not enhanced by vitamin supplements. In fact, megadoses of vitamins may interfere with the delicate balance of other micronutrients and can be toxic as well (3).

ANTIOXIDANTS

Although large doses of vitamins may be counterproductive, recent research has discovered a new function for some vitamins and other micronutrients (3). These vitamins and micronutrients provide protection to cells by working as antioxidants. **Antioxidants** are chemicals that prevent a damaging form of oxygen (called *oxygen free radicals*) from causing damage to the cells. Although free radicals are constantly produced by the body, excess production of these has been implicated in cancer, lung disease, heart disease, and even the aging process (15). If cellular antioxidants can combine with the free radicals as they are produced, the free radicals become neutralized before they cause damage. Therefore, increasing the level of antioxidants may be beneficial to health. Several micronutrients, including vitamins A, E, and C, beta-carotene, zinc, and selenium, have been identified as potent antioxidants.

❂ **IN SUMMARY**

- The intensity of exercise dictates the relative proportions of fat and carbohydrate that are consumed as fuel during exercise.

antioxidants Chemicals that prevent a damaging form of oxygen (called *oxygen free radicals*) from causing destruction to cells. Although free radicals are constantly produced by the body, excess production of these compounds has been implicated in cancer, lung disease, heart disease, and even the aging process.

Nutritional Links
TO HEALTH AND FITNESS

Do Antioxidants Prevent Muscle Injury or Fatigue?

Recent research suggests that the increased muscle metabolism associated with exercise may cause an increase in free radical production (12). Several studies have shown that this increase in free radicals may contribute to fatigue, and perhaps even muscle damage. The obvious question is, Do active individuals need to increase their consumption of antioxidants?

Several preliminary studies have indicated a positive role for antioxidants, primarily vitamin E, in neutralizing exercise-produced free radicals. In fact, recent reports have demonstrated a reduction in muscle damage following administration of antioxidants (12). Several researchers have suggested that an additional 400 I.U. of vitamin E be consumed daily to protect against free radical damage. However, you should consult a nutritionist before consuming more than the RDA of fat-soluble vitamins. Remember: Fat-soluble vitamins are stored in the body, and their accumulation may lead to toxicity.

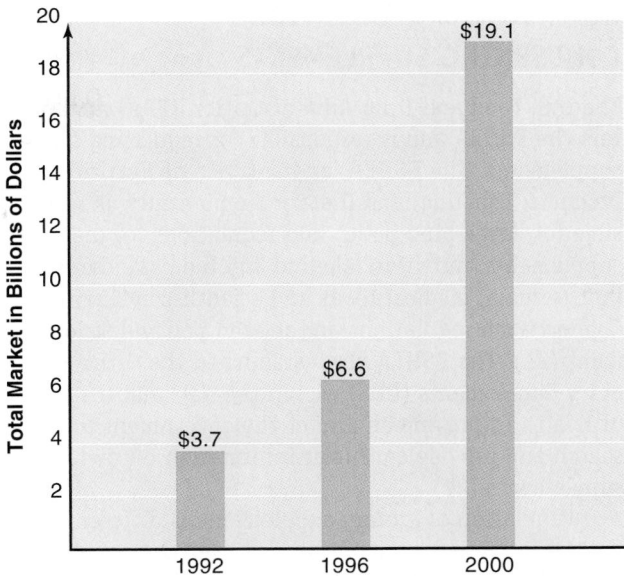

FIGURE 7.10
The steady growth in the use of dietary supplements in the United States. The growing popularity of supplements has helped this billion-dollar industry more than triple its sales between 1992 and 2000.

- The extra energy needed for strength training should not come solely from increased protein intake.

- Excess vitamin intake does not improve exercise performance.

- Antioxidants are chemicals that prevent oxygen free radicals from combining with cells and damaging them. To date, vitamins A, E, and C, beta-carotene, zinc, and selenium have been identified as potent antioxidants.

☀ Do Supplements Provide an Edge for Health and Performance?

What are supplements? Should I take them? Are they safe? Millions of people concerned about health, disease prevention, and exercise performance are asking these questions. Over the past decade the use of nutritional and pharmaceutical supplements has become common in the United States. The search for a speedy path to health, wellness, and fitness led Americans to double what they spent on dietary supplements during 1991–1996 to over $6 billion (Figure 7.10). In the

following sections we examine what supplements are, how they are regulated, and which ones might have the potential to be beneficial.

WHAT IS A DIETARY SUPPLEMENT?

Due to the widespread marketing of dietary supplements over the past two decades, Congress has intervened by defining the term *dietary supplement*. According to the Dietary Supplement Health and Education Act (DSHEA) of 1994, a dietary supplement:

- is a product (other than tobacco) that is intended to supplement the diet and bears or contains one or more of the following dietary ingredients: a vitamin, a mineral, an herb, or other botanical; an amino acid; a dietary substance for use by humans to supplement the diet by increasing the total daily intake; or a concentrate, metabolite, constituent, extract, or combinations of these ingredients.

- is intended for ingestion in pill, capsule, tablet, or liquid form.

- is not represented for use as a conventional food or as the sole item of a meal or diet.

- is labeled as a "dietary supplement."

- includes products such as an approved new drug, certified antibiotic, or licensed biologic that was marketed as a dietary supplement or food before approval, certification, or license (unless the Secretary of Health and Human Services waives this provision).

GOVERNMENT REGULATIONS CONCERNING SUPPLEMENTS

The U.S. Food and Drug Administration (FDA) administers the DSHEA and is responsible for regulating dietary supplements. The DSHEA, or the Office of Nutritional Products, Labeling, and Dietary Supplements, is responsible for developing policy and regulations for dietary supplements, nutrition labeling and food standards, infant formula, medical foods and scientific evaluation to support such regulations and related policy development (21). The DSHEA also established the Office of Dietary Supplements (ODS) within the National Institutes of Health to provide an arm of the government to research and provide consumer information on dietary supplements (21).

Regulation of dietary supplements is different from that of foods and prescription and over-the-counter drugs. The DSHEA dictates that manufacturers, not the government, are responsible for the safety of supplements. Moreover, supplement manufacturers are not required to get FDA approval before they market their products.

The DSHEA allows supplement manufacturers to claim effects on the "structure or function" of the body, but disallows claims concerning the treatment, prevention, cure, or diagnosis of disease. The FDA instituted the "structure/function rule" in 2000 to distinguish disease claims, which require that evidence of safety and benefit be demonstrated to the FDA before marketing, from structure/function claims, which have no such requirement. The rule prohibits both express disease claims (such as "prevents heart disease") and implied disease claims (such as "prevents bone fragility in post-menopausal women") without prior FDA review. However, the rule permits health-maintenance claims (such as "maintains healthy bones"), other claims not related to disease (such as "for muscle enhancement"), and claims for the relief of common minor symptoms associated with life stages (such as "for common symptoms of PMS").

Since its initial release, the rule has been modified both to expand the number of acceptable structure/function claims and to narrow the definition of "disease" to disallow structure/function claims pertaining to aging, pregnancy, menopause, and adolescence. Under the DSHEA, supplement manufacturers are required to keep on file substantiation of any structure/function claims they make. Keep in mind, however, the FDA neither examines nor substantiates the "legitimacy" of this documentation. Manufacturers must also include on their labels a disclaimer stating that their dietary supplements are not drugs and received no FDA approval before marketing. Additionally, manufacturers must notify the FDA of a product claim within 30 days of marketing it. All this means that dietary supplements are not well regulated. The consumer is responsible for determining whether a given supplement is needed or safe.

THE ROLE OF SUPPLEMENTATION IN A HEALTHFUL DIET

The FDA estimates that more than 25,000 products are available as dietary supplements. It is important to note that there is no scientific evidence to validate most of the claims that supplements improve health or exercise performance. Table 7.11 lists and evaluates a few of the more popular supplements currently marketed for improving health and enhancing exercise performance.

Our knowledge of the relationship between diet and disease points out the importance of micronutrients and macronutrients, as well as the need to ensure adequate nutrient consumption while avoiding dietary excesses. However, not much is known about newly discovered, unclassified, and naturally occurring micronutrient components of food and the subsequent effects on health and disease. For example, several studies have identified numerous plant compounds, called phytochemicals, that when ingested by humans in small amounts may protect against a variety of diseases. (See Nutritional Links to Health and Fitness, p. 204.) We still don't know whether phytochemicals, in the large amounts typically present in supplements, are safe or effective. Given our current incomplete knowledge, eating a wide variety of foods and avoiding excesses or imbalances that can potentially result from relying too much on dietary supplements are the best ways to obtain adequate amounts of beneficial food constituents. As previously explained, following the Dietary Guidelines for Americans (7) and the recommendations of the eating-right pyramid can help you consume a variety of foods, which reduces the risks of both inadequate and excessive dietary intake.

☀ IN SUMMARY

- The use of dietary supplements has grown tremendously over the last decade, with Americans spending over $6 million a year on the products.

- The FDA defines a dietary supplement as a product that contains a vitamin, mineral, herb, or other botanical, an amino acid, a dietary substance for use by humans to supplement the diet by increasing the total daily intake, or a concentrate, metabolite, constituent, extract, or combinations of these ingredients. The FDA mandated that the supplement should be in pill, capsule, tablet, or liquid form and labeled as a supplement.

- Regulations also mandate that the only claims that can be made about the supplement must relate to effects on "structure or function" of the body.

TABLE 7.11
Comparison of Dietary Supplements

Supplement	Origin	Benefits Claimed	Evidence of Effectiveness
Androstenedione	Made by the body as part of testosterone production	Enhances the production of testosterone and causes an increase in muscle mass	Evidence suggests that it does not increase testosterone, and it may increase female hormones in men.
Antioxidants	Produced by cells to protect against free radical production. Some vitamins, minerals, and other chemicals in foods also have antioxidant properties.	Buffer free radical damage, which could help prevent fatigue and/or muscle damage during exercise. Also, could help protect against some diseases.	No evidence to suggest enhancement of exercise performance. Some evidence to suggest a benefit in preventing damage to tissues. Growing evidence to suggest benefits in fighting many conditions such as cancer, heart and lung disease, and aging.
Caffeine	Compound found in coffee, cola, candy, stimulants, weight-loss products.	Used to increase muscle fiber activation to increase strength, or to increase fat metabolism and endurance.	Increases endurance in events lasting greater than 20 min. No consistent effects on strength.
Carbohydrates	Component of most food. Usually found as a dietary supplement in the form of beverages or bars.	Increase in stored glucose in muscle and liver and increase in endurance.	Improves endurance in events longer than 90–120 minutes. Also helps restore glucose after exercise.
L-Carnitine	Made by the body and ingested in meat products.	Increases transport of fat in cells, reduces lactate accumulation.	Carnitine is in adequate supply in the cells, and additional amounts provide no benefit before, during, or after exercise.
Chromium picolinate	Chromium is a trace element found in several foods; picolinate is added to supplements to aid absorption in the gut.	Helps insulin action and is thought to aid glucose metabolism, blood fats, and have anabolic effects.	No good evidence for any benefits. *Side effects: Stomach upset, anemia, genetic damage, kidney damage.*
Coenzyme Q-10	Made by the body as a component of the biochemical pathway that makes ATP.	Enhances ATP production.	No evidence suggests a benefit during or after exercise.
Creatine	Made by the body and also obtained by eating meat products.	Decreases fatigue in short, intense exercise. Increases muscle size and strength.	Increases endurance in short, intense exercise. Causes water gain in muscle but not increases in strength.
Echinacea	Herbal supplement.	Reduces duration of colds, boosts immune system, heals wounds.	Some evidence suggests it may be beneficial for these conditions. *Side effects: Uncommon, but possible GI upset, chills, nausea.*
Ginkgo Biloba	Extracts of dried leaves of *Ginkgo* plant.	Used for antioxidant properties and to improve blood flow and memory.	Does have antioxidant properties that may be beneficial in improving blood flow, improving neural function, and reducing production of stress hormones. *Side effects: nausea, headache, dizziness, skin rash, hemorrhage if used with blood thinners.*
B-Hydroxy Methyl Butyate (HMB)	By-product of amino acid breakdown. Also ingested in some food.	Inhibition of protein breakdown.	Scant evidence suggests some increase in muscle mass.
Ribose	Naturally occurring sugar that is now mass produced.	Used to delay fatigue during high-volume type training.	Much evidence to suggest benefits in heart muscle but very little evidence for effects on skeletal muscle.
St. John's Wort	Plant extract.	Used to treat depression and external wounds, burns, and muscle aches.	Some evidence suggests that it is beneficial for treating these conditions.

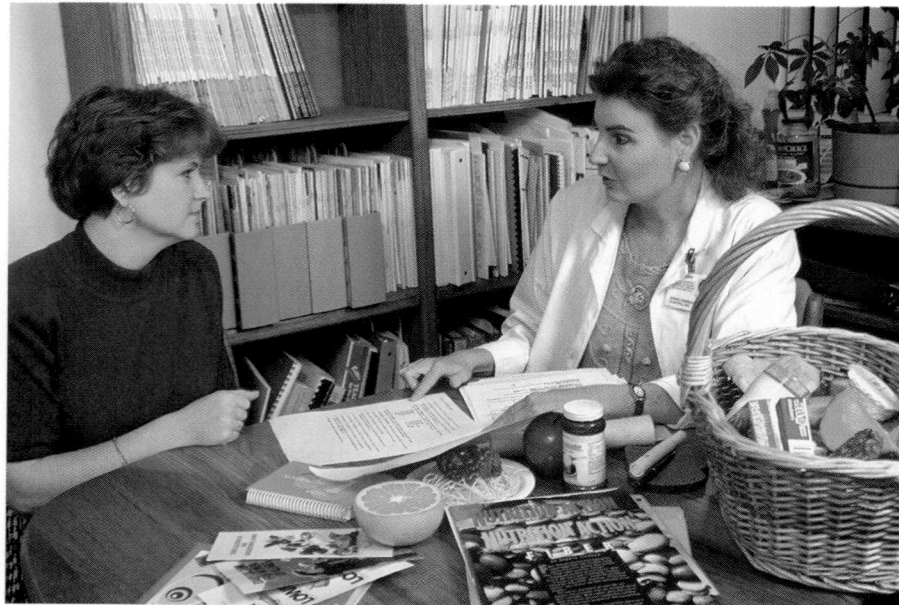

Many considerations such as age, gender, and activity level must be assessed in determining vitamin requirements. Consult a registered dietician or physician when considering any dietary supplementation.

Nutritional Links
TO HEALTH AND FITNESS

Do Phytochemicals Protect Against Disease?

Besides nutrients, plant foods—legumes, vegetables, fruits, and whole grains—contain a whole other "crop" of chemicals called *phytochemicals* (*phyto* means "plant"). These substances, which plants produce naturally to protect themselves against viruses, bacteria, and fungi, may help protect us from diseases as well.

Phytochemicals include hundreds of naturally occurring substances, including carotenoids, flavenoids, indoles, isoflavones, capsaicin, and protease inhibitors. And just as occurs with vitamins and minerals, different plant foods contain different kinds and amounts of phytochemicals.

Even though the exact ways phytochemicals promote health are not yet clear, certain phytochemicals appear to protect against some cancers, heart disease, and other chronic health conditions. Research into their roles is ongoing, so stay tuned! Until more is known, the nutrition bottom line still applies: Eat a wide variety of fruits, vegetables, legumes, and whole grains, and count on food, not diet supplements, to get the nutrients your body needs. That way, you'll reap the potential benefits of the many phytochemicals found in all kinds of plant foods.

Source: Heber, D. Vegetables, fruits and phytoestrogens in the prevention of diseases. *Journal of Postgraduate Medicine* 50(2): 145–149, 2004.

- Manufacturers can make no claims about the effects of a supplement on disease.
- Because dietary supplements are poorly regulated, consumers should be cautious when choosing and using such supplements. When doubts about a product arise, a nutritionist should be consulted.
- Supplements should never be relied on as major sources of dietary nutrients.

☀ Current Topics in Food Safety

Many aspects of nutrition, such as food safety, have significant effects on health. In recent years there have been increased reports of illness and death due to improperly stored and prepared foods. Let's examine some of the latest suggestions for improving food safety.

FOODBORNE INFECTIONS

According to the Institute of Food Technologists, approximately 80 million cases of foodborne bacterial disease occur each year. These illnesses produce nausea, vomiting, and diarrhea from 12 hours to 5 days after infection (8). The severity of the illness depends on the microorganism ingested and the victim's overall health. Indeed, foodborne infections can be fatal in people with compromised immune systems or those in ill health.

One of the most common types of food poisoning is caused by the bacterium *Salmonella*. It is usually found in undercooked chicken, eggs, and processed meats. A relatively uncommon but sometimes fatal form of food poisoning is *botulism,* which usually results from im-

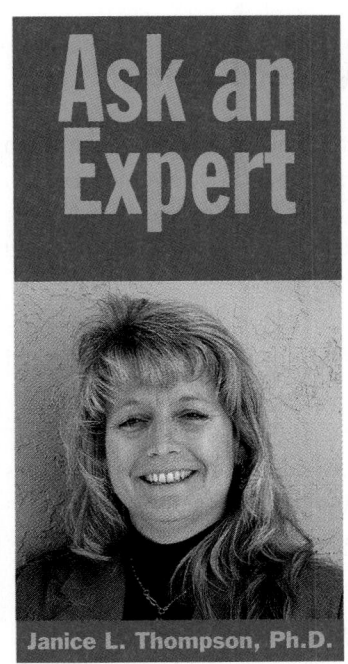

Janice L. Thompson, Ph.D.

Nutrition, Exercise, and Metabolism

Dr. Thompson is an internationally renowned researcher in the Department of Internal Medicine at the University of New Mexico. She is best known for her work describing the interactions of nutrition and physical activity on chronic diseases. She has published many scientific papers, books, and book chapters related to diet, nutrition, and exercise. In the accompanying interview, Dr. Thompson addresses several hot topic questions related to diet and exercise.

Q: There are hundreds of supplements on the market for replenishment of protein and carbohydrates after exercise. Is there any benefit to this type of supplement over the normal diet?

A: Active people need to eat a relatively high carbohydrate diet, or at least 60% of total energy as carbohydrate. Very little protein is used for energy during exercise; however, protein supports the growth and repair of body tissues and helps recovery from exercise. Unless you are exercising more than 60 to 90 minutes each day at a high training intensity, you probably do not need to consume supplements. If you do eat a "normal" diet, you should consume enough carbohydrate and protein to support exercise and recovery from exercise. Women and men who are dieting, highly active people who do not eat a balanced diet, and athletes who train many hours each day are at risk for getting too little carbohydrate and protein and may benefit from supplements.

Q: Weight-training is my primary means of activity. I am concerned that I may not be getting enough protein in my diet. Should I supplement my diet with a protein powder?

A: One of the most prevalent myths in the strength training world is that people who lift weights have very high protein needs. In reality, studies of strength athletes show that they need 1.6 to 1.7 grams of protein each day for every kilogram of body weight, about two times the current protein recommendation for the average adult. Endurance athletes also need more protein than the average person, requiring about 1.2 to 1.4 grams of protein each day for every kilogram of body weight. Most people in the United States eat at least two times the recommendation for protein in their normal diet with no effort, so supplementing your diet with protein powder is not necessary.

Q: I have seen a great deal written about phytochemicals. What are they? Should I be concerned about getting enough in my diet?

A: Phytochemicals are substances found in plants that may protect us against diseases such as heart disease and cancer and are naturally found in fruits, vegetables, grains, legumes, seeds, soy, and green tea. The study of phytochemicals is still new, and we do not yet know the complete story on how these substances can prevent disease. Although we have started to study hundreds of these substances, there could be thousands remaining in food yet to be discovered. Your best approach is to eat more fruits and vegetables, at least two fruits and three vegetables each day.

Nutritional Links

How to Handle Take-out Food Safely

Whether from restaurants, supermarkets, or quick-service establishments, take-out foods have become a part of our way of life. But in order to avoid foodborne illnesses, these foods must be handled with care. The next time your order take-out, keep the following recommendations in mind.

FOR HOT FOODS:

- Hot foods must be kept above 140°F. First, make sure the food is hot when you pick it up or it's delivered. You can cover food with foil (to keep it moist) and keep it warm—140°F or above—in the oven (check the food's temperature with a meat thermometer). Using a crockpot is another option for some foods. It's best to eat food within 2 hours of preparation.

- If the food won't be eaten for more than 2 hours, refrigerate in shallow, covered containers. Before serving, reheat it in an oven to 165°F or until it's hot and steaming. If you prefer, reheat food in a microwave oven—cover and rotate—and then let it stand for 2 minutes to ensure thorough, even heating.

FOR COLD FOODS:

- Cold foods must be kept at 40°F or below.

- If cold take-out foods are not eaten right away, refrigerate them as soon as possible. Transport and store cold foods in chilled, insulated coolers.

- Discard any foods kept at room temperature for more than 2 hours. If conditions are warmer than 90°F, toss the food after only 1 hour.

- Keep deli platters that stay out—as is the practice in buffet dining—on bowls of ice.

Source: Duyff, R. L. *The American Dietetic Association's Complete Food and Nutrition Guide.* Minnetonka, MN: Chronimed Publishing, 1996.

---

proper home-canning procedures. Use the following guidelines for preventing food poisoning:

- Clean food thoroughly. Wash all produce and raw meats, and make sure cans show no sign of leaks or bulges.
- Drink only pasteurized milk.
- Don't eat raw eggs.
- Cook chicken thoroughly.
- Cook pork to an internal temperature of 170°F to kill parasites called trichina.
- Cook all shellfish thoroughly; steaming them open may not be sufficient.
- Be wary of raw fish; it may contain parasitic roundworms. Keep fish frozen and cook until well done.
- Wash utensils, plates, cutting boards, knives, blenders, and other cooking equipment with soap and very hot water after preparing raw poultry.

organic Refers to foods that are grown without pesticides.

FOOD ADDITIVES

Food additives are substances added to food to lengthen its storage time, change its taste or color, or otherwise make it more appealing. Although they can provide these benefits, they may also pose a risk. One example is nitrites, which are found in foods such as bacon, sausages, and lunch meats. Nitrites inhibit spoilage and prevent botulism, but they also form cancer-causing agents (nitrosamines) in the body.

ORGANICALLY GROWN FOODS

Each year, over one million pounds of commercial pesticides are used in the United States. Although these chemicals can save crops from disease and pests, they may also endanger human health. In recent years, many people have begun to purchase organically grown foods. **Organic** in this context refers to foods that are grown without the use of pesticides. Organically grown foods are more expensive than foods commonly supplied by supermarkets.

In the near future, look for new genetics techniques in biology to spawn a new world of pest- and insecticide-free foods. These new techniques combine the genetic material from various plants, in an effort to produce strains of high-yield crops that are resistant to diseases and pests, high in nutritional quality, and free of chemicals. Whether these new plants will live up to expectations remains to be seen.

Detecting Supplement Fraud

Most of the dietary supplements on the market today are useless. Advertisements for fraudulent products are everywhere—in newspaper and magazine ads, on TV "infomercials," on the Internet, and accompanying products sold in stores and through mail-order catalogues. And consumers, in their desire to cure an ailment, improve their well-being, or improve athletic performance, respond by spending billions of dollars each year on fraudulent health products. The products they buy often do nothing more than cheat them out of their money or steer them away from products that have been proven useful. Some supplement products may do more harm than good.

How can you avoid being scammed by the maker of a worthless supplement? Marketers have sophisticated ways of making their products attractive to potential buyers, but you can protect yourself by learning about marketing ploys. Beware of the following techniques, claims, or catch-phrases:

- **The product "does it all."** Be suspicious of any supplement that claims to have multiple benefits. No one product is likely to be capable of so great a range of effectiveness.

- **The product is supported by personal testimonials.** Testimonials are quite often simply stories that have been passed from person to person, and sometimes they are completely made up. Because testimonials are difficult to prove, they may be a "tip" to the possibility of fraud.

- **The product provides a "quick fix."** Be skeptical of products that claim to produce immediate results. Among the tip-offs are ambiguous language like "provides relief in days" or "you'll feel energized immediately." Unscrupulous marketers use such phrases to protect themselves against any subsequent legal action.

- **The product is "natural."** The term *natural,* which is clearly an attention-grabber, suggests that the product is safer than conventional treatments. However, *any* product—whether synthetic or natural—that is potent enough to produce a significant physiological effect is potent enough to cause side effects.

- **The product is "a new, time-tested treatment."** A product is usually one or the other, but be suspicious of any product that claims to be both a breakthrough and a decades-old treatment. If a product that claims to be an "innovation," an "exclusive product," or a "new discovery" were really so revolutionary, it would be widely reported in the media and pre-scribed by health professionals, not featured in obscure ads.

- **Your "satisfaction is guaranteed."** Money-back guarantees are often empty promises. To evade cheated customers, scam artists move often, rarely staying in one place for long. And the makers of this claim know most people won't go to all the trouble involved in trying to get a refund of only $9.95 or so.

- **The product's ads contain meaningless medical jargon.** The use of scientific-sounding terms as "aerobic enzyme booster" may seem impressive and may even contain an element of truth, but these terms likely cover up a lack of scientific data concerning the product.

Always ask yourself, Does this claim seem too good to be true? If it does, then the product is probably a fraud. If you're still not sure, talk to your doctor or other health professional. The Better Business Bureau or your state attorney general's office can tell you whether other consumers have lodged complaints about a product or its marketers. If a product is promoted as being helpful for a specific condition, check with the appropriate professional group—for example, consult the American Heart Association about products that claim some effectiveness concerning heart disease.

IRRADIATED FOODS

Irradiation is the use of radiation (high-energy waves or particles, including radioactivity and X-rays) to kill microorganisms that grow on or in food. When radioactivity is used, the food does not become radioactive; instead the irradiation serves to prolong the shelf life of the food (16). Indeed, irradiated food can be stored for years in sealed containers at room temperature without spoiling. In addition, irradiation can delay the sprouting of vegetables such as potatoes and onions and delay the ripening of fruits such as bananas, mangoes, tomatoes, pears, and avocados. This can result in significant cost savings.

Are these irradiated foods safe to eat? Currently, the best answer is a qualified "yes." All research indicates that the foods are safe and nutritional content is maintained, but only limited data exist (16). In addition, most studies have used very low radiation levels to irradiate foods. This raises the question, "What is a safe level of radiation for the treatment of foods?"

ANIMALS TREATED WITH ANTIBIOTICS AND HORMONES

In recent years, consumers have grown suspicious of eating meat from animals that have been treated with antibiotics to prevent infections. Concern has developed because of the possibility that eating such meat could lead to the development of antibiotic-resistant bacteria in humans. At present, a definitive answer to this issue is not available.

Another recent concern has been the use of hormones to increase production of meat and milk. Most notably, a form of growth hormone, bovine somatotropin, has been used to increase milk production in dairy cows. Some people fear that the presence of hormones in food may result in health problems that have not yet been determined. Many supermarkets are restricting the sale of milk produced with the aid of hormone supplements.

☀ IN SUMMARY

- Proper food storage and preparation are the keys to preventing food poisoning. Select foods that appear clean and fresh; keep foods cold or frozen to prevent bacteria from growing; clean fresh fruits, vegetables, and meats (especially chicken) thoroughly; cook all meats thoroughly; order meats well done when dining out.

- Consumption of organically grown foods may be beneficial if you are concerned about pesticides used to grow grains, fruits, and vegetables.

- Future use of food irradiation and genetic manipulation of plants and animals will likely increase yield and enhance safety of food.

Summary

1. Nutrition is the study of food and its relationship to health and disease. The current primary problem in nutrition in industrialized countries is overeating.

2. A well-balanced diet is composed of approximately 58% complex carbohydrates, 30% fat, and 12% protein. These macronutrients are also called the fuel nutrients, because they are the only substances that can be used as fuel to provide the energy (calories) necessary for bodily functions.

3. Carbohydrate is a primary fuel used by the body to provide energy. The calorie is a unit of measure of the energy value of food or the energy required for physical activity.

4. Simple carbohydrates consist of a single sugar (glucose, fructose, sucrose) or two sugars linked together (galactose, lactose, and maltose).

5. The complex carbohydrates consist of starches and fiber. Starches are composed of chains of simple sugars. Fiber is a nondigestible but essential form of complex carbohydrates contained in whole grains, vegetables, and fruits.

6. Fat is an efficient storage form for energy, because each gram contains over twice the energy content of 1 gram of either carbohydrate or protein. Fat can be derived from dietary sources or formed from excess carbohydrate and protein consumed in the diet. Fat is stored in the body in adipose tissues located under the skin and around internal organs. Fats are classified as either simple, compound, or derived. The triglycerides are the most notable of the simple fats. Fatty acids, the basic structural unit of triglycerides, are classified as either saturated or unsaturated, depending on their chemical structures. For nutritional considerations, the most important of the compound fats are the lipoproteins. Cholesterol is the best example of the class of fats called derived fats.

7. The primary role of protein consumed in the diet is to serve as the structural unit for building and repairing cells in all tissues of the body. Protein

consists of amino acids made by the body (11 non-essential amino acids) and those available only through dietary sources (nine essential amino acids).

8. Vitamins serve many important functions in the body, including regulation of growth and metabolism. The class of water-soluble vitamins consists of several B-complex vitamins and vitamin C. The fat-soluble vitamins are A, D, E, and K.

9. Minerals are chemical elements contained in many foods. Like vitamins, minerals serve many important roles in regulating body functions.

10. Approximately 60–70% of the body is water. Water is involved in all vital processes in the body and is the nutrient of greatest concern to the physically active individual. In addition to the water contained in foods, it is recommended that an additional 8–10 cups of water be consumed daily.

11. The basic goals of developing good nutritional habits are to maintain ideal body weight; eat a variety of foods, following the "eating-right pyramid" model; avoid consuming too much fat, saturated fat, and cholesterol; eat foods with adequate starch and fiber; avoid consuming too much simple sugar; avoid consuming too much sodium; and if you drink alcohol, do so in moderation.

12. The general rule for meeting the body's need for macronutrients is that an individual should consume approximately 58% of needed calories in carbohydrates (48% complex carbohydrates and 10% simple sugars), 30% or less in fats (approximately 10% saturated and 20% unsaturated fats), and 12% in proteins.

13. In order to have a healthy diet, fats (especially saturated or animal fats), cholesterol, salt, sugar/corn syrup, and alcohol should be minimized.

14. The intensity of exercise dictates the relative proportions of fat and carbohydrate that are consumed as fuel during exercise. In general, the lower the intensity of exercise, the more fat is used as a fuel. Conversely, the greater the intensity of exercise, the more carbohydrate is used as a fuel.

15. Antioxidants are nutrients that prevent oxygen free radicals from combining with cells and damaging them. The micronutrients that have been identified as potent antioxidants are vitamins E and C, beta-carotene, zinc, and selenium.

16. Food storage and preparation is key to the prevention of food poisoning. Select foods that appear clean and fresh; keep foods cold or frozen to prevent bacteria from growing; thoroughly clean fresh fruits, vegetables, and meats (especially chicken); cook all meats thoroughly, and order well-done meats when dining out.

Study Questions

1. What is the role of carbohydrates in the diet?
2. List the major food sources of dietary carbohydrates.
3. List the various subcategories of carbohydrates.
4. Compare the three classes of fats.
5. Define *triglyceride* and discuss its use in the body.
6. Distinguish between saturated and unsaturated fatty acids.
7. What are omega-3 fatty acids?
8. Discuss the role of protein in the diet.
9. Distinguish between essential and nonessential amino acids.
10. What are the classes of vitamins, and what is the role of vitamins in body function?
11. Outline the role of minerals in body function.
12. Discuss the importance of water in the diet.
13. What approximate proportions of carbohydrate, fat, and protein in the diet are recommended daily?
14. Discuss the "eating-right pyramid" and its role in the selection of foods for the diet.
15. How many calories are contained in 1 gram of carbohydrate, fat, and protein, respectively?
16. Discuss the special need for carbohydrate in an individual who is engaging in an exercise training program.
17. Discuss the special need for protein for an individual who is engaging in an exercise training program.
18. Define the following:
    antioxidants
    calorie
19. What is the potential role of antioxidants in the diet?
20. Discuss the impact of the following on heart disease:
    high-density lipoproteins (HDL cholesterol)
    low-density lipoproteins (LDL cholesterol)
21. Define "dietary supplement" and give an example.
22. Discuss the "structure/function" rule pertaining to dietary supplements.
23. How does the FDA "police" the marketing of dietary supplements?
24. Compare and contrast dietary supplementation with a good, well-rounded diet.

Suggested Reading

Block, G. Junk foods account for 30% of caloric intake. *Journal of Food Composition and Analysis* 17:439–447, 2004.

Heber, D. Vegetables, fruits and phytoestrogens in the prevention of diseases. *Journal of Postgraduate Medicine* 50(2):145–149, 2004.

Kant AK. Dietary patterns and health outcomes. *Journal of the American Dietetic Association* 104(4):615–35, 2004.

Maughan, R. J., D. S. King, and T. Lea. Dietary supplements. *Journal Sports Sciences* 22(1):95–113, 2004.

Spriet, L. L., M. J. Gibala. Nutritional strategies to influence adaptations to training. *J Sports Sci.* 22(1):127–41, 2004.

Srinath R. K. and M. B. Katan. Diet, nutrition and the prevention of hypertension and cardiovascular diseases. *Public Health and Nutrition* 7(1A):167–86, 2004.

Thompson, Janice and Manore, Melinda. *Nutrition: An Applied Approach.* San Francisco, CA: Benjamin Cummings, 2005.

Willett, W. C. and M. J. Stampfer. Rebuilding the food pyramid. Annual Editions: *Nutrition 2004/2005.* McGraw-Hill, IO, p. 11–16, 2004.

Wood, O. B., and C. M. Bruhn. Position of American Dietetic Association: Food irradiation. *Journal of the American Dietetic Association* 100(2):246–253, 2000.

Position of the American Dietetic Association, Dietitians of Canada, and the American College of Sports Medicine: Nutrition and athletic performance. *Journal of the American Dietetic Association* 100(12):1543–1556, 2000.

For links to the web sites below visit The Total Fitness and Wellness Website at www.aw-bc.com/powers.

About.com

Provides information about many aspects of fitness, health benefits of exercise, and wellness.

Center for Food Safety and Applied Nutrition

Home page for the FDA office of supplement regulation. Great information on food safety and supplements.

Dietary Supplements

Web site of the Office of Dietary Supplements division of the National Institutes of Health. Provides the latest information on the benefits and safety of dietary supplements, research and news.

The Food and Nutrition Board

Part of the National Academy of Sciences whose mission is to establish principles and guidelines of adequate dietary intake.

International Bibliographic Information on Dietary Supplements (IBIDS)

The International Bibliographic Information on Dietary Supplements (IBIDS) NIH, Office of Dietary Supplements is a database of published, international, scientific literature on dietary supplements, including vitamins, minerals, and botanicals.

MEDLINE Plus Health Information: Vitamin and Mineral Supplements

MEDLINE Plus Health Information is a service of the National Library of Medicine, National Institutes of Health, that provides information on health topics, including vitamin and mineral supplements.

FDA Dietary Supplement Questions and Answers.

Provides information about what dietary supplements are, and how they are regulated, including the labeling and claims that can be made for supplements.

NUTRITION.GOV

A new federal resource that provides easy access to all online federal government information on nutrition, including dietary supplements.

Glycemic Index

Information on the Glycemic Index (GI) of foods, latest GI data, GI books, GI testing services, and information on the GI symbol program.

MEDLINEplus

Contains a wealth of up-to-date, quality nutrition information from the world's largest medical library, the National Library of Medicine at the National Institutes of Health. MEDLINEplus is for anyone with a nutrition or medical question.

Food and Drug Administration

In the summer of 2001, the FDA began publishing a quarterly newsletter titled "Dietary Supplement and Food Labeling Electronic Newsletter." The newsletter's goal is to provide interested parties access to key information and updates about regulatory actions related to food labeling, nutrition, and dietary supplements, as well as educational materials and important announcements. To subscribe to the letter, visit the link.

Nutrition Café

Contains several intriguing nutritional games, including one in which you build a meal from the menu and then get nutritional information about your selections.

FoodSafety

Gateway to government food safety information. Includes news and safety alerts, consumer advice, national food safety programs, and food-borne pathogens.

Ask the Dietician

Presents sound nutritional advice on many diet-related questions. Includes an excellent "Health Body Calculator" for formulating diet and exercise programs.

USDA Center for Nutrition Policy and Promotion

Provides governmental guidelines for diets and use of the Food Guide Pyramid.

USDA Food Safety Publications

Contains articles about all aspects of safety in food preparation, storage, and handling.

Fast Food Finder

Enables you to search for desired fast food (by restaurant or food) and find nutritional information.

Fat-Free Recipe Center

Contains a large collection of fat-free recipes.

Veggies Unite! On-line guide to vegetarianism

Includes recipes, books, articles, and discussions.

American Dietetic Association

Presents nutritional resources, FAQs, links, and more.

Crunch Your Numbers

When it comes to health, everything really does add up. So here are 34 fun, easy-to-use calculators. Learn your ideal weight, determine your protein needs, assess your heart rate, determine how many calories your favorite sport will burn and more.

References

1. Guyer, B., M. A. Freedom, D. M. Strobino, and E. J. Sordik. Annual summary of vital statistics: Trends in the health of Americans during the 20th century. *Pediatrics* 106(6): 1307, 2000.

2. Mokdad, A. H., J. S. Marks, D. F. Stroup, and J. L. Gerberding. Actual causes of death in the United States, 2000. *Journal of the American Medical Association* 291(10):1238–1245, 2004.

3. Wardlaw, G. M., J. Hampl, and R. DiSilvestro. *Perspectives in Nutrition.* Columbus, OH; McGraw-Hill, 2003.

4. Tucker, K. L. *Dietary Intake and Coronary Heart Disease: A Variety of Nutrients and Phytochemicals Are Important. Current Treatment Options in Cardiovascular Medicine* 6(4):291–302, 2004.

5. Dragsted, L. O., A. Pedersen, Hermetter, S. Basu, M. Hansen, G. R. Haren, M. Kall, V. Breinholt, J. J. Castenmiller, J. Stagsted, J. Jakobsen, L. Skibsted, S. E. Rasmussen, S. Loft, and B. Sandstrom. The 6-a-day study: Effects of fruit and vegetables on markers of oxidative stress and antioxidant defense in healthy nonsmokers. *American Journal of Clinical Nutrition* 79(6):1060–72, 2004.

6. Powers, S., and E. Howley. *Exercise Physiology: Theory and Application to Fitness and Performance,* 4th ed. Dubuque, IA: McGraw-Hill, 2001.

7. National Academy of Sciences. *Dietary Reference Intakes: Applications in Dietary Assessment.* Washington, DC: National Academy Press, 2001.

8. Donatelle, R. J. *Access to Health,* 8th ed. Pearson Education, Inc., publishing as Benjamin Cummings. San Francisco, 2004.

9. Jones, N. L., and K. J. Killian. Exercise limitation in health and disease. *New England Journal of Medicine* 343(9):632–641, 2000.

10. Tipton, K. D., and R. R. Wolfe. Exercise, protein metabolism, and muscle growth. *International Journal of Sport Nutrition and Exercise Metabolism* 11(1):109–132, 2001.

11. Lemon. P. W., J. M. Berardi, and E. E. Noreen. The role of protein and amino acid supplements in the athlete's diet: does type or timing of ingestion matter? *Current Sports Medicine Reports* 1(4):214–21, 2002.

12. Powers, S. K., K. C. DeRuisseau, J. Quindry, and K. L. Hamilton. Dietary antioxidants and exercise. *Journal of Sports Sciences* 22(1):81–94, 2004.

13. Kanter, M. Free radicals and exercise: Effects of nutritional antioxidant supplementation. *Exercise and Sports Sciences Reviews* 23:375–398, 1995.

14. Lukaski, H. C. Vitamin and mineral status: Effects on physical performance. *Nutrition* 20(7-8):632–644, 2004.

15. Young, I. S., and J. V. Woodside. Antioxidants in health and disease. *Journal of Clinical Pathology* 54(3):176–186, 2001.

16. Meng, J., and M. P. Doyle. Emerging issues in microbiological food safety. *Annual Reviews of Nutrition* 17:255–275, 1997.

17. FDA Consumer magazine. *Revealing Trans Fat.* Pub No. FDA04-1329C. September-October, 2003.

18. Kok, F. J., and D. Kromhout. Atherosclerosis epidemiological studies on the health effects of a Mediterranean diet. *European Journal of Nutrition* 43 Suppl 1:I2–I5, 2004.

19. Brand-Miller, J. C. Glycemic load and chronic disease. *Nutrition Reviews* 61(5 Pt 2):S49–55, 2003.

20. Schlosser, E. *Fast Food Nation: The Dark Side of the All-American Meal.* New York: Houghton Mifflin, 2001.

21. Realignment: CFSAN'S Office of Nutritional Products, Labeling, and Dietary Supplements. Press Release, February, 2003. *FDA/Center for Food Safety & Applied Nutrition.* Rockville, MD. http://www.cfsan.fda.gov/~dms/supplmn.html

Diet Analysis

NAME _____ DATE _____

The purpose of this exercise is to analyze eating habits during a 3-day period.

DIRECTIONS

For a 3-day period (two weekdays and one weekend day), eat the foods that typically constitute your normal diet. At the end of each day, record on the following chart the foods eaten for that day and the amounts of the listed nutrients contained in each. Most packaged foods now have the amounts of the nutrients listed on the package. See the appendix for the listings of the nutrients contained in various foods. Total the values for each nutrient at the bottom of the chart. Transfer the total to the next chart. At the end of the 3-day period, total the daily values and divide by 3 to get the average dietary intake for each of the nutrients analyzed. Compare your average intake for each of the nutrients with those recommended at the bottom of the page for your sex and age group. Remember that this analysis is only as representative of your normal diet as the foods you eat over the 3-day period.

WRITE-UP

In the space provided, list the strengths and weaknesses in your diet and discuss the steps that can be taken to improve it.

(continued on next page)

Daily Nutrient Intake

NAME: _____

DATE: _____

Foods	Amount	kcals (total)	kcals from fat	Protein (gm)	CHO (gm)	Fiber (gm)	Fat (gm)	Fat % (kcal)	Sat. Fat (gm)	Chol. (mg)	Sodium (mg)	Vit. A (I.U.)	Vit. C (mg)	Calcium (mg)	Iron (mg)	Vit. B$_1$ (mg)	Vit. B$_2$ (mg)	Niacin (mg)
Totals																		

Look in your Behavioral Change Log Book for an additional three-day nutrient intake log.

Three-Day Nutrient Summary

Day	kcals Total	kcals from Fat	Protein (gm)	CHO (gm)	Fiber (gm)	Fat (gm)	Fat % (kcal)	Sat. Fat (gm)	Chol. (mg)	Sodium (mg)	Vit. A (I.U.)	Vit. C (mg)	Calcium (mg)	Iron (mg)	Vit. B$_1$ (mg)	Vit. B$_2$ (mg)	Niacin (mg)
One																	
Two																	
Three																	
Totals																	
Average																	

RECOMMENDED DIETARY ALLOWANCES*

- Kcal (total daily energy expenditure) is body weight multiplied by kcals per pound per day:

$$\text{Body weight in lbs} \times \frac{\text{kcals per lb per day}}{\text{(from Table 8.1)}} = \text{kcal total (total daily energy expenditure)}$$

- Kcals from fat should be less than 30% of total calories per day:

$$30\% \ (0.3) \times \frac{\text{kcals per day}}{} = \text{recommended } \underline{\textbf{MAXIMUM}} \text{ kcals from fat}$$

- Protein intake is 0.8 gm per kg of body weight (0.36 gm per lb). (Pregnant women should add 15 gm, and lactating women should add 20 gms):

$$0.36 \ \text{gm} \times \frac{\text{body weight in lbs}}{} = \text{recommended protein intake}$$

- Carbohydrate intake should be more than 58% of total calories per day:

$$58\% \ (0.58) \times \frac{\text{kcals per day}}{} = \text{recommended carbohydrate intake}$$

Fat <30% of diet; Fiber ~30% of diet; Saturated fat <10% of diet; Cholesterol <300 mg.; Sodium <3000 mg

*See Table 7.7 on pp. 188 and 189 for information on vitamin and mineral RDA values.

Setting Goals for a Healthy Diet

NAME _____ DATE _____

Now that you have reviewed your diet in Lab 7.1, reflect on what you learned from that exercise. List the 3 principle things you learned about your diet below:

1. _____

2. _____

3. _____

Check the appropriate boxes in the table below to indicate the changes that you think you need to make to create a healthier diet in the future.

	Increase	Decrease	Keep the Same
Calories			
Carbohydrates			
Fat			
Protein			
Vitamins			
Minerals			

Based upon your selections above, set goals for changing your diet in the space below:

Goal 1 _____

_____

Goal 2 _____

_____

Goal 3 _____

_____

Goal 4 _____

_____

Construct a New Diet

NAME _____ DATE _____

The purpose of this exercise is to construct a new diet using the principles outlined in Chapter 7.

DIRECTIONS

After completing Laboratory 7.1, you should have a general idea of how your diet may need modification. Follow the example given in Table 7.10 and the discussion in the text to choose foods to construct a new diet that meets the recommended dietary goals presented in this chapter. Fill in the blanks on the following chart with the requested information obtained from Appendices B and C or package labels. Use the totals for each column and the RDA for each nutrient in Laboratory 7.1 or Table 7.6 to determine your percent of RDA for each nutrient.

	Kcal (g)	Fat (g)	Sat. Fat (g)	Chol (mg)	Sod. (mg)	CHO (g)	Pro (g)	Vit A (I.U.)	Vit C (mg)	Ca (mg)	Iron (mg)	GI	GL
Breakfast													
Lunch													
Dinner													
Totals													
RDA	*	<30%	<10%	<300	3000	>58%	**	1000	60	1200	12		<120
% of RDA													

* See Chapter 8 for determination of kcal requirements.

**Protein intake should be 0.8 g/kg of body weight (0.36 g/lb). Pregnant women should add 15 g, and lactating women should add 20 g.

*See "A Closer Look—How low carb foods fit in your diet" on p. 196 to calculate glycemic load (GL).

For a complete list of the glycemic index of various foods, visit http://www.glycemicindex.com/

Assessing Nutritional Habits

NAME _____ DATE _____

Read the following scenarios and select which option applies to you. Score your answers according to the instructions at the end.

1. You don't have time to make dinner so you run out to get "fast food." What do you get?

    a. chicken breast sandwich

    b. supersized burger

2. You go to a movie, find yourself hungry, and cannot resist a snack. Which do you buy?

    a. popcorn

    b. candy

3. You're late for work and realize you forgot breakfast. You decide to stop and grab something to eat. What do you pick up?

    a. a muffin

    b. a sausage biscuit

4. You decide to go out for a nice dinner at an Italian restaurant. What do you order?

    a. linguine with clam sauce

    b. fettucine alfredo

5. It's 3 p.m. and you didn't have much lunch and need an afternoon snack. What do you reach for?

    a. an apple

    b. M&Ms

6. You stop for ice cream. Which do you pick?

    a. sorbet, sherbet, or ices

    b. regular ice cream

7. What kind of cake would you normally choose to eat?

    a. muffin, banana bread, or carrot cake

    b. chocolate cake with frosting

8. What do you use to stir fry vegetables?

    a. olive oil

    b. margarine

(continued on next page)   **221**

9. Which of the following salty snacks would you prefer?

    a. I don't eat salty snacks.

    b. popcorn or reduced-fat potato chips

10. You want cereal for breakfast. You would choose:

    a. Cream of Wheat or Corn Flakes

    b. regular granola

INTERPRETATION

If you answered "b" to any of the above questions, you chose foods that are high in calories, fat, or sugar. Follow the eating-right pyramid to determine better choices for your diet.

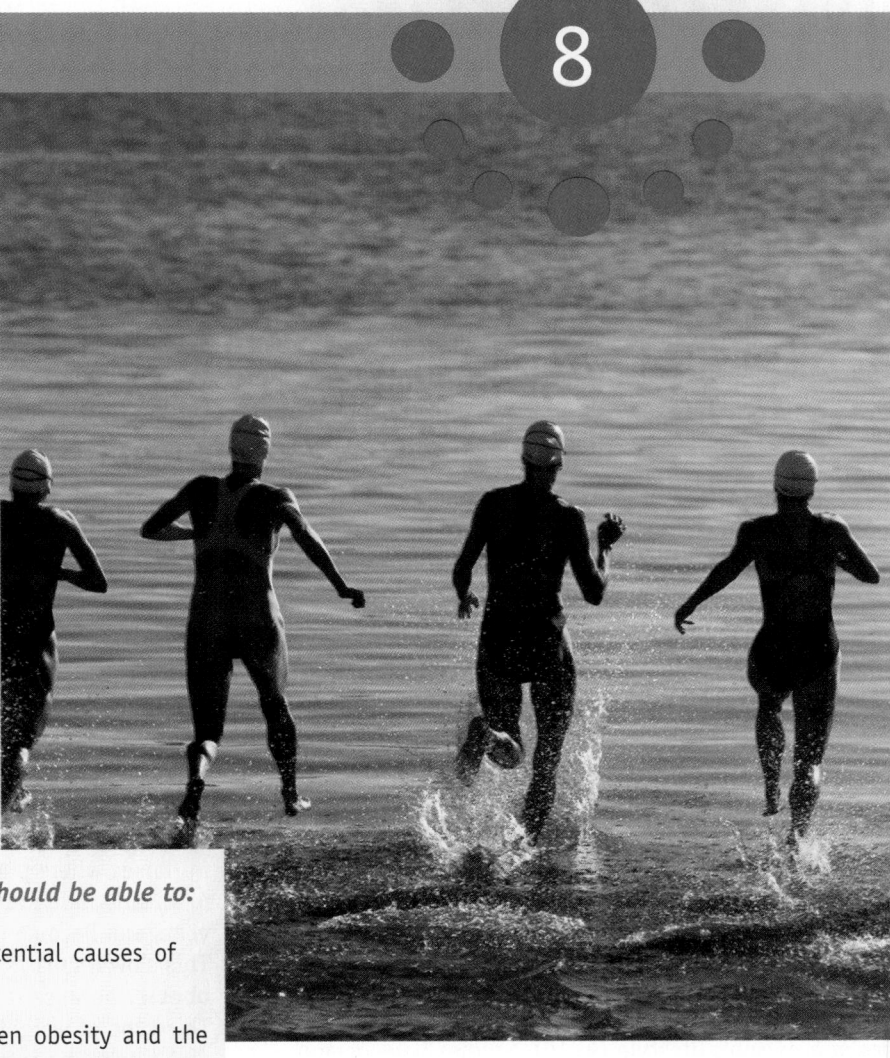

8

Exercise, Diet, and Weight Control

After studying this chapter, you should be able to:

1. Define obesity and discuss potential causes of obesity.

2. Explain the relationship between obesity and the risk of disease.

3. Explain the concept of optimal body weight.

4. Discuss the energy balance theory of weight control.

5. Explain the roles of resting metabolic rate and exercise metabolic rate in determining daily energy expenditure.

6. Outline a simple method to estimate your daily caloric expenditure.

7. List and define the four basic components of a weight loss program.

8. Discuss several weight loss myths.

9. Describe the eating disorders anorexia nervosa and bulimia.

10. Discuss strategies to gain body weight.

Millions of people in the United States believe they are too fat. This is evidenced by the fact that 30–40% of adult women and 20–25% of adult men are currently trying to lose weight (1). Interest in weight loss has opened the door to numerous commercial weight loss programs and a billion-dollar industry. Many commercial weight loss programs advertise that they are highly successful in promoting individual weight loss. Unfortunately, research demonstrates that if no other treatment is given, only 5% of individuals maintain the weight loss for 5 years after completion of the program (2).

A key element in any weight loss program is education. This chapter, therefore, provides a general overview of body fat control. Specifically, we will discuss the principles of determining an ideal body weight for health and fitness; ways to achieve loss of body fat, using a combination of diet, exercise, and behavior modification; and the principles involved in maintaining a desirable body weight throughout life. We begin with an overview of body weight gain and an introduction to obesity.

☀ Obesity

Obesity is a term applied to individuals with a high percentage of body fat, generally over 25% for men and over 30% for women (3–7). Obesity is a major health problem in the United States, and numerous diseases have been linked to being too fat (A Closer Look, p. 225). Current estimates for the United States suggest that over 65 million people meet the criteria for obesity (1, 8).

What causes obesity? There is no single answer. Obesity is related to both genetic traits and characteristics of a person's lifestyle (9, 10). Studies have demonstrated that children of obese parents have a greater potential to become obese than children of nonobese parents (10). Further, adopted children with low genetic potential for obesity have a greater chance of becoming obese if their adoptive parents are obese (10).

The link between genetics and obesity is poorly understood. Researchers continue to search for specific genes that could influence body fatness (Fitness and Wellness for All, p. 226). In contrast, the tie between lifestyle and obesity is well defined. Nutritional studies have demonstrated that families consuming high-fat meals have a greater risk of obesity than families who eat low-fat diets (4, 5, 9). Similarly, children raised in

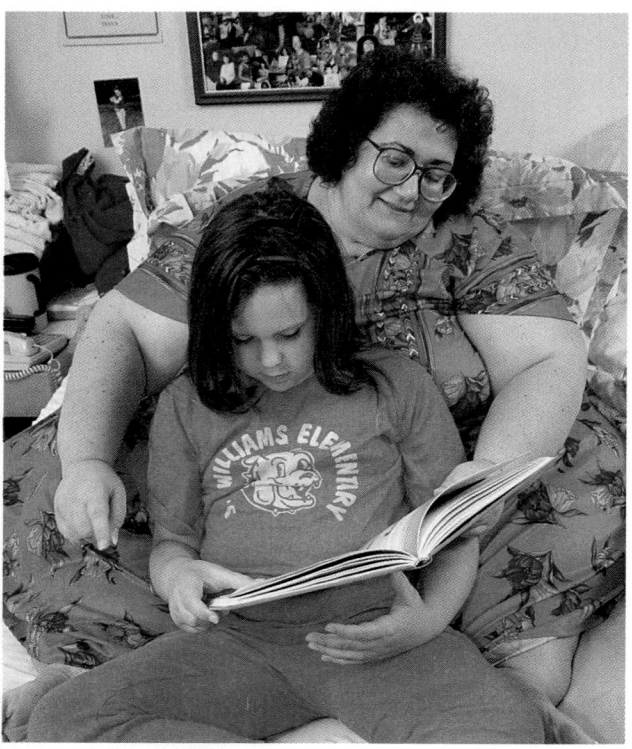

Obesity tends to run in families.

households where physical activity is not encouraged have a greater potential for obesity than children reared in homes where physical activity is encouraged (4, 11).

Many individuals may gradually add fat over the years and become obese at some point in their lives. This slow increase in body fat is often called **creeping obesity** because it gradually "creeps up" on us (12). This type of weight gain is usually attributed to poor diet (including increased food intake) and a gradual decline in physical activity (12). Figure 8.1 illustrates the process of creeping obesity over a 5-year period. In this example, the individual is gaining one-half pound of fat per month (6 pounds per year), resulting in a total weight gain of 30 pounds over 5 years.

News sources frequently report that the obesity rate in America is the highest in the world and continues to grow. The reports are based on studies indicating that the number of obese or overweight people in the United States has increased by 40% in the last 20 years (43). Indeed, the percent of Americans that were obese or overweight in 1980 was 46%; this percentage has grown to 65% in 2000. Despite the sounding of the alarm in recent years, a new study reveals that the level of obesity in the United States has remained steady since 1999 (44). This is the good news. Nonetheless, the bad news is that 65% of all Americans are either obese or overweight and there is no evidence that the prevalence of obesity is decreasing in adults or children (44). Therefore, obesity continues to be a major threat to wellness in the United States.

---

obesity A term applied to individuals with a high percentage of body fat, generally over 25% for men and over 30% for women.
creeping obesity A slow increase of several years.

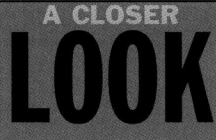

A CLOSER LOOK

Obesity and the Risk of Disease

Obesity increases the risk of developing at least 26 diseases (8, 12, 13), among the most serious of which are heart disease, colon cancer, hypertension (high blood pressure), kidney disease, arthritis, and diabetes (12). For example, obesity increases the risk of heart attack by 60–80% (14). Further, a high correlation exists between the onset of type II diabetes and body fatness; over 80% of type II diabetics are obese (1). In light of

this strong link between obesity and disease, the National Institutes of Health has estimated that obesity directly accounts for 15–20% of the deaths in the United States (13).

Even though the biological link between obesity and a specific disease is not always clear, new research has linked obesity to diabetes via a hormone called resistin (15). This hormone, which is produced by fat cells and released into the blood,

inhibits glucose uptake into cells. Thus it is not surprising that obese individuals, who have a large number of fat cells, also have high blood levels of resistin. The resulting inhibition of glucose uptake into cells produces high blood sugar (hyperglycemia) and type II diabetes.

Obesity may also contribute to emotional disorders in individuals (particularly adolescents and young adults) whose negative feelings about their body image and being overweight lowers their self-esteem and thus reduces their quality of life.

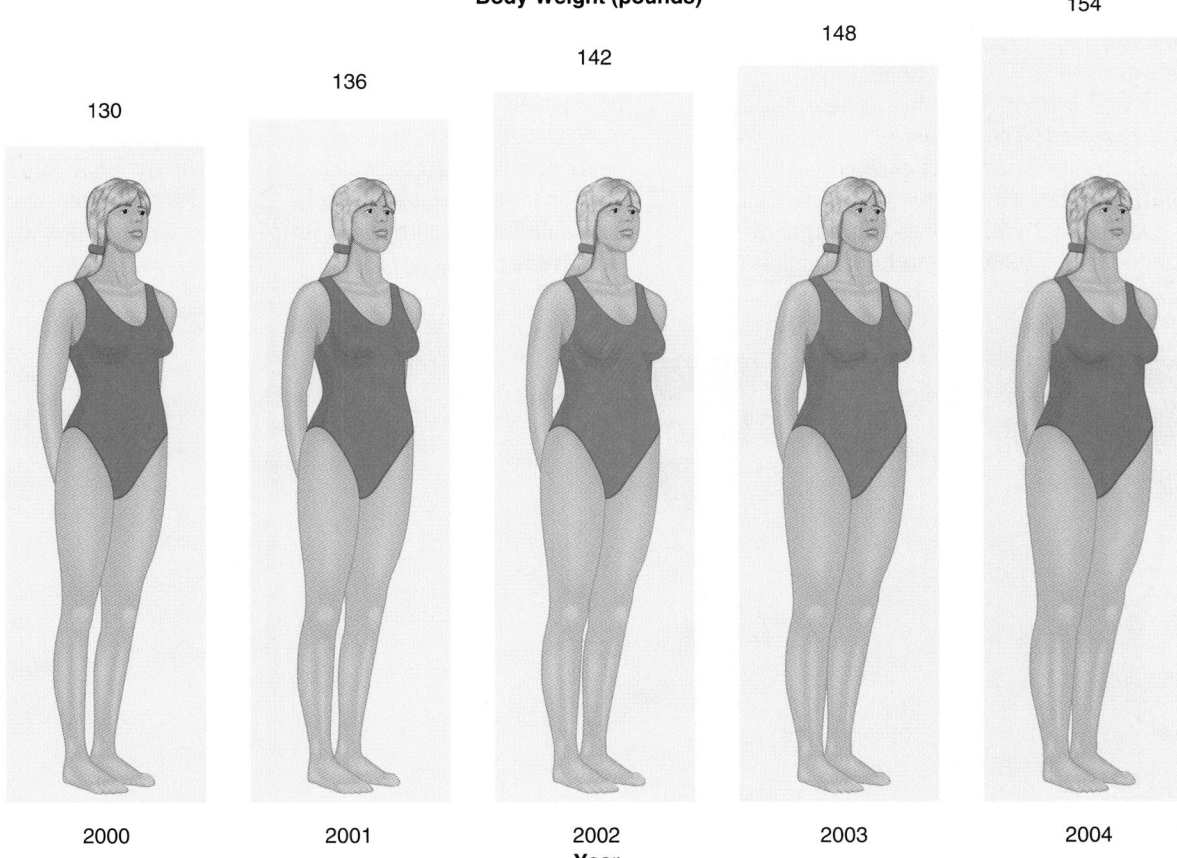

Body Weight (pounds)

130   136   142   148   154

2000   2001   2002   2003   2004

Year

FIGURE 8.1
The concept of creeping obesity.

The Search for Obesity-Related Genes

Even though obese individuals are found in every segment of the U.S. population, certain subsets of Americans experience the greatest prevalence of obesity. For example, compared to the U.S. population as a whole, the risk of becoming obese is greatest among Mexican-American women, African-American women, some Native Americans (for example, Pima Indians), and children from low-income families. The high prevalence of obesity in these populations places individuals in those groups at the greatest risk of developing obesity-related diseases.

Research efforts to understand the roles of genetics in the high prevalence of obesity in these populations are expanding. One large investigation, called the Heritage Family Study, is searching for the genes responsible for both obesity and weight loss (22). Results from this and other genetics studies are expected to provide important information for developing programs that can prevent and treat obesity in high-risk populations.

⚙ Regional Fat Storage

Recall from Chapter 2 that much of our body fat is stored beneath the skin (Figure 8.2). The fact that different people can have very different regional patterns of fat storage is well known. What factor determines where body fat is stored? The answer is genetics. We inherit specific fat storage traits that determine the regional distribution of fat. This occurs due to the fact that fat cells are unequally distributed throughout the body. For example, many men have a high number of fat cells in the upper body, which results in a predominance of fat storage within the abdominal area (i.e., waist area). In contrast, most women contain a high number of fat cells in the lower body, resulting in fat storage in the waist, hips, and thighs. As we have seen, people who carry body fat primarily in the abdominal or waist area are at greater risk for development of heart disease than are those who store body fat in the hips or lower part of the body. Therefore, obtaining a desirable body weight with proper fat distribution is a primary health goal (1,16).

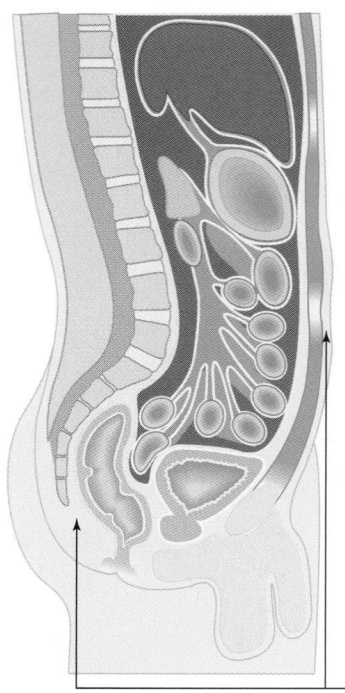

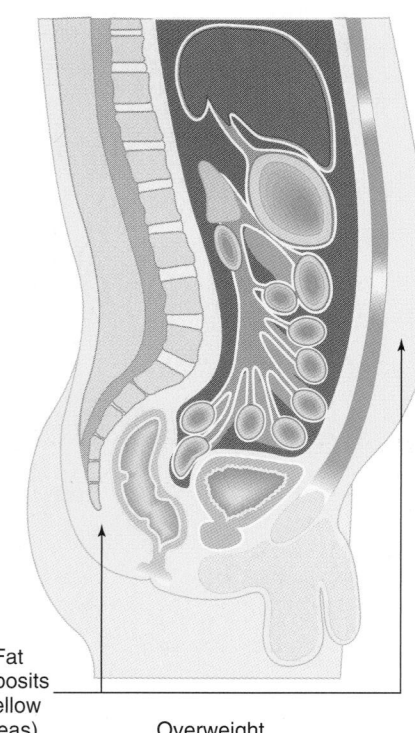

Average Weight

Fat Deposits (yellow areas)

Overweight

FIGURE 8.2
The sites of fat storage. Much of our body fat (shown in yellow) is stored directly beneath the skin.

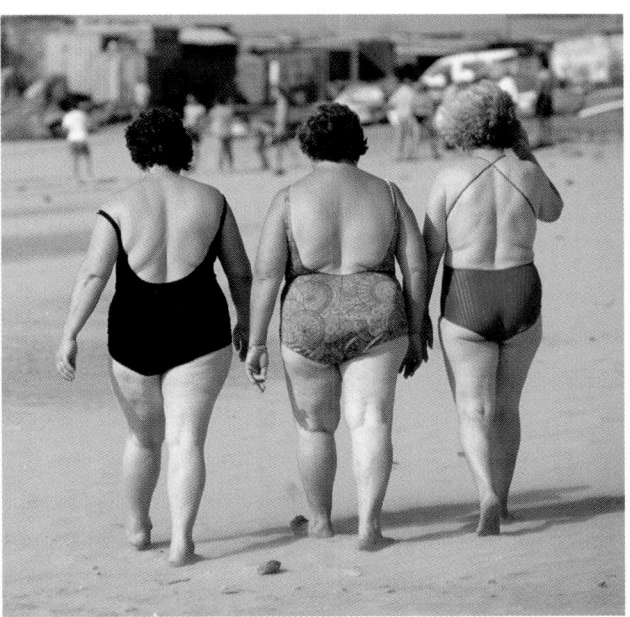

Fat storage in women tends to be in the lower body.

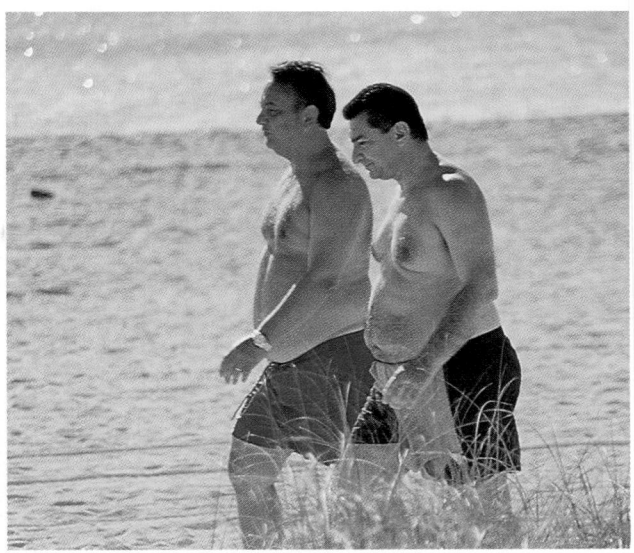

Men tend to store body fat in the upper body.

✺ Optimal Body Weight

Almost everyone has an idea about how much they should weigh for optimal physical appearance. However, a key question is, "What is my optimal body weight for health and fitness?" Although researchers disagree on the answer to this question, some guidelines are available. In general, optimal body fat for health and fitness in men ranges from 10–20%, whereas the optimal range of body fat for women is 15%–25% (11, 17–21) (Figure 8.3). These ranges allow for individual differences in physical activity and appearance and are associated with limited risk of the diseases linked to body fatness.

OPTIMAL BODY WEIGHT BASED ON PERCENT FAT

A variety of methods and equipment is available for estimating body fat composition, including the skinfold caliper technique discussed in Chapter 2. (For a brief review of what's available on the market, see Fitness-Wellness Consumer, p. 228). Once we know how to compute percent body fat and the optimal range of body fat, how can we determine the desired range of body weight? Consider the following example of a male college student who has 25% body fat and weighs 185 pounds. What is the optimal range of body weight for health and fitness in this individual? The calculations can be done in two simple steps:

Step 1: Compute fat-free weight—that is, the amount of total body weight contained in bones, organs, and muscles:

$$\text{Total body weight} - \text{fat weight} = \text{fat-free weight}$$
$$100\% \quad - \quad 25\% \quad = \quad 75\%$$

This means that 75% of total body weight is fat-free weight. Therefore, the fat-free weight for this student is

$$75\% \times 185 \text{ pounds} = 138.8 \text{ pounds}$$

Step 2: Calculate the optimal weight (which for men is 10–20% of total body weight): The formula to compute optimum body weight is

$$\text{Optimum weight} = \text{fat-free weight} \div (1 - \text{optimal \% fat})$$

Note that % fat should be expressed as a decimal. Thus, for 10% body fat,

$$\text{Optimum weight} = 138.8 \div (1 - 0.10) = 154.2 \text{ pounds}$$

For 20% body fat,

$$\text{Optimum weight} = 138.8 \div (1 - 0.20) = 173.5 \text{ pounds}$$

Hence, the optimal body weight for this individual is between 154.2 and 173.5 pounds. Laboratory 8.1 on p. 249 provides the opportunity to compute your optimal body weight, using both percent body fat and body mass index (introduced in Chapter 2).

✺ IN SUMMARY

- Obesity refers to individuals with a high percentage of body fat, generally over 25% for men and over 30% for women.

- Much of an individual's body fat is stored directly beneath the skin. The different regional patterns of fat storage in different individuals result from genetic differences.

- The ranges of optimal body fat for health and fitness are 10–20% for men and 15–25% for women.

Commercial Devices for Measuring Body Composition

Public interest in measuring body fat has prompted several companies to develop and sell a variety of devices, which range in price from under $20 to over $30,000. As discussed in Chapter 2, one of the least expensive and most accurate techniques involves measuring fat beneath the skin using skinfold calipers.

Several companies sell high-quality metal calipers that maintain a standard amount of tension when the calipers are closed up around the skinfold (cost: generally above $300). Such standardized tension is critical to the accurate measurement of skinfold thickness. In contrast, some companies market plastic calipers (cost: $20–$50), some of which generate too much or too little tension when in use. Therefore, before you purchase a lower-cost plastic caliper, do some homework and choose calipers that have been scientifically proven to provide accurate skinfold measurements.

Several companies are also marketing bathroom scales that contain electronic instruments designed to estimate body fat rapidly and noninvasively (cost: $70–$2500). Most of these devices use the principle of bio-electric impedance analysis (BIA) and measure the conductance of electricity in your body. Put simply, because fat-free (lean) tissues (such as skeletal muscle) contain large amounts of electrolytes (such as sodium and potassium) and water, lean tissue is a good conductor of electricity. In contrast, fat contains limited water and therefore is a poor conductor of electricity. Accordingly, an individual with a high percentage of body fat conducts electricity more poorly than someone with a lower percentage of body fat. These instruments are calibrated to estimate the amount of lean tissue in the body based on the electrical conductance they measure.

But are BIA devices accurate? Unfortunately, a direct answer to this question is not available, but it's clear that some of them are more accurate than others. Before you purchase any BIA device for home use, consult some of the excellent published reviews on BIA, including Going and Davis (2001) (cited in Suggested Readings at the end of this chapter).

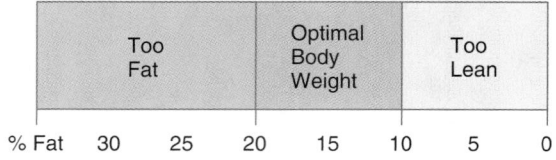

Men

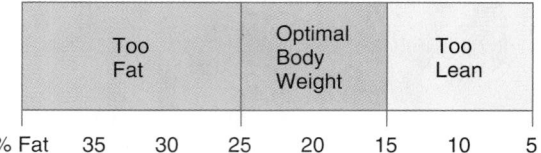

Women

FIGURE 8.3
The concept of ideal body weight based on a desirable percent of body fat.

 Physiology of Weight Control

Before we discuss how to begin a weight loss program, let's outline some key physiological concepts associated with weight loss. Although the details of how body fat stores are regulated are beyond the scope of this text, Figure 8.4 on p. 230 presents a simplified overview of the processes involved. Simply stated, body fat stores are regulated by two factors: (1) the rate at which fat is synthesized and stored, and (2) the rate at which energy is expended and fat is metabolized (broken down). In general, fat stores increase when energy intake exceeds energy expenditure, and decrease when energy expenditure exceeds energy intake. Note in Figure 8.4a that an increase in energy intake in response to increased appetite leads to increases in fat synthesis and storage. In contrast, fat stores are reduced when fat is broken down for use as a source of energy for the body (Figure 8.4b).

We discuss energy expenditure and fat metabolism later in this chapter; here the focus is on the rate of energy intake. Because the key factor determining the rate of energy intake is appetite, it is not surprising that the factors that regulate hunger are the subjects of intense research. In 1994, scientists discovered in fat cells a new gene, called the obese (Ob) gene, that produces the hormone leptin, which appears to depress appetite by acting on areas of the brain that control hunger (23). Research revealed that obese mice had very low blood levels of leptin, and when obese mice injected with leptin became lean, researchers became hopeful that leptin might become a cure for obesity in humans. However, those hopes were dashed when it was later discovered that many obese people produce abnormally high levels of leptin, and that leptin is but one of several interacting chemicals involved in appetite (23). Perhaps ongoing research will soon provide a clearer picture of what controls appetite.

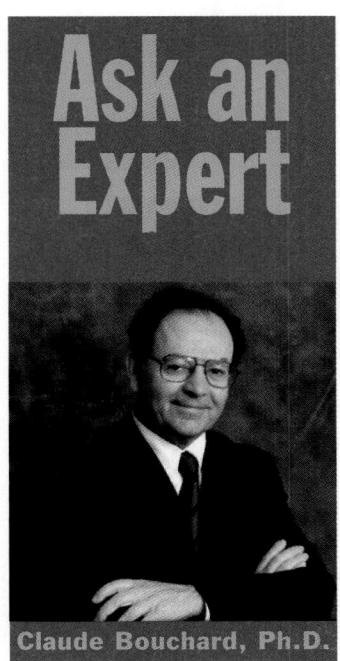

Ask an Expert

Claude Bouchard, Ph.D.

Obesity and Weight Loss

Dr. Bouchard is professor and Director of the Pennington Biomedical Research Institute at Louisiana State University School of Medicine. Dr. Bouchard is an internationally known expert regarding the cause and treatment of obesity. Indeed, Dr. Bouchard has published many scientific papers, books, and book chapters related to physical activity, diet, genetics. and weight loss. In the following interview, Dr. Bouchard addresses several hot topic questions related to obesity and weight loss.

Q: Having a low resting metabolic rate is generally accepted as a major contributing factor to obesity. Based on current research, what percent of obese individuals actually suffer from an abnormally low resting metabolic rate?

A: There is no universal agreement on the notion that a low resting metabolic rate is a cause of obesity. The hypothesis is supported by a study on Pima Indians but is not supported in several other reports. It is unlikely that a low resting metabolic rate is an important cause of the predisposition to become obese over time. Most likely, low resting metabolic rate plays only a minor role in the cause of obesity.

Q: How important is daily exercise in the prevention and treatment of obesity?

A: A low level of daily energy expenditure from physical activity is one of the factors contributing to the current epidemic of overweight and obesity cases. Over the last century we have continued to consume about the same number of calories in the presence of a decreasing level of energy expenditure as a result of major changes in transportation, work environment, household and other chores, as well as in discretionary time. As a result of decreasing energy expenditure, a growing number of people are gaining body fat (weight) until their weight reaches a new level that matches energy balance. The only way to prevent this weight gain is to reduce calorie intake or to become physically active. A reasonable volume of weekly physical activity, say about 200 min per week, is an excellent way to prevent unwarranted weight gain.

Q: You are currently the principal investigator of a very important research study aimed at determining the role of genetics in obesity. What are some of the most important findings of this work?

A: The main finding is that obesity is seldom caused by one simple deficiency in one specific gene. A genetic predisposition to obesity is generally brought about by multiple deficiencies of multiple genes. In other words, the genetic predisposition to gain weight for prolonged periods of time is not the prime determinant of obesity. In most cases, the predisposition can be opposed by reducing calorie intake and increasing calorie expenditure.

In the last several decades, three primary approaches to weight loss have emerged: the energy balance concept of weight control, the fat deficit concept of weight control, and the low carbohydrate diet approach to weight control. Let's examine the theory behind each of these three concepts.

ENERGY BALANCE CONCEPT OF WEIGHT CONTROL

The energy balance theory of weight control is simple and can be illustrated by the energy balance equation (Figure 8.5). To maintain a constant body weight, your food energy intake (expressed in calories) must equal

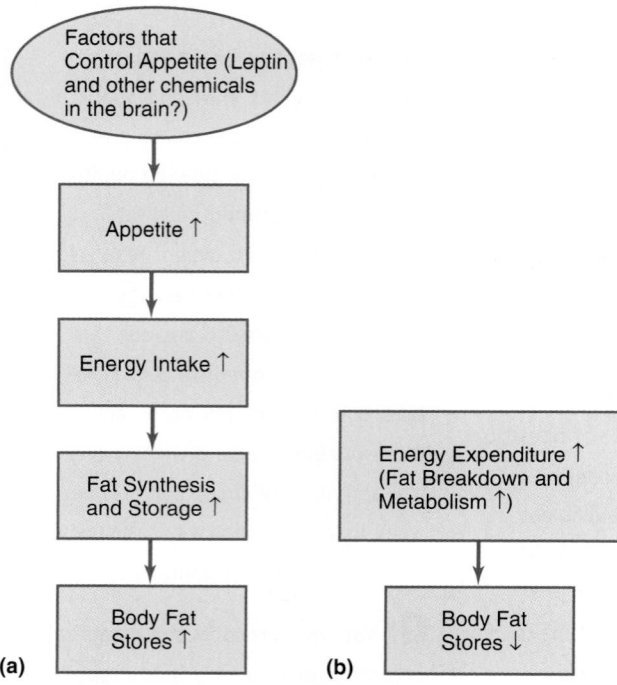

(a) **(b)**

FIGURE 8.4
Regulation of body fat stores.

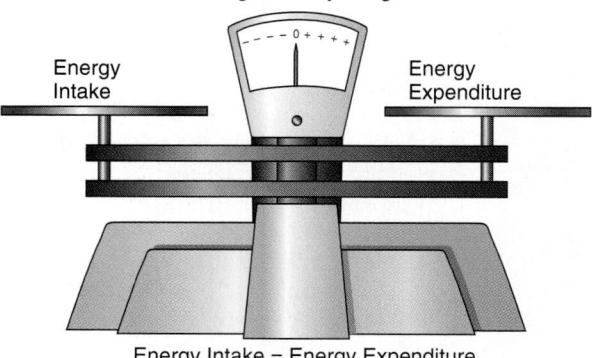

(a) Isocaloric Balance

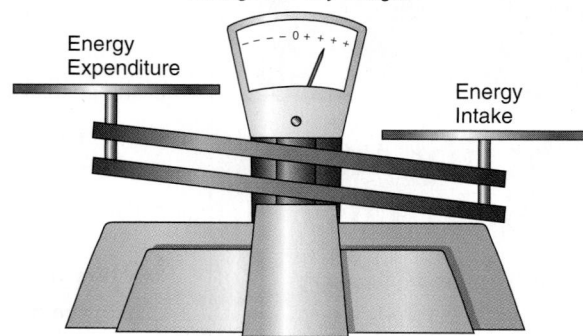

(b) Positive Balance

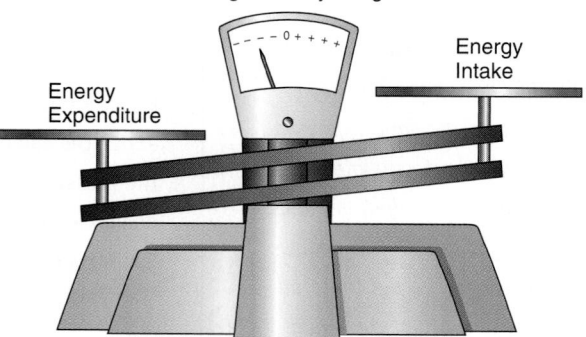

(c) Negative Caloric Balance

FIGURE 8.5
The concept of energy balance. a) Isocaloric balance; b) a positive caloric balance; and c) a negative caloric balance

your energy expenditure, a condition called **isocaloric balance** (Figure 8.5a). If you consume more calories than you expend, you gain body fat. Consuming more calories than you expend results in a **positive caloric balance** (Figure 8.5b). Finally, if you expend more calories than you consume, you lose body fat and have a **negative caloric balance** (Figure 8.5c).

From the energy balance equation presented in Figure 8.5, you might conclude that weight gain can be prevented by either decreasing your energy (food) intake or increasing your energy (exercise) expenditure. In practice, good weight loss programs include both a reduction in caloric intake and an increase in caloric expenditure achieved through exercise (7, 21, 24, 25).

ENERGY EXPENDITURE Estimating your daily energy expenditure is a key factor in planning a weight loss program and adjusting the energy balance equation. The daily expenditure of energy involves both the resting metabolic rate and exercise metabolic rate. Let's examine each of these individually.

isocaloric balance Condition when food energy intake equals energy expenditure.
positive caloric balance Condition when more calories are consumed than are expended.
negative caloric balance Condition when more calories are expended than are consumed.

TABLE 8.1
Estimation of Daily Caloric Expenditure Based on Body Weight and Physical Activity
To compute your estimated daily caloric expenditure, multiply your body weight in pounds by the calories per pound that corresponds to your activity level.

Activity Level	Description	Calories per Pound of Body Weight Expended during a 24-hour Period
1	Very sedentary (restricted movement, such as a patient confined to a house)	13
2	Sedentary (most U.S. citizens; light work or office job)	14
3	Moderate activity (many college students; some daily activity and weekend recreation)	15
4	Very physically active (vigorous activity at least 3–4 times/week)	16
5	Competitive athlete (daily activity in high-energy sport)	17–18

Resting metabolic rate (RMR) is the amount of energy expended during all sedentary activities. That is, RMR includes the energy required to maintain necessary bodily functions (called the basal metabolic rate) plus the additional energy required to perform such activities as sitting, reading, typing, and digestion of food. The RMR is an important component of the energy balance equation because it represents approximately 90% of the total daily energy expenditure in sedentary individuals (26). Resting metabolic rate is influenced by a variety of factors including age and the amount of lean body mass that an individual possesses. For example, resting metabolic (expressed per pound of body weight) is generally higher in growing children compared to adults. Moreover, resting metabolic rate declines with advancing age. Finally, resting metabolic rate is elevated in individuals with a low percentage of body fat and high lean mass (i.e., high levels of muscularity). The physiological explanation for this observation is that the energy required to maintain muscle tissue is greater than the cost of maintaining fat tissue (55). Recall that the importance of resting metabolic rate on obesity was discussed earlier in the Ask an Expert box feature on Obesity and Weight Loss.

Exercise metabolic rate (EMR) represents the energy expenditure during any form of exercise (walking, climbing steps, weight lifting, and so on). In sedentary individuals, EMR constitutes only 10% of the total daily energy expenditure. By comparison, EMR can account for 20–40% of the total daily energy expenditure in active individuals (26). For example, during heavy exercise, EMR may be 10–20 times greater than RMR (21). Therefore, increased daily exercise results in an increase in the EMR and is a key factor in weight control programs.

ESTIMATING DAILY ENERGY EXPENDITURE Dieting is widespread in the United States as people try to reduce body fat by decreasing energy intake. The obvious goal of dieting is to consume less energy than is expended and therefore create a negative energy balance and resulting weight loss. The first step in this process is to estimate your daily caloric expenditure. One of the simplest ways to do so is presented in Table 8.1, which provides estimates of daily caloric energy expenditure based on body weight and physical activity. For example, let's compute the estimated daily caloric expenditure for a college-age woman whose body weight is 120 pounds and who is involved in only moderate physical activity on weekends. Using Table 8.1, we locate her activity level on the left (i.e., level 3) and her estimated calories expended per pound of body weight (15 calories per pound per day) in the right-hand column. To calculate her total daily energy expenditure, we multiply her body weight by her caloric expenditure:

$$\text{Daily caloric expenditure} = 120 \text{ pounds} \times 15$$
$$\text{calories/pound/day} = 1800 \text{ calories/day}$$

Do this same calculation for your own daily caloric expenditure. If you need to lose weight, you are now prepared to create a negative energy balance by reducing your energy intake. Note that after losing 5 pounds of body weight, you should recalculate your estimated caloric expenditure; this is necessary because the weight loss results in a lower daily energy expenditure (Laboratory 8.2, p. 251).

---

resting metabolic rate (RMR) The amount of energy expended during all sedentary activities.
exercise metabolic rate (EMR) The energy expenditure during any form of exercise.

(a) Positive Fat Balance

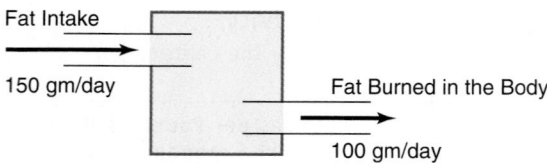

Fat Intake > Fat Metabolism (weight gained)

(b) Iso Fat Balance

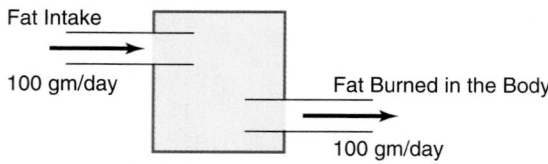

Fat Intake = Fat Metabolism (no weight gained)

(c) Negative Fat Balance

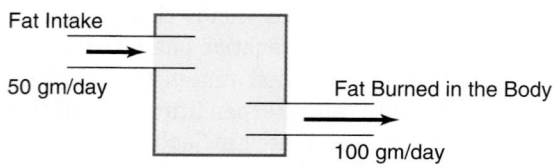

Fat Intake < Fat Metabolism (weight loss)

FIGURE 8.6
Importance of a low-fat diet in creating a fat deficit and promoting weight loss.

FAT DEFICIT CONCEPT OF WEIGHT CONTROL

The general concept that weight loss occurs due to a negative caloric balance is straightforward and easy to understand. Nonetheless, recent evidence suggests that creating a fat deficit is an important factor in weight loss that is often overlooked (27). For instance, it is now accepted that dietary fat is more easily stored as body fat than are either carbohydrates or protein (27). This occurs because dietary fat is not used as a body fuel as rapidly as is carbohydrate or protein. For example, if eating large amounts of carbohydrates or protein creates a positive caloric balance, some of the excess calories are used to repair body tissues, replace body carbohydrate stores, or provide body energy. In contrast, if excess calories are consumed as fat, they are likely to be stored as body fat (27).

The importance of a low-fat diet in weight control can best be illustrated by the fact that body fat gain is a result of a continual imbalance of fat intake and fat metabolism (fat burned in the body). In other words, if you ingest more fat than you burn during the day, you gain fat and weight (Figure 8.6a). It follows that if you consume and burn equal amounts of fat, your fat weight remains constant (Figure 8.6b). Finally, if you burn more fat than you consume (a fat deficit), you lose body fat and weight (Figure 8.6c). Thus, losing

body fat involves not only creating an energy deficit; your diet must provide a caloric deficit that also results in a fat deficit. We will discuss how to design a diet plan that is low in fat and calories shortly.

LOW CARBOHYDRATE DIETS AND WEIGHT LOSS

Almost everyone has heard about the many popular diet books that proclaim the secret to losing weight is a low carbohydrate diet. Indeed, several low carbohydrate diet books have become best sellers during the past 10 years. So, given the hype about low carbohydrate diets, is there a physiological basis to support the argument that diets low in carbohydrates (and calories) provide superior weight loss compared to other diet plans?

Before we begin a discussion of the physiological basis of why low carbohydrate diets may be effective in weight loss, it is important to appreciate that, identical to all other successful weight loss plans, low carbohydrate diets must result in a caloric deficit for an individual to lose body fat. With this fact established, is there a beneficial weight loss effect of consuming a low calorie diet that is also low in carbohydrates?

Proponents of low carbohydrate diets argue that these diets have two major advantages over conventional diet plans (45, 49). First, eating high carbohydrate foods promotes the use of carbohydrate as fuel and reduces the rate of fat metabolism. This argument is supported experimentally and the physiology to explain this claim is as follows. Consuming high carbohydrate foods promotes an increase in the hormone, insulin. High insulin levels are counter-productive to weight loss because insulin stimulates both fat storage and a reduction in the use of fat as a body fuel (21, 49).

The second argument in favor of low carbohydrate diets is that high carbohydrate foods are less satiating than foods containing high levels of proteins or fats (49). Therefore, low carbohydrate diets may promote satiety, reduce overall caloric intake, and assist in achieving a negative caloric balance. While evidence exists to support this argument, low-carbohydrate diets do not suppress appetite in all people.

Low carbohydrate diets that create a caloric deficit do result in weight loss, and it is arguable that these diets may have advantages over conventional weight loss programs. Nonetheless, the long-term effectiveness and safety of low carbohydrate diets is still in question. See A Closer Look on p. 233 for more details on low carbohydrate diets.

WHAT IS A SAFE RATE OF WEIGHT LOSS?

Before we discuss how to design a weight loss program, we should address two general points about weight loss. First, the maximum recommended rate for weight loss

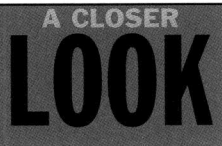

More Details on Low-Carbohydrate Diets and Weight Loss

Many different types of low-carbohydrate diets have been popularized over the years. Names of low carbohydrate diets include the Zone diet, Atkins New Diet Revolution, Calories Don't Count, Sugar Busters, Scarsdale diet, and the South Beach diet. New ones continue to be introduced but essentially they are all the same diet. That is, any diet low in carbohydrates will promote physiological responses similar to other low calorie diets.

Low carbohydrate diets were first introduced in the 1970s and have enjoyed a recent surge in popularity due to the initial weight loss that occurs with low carbohydrate diets. A common sales pitch for these diets is "you never feel hungry" and "you will lose weight fast." Both claims are true but can be misleading. For example, loss of appetite does occur in some people with a low carbohydrate diet but it does not occur in everyone. Further, although it is true that most people

lose body weight rapidly after beginning a low carbohydrate diet, this initial weight loss is not fat loss. Indeed, a low-carbohydrate diet results in a reduction of body water stores and this water loss explains the rapid weight loss observed in these diets. Importantly, the water can be regained after a normal diet is resumed causing some people on low carbohydrate diets to regain weight that voids their initial weight loss (21,52).

Are low carbohydrate diets superior to conventional low fat diets in promoting weight loss? This is a difficult question to answer but recent studies suggest that low carbohydrate diets and low fat diets result in approximately equal weight loss over a 3- to 12-month period (46, 47). Because of the limited number of long-term studies, most scientists agree that more studies are required to determine which diet approach is superior for long-term weight loss.

Nonetheless, current evidence suggests that both dietary approaches to weight loss are effective.

Are low carbohydrate diets safe for long-term use? Unfortunately, the answer to this question is currently unknown. It has been argued that health hazards may accompany low carbohydrate diets. For example, some low carbohydrate diets have been associated with high blood cholesterol, hypoglycemia, and other metabolic disorders. These observations suggest that low carbohydrate diets can be dangerous. While it is true that some low carbohydrate (and high fat diets) can lead to high blood cholesterol, a recent study reveals that a low carbohydrate diet with relatively low fat does not elevate blood cholesterol levels and promote cardiovascular risk factors (47). Nonetheless, while evidence is accumulating in favor of low carbohydrate diets, the safety and effectiveness of a low carbohydrate/high protein diet needs further long-term study before firm recommendations can be made (45, 49).

---

is 1 to 2 pounds per week. Diets resulting in a weight loss of more than 2 pounds per week are associated with a significant loss of lean body mass (i.e., muscle and body organs). In general, a weight loss goal of 1 pound per week is a safe and reasonable goal. The negative energy balance required to lose 1 pound per week is approximately 3500 calories. Therefore, a negative energy balance of 500 calories per day would theoretically result in a loss of 1 pound of fat per week (3500 calories/week ÷ 7 days/week = 500 calories/day).

A second general point about weight loss is that the rate of loss during the first several days of dieting will be greater than later in the dieting period. This is true because at the onset of a diet, in addition to fat loss there is an initial reduction in body carbohydrate and water stores, which also results in some weight loss (21). Further, some lean tissue, such as muscle, may also be lost during the beginning of any diet; the caloric content of lean tissue is less than fat. Therefore,

more than 1 pound will be lost during the first 3500-calorie deficit. However, as the diet continues, weight loss will occur at a slower rate. This fact should not discourage you, because subsequent weight loss will be primarily from body fat stores. Sticking with your weight plan for several weeks will result in a significant fat loss, and you will like the associated changes.

WHERE ON THE BODY DOES FAT REDUCTION OCCUR?

A key weight loss question is, "Where on the body do changes occur when fat is lost?" The answer is that most weight loss occurs in body areas that contain the greatest fat storage. Figure 8.7 illustrates this point in a study of obese women who completed a 14-week weight loss program that resulted in each participant losing approximately 20 pounds of fat (28). At the beginning of the study, regional fat storage was assessed using skinfold measurements, and it was determined

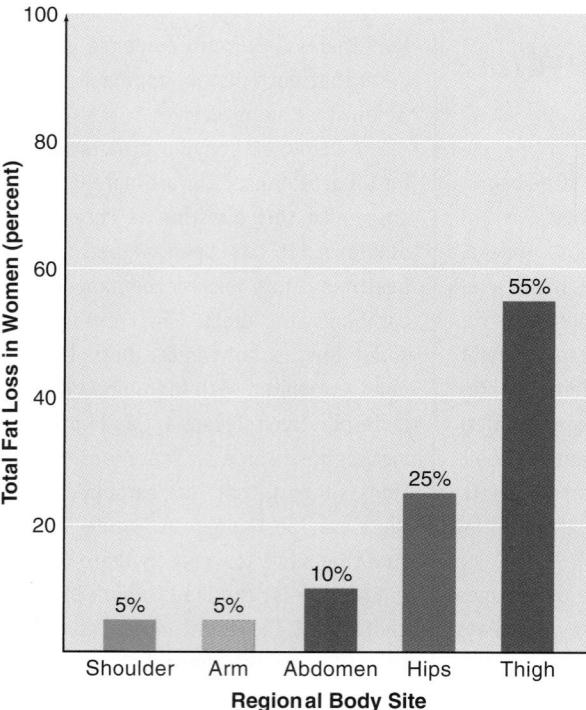

FIGURE 8.7
Fat Loss from different areas of the body in women. In both sexes, fat is lost from those areas that store the most fat.
Source: Data from King, M., and F. Katch. Changes in body density, fat folds, and girths at 2.3 kg increments of weight loss. *Human Biology* 58:709, 1986.

that the largest percentage of fat was stored in the thighs, hips, and abdomen. At the completion of the study, regional fat storage was reassessed to determine where the fat loss occurred. Approximately 90% of the fat loss occurred in the body regions with the highest fat storage (Figure 8.7). This is good news because most people want to lose fat from those areas.

☀ IN SUMMARY

- To maintain a constant body weight, your food energy (caloric) intake must equal your caloric expenditure; this is called an isocaloric balance.
- Consuming more calories than you expend results in a positive caloric balance and weight gain.
- Consuming fewer calories than you expend results in a negative caloric balance and weight loss.
- Daily energy expenditure can be estimated by considering both your resting metabolic rate and your exercise caloric expenditure.
- While it is true that weight loss generally occurs due to a caloric deficit, new evidence also indicates that creating a fat deficit is another essential factor in the loss of body fat. A fat deficit is created when the amount of fat burned in the body exceeds the dietary intake of fat.

☀ Establishing a Successful Weight Loss Program

With proper knowledge and motivation, almost anyone can design a weight loss program. The four basic components of a comprehensive weight control program are establishment of weight loss goals; a reduced caloric diet stressing balanced nutrition, high carbohydrate intake, and low fat intake; an exercise program designed to increase caloric expenditure and maintain or increase muscle mass; and a behavior modification program aimed at changing eating habits that contribute to weight gain.

WEIGHT LOSS GOALS

The establishment of weight loss goals is a key component of any weight loss program. The first step is to decide where your percent body fat should be within the optimal range (10–20% for men, 15–25% for women). Many people who are beginning a comprehensive weight loss program choose a long-term weight loss goal that will place them in the middle of the optimal weight range (15% body fat for men, 20% body fat for women). After choosing your long-term goal, it is also useful to establish short-term weight loss goals—usually expressed in the number of pounds lost per week (A Closer Look and Laboratory 8.3 on p. 253).

ROLE OF DIET IN WEIGHT LOSS

Bookstore shelves are filled with diet books, and television and radio advertisements promote "miracle" diets. While some of these diets may promote weight loss, many do not provide balanced nutrition. When assessing new diets, a general rule of thumb is to avoid fad diets that promise fast and easy weight loss (Nutritional Links to Health and Fitness, p. 236). If you have concerns about the safety or effectiveness of a published diet, you can either contact your local branch of the American Dietetic Association for information or approach a dietitian at a hospital or college. By learning the basic nutrition principles contained in this chapter and in Chapter 7, you should be able to critically evaluate most diet plans.

Table 8.2 presents a brief summary of some of the major types of diets used in weight loss programs (21). Any safe and nutritionally sound diet should adhere to the following guidelines (4–7, 12, 19, 30):

- The diet should be low in calories but provide all the essential nutrients the body requires.
- The diet should be low in fat (less than 30% of total calories) in complex carbohydrates. Remember, a diet low in fat and calories is essential to

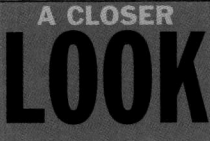

Short-Term and Long-Term Weight Loss Goals

Short-term weight loss goals are designed to provide weight loss targets that can be achieved within a 2- to 4-week period. For example, an initial short-term weight loss goal might be to lose 2 pounds during the first 2 weeks of your weight loss program. Achievement of each short-term goal provides the motivation to establish another short-term goal and continue the weight loss program. (See the box figure.)

Long-term weight loss goals generally focus on reaching the desired percent of body fat. For instance, a long-term goal for a male college student might be to reach 15% body fat within the first year of his weight loss program. After reaching this long-term goal, his objective then becomes the maintenance of this desired body composition.

The relationship between short-term and long-term weight loss goals

Weight Loss Goals

↓

Short-Term Goal 1

↓

Short-Term Goal 2

↓

Short-Term Goal 3

↓

Long-Term Goal

TABLE 8.2
Examples of Weight Loss Diets

Type of Diet	Description/Comments	Recommended?
Low carbohydrate	High protein and may also contain high fat content; well-designed diets can be nutritionally balanced	With caution*
Low calorie liquid diet	Although nutritionally balanced, these diets are typically monotonous and unsatisfying	No
Very-low calorie diet	Provides 300–600 calories/day; nutritionally unbalanced and unsafe for long-term use	No
Balanced low calorie diet	Can be nutritionally balanced and safe for long-term use; typically provides a 500–1000 calorie/day deficit	Yes

* Long-term use of low carbohydrate diets require additional study before a firm recommendation can be made (see text for more details).

---

creating fat loss. Establishing a diet that creates a negative caloric balance with less than 30% of the total calories coming from fat will ensure that each day you metabolize more fat than you take in.

- The diet should contain a variety of foods to appeal to your tastes and to prevent hunger between meals.

- The diet should be compatible with your lifestyle, and the foods should be easily obtainable.

- The diet should be a lifelong diet; that is, it should be one that you can follow for the remainder of your life. This type of diet greatly increases your chances of maintaining an ideal weight in the future.

- The diet should provide foods that adhere to the principles of eating for health.

In addition to these diet guidelines, here are some helpful reminders (some of which were covered in Chapter 7) for planning a successful balanced diet:

- Avoid high-calorie, low-nutrient foods such as those high in sugar (e.g., candy bars, cookies). Instead, select low-calorie, nutrient-dense foods such as fruits, vegetables, and whole-grain breads.

- Reduce the amount of fat in your diet. High-fat foods are high in calories. For example, eat less butter and choose meats that are low in fat, such as lean cuts of beef, chicken, and fish. Avoid fried foods; broil, bake, or microwave your food. If you must use oil in your cooking, use monosaturated oils such as olive oil or peanut oil.

Nutritional Links
TO HEALTH AND FITNESS

Frequently Asked Questions About Weight-Loss Diets

What types of weight loss diets are considered "Fad diets"?

A diet is considered a "Fad" if it gains fame but then the popularity fades quickly when consumers realize that the diet does not perform as advertised. Numerous "Fad" diets currently exist and these diets come and go. Consumers can quickly evaluate the validity of a "Fad" weight loss diet in the following way. In general, any diet plan that claims to provide weight loss without using exercise and/or a reduction in caloric intake will not result in the loss of body fat. An example of a Fad diet is the grapefruit diet. Many myths have circulated about the value of consuming large quantities of grapefruit to promote weight loss. One of these myths suggests that eating highly acidic grapefruit dissolves fat and results in a rapid loss of body weight. Although eating citrus fruits as a part of healthy diet is a good idea, there is nothing magical about grapefruit that promotes fat loss. In fact, there are no magical foods that assist in weight loss. Therefore, consumers should be wary of any "Fad" diet that promises weight loss without providing a caloric deficit by reducing calorie intake.

What is the "glycemic index" of foods?

The "glycemic index" is a measure of how much insulin is released when a particular type of food is consumed. For example, foods that produce the highest release of insulin are assigned a high glycemic index. Since insulin release promotes fat storage in the body, proponents of low carbohydrate diets argue that people should avoid foods with a high glycemic index.

What are high protein diets and do they differ from low carbohydrate diets?

High protein diets are essentially low carbohydrate diets that emphasize consuming high levels of proteins. Most high protein diets recommend consuming large quantities of protein in unrestricted amounts. It follows that a diet that is high in protein results in a low carbohydrate intake. Therefore, any high protein diet would also be a low carbohydrate diet.

A health concern associated with high protein diets is that these diets often result in the consumption of large quantities of red meat, eggs, and cheese. Therefore, high protein diets may also be high fat diets. A high fat diet can result in elevated blood levels of cholesterol and therefore an increased risk of cardiovascular disease. Moreover, a high fat diet has been associated with an increased risk of certain cancers. For this reason, the World Cancer Research Fund recommends against the use of any high protein diet.

Can caloric restriction slow aging and increase longevity?

The practice of caloric restriction involves consuming a balanced diet but restricting your caloric intake by approximately 20 to 40 percent below the level of energy consumed in freely chosen diet. This practice has been shown to extend life span in a variety of animal species including rats, mice, and worms (53). However, whether prolonged caloric restriction increases life span or reduces the rate of aging in humans is unknown (53). For more information on this topic see Heilbronn and Ravussin (2003) in the suggested readings list.

What role does dietary calcium and diary products have on weight management?

New evidence suggests that dietary calcium from diary products may play an important role in weight management. The proposed mechanism relates to the fact that calcium plays a key role in fat metabolism and the storage of fat (54). Specifically, a diet high in calcium from diary products has been shown to promote fat metabolism, inhibit fat synthesis, and therefore, increase the loss of body fat (54). These concepts have been confirmed by epidemiological data and recent clinical studies indicating that diets high in diary products (> 3 servings per day) accelerate fat loss compared with diets low in dairy products (54). While these results are promising, additional studies are required to confirm the argument that increased calcium via diary products is a useful adjunct to a weight loss program.

- Although dairy products are excellent sources of protein, they may be high in calories unless the fat has been removed. Use nonfat or low-fat milk, low-fat cottage cheese, and similar products.
- Select fresh fruits and vegetables whenever possible, and avoid fruits that are canned in heavy syrup.
- Limit salt intake. Use herbs and other seasonings as substitutes for salt.
- Drink fewer alcoholic beverages. Alcoholic beverages are low in nutrients and high in calories.
- Eat three meals per day, and do not snack in between.

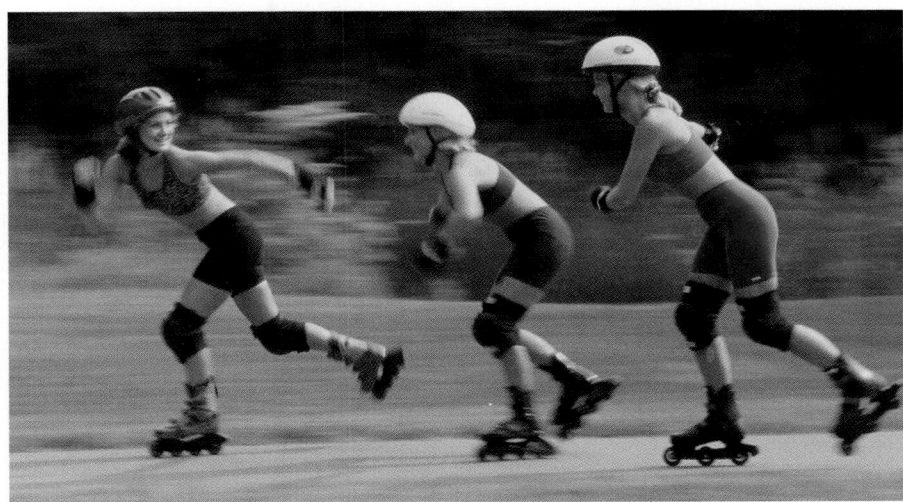

Exercise is a key component to any weight loss program.

Remember that a negative energy balance of 500 calories/day will result in a weight loss of approximately 1 pound per week. The key to maintaining a caloric deficit of 500 calories/day is careful planning of meals and accurate calorie counting.

EXERCISE AND WEIGHT LOSS

Exercise plays a key role in weight loss for several reasons (25, 31, 50). First, increased physical activity elevates your daily caloric expenditure and therefore assists you in creating a negative energy balance. Second, regular cardiorespiratory exercise training improves the ability of skeletal muscles to burn fat as energy. Third, regular resistance exercise (such as weight training) can reduce the loss of muscle that occurs during dieting. This is important because your primary goal in dieting is not to lose muscle mass but to promote fat loss. Finally, increasing your muscle mass by weight training results in an increased resting metabolic rate, which further aids in weight loss (33).

What type of exercise should be performed to assist in weight loss? A sound recommendation is that both cardiorespiratory training (i.e., running, cycling, swimming, and so on) and strength training be performed while dieting. (See A Closer Look on p. 239 for some details about the relationship between exercise and fat metabolism.) The combination of these two types of training will maintain cardiorespiratory fitness and reduce the loss of muscle.

How much exercise must be performed during a weight loss program? In general, exercise sessions designed to promote weight loss should expend in excess of 250 calories. Further, it is recommended that the negative caloric balance should be shared equally by exercise and diet. For instance, if an individual wishes to achieve a 500-calorie/day deficit, this should be done by increasing energy expenditure (exercise) by 250 calories/day and by decreasing caloric intake by 250 calories.

Although intensity of exercise is an important factor in improving cardiorespiratory fitness, it is the total amounts of energy expended and fat burned that are important in weight loss. Some authors have argued that low-intensity prolonged exercise is better than short-term high-intensity exercise (e.g., sprinting 50 yards) in burning fat calories and promoting weight loss (34, 35). However, recent evidence clearly demonstrates that both high- and low-intensity exercise can promote fat loss (21). Nonetheless, for the sedentary or obese individual, low-intensity exercise is the proper choice because it can be performed for longer time periods and results in an increase in the ability of skeletal muscle to metabolize fat as an energy source (21, 36). A brief discussion of the energy cost of various activities follows.

Table 8.3 contains estimates of the caloric costs of several types of physical activities. To compute your caloric expenditure (per minute) during an activity, simply multiply your body weight in kilograms (2.2 pounds = 1 kilogram) by the values in the Cal/min./kg column in Table 8.3 and by the exercise time. For example, suppose a 70-kilogram (kg) individual plays 20 minutes of handball. How many calories did he or she expend during the time of play? The total estimated caloric expenditure is computed as follows:

$$\text{Caloric expenditure} = 70 \text{ kg} \times 0.1603 \text{ calories/kg/min} \times 20 \text{ min} = 224 \text{ calories}$$

EXERCISE AND APPETITE

A common question is, Does exercise increase appetite? Although the high-intensity training programs used by many athletes may increase appetite, it is generally believed that when a moderate exercise program is intro-

TABLE 8.3
Energy Costs for Selected Sporting Activities

	Cal/min./kg	Cal/min.[*]	METs[**]
Archery (American Round)	0.0412	2.8	2.3
Bowling (with three other bowlers)	0.0471	3.2	2.7
Golf (playing in a foursome)	0.0559	3.8	3.2
Walking (17-min. mile on a grass surface)	0.0794	5.4	4.5
Cycling (6.4-min. mile)	0.0985	6.7	5.6
Canoeing (15-min. mile)	0.1029	7.0	5.8
Swimming (50-yd./min.)	0.1333	9.1	7.6
Running (10-min. mile)	0.1471	10.0	8.0
Cycling (5-min. mile)	0.1559	10.6	8.5
Handball (singles)	0.1603	10.9	9.1
Skipping rope (80 turns/min.)	0.1655	11.3	9.5
Running (8-min. mile)	0.1856	12.6	10.0
Running (6-min. mile)	0.2350	16.0	12.8

[*]*These values are for a 150-lb (68-kg) person.*

[**]*1 MET equals your resting metabolic rate.*

Source: From Getchell, B., 1992. Physical Fitness: A Way of Life. Copyright © 1992. Reprinted with permission from Benjamin Cummings.

duced to sedentary or obese individuals, appetite does not increase (37). In fact, moderate exercise training may diminish appetite (37).

BEHAVIOR MODIFICATION

Research demonstrates that behavior modification plays a key role in both achieving short-term weight loss and maintaining weight loss over the years (4–7). **Behavior modification** is a technique used in psychological therapy to promote desirable changes in behavior. The rationale behind it is that many behaviors are learned. For example, attending movies at the theater elicits, in many people, a response of eating popcorn and candy. Because these types of responses are learned, they can also be eliminated (unlearned). In regard to weight control, behavior modification is used primarily to reduce or (ideally) eliminate social or environmental stimuli that promote overeating.

The first step in a diet-related behavior modification program is to identify those social or environmental factors that promote overeating. This can be done by keeping a written record of daily activities for 1 or 2 weeks to identify factors associated with

consumption of high-calorie meals. In recording your daily eating habits, consider the following social or environmental factors (12):

- *Activities.* What activities are associated with eating? You may find a correlation between specific types of activities, such as watching TV and eating snacks.
- *Emotional behavior before or during eating.* What emotions are associated with eating? For instance, do you overeat when you are depressed or under stress? (Overeating is defined as the consumption of high-calorie meals that leads to a positive calorie balance).
- *Location of meals.* Where do you eat? Are specific rooms associated with snacks?
- *Time of day and level of hunger.* Do you eat at specific times of the day? When you eat, are you always hungry?
- *People involved.* With whom do you eat? Are specific people associated with periods of overeating?

After identifying the factors that influence your eating behavior, start a program aimed at correcting those behaviors that contribute to weight gain. The following weight control techniques have been used successfully for many years. Although it is not essential to use each of them, adhering to many will make weight control easier (12).

behavior modification A technique used in psychological therapy to promote desirable changes in behavior.

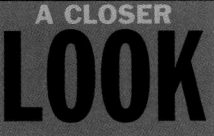

What Intensity of Aerobic Exercise Is Best for Burning Fat?

Many people assume that the intensity of aerobic exercise (running, cycling, and so on) must be maintained at a low level if fat is to be burned as fuel, and it is true that fat is a primary fuel source during low-intensity exercise. But as the figure in this box shows, the total amount of fat burned during exercise varies with the intensity of exercise, and for a given exercise duration, more total fat is metabolized during moderate-intensity exercise. Therefore, moderate-intensity exercise (that is, approximately 50% $\dot{V}O_{2max}$) is typically the optimal intensity of exercise for burning the most fat during an endurance exercise workout. For more details on this topic, see reference 32 in the References list at the end of this chapter.

Source: Coyle, E. Fat metabolism during exercise. *Sports Science Exchange* (Gatorade Sports Science Institute) 8:6, 1995.

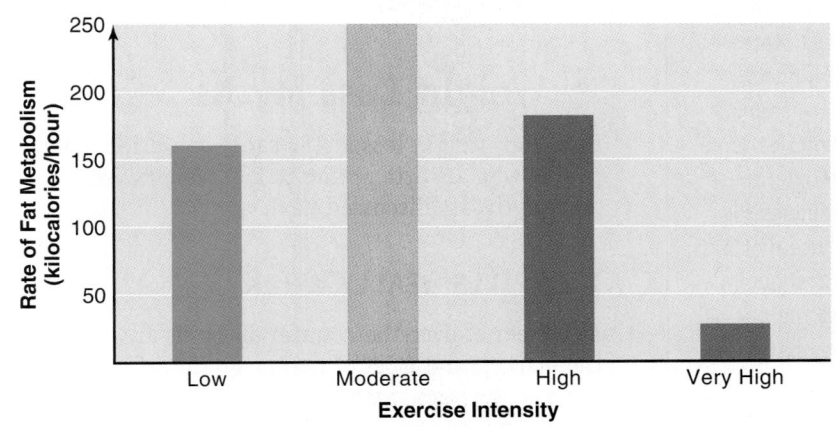

The rates of fat metabolism at low-intensity (20% $\dot{V}O_{2max}$), moderate-intensity (50% $\dot{V}O_{2max}$), high-intensity (80% $\dot{V}O_{2max}$), and very-high intensity (100% $\dot{V}O_{2max}$) exercise. While this figure is not intended to reveal any "ideal" exercise intensity for all individuals, it indicates that moderate-intensity exercise is often optimal for maximizing the amount of fat metabolized during exercise.

- *Make a personal commitment to losing weight.* This is the first step toward behavior modification and weight loss. The establishment of realistic short-term and long-term weight loss goals assists in maintaining a lifelong commitment to weight control.

- *Develop healthy low-calorie eating patterns.* Avoid eating when you are not hungry. Learn to eat slowly and only while sitting at the table. Finally, keep food quantities to the minimum amount within your caloric guidelines.

- *Avoid social settings where overeating is encouraged.* If you go to parties where high-calorie foods are served, don't go to these functions hungry. Eat a low-calorie meal before going.

- *Avoid snacking.* If snacks must be eaten, eat low-calorie foods such as carrots or celery.

- *Engage in daily exercise.* Regular exercise that uses large-muscle groups can play an important role in increasing your daily caloric expenditure and can therefore assist in weight control.

- *Reward yourself for successful weight loss with non-food rewards.* Rewards or positive feedback are an important part of behavior modification. For example, after reaching part of your weight loss goal, reward yourself by doing something you like to do (going to the beach, going hiking, or buying a new CD.)

- *Think positively.* Avoid negative thinking about how difficult weight loss can be. Positive thinking promotes confidence and maintains the enthusiasm necessary for a lifetime of successful weight control.

☀ IN SUMMARY

- Designing and executing a successful weight loss program requires knowledge and motivation.

- Establishing weight loss goals is a key component of any weight loss program.

- A safe and nutritionally sound diet should adhere to the guidelines of good nutrition.

- Both exercise and behavior modification play a key role in weight loss.

Lifetime Weight Control

The good news about weight loss is that anybody with the proper motivation can lose body fat. The bad news is that there is no simple way of losing body fat and keeping the fat off forever. Weight control over the course of a lifetime is only accomplished by the proper combination of diet, exercise, and behavior modification. The key factors in long-term weight control are a positive attitude toward weight control, regular exercise, and a personal commitment to maintaining a desired body composition.

Like many other facets of personal or professional life, weight control has its ups and downs. Be prepared for occasional setbacks. For instance, gaining weight during holiday periods is common and experienced by everyone at some time. When this type of weight gain occurs, avoid self-criticism, quickly reestablish your personal commitment to a short-term weight loss goal,

spot reduction The false notion that exercise applied to a specific region of the body will result in fat loss in that region.

and develop a new diet and exercise plan to lose the undesired fat. Remember, any amount of weight gain can be lost by applying the principles discussed in this chapter.

Finally, the importance of family and friends in lifetime weight control cannot be overemphasized. Their encouragement and support can both assist you in maintaining good eating habits and provide the needed support to sustain a lifetime commitment to exercise. It is much easier to lose weight if your close associates are trying to help you achieve your goals rather than tempting you to eat improperly. Therefore, surround yourself with friends that support you in your weight control goals.

Weight Loss Myths

Numerous weight loss myths cause confusion among people who are attempting to lose weight. Several common myths are discussed next.

DIET PILLS REALLY WORK

A number of over-the-counter diet pills are available on the market, and most of them contain caffeine and other mild stimulants (Fitness-Wellness Consumer, above left). Unfortunately, none of these products has been scientifically shown to assist in achieving safe and permanent weight loss. One study of individuals using commercially available diet pills reported that fewer than 3% of users lost weight and retained this weight loss longer than 12 months (2).

SPOT REDUCTION CAN OCCUR

The notion that exercise applied to a specific region of the body will result in fat loss in that region is called **spot reduction.** Will performing sit-ups, for example, result in a reduction in abdominal fat? Unfortunately, the answer is "no." To date, there is no scientific evidence to show that exercise promotes fat loss in local regions of the body (38). As we have seen, the evidence suggests that when a caloric deficit exists, fat loss will occur from the largest sites of fat stores and not from specific areas (28).

EATING BEFORE BEDTIME MAKES YOU FATTER

Some people believe that eating immediately prior to going to bed at night results in a greater fat gain than if the same meal were consumed during the day. These rumors are probably unfounded. Although eating a late-night meal or snack might not be a good dietary

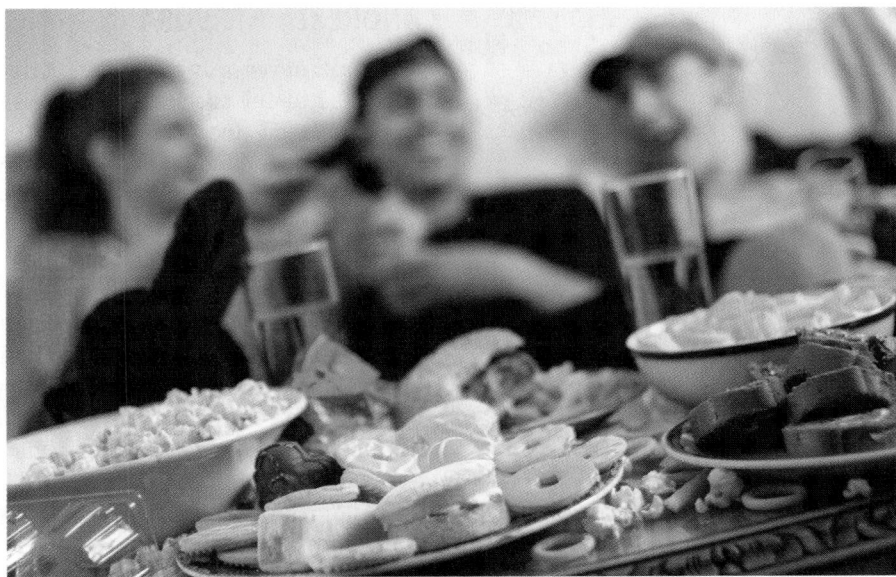

At parties or social gatherings, try to avoid high calorie snack foods.

habit, this practice does not result in a greater weight gain than if the same meal had been consumed at another time during the day. Remember, it is the total daily caloric intake that determines fat gain, not the timing of the meal (4, 5).

CELLULITE IS A SPECIAL TYPE OF FAT

It is commonly believed that two kinds of body fat exist: cellulite and regular fat (19). The term **cellulite** refers to the "lumpy" hard fat that often gives skin a dimpled look. In reality, cellulite is just plain fat, not a special type of fat. The "dimpled" appearance comes from fat accumulating into small clusters beneath the skin.

Some health spas have advertised that vigorous massages provided by machines can remove cellulite and improve the appearance of your skin. Nonetheless, no scientific evidence exists that massage techniques are effective in promoting body fat loss or altering skin appearance.

FAT-DISSOLVING CREAMS ARE EFFECTIVE

Over the years, numerous companies have marketed "weight loss creams" that are claimed to cause spot reduction of fat when applied to the skin. This is an attractive idea, as evidenced by the fact that companies have made millions of dollars from selling these products. Despite the boastful claims made by manufacturers, only limited scientific evidence suggests that these creams are effective in promoting fat loss.

SAUNAS, STEAMBATHS, AND RUBBER SUITS CAN AID IN LONG-TERM WEIGHT LOSS

Another myth related to the loss of body fat is the notion that sitting in saunas or steambaths and/or running in a rubber suit melts body fat. Although saunas and steambaths do temporarily increase your metabolic rate, they do not melt away fat, nor do they significantly contribute to weight loss (7). For similar reasons, exercising in a rubber suit does not promote greater fat loss than would be achieved by performing the same exercise in comfortable clothes.

These three methods do result in body water loss due to sweating, however. The accompanying body weight loss has been believed by some to be a loss of fat, but this is not the case. The weight temporarily lost in this way is regained as soon as body water is restored to normal levels.

Using saunas or steambaths and exercising while wearing a rubber suit may increase body temperature well above normal. This puts additional stress on the heart and circulatory system and could increase the risk of cardiac problems for older individuals or anyone with heart problems.

---

cellulite The "lumpy" hard fat that often gives skin a dimpled look. Cellulite is just plain fat and not a special category of fat.

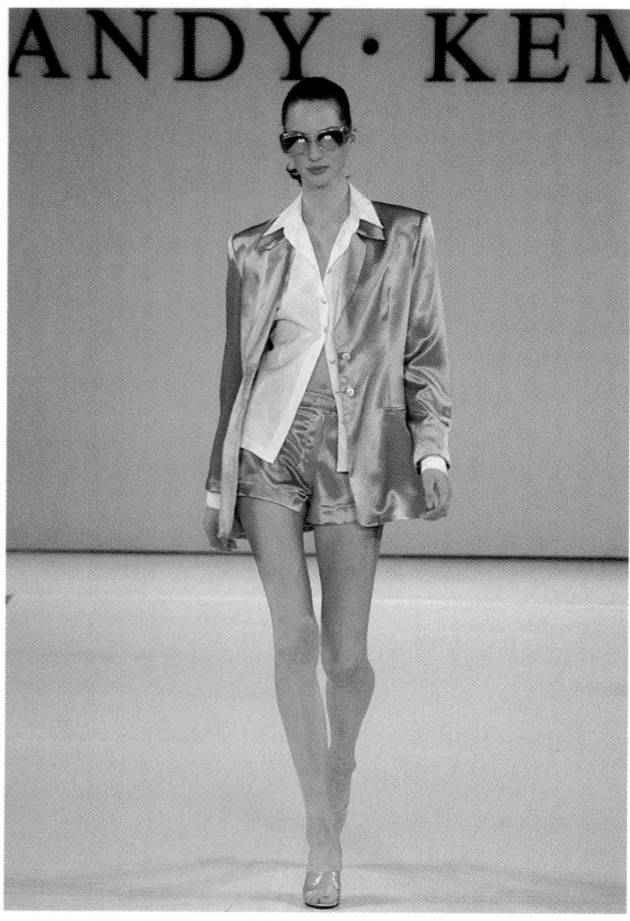

There are enormous societal pressures to be lean.

☀ Eating Disorders

The low social acceptance of individuals with a high percentage of body fat and an emphasis on having the "perfect" body have increased the incidence of eating disorders. Two of the more common ones that affect young adults are anorexia nervosa and bulimia. Because of the relatively high occurrence of both disorders in female college students, we will discuss both the symptoms and health consequences of each.

---

anorexia nervosa A common eating disorder that is unrelated to any specific physical disease. The end result of extreme anorexia nervosa is a state of starvation in which the individual becomes emaciated due to a refusal to eat.

bulimia An eating disorder that involves overeating (called *binge eating*) followed by vomiting (called *purging*).

ANOREXIA NERVOSA

Anorexia nervosa is a common eating disorder that is unrelated to any specific physical disease. The end result of extreme anorexia nervosa is a state of starvation in which the individual becomes emaciated due to a refusal to eat. The psychological cause of anorexia nervosa is unclear, but it seems to be linked to an unfounded fear of fatness that may be related to familial or societal pressures to be thin (12).

The incidence of this eating disorder has grown in recent years. Individuals with the highest probability of developing anorexia nervosa are upper-middle-class young women who are extremely self-critical. It is estimated that the incidence of anorexia nervosa is as high as one of every 200 adolescent girls (39, 40).

Anorexics may use a variety of techniques to remain thin, including starvation, exercise, and laxatives. The effects of anorexia include excessive weight loss, cessation of menstruation, and, in extreme cases, death. Because anorexia is a serious mental and physical disorder, medical treatment by a team of professionals (physician, psychologist, nutritionist) is needed to correct the problem. Treatment may require years of psychological counseling and nutritional guidance. The first step in seeking treatment for anorexia is recognizing a problem exists. The following are common symptoms of anorexia:

- An intense fear of gaining weight or becoming obese
- Feeling fat even at normal or below-normal body fatness because of a highly distorted body image
- In women, the absence of three or more menstrual cycles
- The possible development of odd behaviors concerning food; for example, the preparation of elaborate meals for others but of only a few low-calorie foods for their own consumption

BULIMIA

About 50% of all anorexics eventually come to suffer **bulimia,** which is overeating (called *binge eating*) followed by vomiting (called *purging*). In essence, bulimics repeatedly ingest large quantities of food and then force themselves to vomit in order to prevent weight gain. Bulimia may result in damage to the teeth and the esophagus due to frequent vomiting of stomach acids. Like anorexia nervosa, bulimia is most common in young women, has a psychological origin, and requires professional treatment when diagnosed. Several authors have indicated that the prevalence of bulimia may be as low as 1% or as high as 20% among U.S. girls and women aged 13 to 23 years (39, 40).

Most bulimics look "normal" and are of normal weight. However, even when their bodies are slender, their stomachs may protrude due to being stretched by frequent eating binges. Other common symptoms of bulimia include the following (41):

- Recurrent binge eating
- A lack of control over eating behavior
- Regular self-induced vomiting and use of diuretics or laxatives
- Strict fasting or use of vigorous exercise to prevent weight gain
- Averaging two or more binge-eating episodes a week during a 2- to 3-month period
- Overconcern with body shape and weight

Although maintaining an optimal body composition is a primary health goal, eating disorders are not appropriate means of weight loss. If you or any of your friends exhibit one or more of the symptoms cited here, please seek professional advice and treatment.

☀ IN SUMMARY

- Numerous weight loss myths add to confusion about weight loss.
- Even though many nonprescription diet pills are available, research indicates that the diet pill approach to weight loss is not successful for most people.
- Research indicates that exercise applied to a specific region of the body will not result in a "spot reduction" of body fat.
- The prevalence of two common eating disorders, anorexia nervosa and bulimia, is relatively high among female college students in the United States.

☀ Exercise and Diet Programs to Gain Weight

The major focus of this chapter has been how to lose body fat. However, a small number of people, who consider themselves to be too thin, want to gain body weight. Both men and women can suffer from self-image problems if they feel they are too skinny. Although current social attitudes stress leanness in women, many women agree that some degree of body curvature is desirable. Also, many men want a muscular body because of the improved self-image that comes with increased muscularity (12).

Body weight gain can be achieved in two ways. First, you can create a positive caloric balance and a positive fat balance and gain additional body fat.

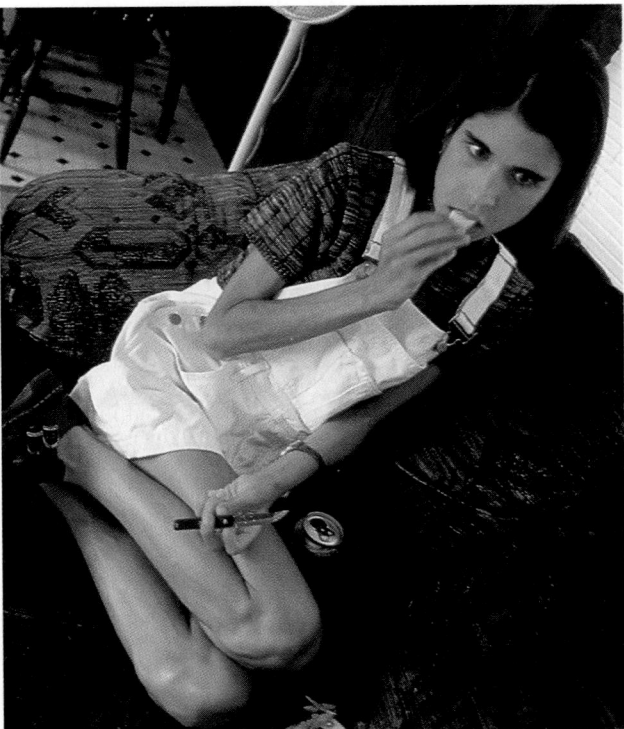

People with anorexia often have distorted body images.

Second, you can increase your body weight by increasing your muscle mass through a weight-training program. Let's discuss each of these types of body weight gain.

GAINING BODY FAT

Before deciding to gain body fat, you should determine if your current body composition is within the desired range (Chapter 2). If your percent body fat is below the recommended range (fewer than 8% of people fall into this category), it may be desirable for you to add body fat to reach the optimal percent body fat. Nonetheless, before looking at a dietary means for gaining fat, you should examine the cause of your being too lean (12).

Several lifestyle problems could contribute to a low percentage of body fatness (12). For example, are you getting enough sleep? If not, you may be burning large amounts of energy and creating a negative caloric balance. Do you drink large amounts of coffee? Coffee can influence body weight in two ways. First, more than three to five cups of coffee can reduce your appetite. Second, consumption of coffee or other caffeine-containing beverages increases your resting metabolism for several hours. Further, do you skip meals? Failing to eat regularly may result in a negative caloric balance and fat loss. Finally, do you have an eating disorder?

If lifestyle is not the problem, consult with your physician to rule out the possibility that the cause of

Nutritional Links

Do Protein Supplements Have a Role in Promoting Muscle Growth?

Many of the numerous nutritional products that are advertised as "wonder drugs" for promoting muscle growth are high-protein (and often high-calorie) drinks. But are they effective? There is no scientific evidence to support the notion that any of these products result in increases in muscular size or strength. The only proven and safe method of building muscle mass is regular weight training coupled with a nutritionally sound diet. (See reference 21 for a review of this topic.)

But do you even need such high intakes of protein to promote muscle growth? Although consumption of small quantities of high-protein drinks may not be harmful, if you are eating a typical U.S. diet you don't need to increase your protein intake to achieve muscle growth (12, 21). Here's why: To achieve normal growth and development, the RDA for protein is 0.8 gram per kilogram (kg) of body weight, which means that a 70-kg man needs 56 grams of protein per day (70 kg 3 0.8 gram/kg/day 5 56 grams/day). But because the average daily U.S. diet contains about 100 grams of protein, which is well above the RDA, no protein supplementation is needed to promote muscle growth.

your low body fat is hormonal imbalances or other diseases that influence body weight. After discussing with your physician your desire to gain fat and obtaining medical clearance to do so, consider the following recommendations:

1. Establish a weight gain goal that will place you at the low end of the recommended percent body fat range.

2. Create a positive caloric balance. This is accomplished by increasing your total caloric intake to exceed your daily expenditure. A positive caloric balance of 500 calories per day will generally result in a weight gain of 1 pound of fat per week, a reasonable goal.

3. To create a positive caloric balance, compute your daily caloric expenditure, and increase your caloric intake to exceed expenditure. When creating a positive caloric diet, use the basic principles of

nutrition discussed in Chapter 7. That is, increase your total caloric intake by using the "eating-right pyramid," so that you adhere to the recommended guidelines for fat, carbohydrate, and protein intake.

4. Consult a physician and a nutritionist. Although anyone can gain weight while eating a positive caloric diet, the safest means of gaining body fat is with the assistance of these professionals.

GAINING MUSCLE MASS

If your percent of body fat is within the recommended range and you wish to increase your body mass, your goal should be to gain muscle mass, not fat. Unfortunately, there are no over-the-counter products or shortcuts for gaining muscle (Nutritional Links to Health and Fitness). The key to gaining muscle mass is a program of rigorous weight training combined with the increase in caloric intake needed to meet the increased energy expenditure and energy required to synthesize muscle. Exercise programs designed to improve muscular strength and size are discussed in Chapter 5 and are not addressed here. The focus here is on the dietary adjustments needed to optimize gains in muscle mass. Again, in order to gain muscle mass, you need to create a small positive caloric balance to provide the energy required to synthesize new muscle protein. Nonetheless, before we provide dietary guidelines, let's discuss how much energy is expended during weight training, and how much energy is required to promote muscle growth.

How much energy is expended during weight training? Energy expenditure during routine weight training is surprisingly small. For instance, a 70-kg man performing a 30-minute weight workout probably burns fewer than 70 calories (12). The reason for this low caloric expenditure is that during 30 minutes in the weight room, the average person spends only 8 to 10 minutes actually lifting weights; much time is spent in recovery periods between sets.

How much energy is required to synthesize 1 pound of muscle mass? Current estimates are approximately 2500 calories, of which about 400 calories (100 grams) must be protein (12). To compute the additional calories required to produce an increase in muscle mass, you must first estimate your rate of muscular growth. This is difficult because the rate of muscular growth during weight training varies among people. While relatively large muscle mass gains are possible in some individuals, studies have shown that most men and women rarely gain more than 0.25 pound of muscle per week during a 20-week weight training program (3 days/week, 30 minutes/day). If we assume that the average muscle gain is 0.25 pound per week and that 2500 calories are required to synthesize one pound of muscle, a positive caloric balance of less than 100 calories per day is needed to promote muscle growth (0.25 pound/week × 2500 calories/pound = 625 calories/week; therefore, 625 calories/week ÷ 7 days/week = 90 calories/day).

What are the dietary guidelines for gaining muscle mass? The major adjustments in diet are an increased caloric intake and assurance that you are obtaining adequate amounts of dietary protein. If you follow the dietary guidelines discussed in Chapter 7 while producing a positive caloric balance, your diet will contain enough protein to support an increase in muscle mass. When planning your diet, consider the following points:

- To increase your caloric intake, use the "eating-right pyramid" presented in Chapter 7. This will ensure that your diet meets the criteria for healthful living and provides adequate protein for building muscle.

- Avoid intake of high-fat foods, and limit your positive caloric balance to approximately 90 calories per day. Increasing your positive caloric balance above this level will not promote a faster rate of muscular growth but will result in increased body fat.

- If you discontinue your weight-training program, lower your caloric intake to match your daily energy expenditure.

☀ IN SUMMARY

- Gaining body fat can be achieved by creating a positive caloric balance. Before deciding to gain body fat, you should consider whether your current body composition is within your desired range.
- Gaining muscle mass cannot be attained by over-the-counter products alone; it must be achieved by combining exercise with proper nutrition.

Summary

1. Millions of people in the United States carry too much body fat for optimal health.
2. Obesity is defined as a high percentage of body fat—that is, over 25% for men and over 30% for women.
3. Obesity is linked to many diseases, including heart disease, diabetes, and hypertension.
4. The optimal percent body fat for health and fitness is believed to be 10–20% for men and 15–25% for women.
5. The energy balance theory of weight control states that to maintain your body weight, your energy intake must equal your energy expenditure.
6. Evidence suggests that creating a fat deficit is an essential factor in weight loss. This is because dietary fat is more easily stored as body fat than are either carbohydrate or protein. The importance of a low-fat diet in weight control is illustrated by the fact that body fat gain results when fat intake continually exceeds fat metabolism.
7. Total daily energy expenditure is the sum of resting metabolic rate and exercise metabolic rate.
8. The four basic components of a comprehensive weight control program are weight loss goals; a reduced-calorie diet stressing balanced nutrition; an exercise program designed to increase caloric expenditure and maintain muscle mass; and a behavior modification program designed to modify those behaviors that contribute to weight gain.

9. Weight loss goals should include both short-term and long-term goals.
10. Numerous weight loss myths exist. This chapter has discredited weight loss myths concerning diet pills, spot reduction, grapefruit diets, cellulite reduction, and the use of saunas, steam baths, and rubber exercise suits.
11. Two relatively common eating disorders, anorexia nervosa and bulimia, are serious medical conditions that require professional treatment.
12. Weight training and a positive caloric balance are required to produce increases in muscle mass.

Study Questions

1. What is obesity? What diseases are linked to obesity?
2. Discuss several possible causes of obesity.
3. Discuss the concept of optimal body weight. How is optimal body weight computed?
4. Explain the roles of resting metabolic rate and exercise metabolic rate in determining total caloric expenditure. Which is more important in total daily caloric expenditure in a sedentary individual?
5. Outline a simple method for computing your daily caloric expenditure. Give an example.
6. List the four major components of a weight loss program.

7. Discuss the weight loss myths concerning the following: spot reduction; grapefruit diet; eating before bedtime; cellulite reduction; and saunas, steam baths, and rubber suits.

8. Define the eating disorders anorexia nervosa and bulimia.

9. Discuss the role of behavior modification in weight loss.

10. Define the following terms:
    energy balance theory of weight control
    isocaloric balance
    negative caloric balance
    positive caloric balance

11. Explain the fat deficit concept of weight control.

12. Compare exercise metabolic rate with resting metabolic rate.

13. What is cellulite?

14. How does creeping obesity occur?

15. Discuss the process of combining diet and exercise to increase muscle mass.

Suggested Reading

Acheson, K. Carbohydrate and weight control: Where do we stand? *Current Opinion in Clinical Nutrition and Metabolic Care* 7:485–492, 2004.

Buchholz, A., and D. Schoeller. Is a calorie a calorie? *American Journal of Nutrition* 79:899–906S, 2004.

Heilbronn, L., and E. Ravussin. Calorie restriction and aging: Review of the literature and implications for studies in humans. *American Journal of Clinical Nutrition* 78:361–369, 2003.

Jakicic, J. et al. Appropriate intervention strategies for weight loss and prevention of weight regain for adults. (ACSM Position Stand). *Medicine and Science in Sports and Exercise* 33:2145–2156, 2001.

Powers, S., and E. Howley. *Exercise Physiology: Theory and Application to Fitness and Performance,* 5th ed. McGraw-Hill, St. Louis, Mo. 2004.

Stein, C., and G. Colditz. The epidemic of obesity. *Journal of Clinical Endocrinology and Metabolism* 89:2522–2525, 2004.

For links to the web sites below visit The Total Fitness and Wellness Website at www.aw-bc.com/powers.

American Dietetic Association

Contains articles about nutrition and fad diets.

Nutrition with Rick Hall

Provides links to over 700 health, weight loss, and nutrition-related websites.

References

1. Atkinson, R. Treatment of obesity. *Nutritional Reviews* 50:338–345, 1992.

57. National Institutes of Health technology assessment conference statement: Methods for voluntary weight loss and control. *Nutritional Reviews* 50:340–345, 1992.

2. Wadden, T., J. Sternberg, K. Letizia, A. Stunkard, and G. Foster. Treatment for obesity by very low calorie diet, behavior therapy, and their combination: A five year prospective. *International Journal of Obesity* 13(Suppl. 2):39–46, 1989.

3. Roitman, J. (Editor). *ACSM'S Resource Manual for Guidelines for Exercise Testing and Prescription.* Philadelphia: Lippincott 2001.

4. Bjorntorp, P., and B. Brodoff, eds. *Obesity.* Philadelphia: Lippincott, 1992.

5. Perri, M., A. Nezu, and B. Viegener. *Improving the Long-term Management and Treatment of Obesity.* New York: John Wiley and Sons, 1992.

6. Stefanik, M. Exercise and weight control. In *Exercise and Sport Science Reviews,* J. Holloszy, ed. Baltimore: Williams and Wilkins, 1993.

7. Stunkard, A., and T. Wadden, eds. *Obesity: Theory and Therapy.* New York: Raven Press, 1993.

8. Kuczmarski, R. Prevalence of overweight and weight gain in the United States. *American Journal of Clinical Nutrition* 55:495s–502s, 1992.

9. Bouchard, C., A. Tremblay, J. Despres, et al. The response to long-term overfeeding in identical twins. *New England Journal of Medicine* 322:1477–1482, 1990.

10. Stunkard, A., T. Sorensen, C. Hanis, et al. An adoption study of human obesity. *New England Journal of Medicine* 314:193–198, 1986.

11. Howley, E., and B. D. Franks. *Health Fitness: Instructors Handbook.* Champaign, IL: Human Kinetics, 1997.

12. Williams, M. *Lifetime Fitness and Wellness.* Dubuque, IA: Wm. C. Brown, 1996.

13. Van Itallie, T. Health implications of overweight and obesity in the United States. *Annals of Internal Medicine* 103:983–988, 1985.

14. Health implications of obesity: National Institutes of Health consensus development conference. *Annals of Internal Medicine* 103:977–1077, 1985.

15. Steppan, C. M., et al. The hormone resistin links obesity to diabetes. *Nature* 409:307–312, 2001.

16. Bouchard, C., R. Shepherd, T. Stephens, J. Sutton, and B. McPherson, eds. *Exercise, Fitness, and Health: A Consensus of Current Knowledge.* Champaign, IL: Human Kinetics, 1990.

17. Hockey, R. *Physical Fitness: The Pathway to Healthful Living,* 8th ed. St. Louis: Times Mirror/Mosby, 1996.

18. Getchell, B. *Physical Fitness: A Way of Life,* 5th ed. Needham Heights, MA: Allyn and Bacon, 1998.

19. Corbin, C., G. Welk, R. Lindsey, and W. Corbin. *Concepts of Physical fitness.* St. Louis: McGraw-Hill, 2003.

20. Pollock, M., and J. Wilmore. *Exercise in Health and Disease,* 3rd ed. Philadelphia: W. B. Saunders, 1999.

21. Powers, S., and E. Howley. *Exercise Physiology: Theory and Application to Fitness and Performance,* 4th ed. St. Louis: McGraw-Hill, 2004.

22. Changnon, Y. C., et al. Genomic scan for genes affecting body composition before and after training in Caucasions from HERITAGE. *Journal of Applied Physiology* 90:1777–1787, 2001.

23. Frubeck, G., J. Gomez-Amrosi, F. Muruzabal, and M. Burrell. The adipocyte: A model for integration of endocrine and metabolic signaling in energy metabolism regulation. *American Journal of Physiology* 280:E827–E847, 2001.

24. Bailey, J., R. Barker, and R. Beauchene. Age-related changes in rat adipose tissue cellularity are altered by dietary restriction and exercise. *Journal of Nutrition* 123: 52–58, 1993.

25. Blair, S. Evidence for success of exercise in weight loss control. *Annals of Internal Medicine* 119:702–706, 1993.

26. Poehlman, E. A review: Exercise and its influence on resting energy metabolism in man. *Medicine and Science in Sports and Exercise* 21:515–525, 1989.

27. Jequier, E. Body weight regulation in humans: The importance of nutrient balance. *News in Physiological Sciences* 8:273–276, 1993.

28. King, M., and F. Katch. Changes in body density, fatfolds, and girths at 2.3 kg increments of weight loss. *Human Biology* 58:709,1986.

29. Sizer, F., and E. Whitney. *Nutrition: Concepts and Controversies.* New York: West/Wadsworth, 1997.

30. AHA Dietary Guidelines. Revision 2000: A statement for healthcare professionals from the nutrition committee of the American Heart Association. *Circulation* 102:2284–2299, 2000.

31. Ross, R., J. Freeman, and I. Janssen. Exercise alone is an effective strategy for reducing obesity and related comorbidities. *Exercise and Sport Sciences Reviews* 28(4):165–170, 2000.

32. Coyle, E. Fat metabolism during exercise. *Sports Science Exchange* (Gatorade Sports Science Institute) 8:6, 1995.

33. Broeder, C., K. Burrhus, L. Svanevik, and J. Wilmore. The effects of either high intensity resistance or endurance training on resting metabolic rate. *American Journal of Clinical Nutrition* 55:802–810, 1992.

34. Bailey, C. *The New Fit or Fat.* Boston: Houghton Mifflin, 1991.

35. Romijn, J., E. Coyle, L. Sidossis, et al. Regulation of endogenous fat and carbohydrate metabolism in relation to exercise and duration. *American Journal of Physiology* 265:E380–E391, 1993.

36. Tremblay, A., S. Coveney, J. Despres, A. Nadeau, D. Prud'homme. Increased resting metabolic rate and lipid oxidation in exercise-trained individuals: Evidence for a role of beta-oxidation. *Canadian Journal of Physiology and Pharmacology* 70:1342–1347, 1992.

37. Mayer, J., N. Marshall, J. Vitale, J. Christensen, M. Mashayekhi, and F. Stare. Exercise, food intake, and body weight in normal rats and genetically obese adult mice. *American Journal of Physiology* 177:544–548, 1954.

38. Gwinup, G., R. Chelvam, and T. Steinberg. Thickness of subcutaneous fat and activity of underlying muscles. *Annals of Internal Medicine* 74:408–411, 1971.

39. Andersen, A. Anorexia nervosa and bulimia. *Journal of Adolescent Health Care* 4:15–21, 1983.

40. Borgen, J., and C. Corbin. Eating disorders among female athletes. *Physician and Sports Medicine* 15:89–95, 1987.

41. Leeds, M. *Nutrition for Healthy Living.* Boston: WCB-McGraw-Hill, 1998.

42. Buchholz, A., and D. Schoeller. Is a calorie a calorie? *American Journal of Nutrition* 79:899–906S, 2004.

43. Stein, C., and G. Colditz. The epidemic of obesity. *Journal of Clinical Endocrinology and Metabolism* 89:2522–2525, 2004.

44. Hedley, A., C. Ogden, C. Johnson, M. Carroll, L. Curtin, and K. Flegal. Prevalence of overweight and obesity among US children, adolescents, and adults, 1999–2002. *Journal of American Medical Association* 16:2847–2850.

45. Acheson, K. Carbohydrate and weight control: Where do we stand? *Current Opinion in Clinical Nutrition and Metabolic Care* 7:485–492, 2004.

46. Meckling, K., C. O'Sullivan, and D. Saari. Comparison of a low-fat to a low-carbohydrate diet on weight loss, body composition, and risk factors for diabetes and cardiovascular disease in free-living, overweight men and women. *Journal of Clinical Endocrinology and Metabolism* 89:2717–2723, 2004.

47. Stern, L. et al. The effects of low-carbohydrate versus conventional weight loss diets in severely obese adults: One-year follow-up of a randomized trial. *Annals of Internal Medicine* 140:778–785, 2004.

48. Foster, G., et al. A randomized trial of low-carbohydrate diet for obesity. *New England Journal of Medicine* 348:2082–2090, 2003.

49. Saris, W. Sugars, energy metabolism, and body weight control. *American Journal of Nutrition* 78: 850–857S, 2003.

50. Jakicic, J. et al. Appropriate intervention strategies for weight loss and prevention of weight regain for adults. (ACSM Position Stand). *Medicine and Science in Sports and Exercise* 33:2145–2156, 2001.

51. Vermunt, S., W. Pasman, G. Schaafsma, and F. Kardinaal. Effects of sugar intake on body weight: A review. *Obesity Reviews* 4:91–99, 2003.

52. Foster, G. et al. A randomized trial of a low-carbohydrate diet for obesity. *New England Journal of Medicine* 348:2082–2090, 2003.

53. Heilbronn, L., and E. Ravussin. Calorie restriction and aging: Review of the literature and implications for studies in humans. *American Journal of Clinical Nutrition* 78:361–369, 2003.

54. Zemel, MB. Role of calcium and diary products in energy partitioning and weight management. *American Journal of Clinical Nutrition* 79:907S–912S, 2004.

55. Powers, S., and E. Howley. *Exercise Physiology: Theory and Application to Fitness and Performance.* 5th ed. St. Louis: McGraw-Hill, 2004.

Determining Ideal Body Weight Using Percent Body Fat and the Body Mass Index

NAME _____ DATE _____

There are a number of different ways to compute an ideal body weight. In Chapter 2 we discussed percent body fat (estimated from skinfold measurements). Method A of this laboratory enables you to compute and record your ideal body weight using the percent body fat method. Method B enables you to calculate and record your ideal body weight using the body mass index procedure (Chapter 2). Choose one of these techniques and complete the appropriate section.

METHOD A: COMPUTATION OF IDEAL BODY WEIGHT USING PERCENT BODY FAT

STEP 1: CALCULATE FAT-FREE WEIGHT

100% − your percent body fat estimated from skinfold measurement
= _____ % fat free weight.

Therefore,

_____ % fat-free weight expressed as a decimal × your body weight in pounds
= _____ pounds of fat-free weight.

STEP 2: CALCULATE OPTIMAL WEIGHT

Remember: Optimal body fat ranges are 10–20% for men and 15–25% for women.

Optimal weight = fat-free weight/(1.00 − optimal %fat), with optimal %fat expressed as a decimal. Therefore, the low and high optimal weight ranges for your gender are

For low %fat: Optimal weight = _____ pounds

For high %fat: Optimal weight = _____ pounds

(continued on next page)

METHOD B: COMPUTATION OF IDEAL BODY WEIGHT USING BODY MASS INDEX (BMI)

The BMI uses the metric system. Therefore, you must express your weight in kilograms (1 kilogram = 2.2 pounds) and your height in meters (1 inch = 0.0254 meters).

STEP 1: COMPUTE YOUR BMI

BMI = body weight (kg)/(height in meters)^2

Your BMI = _____

STEP 2: CALCULATE YOUR IDEAL BODY WEIGHT BASED ON BMI*

The ideal BMI is 21.9 to 22.4 for men and 21.3 to 22.1 for women. The formula for computing ideal body weight using BMI is

ideal body weight (kilograms) = desired BMI × (height in meters)^2

Consider the following example as an illustration of the computation of ideal body weight. A man who weighs 60 kilograms and is 1.5 meters tall computes his BMI to be 26.7. His ideal BMI is between 21.9 and 22.4; therefore, his ideal body weight range is

ideal body weight = 21.9 × 2.25 = 49.3 kilograms
ideal body weight = 22.4 × 2.25 = 50.4 kilograms

Now complete this calculation using your values for BMI.

My ideal body weight range using the BMI method is _____ to _____ kilograms.

*Note: BMI may not be a good method to determine ideal body weight for a highly muscled individual.

Estimating Daily Caloric Expenditure and the Caloric Deficit Required to Lose 1 Pound of Fat Per Week

NAME _____ DATE _____

PART A. ESTIMATION OF YOUR DAILY CALORIC EXPENDITURE

Using Table 8.1, compute your estimated daily caloric expenditure.

Estimated daily caloric expenditure = _____ calories/day.

PART B. CALCULATION OF CALORIC INTAKE REQUIRED TO PROMOTE 1 POUND PER WEEK OF WEIGHT LOSS

Recall that 1 pound of fat contains approximately 3500 calories. Therefore, a negative caloric balance of 500 calories per day will result in a weight loss of 1 pound per week. Use the following formula to compute your daily caloric intake to result in a daily caloric deficit of 500 calories.

estimated daily caloric expenditure − 500 calories (deficit)
= daily caloric intake needed to produce a 500-calorie deficit

In the space provided, compute your daily caloric intake needed to produce 1 pound per week of weight loss.

_____ (estimated caloric expenditure) −

___ − 500 ___ (caloric deficit)

= _____ target daily caloric intake

Weight Loss Goals and Progress Report

NAME _____ DATE _____

In the spaces provided, record your short-term and long-term weight loss goals. Then keep a record of your weight loss progress on the chart.

    Ideal body weight (range): _____

    Short-term weight loss goal: _____ (pounds/week)

    Long-term weight loss goal: _____ pounds

Week No.	Body Weight	Date	Weight Loss
1			
2			
3			
4			
5			
6			
7			
8			
9			
10			
11			
12			
13			
14			
15			
16			
17			
18			
19			
20			
21			
22			
23			
24			

(continued on next page)

Week No.	Body Weight	Date	Weight Loss
25			
26			
27			
28			
29			
30			
31			
32			
33			
34			
35			
36			
37			
38			
39			
40			

Assessing Body Image

NAME _____ DATE _____

Respond to the questions below to assess your body image.

Where do you get your ideas about the "ideal body"? If more than one applies, how do they rank?

    a. TV/movies

    b. friends

    c. parents

    d. athletes

What other sources contribute to your image of the "ideal body"?

_____

_____

_____

Fill in the blanks to complete the following statements about your body image. Use extra paper if needed.

    1. I like _____ about my body.

    2. I dislike _____ about my body.

    3. When I eat a big meal, I feel _____

    4. When I look in the mirror, I see _____

    5. I like/dislike (circle one) shopping for clothes because _____

       _____

    6. I feel self-conscious when _____

       _____

    7. Compared to others, I feel my body is _____

    8. In the presence of someone I find attractive, I feel _____

    9. I feel that my appearance is _____

    10. One word to describe my body is _____

(continued on next page)

INTERPRETATION

Now review your answers to the previous questions and think about whether they are positive or negative. To improve a negative body image, keep the following strategies in mind:

1. Focus on good physical health. Engage in physical activities that you enjoy.

2. Remember that your self-worth is not dependent on how you look.

3. Avoid chronic, restrained dieting.

4. Find aspects to appreciate in yourself besides an idealized body.

What Triggers Your Eating?

NAME _____ DATE _____

There are many things that cause us to eat. Usually, just by identifying the triggers that cause you to eat, you can develop a strategy to counter those habits. Use the questions below to determine your motivation for eating.

For each question, record a "Yes" or "No" in the blank.

Emotional

1. I cannot lose weight and keep it off. _____

2. My eating is out of control. _____

3. Even if I'm not hungry, I eat. _____

4. I eat when stressed or upset. _____

5. Food gives me great pleasure and I use it as a reward. _____

6. Eating is usually on my mind. _____

7. My eating causes problems with weight management. _____

8. I go on eating "binges" or find myself eating constantly. _____

9. My eating habits cause me embarrassment. _____

10. I use food to help me cope with feelings. _____

Social

11. I eat whenever others around me are eating. _____

12. If anyone offers food, I take it. _____

13. Whenever I am in a stressful social situation, I want to eat. _____

14. Whenever I am in a relaxed social situation, I want to eat. _____

15. I eat more in a social setting than I do at home. _____

16. I eat less when others are around to see me. _____

17. In a social setting, the amount of food I eat depends on the group of people. _____

18. I eat different foods in a social setting than I do at home. _____

(continued on next page)

Environmental

19. I eat more at restaurants that I do at home. _____

20. I eat less at restaurants than I do at home. _____

21. If I smell food I can't resist the urge to eat. _____

22. If I walk by a restaurant or bakery I can't resist the urge to eat. _____

23. I like to eat while reading or watching TV. _____

24. I find food comforting in different environmental conditions, such as on a rainy day or in cold weather. _____

25. I find food comforting when I am in unfamiliar surroundings. _____

26. If I am outdoors, I feel like I can eat more. _____

INTERPRETATION

Insignificant influence: If you answered "Yes" to 1 question within a section or less than 6 questions total, weight management is probably relatively easy for you.

Some influence: If you answered "Yes" to 2 questions within a section or 6–9 questions total, there are issues that are complicating your weight management. It might help to talk with a health care professional while developing a weight management plan.

Significant influence: If you answered "Yes" to 3 questions within a section or 10–13 questions total, there are several issues affecting your weight management plan. Speaking with a health care professional or counselor can help you deal with issues that trigger your eating.

Severe influence: If you answered "Yes" to 4 or more questions within a section or 14 or more questions total, there are many issues that complicate your weight management. Counseling and speaking with a health care professional will help you to develop a weight management plan.

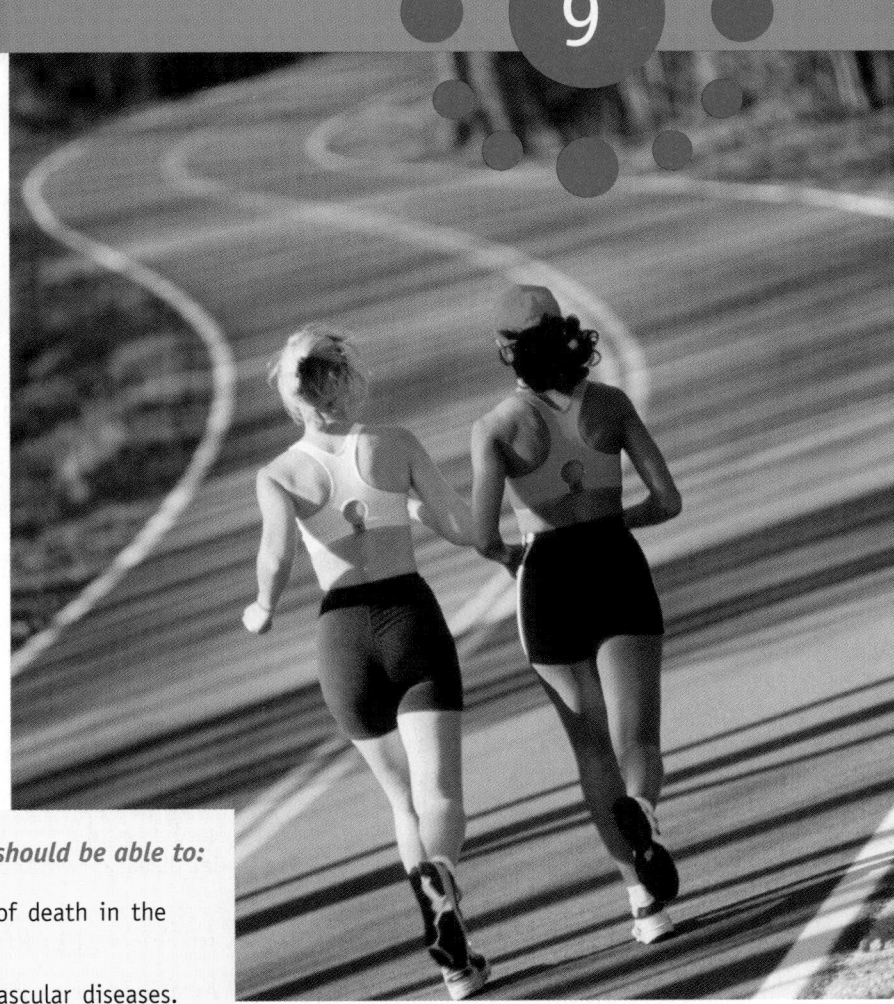

9

Prevention of Cardiovascular Disease

After studying this chapter, you should be able to:

1. Name the number one cause of death in the United States.

2. Identify four common cardiovascular diseases.

3. Discuss the major and contributory risk factors associated with the development of coronary heart disease.

4. Identify the coronary heart disease risk factors that can be modified by lifestyle alterations.

5. List the steps involved in reducing your risk of coronary heart disease.

6. Describe the link between dietary sodium and hypertension.

7. Identify the total blood cholesterol levels associated with low, moderate, and high risk of developing coronary heart disease.

8. Discuss the relationship between diet and elevated blood cholesterol levels.

ardiovascular diseases are a major health problem around the world and account for millions of deaths each year. The incidence of cardiovascular disease is greatest in industrialized countries, and the United Stated has one of the world's highest death rates (1). Although it is impossible to place a dollar value on human life, the economic cost of cardiovascular disease in the United States is great (Figure 9.1). Estimates of lost wages and medical expenses exceed 95 billion dollars every year (1); therefore, developing a national strategy to reduce the risk of cardiovascular disease is a major heath priority. This chapter focuses on lifestyle changes (e.g., exercise and diet) that can reduce your risk of cardiovascular diseases. Let's begin our discussion with an overview of cardiovascular disease in the United States.

☀ Cardiovascular Disease in the United States

Although public awareness is currently more focused on diseases such as cancer and AIDS, **cardiovascular disease**—any disease that affects the heart or blood vessels—remains the number one cause of death in the United States, accounting for nearly one of every two deaths. Current data indicate that over 60 million adults have one or more forms of cardiovascular disease and that approximately 1 million people die annually from cardiovascular disorders (1). Equally alarming is the fact that cardiovascular disease is not restricted to the elderly. It is the leading cause of death in men between the ages of 35 and 44 (1). Although the death rate from cardiovascular disease has always been higher for men than for women, the incidence of cardiovascular disease in women has increased dramatically in recent years (1). (See Fitness and Wellness for All for a brief discussion of the segments of the population at greatest risk of cardiovascular disease.) Fortunately, it is possible to reduce your risk of developing cardiovascular disease, but before discussing how to do this, we will define the major types of cardiovascular disease.

> **cardiovascular disease** Any disease that affects the heart or blood vessels.
>
> **arteriosclerosis** A group of diseases characterized by a narrowing or "hardening" of the arteries. The end result of any form of arteriosclerosis is that blood flow to vital organs may be impaired due to progressive blockage of the artery.
>
> **atherosclerosis** A special type of arteriosclerosis that results in arterial blockage due to buildup of a fatty deposit (called *atherosclerotic plaque*) inside the blood vessel.

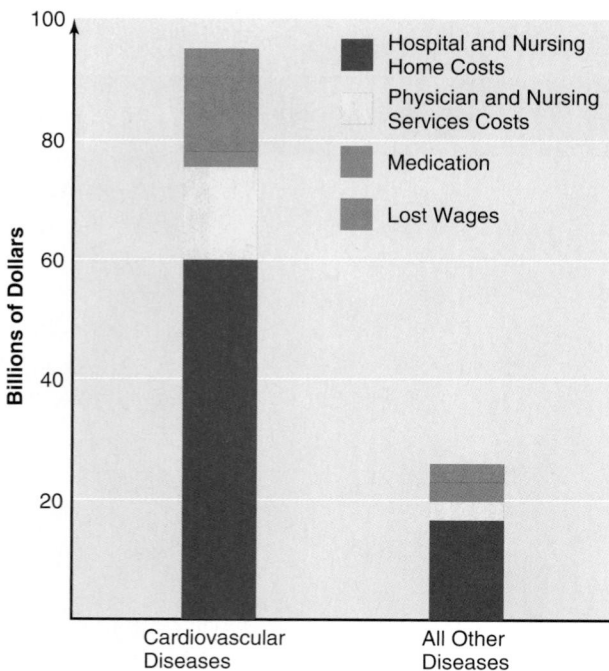

FIGURE 9.1
Annual economic costs of cardiovascular diseases and all other diseases in the United States.

☀ Cardiovascular Diseases

Although literally hundreds of diseases impair normal cardiovascular function, only four common cardiovascular diseases warrant discussion here.

ARTERIOSCLEROSIS

Arteriosclerosis is not a single disease but rather a group of diseases characterized by a narrowing or "hardening" of the arteries. The end result of any form of arteriosclerosis is that blood flow to vital organs may be impaired due to progressive blockage of the artery. **Atherosclerosis** is a special type of arteriosclerosis that results in arterial blockage due to buildup of a fatty deposit (called *atherosclerotic plaque*) inside the blood vessel. This plaque deposit is typically composed of cholesterol, cellular debris, fibrin (a clotting material in the blood), and calcium. Atherosclerosis is a progressive disease that begins in childhood, and symptoms appear later in life. Figure 9.2 illustrates the progression of arterial blockage caused by atherosclerosis. Note that atherosclerosis is not an "all or none" disease but occurs in varying degrees, with some arteries exhibiting little blockage and others exhibiting major obstruction. Development of severe atherosclerosis within arteries supplying blood to the heart is the cause of almost all heart attacks.

Who Is at Greatest Risk of Cardiovascular Disease?

Ethnicity, gender, age, and socioeconomic status can all affect an individual's risk of developing cardiovascular disease, and these factors explain why cardiovascular disease is more prevalent in certain segments of the U.S. population. African Americans, for example, are at greater risk of developing hypertension (or high blood pressure, one form of cardiovascular disease) compared to the U.S. population as a whole. Similarly, Native Americans and people of Latino heritage have higher prevalences of diabetes, an important contributory risk factor for cardiovascular disease. Between the ages of 20 and 65, men are at greater risk than women for developing cardiovascular disease. Finally, individuals who earn low incomes experience higher incidences of both heart disease and obesity (a contributory risk factor for heart disease).

CORONARY HEART DISEASE

Coronary heart disease is the major disease of the cardiovascular system. **Coronary heart disease (CHD),** also called *coronary artery disease,* is the result of atherosclerotic plaque forming a blockage of one or more coronary arteries (the blood vessels supplying the heart; Figure 9.3). When the degree of blockage of a major coronary artery reaches 75%, the resulting lack of blood flow to the working heart muscle causes chest pain. This type of chest pain, called *angina pectoris,* occurs most frequently during exercise or emotional stress (2).

Severe blockage of coronary arteries may result in a blood clot forming around the layer of plaque. When this happens, a complete blockage of heart blood flow occurs, resulting in a **heart attack** (also called a **myocardial infarction**). Figure 9.4 illustrates what happens during a heart attack caused by complete blockage of the left coronary artery. The end result is the death of heart muscle cells in the left ventricle; the severity of the heart attack is judged by how many heart muscle cells are damaged. A "mild" heart attack may only damage a small portion of the heart, whereas a "major" heart attack may destroy a large number of heart muscle cells. Because the number of heart muscle cells destroyed during a heart attack determines the patient's chances of recovery, recognizing the symptoms of a heart attack and getting prompt medical attention are crucial (A Closer Look, p. 263).

STROKE

It is estimated that each year 2 million Americans suffer a stroke (1). A **stroke** occurs when the blood supply to the brain is reduced for a prolonged period of time. A common cause of stroke is blockage (due to atherosclerosis) of arteries leading to the brain (Figure 9.5). However, strokes can also occur when a cerebral (brain)

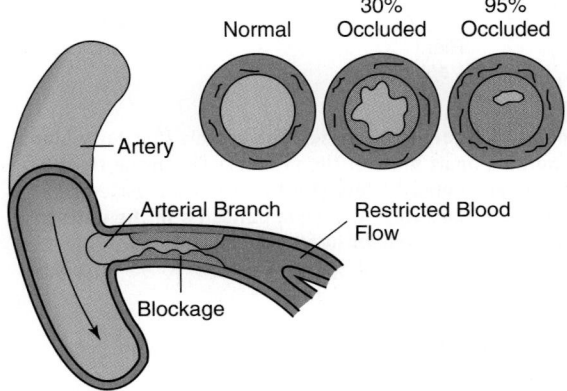

FIGURE 9.2
Progressive stages of atherosclerosis. The three cross-sections show (from left to right) a "normal" artery that has no blockage, and two arteries that have 30% and 95% blockage, respectively, due to the progressive buildup of atherosclerotic plaque within them.

blood vessel ruptures and disturbs normal blood flow to that region of the brain.

Similar to a heart attack, which results in death of heart cells, a stroke results in death of brain cells. The severity of the stroke may vary from slight to severe,

coronary heart disease (CHD) Also called *coronary artery disease;* CHD is the result of atherosclerotic plaque forming a blockage of one or more coronary arteries (the blood vessels supplying the heart).
heart attack Stoppage of blood flow to the heart resulting in the death of heart cells; also called *myocardial infarction.*
stroke Brain damage that occurs when the blood supply to the brain is reduced for a prolonged period of time.

Heart and Coronary Arteries

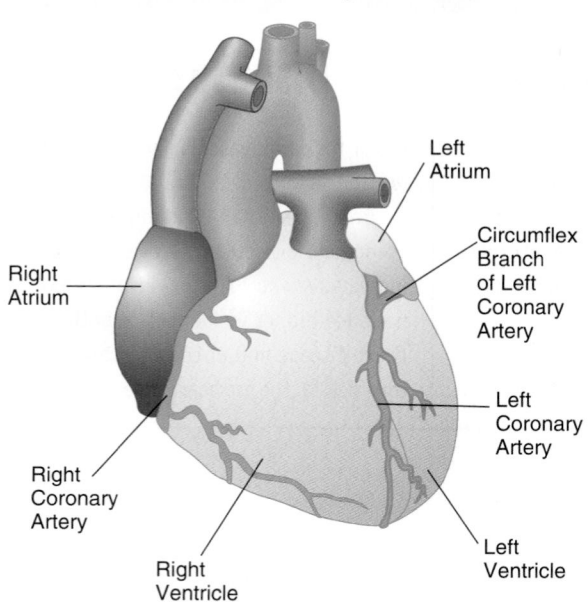

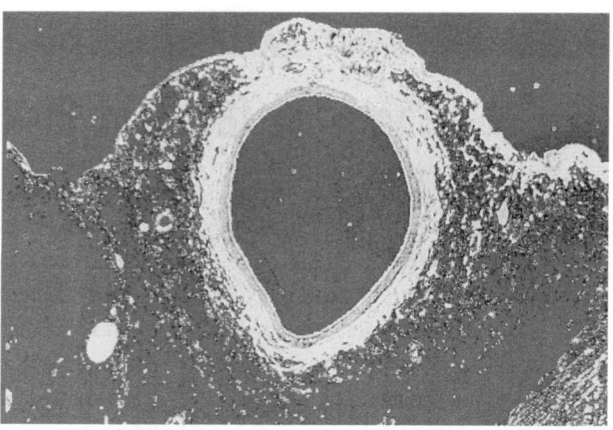

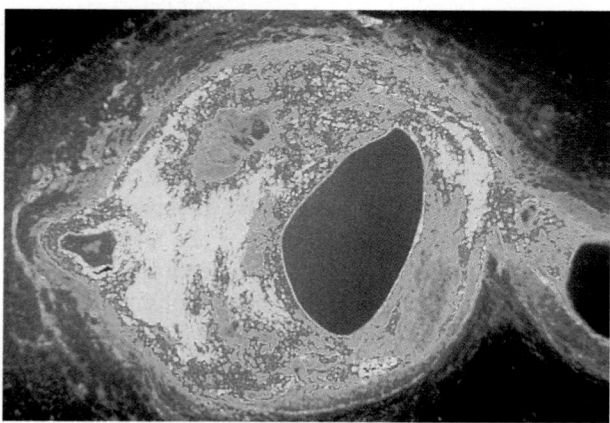

FIGURE 9.3
Locations of the coronary arteries, the vessels that carry blood to the working heart muscle. The photographs on the right show a normal coronary artery (top) and an atherosclerotic coronary artery (bottom). As plaque builds up in the walls of coronary arteries, the risk of heart attack increases.

Source: From Melvin H. Williams, *Lifetime Fitness and Wellness,* 4th ed. Copyright © 1993. Reprinted by permission of the author.

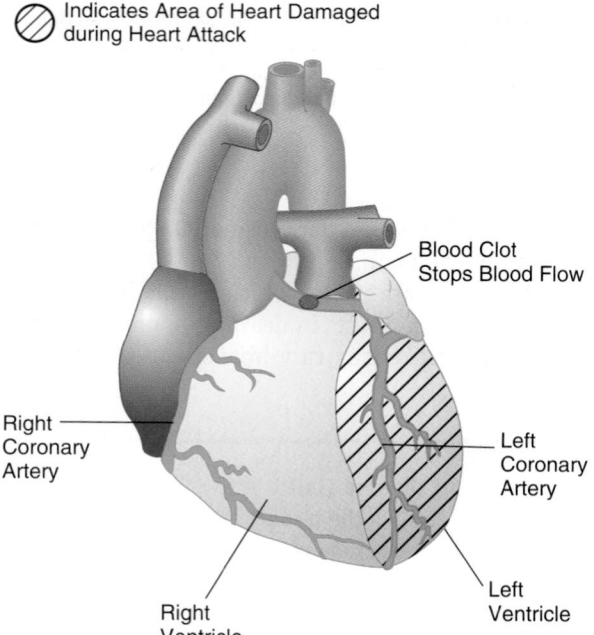

FIGURE 9.4
Effect of a myocardial infarction (heart attack). The cross-hatched area of the heart is damaged due to a stoppage of blood flow during the heart attack.

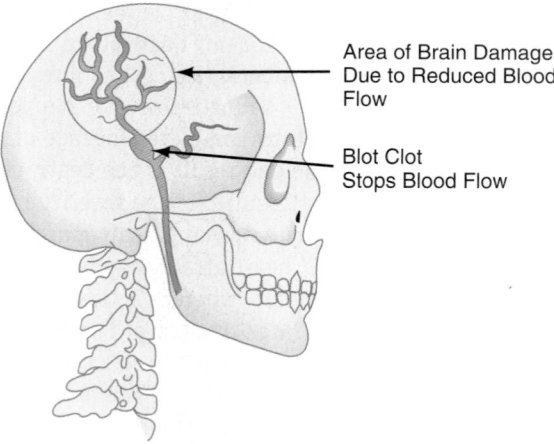

FIGURE 9.5
How blockage of an artery in the brain causes a stroke. Stoppage of blood flow through an artery supplying the brain produces damage to the portion of the brain supplied by that artery (indicated by the circle).

A CLOSER LOOK

Heart Attack: Recognition of Symptoms and Emergency Action

Recognition of heart attack symptoms and knowledge of the appropriate emergency action could save your life or that of someone else. First, here's how to recognize the symptoms of an ongoing heart attack.

WARNING SIGNALS OF A HEART ATTACK

Some of the most common symptoms of a heart attack (2) are

- Mild to moderate pain in your chest that may spread to the shoulders, neck, or arms

- Uncomfortable pressure or sensation of fullness in the chest

- Severe pain in the chest, dizziness, fainting, sweating, nausea, or shortness of breath

Note that not all of these symptoms occur in every heart attack. Therefore, if you or someone you're with experiences any one of these symptoms for 2 minutes or more, follow the emergency procedures described next.

Because 40% of heart attack victims die within the first hour, immediate medical attention is vital to a patient's survival.

WHAT TO DO IN THE CASE OF A HEART ATTACK

If you or someone near you experiences any of the aforementioned symptoms for 2 minutes or longer, call the emergency medical service or get to the nearest hospital that offers emergency cardiac care. If you are trained in cardiopulmonary resuscitation (CPR) and the patient is not breathing or does not have a pulse, call 911 or the emergency medical service in your area, and then start CPR immediately. In any cardiac emergency, rapid action may mean the difference between life and death.

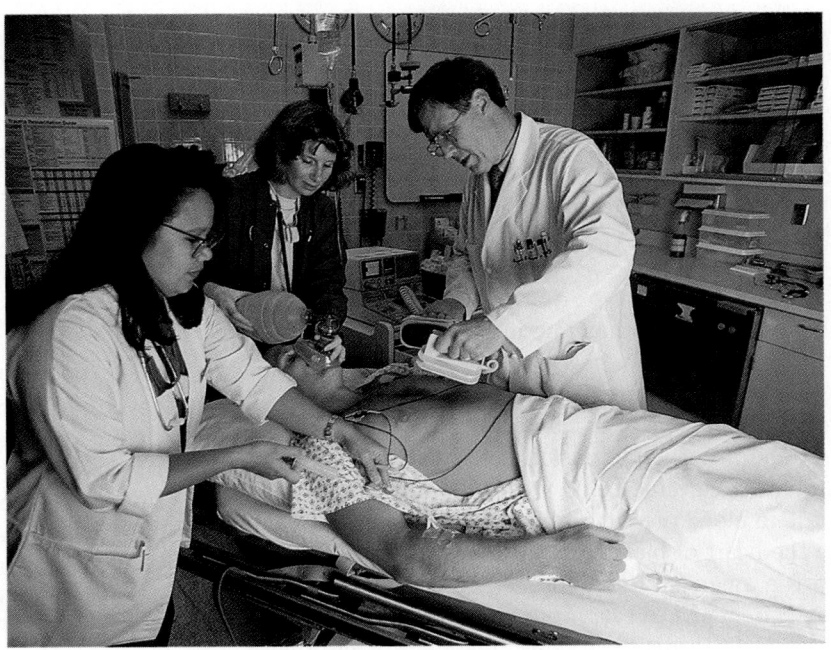

---

depending on the location and the number of brain cells damaged. Minor strokes may involve a loss of memory, speech problems, disturbed vision, and/or mild paralysis in the extremities. In contrast, severe strokes may result in major paralysis or death.

HYPERTENSION

Hypertension is abnormally high blood pressure. Clinically, hypertension is generally defined as a resting blood pressure over 140 mm Hg systolic or 90 mm Hg diastolic (2). Approximately 10% of hypertension cases are caused by a specific disease (such as kidney disease). This type of hypertension is called *secondary hypertension,* because the hypertension is secondary to a primary disease. Nonetheless, in 90% of hypertension

cases, the exact cause of the high blood pressure is unknown; this type of hypertension is called *essential hypertension.*

The prevalence of hypertension in the United States is remarkably high (Figure 9.6). The factors that increase your risk of hypertension include lack of exercise, a high-salt diet, obesity, chronic stress, family history of hypertension, gender (men have a greater risk than women), and race (blacks have a greater risk than whites).

Hypertension is a health problem for several reasons. First, high blood pressure increases the workload on the heart; this may eventually damage the heart muscle's ability to pump blood effectively throughout the body (2). Second, high blood pressure may damage the lining of arteries, resulting in the development of

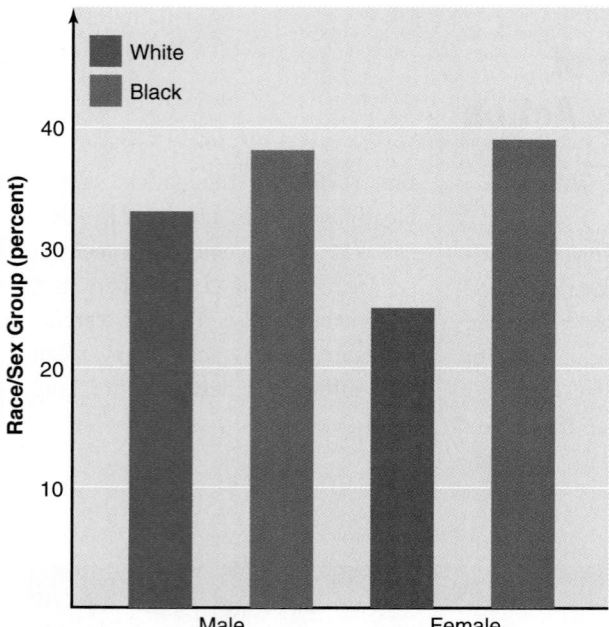

FIGURE 9.6
The prevalence of hypertension in selected groups in the United States.

atherosclerosis and therefore increasing the risk of CHD and stroke (2).

Although exercise causes acute increases in blood pressure, this type of blood pressure elevation is transient and is not hypertension (i.e., hypertension is chronically elevated blood pressure). Further, the increase in blood pressure during exercise does not damage the heart or blood vessels.

The American Heart Association estimates that approximately one of every four people in the United States suffers from hypertension—that is, more than 62 million people (1). Unfortunately, because they lack symptoms, many people are not aware that they are hypertensive. Although severe hypertension may result in headaches and dizziness, these symptoms are often absent. Therefore, without annual medical checkups or blood pressure screenings, hypertension may go undiagnosed for many years. For this reason, hypertension is often called *the silent killer*.

---

major risk factors Factors considered to be directly related to the development of CHD and stroke; also called *primary risk factors*.
contributory risk factors Factors that increase the risk of CHD, but their direct contribution to the disease process has not been precisely determined; also called *secondary risk factors*.

☀ **IN SUMMARY**

- Cardiovascular disease remains the number one cause of death in the United States and in many other developed countries.
- The term *cardiovascular disease* refers to any disease that affects the heart or blood vessels.
- The four major cardiovascular diseases are arteriosclerosis, coronary artery disease, stroke, and hypertension.

☀ Risk Factors Associated with Coronary Heart Disease

In an effort to understand the causes and reduce the occurrence of CHD, researchers have identified a number of major and contributory risk factors that increase the chance of developing both CHD and stroke. **Major risk factors** (also called *primary risk factors*) are factors considered to be directly related to the development of CHD and stroke. In contrast, **contributory risk factors** (also called *secondary risk factors*) are those that increase the risk of CHD, but their direct contribution to the disease process has not been precisely determined.

MAJOR RISK FACTORS

Each year the American Heart Association publishes new information concerning the major risk factors associated with the development of CHD and stroke. The most recent list includes cigarette smoking, hypertension, high blood cholesterol levels, physical inactivity, heredity, gender, and increasing age (1) (Figure 9.7). The greater the number of CHD risk factors an individual has, the greater the likelihood that he or she will develop CHD (Figure 9.8). Let's discuss each of the major risk factors for CHD and stroke.

SMOKING It is estimated that over 50 million people in the United States smoke (3). Many U.S. health care workers believe that cigarette smoking is the single largest cause of disease and premature death. Cigarette smoking has been linked to over 30 health problems, including cancer, lung disease, and cardiovascular disease (1–4). In regard to smoking and cardiovascular disease, a smoker's risk of developing CHD is more than twice that of a nonsmoker (1) (Figure 9.8). Smoking is also considered the biggest risk factor for sudden cardiac death (i.e., sudden death due to cardiac arrest, a heart attack, or irregular heartbeats). In addition, smoking promotes the development of atherosclerosis in peripheral blood vessels (arterial blockage in the arms or legs). Finally, smokers who have a heart attack are more likely to die suddenly (within an hour after the attack) than are nonsmokers.

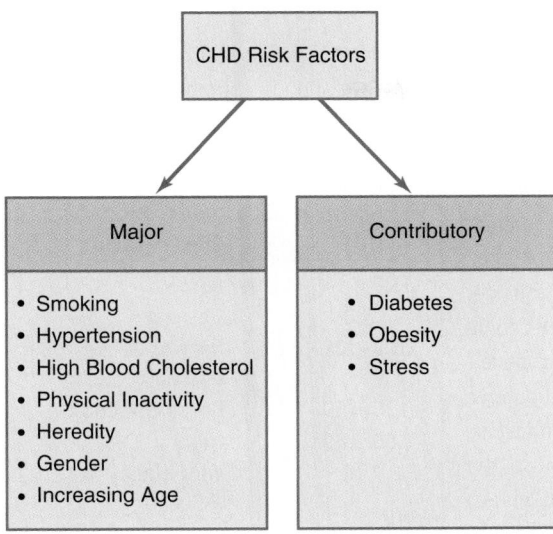

FIGURE 9.7
Coronary heart disease risk factors.

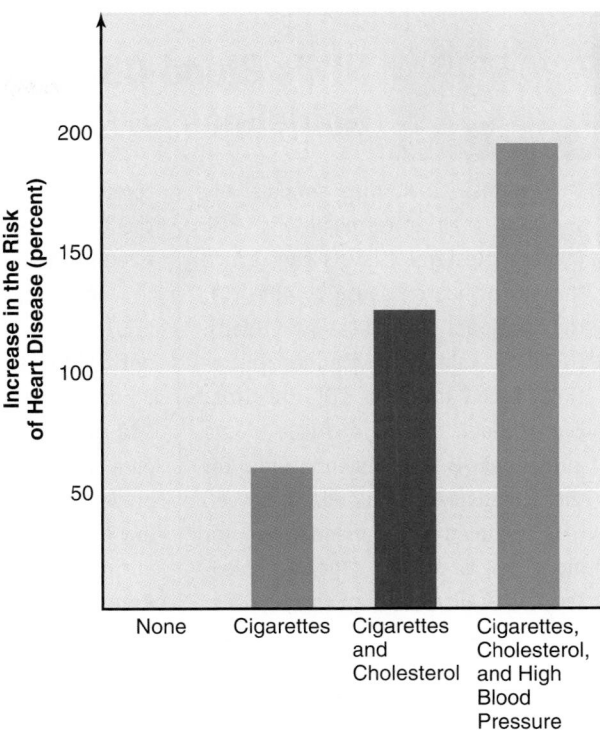

FIGURE 9.8
The effects of multiple risk factors for coronary heart disease. Your risk of developing CHD increases as the number of risk factors increases.

Is the risk of cardiovascular disease increased for nonsmokers who breathe in "secondhand" cigarette smoke? Unfortunately, the answer is "yes." Numerous studies have concluded that passive inhalation of cigarette smoke can increase the risk for both cardiovascular and lung disease (3). This has prompted the banning of smoking in many public places, including airplanes, restaurants, and shopping malls.

Cigarette smoking can influence your risk of cardiovascular disease in at least four ways. First, cigarette smoke contains the drug nicotine, which increases both heart rate and blood pressure (3). Second, smoking increases your blood's ability to clot; the elevated possibility of a blood clot forming raises your risk of heart attack (3). Third, nicotine also influences the way your heart functions, leading to irregular heart beats (called *arrhythmias*) (3). These arrhythmias can lead to sudden cardiac death. Finally, cigarette smoking increases your chance of developing atherosclerosis by elevating the amount of cholesterol in the blood and encouraging fat deposits in arterial walls (3).

When people stop smoking, their risk of heart disease rapidly declines. It is believed that within 10 years after quitting smoking, a person's risk of death from CHD is reduced to a level equal to that of someone who has never smoked (1). Strategies to stop smoking are discussed in Chapter 10.

HYPERTENSION   Hypertension is a unique risk factor because it is both a disease and a risk factor for stroke and CHD. As mentioned earlier, hypertension is considered a disease because it forces the heart to work harder than normal, which can eventually damage the heart muscle. As a CHD risk factor, it contributes to the

development of CHD by accelerating the rate of atherosclerosis development (2, 5).

HIGH BLOOD CHOLESTEROL LEVELS   As discussed in Chapter 7, cholesterol is a type of fat that can either be consumed in the diet or synthesized in the body, and it is a primary risk factor for CHD. Indeed, the risk of CHD increases as the blood cholesterol increases.

Because cholesterol is not soluble in blood, it is combined with proteins in the liver so it can be transported in the bloodstream. This combination of cholesterol and protein results in two major forms of cholesterol: **low-density lipoproteins (LDL)** and

low-density lipoproteins (LDL) A combination of protein, triglycerides, and cholesterol in the blood, composed of relatively large amounts of cholesterol. Promotes the fatty plaque accumulation in the coronary arteries that leads to heart disease. The association between elevated total blood cholesterol and the increased risk of CHD is due primarily to LDL. Research has shown that individuals with high blood LDL levels have an increased risk of CHD. Because of this relationship, LDL has been labeled "bad cholesterol."

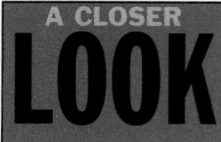

NIH's Blood Cholesterol Guidelines

In response to studies conclusively showing that lowering blood LDL ("bad cholesterol") levels can reduce the risk of heart disease by 40% (6), the National Institutes of Health (NIH) has released guidelines for optimal blood levels of LDL and HDL. Even though the major focus of the guidelines is recommendations for the management of blood LDL levels, NIH included recommendations for blood levels of HDL ("good cholesterol") because HDL can carry choles-

terol away from arteries and back to the liver. The guidelines are summarized in the table in this box.

In short, the guidelines consider LDL levels of 100 mg/dl or lower to be optimal for reducing the risk of developing CHD, whereas LDL levels above 190 mg/dl are considered indicative of a high risk for CHD. Because the presence of HDL can lower LDL levels, low blood levels of HDL can indicate an increased risk of developing CHD. Accordingly, the guidelines consider

blood HDL levels below 40 mg/dl to be low and undesirable in terms of CHD risk.

Cholesterol Concentration mg/dl	Classification
LDL	
< 100	Optimal
100–129	Near or above optimal
130–159	Borderline high
160–189	High
> 190	Very high
HDL	
< 40	Low (undesirable)
> 60	High (very desirable)

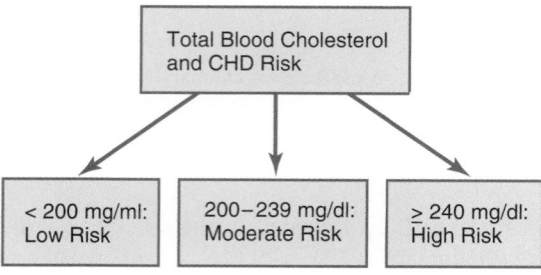

FIGURE 9.9
Total blood cholesterol levels and the CHD risks associated with each.

high-density lipoproteins (HDL). The association between elevated blood cholesterol and CHD is primarily due to LDL: Individuals with high blood LDL levels have an increased risk of CHD, whereas those with high levels of HDL have a decreased risk of CHD (1, 2, 6, 7). Because of these relationships, LDL has been called "bad cholesterol" while HDL has been called "good cholesterol."

---

high-density lipoproteins (HDL) A combination of protein, triglycerides, and cholesterol in the blood, composed of relatively large amounts of protein. Protects against the fatty plaque accumulation in the coronary arteries that leads to heart disease. Research has shown that individuals with high blood HDL levels have a decreased risk of CHD. Therefore, HDL is often called "good cholesterol."

Even though the risk of developing CHD is best predicted from LDL and HDL levels in the blood, measurement of total blood cholesterol (i.e., the sum of all types of cholesterol) also provides a good indication of CHD risk (1, 2, 7). As shown in Figure 9.9, a total blood cholesterol concentration that is less than 200 mg/dl (milligrams per deciliter) indicates a low risk of developing CHD, whereas a concentration that is greater than 240 mg/dl indicates a high CHD risk (2, 7). Unfortunately, because of high-fat diets and lack of exercise, over 21% of people in the United States have total blood cholesterol levels above 240 mg/dl (2).

The National Institutes of Health recently released new guidelines for assessing CHD risks using blood levels of LDL and HDL. For a brief overview of these guidelines, see A Closer Look above.

PHYSICAL INACTIVITY In 1992, the American Heart Association added physical inactivity (defined as a lack of regular exercise) to the list of major risk factors for the development of CHD. The addition of physical inactivity to the list of major risk factors for CHD is based on a large volume of research indicating that the incidence of CHD is higher in people who do not engage in regular physical activity (7–11, 18, 23). Thus, exercise has gained new importance in the prevention of CHD.

The first evidence that physical activity reduces the risk of heart disease was provided over 50 years ago (23). This interesting study compared the rates of CHD between bus conductors and bus drivers in London, England. The conductors are ticket collectors that spend their day walking up and down the stairs of "double-decker" London buses. By contrast, the bus drivers remain seated and are therefore sedentary

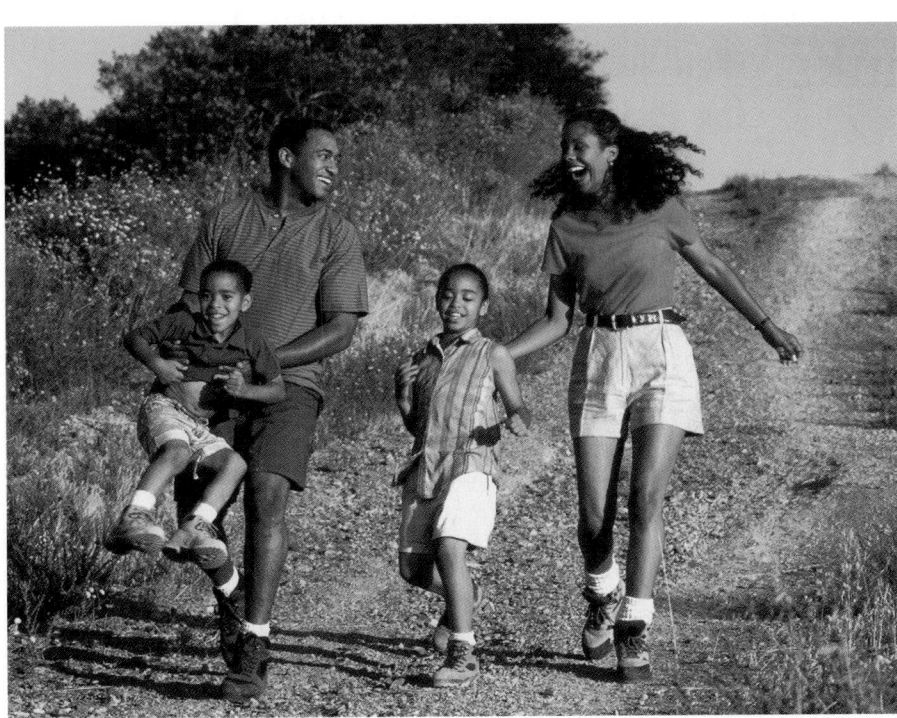

Regular exercise should begin early in life and continue throughout the lifespan.

throughout the workday. This early study demonstrated that the rate of CHD was much higher in the sedentary bus drivers compared to the more physically active conductors. Since this initial study, numerous investigations have consistently reported that regular physical activity reduces the risk of developing CHD (7–11, 18).

Although it is well known that exercise reduces the risk of CHD, the mechanism by which exercise provides protection is unclear. Nonetheless, it seems likely that exercise reduces the risk of CHD by several different pathways including improvements in body weight, blood pressure, lipid profile, and the reduced risk of diabetes (12–14,18, 24). Collectively, these changes can greatly reduce the overall risk of developing CHD.

The relationship between a lack of physical activity and the development of CHD is supported by numerous studies indicating that regular physical activity reduces the risk of cardiovascular mortality independent of other lifestyle modifications (18). A key point to remember is that inactivity as a CHD risk factor is completely under your control and can be eliminated by participation in a regular exercise program. However, to optimally reduce your risk of CHD via exercise, it is important to maintain a regular exercise program throughout the lifespan. More will be said about this important topic in a later section.

HEREDITY It is firmly established that inherited traits can increase your risk of CHD and stroke (1, 2). This means that children of parents with CHD are more likely to develop CHD than are children of parents who do not

have CHD. Current evidence suggests that the familial risk for CHD may be linked to factors such as high blood cholesterol, hypertension, diabetes, and obesity (2).

Race is also a consideration, because African Americans develop hypertension two to three times more often than whites. Therefore, because hypertension increases the chances of developing CHD, African Americans have a greater risk for CHD than do whites. The reason for the high rate of hypertension among African Americans is unknown.

GENDER Men have a greater risk of developing CHD and stroke than do women. Much of the protection against CHD in women is linked to the female sex hormone estrogen, which may elevate HDL cholesterol. Although the risk of CHD increases in women after menopause, it never becomes as great as for men (2).

INCREASING AGE Advancing age increases the risk of developing CHD. The explanation for this observation is that the buildup of arterial plaque is an ongoing process; the longer one lives, the greater the buildup. This is illustrated by the statistic that over 50% of all heart attack victims are 65 or older (1).

CONTRIBUTORY RISK FACTORS

Contributory risk factors are those that increase the risk of CHD, but their direct contribution to the disease process is unclear. You can think of contributory risk factors as those that increase your risk of developing a

Nutritional Links

High Sodium Intake Increases the Risk of Hypertension

A key factor in regulating blood pressure is dietary sodium. High sodium intake results in an elevated blood volume, which promotes higher blood pressure. Therefore, monitoring sodium intake is an important factor in preventing or controlling hypertension.

As mentioned in Chapter 7, sodium (contained in table salt) is a required micronutrient, but the daily requirement for most people is small (less than one-fourth teaspoon or 400 mg). Even athletes or laborers who lose large amounts of water and electrolytes via sweat rarely require more than 1.5 teaspoons (3000 mg) of salt per day. Currently, many U.S. citizens consume more than 6 teaspoons (12,000 mg) of salt per day; clearly, this level of sodium intake is unhealthy and can lead to hypertension.

What is the maximum amount of dietary sodium that the body can tolerate without developing hypertension? Even though a definitive answer

to this question is not available, hypertension is rare in countries where sodium intake is less than 1 teaspoon per day.

The key to lowering your sodium intake is avoiding foods that are high in salt. The table in this box illustrates some common foods that are high in sodium. Take the time to learn which foods contain a lot of sodium and limit your intake of sodium to less than 1 teaspoon per day (14).

Food	Serving Size	Sodium Content (mg)
Bologna	2 oz	700
Cheese		
American	1 oz	305
Cheddar	1 oz	165
Parmesan	1 oz	525
Deviled crab	1	2085
Frankfurter	1	495
Hamburger patty	1 small	550
Pickles (dill)	1 medium	900
Pizza (cheese)	1 slice (14" diameter)	600
Potato chips	20	300
Pretzels	1 oz	890
Salami	3 oz	1047
Soup		
Chicken noodle	1 cup	1010
Vegetable beef	1 cup	1046
Soy sauce	1 tablespoon	1320

major risk factor. At present, the American Heart Association recognizes diabetes, obesity, and stress as contributory risk factors.

DIABETES   As we saw in Chapter 1, diabetes is a disease that results in elevated blood sugar levels due to the body's inability to use blood sugar properly. Diabetes occurs most often in middle age and is common in people who are overweight. In addition to increasing your risk of kidney disease, blindness, and nerve damage, diabetes increases your risk of CHD and stroke. The link between diabetes and CHD is well established; more than 80% of all diabetics die from some form of cardiovascular disease. The role of diabetes in increasing your risk of CHD may be tied to the fact that diabetics often have elevated blood cholesterol levels, hypertension, and are inactive (9).

OBESITY   Compared with individuals who maintain their ideal body weight, obese individuals are more

likely to develop CHD, even if they have no other major risk factors (9). Further, obesity is often associated with elevated blood cholesterol levels and may contribute to hypertension (9).

Of particular interest is the fact that a person's fat distribution pattern affects the risk of CHD. As discussed in Chapter 2, waist-to-hip circumference ratios greater than 1.0 for men and 0.8 for women indicate a significant risk for development of CHD. The physiological reason for the link between CHD and regional fat distribution is not well established but may be due to the fact that people with high waist-to-hip circumference ratios often eat high-fat diets, which elevate blood cholesterol levels.

The fact that obesity is associated with a high incidence of hypertension is well established; however, the exact physiological link between obesity and hypertension is less clear. Possible causes of hypertension in obese individuals include a high-salt diet, which elevates blood pressure, and increased vascular resistance, which results in the need for higher pressure to pump blood to the tissues (2). The role of sodium in promoting hypertension is discussed in Nutritional Links to Health and Fitness, p. 268.

STRESS   Stress increases the risk of CHD; however, the exact link between stress and CHD is unclear and continues to be studied. Nonetheless, it seems likely that stress contributes to the development of several major CHD risk factors. For example, stress may be linked to smoking habits. People under stress may start smoking in an effort to relax, or stress could influence smokers to smoke more than they normally would. Further, stress increases the risk of developing both hypertension and elevated blood cholesterol. The physiological connection between stress and hypertension appears to be the stress-induced release of "stress" hormones, which elevate blood pressure. Currently, it is unclear how stress is linked to high blood cholesterol.

☼ IN SUMMARY

- Researchers have identified several major and contributory risk factors that increase the chance of developing both coronary heart disease (CHD) and stroke.
- Major risk factors for CHD and stroke include smoking, hypertension, high blood cholesterol levels, physical inactivity, heredity, gender, and increasing age.
- Contributory risk factors for CHD and stroke include diabetes, obesity, and stress.

☼ Reducing Your Risk of Heart Disease

Although cardiovascular disease remains the number one killer in the United States, incidence of the disease has declined over the past 30 years (1). This drop is due primarily to people reducing their risk factors for CHD. Table 9.1 contains a list of the major and contributory CHD risk factors discussed earlier in the chapter. Note that four of the seven major risk factors and all three of the contributory factors can be modified by behavior. Therefore, 70% of CHD risk factors can be modified to reduce your risk of developing cardiovascular disease.

How does one implement a CHD risk reduction program? The first step is the identification of your risk status. This can be done by completing Laboratory 9.1 on p. 275 and by carefully examining Table 9.1. The next step is to implement lifestyle changes to modify those CHD risk factors that can be altered.

MODIFICATION OF MAJOR RISK FACTORS

The four major CHD risk factors that can be modified are smoking, hypertension, high blood cholesterol, and physical inactivity. A brief discussion of the importance of modifying these major risk factors follows.

STOP SMOKING AND REDUCE YOUR RISK OF CHD

Smoking cessation is an important way to reduce CHD risk. Indeed, the risk of CHD decreases as soon as

---

TABLE 9.1
Major and Contributory Risk Factors for the Development of Coronary Heart Disease

Risk Factor	Risk Factor Classification	Is Behavior Modification Possible?	Behavior Modification to Reduce Risk
Smoking	Major	Yes	Smoking cessation
Hypertension	Major	Yes	Exercise, proper diet, and reduce stress
High blood cholesterol	Major	Yes	Exercise, proper diet, and medication
Physical inactivity	Major	Yes	Exercise
Heredity	Major	No	
Gender	Major	No	
Increasing age	Major	No	
Diabetes	Contributory	Yes	Proper nutrition, exercise
Obesity	Contributory	Yes	Weight loss, proper nutrition, exercise
Stress	Contributory	Yes	Stress management, exercise

Source: Data from Heart Facts, *American Heart Association, 2004.*

Nutritional Links

Can Antioxidant Vitamins Reduce Your Risk of Coronary Heart Disease?

Free radicals are molecules with an unpaired electron in their outer orbital. While understanding the chemistry of these molecules is not essential,, it is important to know that formation of free radicals can result in "oxidative injury" to cells. This free radical-mediated oxidative injury has been linked to many diseases including CHD. In this regard, research indicates that oxidative injury inside blood vessels is a major contributor to the development of atherosclerosis and CHD. Specifically, oxidative injury in blood vessels promotes the buildup of LDL (bad) cholesterol on arterial walls. Since antioxidant vitamins (e.g., vitamin E and C, and beta carotene) can prevent radical-mediated oxidative injury, it has been reasoned that dietary supplementation with antioxidant vitamins may reduce your risk of CHD (15). Although some studies have reported that antioxidant supplementation reduces the risk of arteriosclerosis, many studies have failed to find that antioxidant supplementation protects against atherosclerosis (25, 26). Moreover, most studies showing protective effects of antioxidants have used vitamin supplements at doses above the recommended dietary allowances (RDA). This has raised concern among many nutritionists, who argue that high doses of these vitamins may result in toxic side effects. Until additional research is performed, the best advice is to eat plenty of fresh fruits and vegetables to obtain as many antioxidants as possible from your diet (15).

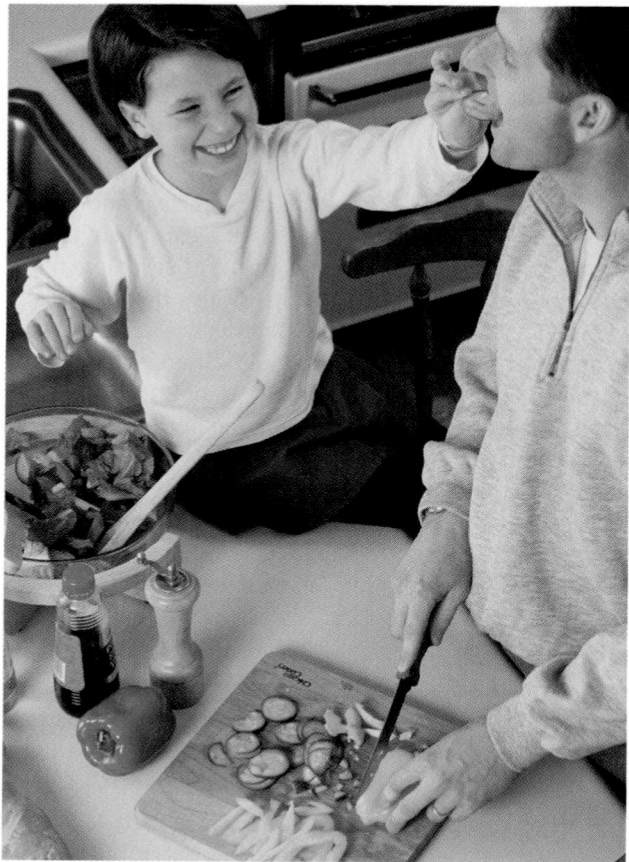

Parents should impress on their children the importance of good dietary habits in preventing cardiovascular disease.

smokers quit. The well-known fitness and wellness expert, Dr. Melvin Williams, offers the following advice on smoking (11): "If you don't smoke, don't start! If you smoke, quit!" Unfortunately, for most people, smoking is a difficult habit to break. Smoking cessation requires major behavior modification to stop smoking and remain smoke free for the rest of your life. See Chapter 10 for a detailed discussion of guidelines to assist in smoking cessation.

LOWER YOUR BLOOD PRESSURE TO REDUCE CHD RISK Hypertension can be combated in several ways. In some instances, medication may be required to

control high blood pressure. However, in many cases of hypertension, exercise and a healthy diet that features low sodium intake can assist in lowering blood pressure (see Nutritional Links to Health and Fitness, p. 268). Since stress can also contribute to hypertension, maintaining low levels of daily stress is also important. The next chapter (Chapter 10) discusses approaches to stress management in detail.

CONTROL OF BLOOD CHOLESTEROL LEVELS IS ESSENTIAL TO REDUCE CHD RISK High blood cholesterol may be lowered by diet, exercise, and drug treatment (2, 14). One of the simplest ways of reducing cholesterol is through diet and exercise. Decreasing your intake of saturated fats and cholesterol may significantly reduce your blood cholesterol levels (see Nutritional Links to Health and Fitness, p. 271). Further, regular exercise has been shown to improve blood lipid profiles in most people. However, if diet and exercise are not effective in lowering your blood lipid levels to a desirable range, cholesterol-lowering drugs are available to assist individuals in lowering their blood cholesterol levels (see A Closer Look, p. 272).

Nutritional Links
TO HEALTH AND FITNESS   **Diet and Blood Cholesterol Levels**

One of the easiest dietary means of reducing your blood cholesterol is to reduce your intake of saturated fat and cholesterol. Saturated fats stimulate cholesterol synthesis in the liver and therefore contribute to elevated blood cholesterol. Saturated fats are found mostly in meats and dairy products; avoiding high intake of these foods can reduce your blood cholesterol levels. The table in this box lists the cholesterol content of selected foods. See Appendix B for a more complete listing.

Food	Serving Size	Cholesterol (mg)	Saturated Fat (g)
Bacon	2 slices	30	0.7
Beef (lean)	8 oz	150	12
Butter	1 tablespoon	32	0.4
Cheese			
American	1 oz	27	5.4
Cheddar	1 oz	30	5.9
Egg	1 (boiled)	113	2.8
Frankfurter	1	30	5.2
Hamburger patty	1 small	68	5.9
Milk (whole)	1 cup	33	5
Milkshake	10 oz	54	8.2
Pizza (meat)	1 slice (14" diameter)	31	8
Sausage	3 oz	42	8.6

REGULAR EXERCISE CAN ELIMINATE INACTIVITY AS A CHD RISK FACTOR   The addition of exercise to your daily routine is an important and simple way to reduce your overall CHD risk. Even modest levels of exercise (e.g., 30 minutes of walking performed three to five times per week) have been shown to reduce the risk of CHD development due to physical inactivity (1, 8–10). In addition, regular aerobic exercise has been shown to modify other CHD risk factors by positively influencing blood pressure, body composition, insulin resistance, and blood cholesterol levels.

While even small amounts of exercise can provide some protection against CHD, studies reveal that the risk of death from CHD decreases as the total physical activity energy expenditure increases from 500 to 3500 kilocalories per week (18). Further, while total energy expenditure from exercise is important in the prevention of CHD, the intensity of exercise is also important. A study of Harvard alumni reported that individuals engaged in regular vigorous exercise (i.e., 50% $\dot{V}O_{2max}$ or higher) were better protected against CHD than people exercising at much lower levels (27). A strong link between exercise intensity and reduction in death from CHD has also been reported by other studies (18).

Remember, "regular" exercise (3 or more days per week) is the key. Indeed, sporadic bouts of exercise (i.e., 3–4 days per month) will not reduce the risk of CHD. Moreover, cessation of exercise will result in a loss of exercise-induced protection from heart disease (19–21). So, make a commitment to a consistent and life-long exercise program today. You heart will love you for it!

MODIFICATION OF CONTRIBUTORY CHD RISK FACTORS

The three contributory CHD risk factors that can be modified are obesity, diabetes, and stress. Body weight loss can be achieved by a combination of diet modification and exercise (Chapter 8). For example, a diet low in calories and fat coupled with an increase in physical activity will help reduce excess body fat. Regular exercise can reduce the risk of developing type II diabetes. Relaxation techniques (discussed in Chapter 10) can help in counteracting the effects of a stressful lifestyle and therefore reduce the risk for development of CHD.

☀ IN SUMMARY

- While heart disease remains the number one killer in the United States, the incidence of heart disease has declined during the past 30 years. This reduction in CHD has occurred because people have modified their behavior to reduce their risk factors for CHD.
- Four major CHD risk factors that can be modified are smoking, hypertension, high blood cholesterol, and inactivity.
- The contributory CHD risk factors that can be modified are obesity, diabetes, and stress.

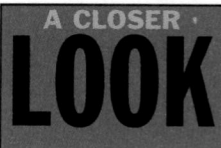

A CLOSER LOOK
Frequently Asked Questions About Exercise, Diet, and Heart Disease

Can dietary modifications or regular exercise slow the progression of atherosclerosis?

Several studies have concluded that a diet low in saturated fat will retard the development of atherosclerotic plaque in blood vessels. Further, regular endurance exercise also slows the progression of atherosclerosis (28). It follows that a lifestyle that includes both regular exercise and a low fat diet would be a good strategy to slow the collection of atherosclerotic plaque in blood vessels.

What if diet and exercise aren't enough to successfully lower my cholesterol to desirable levels?

When diet and exercise alone are not successful in lowering blood cholesterol, drug therapy may help. The most effective and widely tested cholesterol drugs are a class of drugs called "statins" (22). These drugs work by preventing the formation of cholesterol in the liver and also assist in removing cholesterol from the blood. Statins can reduce the bad cholesterol (i.e., LDL) level by 20–45% depending upon the drug used and the dosage (22). While statins have been shown to reduce the risk of atherosclerosis in many people, statins can produce some potentially serious side effects (22). Therefore, if diet and exercise alone cannot successfully lower your cholesterol, you and your physician can decide together if a statin drug is right for you. For more information on the treatment for high cholesterol, consult the National Cholesterol Education Program online at http://www.nhlbi.nih.gov/guidelines/cholesterol/pat_pub.htm.

Some doctors are recommending aspirin to patients to reduce the risk of heart attack. How does aspirin reduce the risk of heart attack?

Extensive research indicates that daily aspirin (80–325 mg/day) can help prevent heart attacks. A heart attack occurs when part of the heart muscle is damaged by a stoppage of blood flow to this region of the heart. Often this occurs when a blood clot blocks arteries that are narrowed by buildup of atherosclerotic plaque. Aspirin helps prevent heart attacks by reducing the risk of blood clots by preventing blood platelets from sticking together.

Despite the benefit of aspirin, taking aspirin daily is not risk free (14). For example, aspirin may be contraindicated for people with bleeding disorders, liver disease, kidney disease, peptic ulcers, or for individuals that are allergic to aspirin. Therefore, consult your family physician before beginning a daily regimen of aspirin.

Can a medical exam identify people at risk for sudden cardiac death during exercise?

Yes, a medical exam can usually identify if individuals are at risk for sudden cardiac death during exercise. Specifically, a medical history and a physical exam from a qualified physician are excellent tools to detect hidden heart disease that could pose a risk for participation in regular exercise.

☀ Lowering Your Risk of Coronary Heart Disease: A Final Word

Regardless of your family history of cardiovascular disease, you can reduce your risk of disease by positively modifying your CHD risk factors. The more changes you make to lower your CHD risk, the better your chances are of preventing cardiovascular disease. Be prepared for occasional backsliding (e.g., eating a high-fat meal); however, when this occurs, quickly regain your focus and return to a healthy lifestyle. Proper CHD risk factor management can add both quality and years to your life. Take action today and lower your CHD risk. See A Closer Look above, for answers to some frequently asked questions about heart disease, diet, and exercise.

Summary

1. Heart disease is the number one cause of death in the United States. Almost one of every two deaths in the United States is due to heart disease.

2. Cardiovascular disease refers to any disease that affects the heart and blood vessels. Common cardiovascular diseases include arteriosclerosis, coronary artery disease, stroke, and hypertension.

3. Coronary risk factors are those that increase your risk for the development of coronary heart disease.

4. Coronary risk factors are classified as either major or contributory. Major risk factors are defined as those that directly increase the risk of coronary

heart disease. Contributory risk factors may increase your chance of developing coronary heart disease by promoting the development of a major risk factor.

5. Major risk factors for the development of coronary heart disease include smoking, hypertension, high blood cholesterol, physical inactivity, heredity, gender, and increasing age.

6. Contributory risk factors for the development of coronary heart disease include diabetes, obesity, and stress.

7. Your risk of developing coronary heart disease can be reduced by modification of the following risk factors: smoking, hypertension, high blood pressure, physical inactivity, obesity, and stress.

Study Questions

1. Identify the number one cause of death in the United States.

2. Define the following terms:
cardiovascular disease
coronary heart disease
coronary artery disease
hypertension

3. List the major and contributory risk factors for the development of coronary heart disease.

4. Discuss the difference between *major* and *contributory* risk factors for the development of coronary heart disease.

5. High-density and low-density lipoproteins have been labeled "good" and "bad" cholesterol, respectively. Explain.

6. Which major coronary heart disease risk factors can be modified?

7. Which contributory coronary heart disease risk factors can be modified?

8. How does a high-salt diet contribute to hypertension?

9. What is the link between diet and blood cholesterol?

10. How does smoking increase your risk of developing cardiovascular disease?

11. How are arteriosclerosis and atherosclerosis related?

Suggested Reading

Eyre, H. et al. Preventing cancer, cardiovascular disease, and diabetes. *Stroke.* 35:1–12, 2004.

Heart and Stroke Facts. American Heart Association. Dallas, Texas. 2004.

Heart Facts 2004: Latino/Hispanic Americans. American Heart Association. Dallas, Texas. 2004.

Heart Facts 2004: All Americans. American Heart Association. Dallas, Texas. 2004.

Heart Disease and Stroke: Statistics-2004 update. American Heart Association. Dallas, Texas. 2004.

Gotto, A. Statins: Powerful drugs for lowering cholesterol. *Circulation.* 105:1514–1516, 2002.

Peterson, J. A. Take ten: 10 ways to protect your heart. *ACSM's Health and Fitness Journal* 4 (2):48, 2000.

Powers, S., S. Lennon, J. Quindry, and J. L. Mehta. Exercise and cardioprotection. *Current Opinion in Cardiology* 17:495–502, 2002.

Powers, S., and E. Howley. *Exercise Physiology: Theory and Application to Fitness and Performance,* 5th edition. St. Louis: McGraw Hill, 2004.

Rauramaa, P. et al. Summaries for patients. Does Aerobic exercise slow progression of atherosclerosis? *Annals of Internal Medicine. Summaries for patients* 140:I-37, 2004

For links to the web sites below visit The Total Fitness and Wellness Website at www.aw-bc.com/powers.

Mayo Clinic Health

Contains wide-ranging information about diet, fitness, and health.

American Medical Association

Contains many sources of information about a wide variety of medical problems, including heart disease.

WebMD

Presents information about a wide variety of diseases and medical problems, including heart disease.

American Heart Association

Contains information about a variety of topics related to both heart disease and stroke.

References

1. American Heart Association. Heart and stroke facts. *Statistical Update.* Dallas: American Heart Association, 2004.

2. Barrow, M. *Heart Talk: Understanding Cardiovascular Diseases.* Gainesville, FL: Cor-Ed Publishing, 1992.

3. American Cancer Society. *Fifty Most Often Asked Questions About Smoking and Health and the Answers.* New York: The American Cancer Society, 1990.

4. American Cancer Society. *1996 Cancer Facts and Figures.* Atlanta: The American Cancer Society, 1993.

5. Pollack, M., and D. Schmidt. *Heart Disease and Rehabilitation.* Champaign, IL: Human Kinetics, 1995.

6. Third report of the National Cholesterol Education Program Expert Panel on Detection, Evaluation, and Treatment of High Blood Cholesterol in Adults. *Journal of the American Medical Association* 285(19):1–19, 2001.

7. Thomas, T., and T. LaFontaine. Exercise, nutritional strategies, and lipoproteins. In *ACSM's Resource Manual for Guidelines for Exercise Testing and Prescription,* 4th ed. J. Roitman, ed. Philadelphia: Lippincott Williams & Wilkins, 2001.

8. Blair, S. N., H. W. Kohl, R. S. Paffenbarger, D. G. Clark, K. H. Cooper, and L. W. Gibbons. Physical fitness and all-cause mortality: A prospective study of healthy men and women. *Journal of the American Medical Association* 262:2395–2401, 1989.

9. Bouchard, C., R. Shephard, T. Stephens, J. Sutton, and B. McPherson. *Exercise, Fitness, and Health: A Consensus of Current Knowledge.* Champaign, IL: Human Kinetics, 1990.

10. Paffenbarger, R. S., R. T. Hyde, A. L. Wing, and C. C. Hsieh. Physical activity, all-cause mortality of college alumni. *New England Journal of Medicine* 314:605–613, 1986.

11. Kohl, H. Physical activity and cardiovascular disease: Evidence for a dose-response. *Medicine and Science in Sports and Exercise* 33(Suppl.):S472–S483, 2001.

12. Wood, P. Physical activity, diet, and health: Independent and interactive effects. *Medicine and Science in Sports and Exercise* 26:838–843, 1994.

13. Durstine, J., and W. Haskell. Effects of training on plasma lipids and lipoproteins. *Exercise and Sport Science Reviews* 22:477–521, 1994.

14. Durstine, J. L., and R. Thompson. Exercise modulates blood lipids and exercise plan. *ACSM's Health and Fitness Journal* 4(4):44–46, 2000.

15. Leeds, M. *Nutrition for Healthy Living.* Boston: WCB-McGraw-Hill, 1998.

16. American Heart Association. *Aspirin and Your Health.* Dallas: American Heart Association, 2000.

17. Rowland, T. Screening for risk of cardiac death in young athletes. *Sports Science Exchange* 12(3):1–5, 1999.

18. Powers, S., S. Lennon, J. Quindry, and J. L. Mehta. Exercise and cardioprotection. *Current Opinion in Cardiology* 17:495–502, 2002.

19. Lennon, S., J. C. Quindry, K. L. Hamilton, J. French, J. Staib, J. L. Mehta, and S. K. Powers. Loss of exercise-induced cardioprotection following cessation of exercise. *Journal of Applied Physiology* 96:1299–1305, 2004.

20. Lennon, S., J. C. Quindry, K. L. Hamilton, J. P. French, J. Hughes, J. L. Mehta, and S. K. Powers. Elevated MnSOD is not required for exercise-induced cardioprotection against myocardial stunning. *American Journal of Physiology* 287:H975–980, 2004.

21. Powers, S., J. C. Quindry, and K. Hamilton. Aging, exercise, and cardioprotection. *Annals of the New York Academy of Sciences* 2004.

22. Gotto, A. Statins: Powerful drugs for lowering cholesterol. *Circulation* 105:1514–1516, 2002.

23. Morris, J., J. Heady, P. Raffle, C. Roberts, and J. Parks. Coronary heart disease and physical activity of work. *Lancet* Ii:1053–1057, 1953.

24. Batty, G., and I-Min Lee. Physical activity and coronary heart disease. *British Medical Journal* 328:1089–1090, 2004.

25. Kinlay, S. et al. Long-term effect of combined vitamin E and C on coronary and peripheral endothelial function. *Journal of American College of Sports Medicine* 18:629–634, 2004.

26. Hasnain, B., and A. Mooradian. Recent trials of antioxidant therapy: What should we be telling our patients? *Cleveland Clinic Journal of Medicine* 71:327–334, 2004.

27. Lee, I., C. Hsich, and R. Paffenbarger. Exercise intensity and longevity in men. The Harvard Alumni Health Study. *Journal of American Medical Association* 273:1179–1184, 1995.

28. Henderson, K., J. Turk, J. Rush, and M. Laughlin. Endothelial function in coronary arterioles from pigs with early stage coronary disease induced by high fat/cholesterol diet: Effect of exercise. *Journal of Applied Physiology* 2004.

Find Your Cholesterol Plan

NAME _____ DATE _____

The following two-step program will guide you through the National Cholesterol Education Program's new treatment guidelines. The first step helps you establish your overall coronary risk; the second uses that information to determine your LDL treatment goals and how to reach them. You'll need to know your blood pressure, your total LDL and HDL cholesterol levels, and your triglyceride and fasting glucose levels. If you're not sure of those numbers, ask your doctor and, if necessary, schedule an exam to get them. (Everyone should have a complete lipid profile every five years, starting at age 20.)

STEP 1: TAKE THE HEART-ATTACK RISK TEST

This test will identify your chance of having a heart attack or dying of coronary disease in the next 10 years. (People with previously diagnosed coronary disease, diabetes, aortic aneurysm, or symptomatic carotid- or peripheral-artery disease already face more than a 20 percent risk; they can skip the test and go straight to Step 2.) The test uses data from the Framingham Heart Study, the world's longest-running study of cardiovascular risk factors. The test is limited to established, major factors that are easily measured. Circle the point value for each of the risk factors shown at right and below.

Age

Years	Women	Men
20–34	–7	–9
35–39	–3	–4
40–44	0	0
45–49	3	3
50–54	6	6
55–59	8	8
60–64	10	10
65–69	12	11
70–74	14	12
75–79	16	13

Total Cholesterol

	AGE 20–39		AGE 40–49		AGE 50–59		AGE 60–69		AGE 70–79	
Mg/dL	Women	Men	Women	Men	Women	Men	Women	Men	Women	Men
<160	0	0	0	0	0	0	0	0	0	0
160–199	4	4	3	3	2	2	1	1	1	0
200–239	8	7	6	5	4	3	2	1	1	0
240–279	11	9	8	6	5	4	3	2	2	1
280+	13	11	10	8	7	5	4	3	2	1

High-Density Lipoprotein (HDL) Cholesterol

Mg/dL	Women and Men
60+	—1
50–59	0
40–49	1
<40	2

Systolic Blood Pressure (the Higher Number)

	TREATED		UNTREATED	
Mm/Hg	Women	Men	Women	Men
<120	0	0	0	0
120–129	1	0	3	1
130–139	2	1	4	2
140–159	3	1	5	2
>159	4	2	6	3

Smoking

AGE 20–39		AGE 40–49		AGE 50–59		AGE 60–69		AGE 70–79	
Women	Men	Women	Men	Women	Men	Women	Men	Women	Men
9	8	7	5	4	3	2	1	1	1

Total Your Points _____

(continued on next page)

Now find your total point score in the men's or women's column at right, then locate your 10-year risk in the far-right column.

Women's Score	Men's Score	Your Ten-Year Risk
<20	<12	<10%
20–22	12–15	10%–20%
>22	>15	>20%

STEP 2: FIND YOUR LOW-DENSITY LIPOPROTEIN (LDL) TREATMENT PLAN

Consult the table below to learn how your overall coronary risk affects whether you need to lower your LDL cholesterol level and, if you do, by how much. First, locate your coronary risk in the left-hand column. (That's based on the 10-year heart-attack risk that you just calculated as well as your coronary risk factors and any heart-threatening diseases you may have.) Then look across that row to see whether you should make lifestyle changes and take cholesterol-lowering medication, based on your current LDL level.

Coronary-Risk Group	Start lifestyle changes if your LCL level is . . . [1]	Add drugs if your LDL level is . . .
Very High 1. Ten-year heart-attack risk risk of 20% or more or 2. history of coronary heart disease, diabetes, peripheral-artery disease, carotid-artery disease, or aortic aneurysm.	100 mg/dl or higher. (Aim for an LDL under 100.) Get retested after 3 months.	130 or higher. (Drugs are optional if your LDL is between 100 and 130.)
High 1. Ten-year heart-attack risk of 10% to 20% and 2. two or more major coronary risk factors.[2]	130 or higher. (Aim for an LDL under 130.) Get retested after 3 months.	130 or higher and lifestyle changes don't achieve your LDL goal in 3 months.
Moderately High 1. Ten-year heart-attack risk under 10% and 2. two or more major coronary risk factors.[2]	Same as above.	160 or higher, and lifestyle changes don't achieve your LDL goal in 3 months.[3]
Low to Moderate 1. One or no major coronary risk factors.[2, 4]	160 or higher. (Aim for an LDL under 160.) Get retested after 3 months.	190 or higher, and lifestyle changes don't achieve your LDL goal in 3 months. (Drugs are optional if your LDL is between 160 and 189.)

1. People who have the metabolic syndrome should make lifestyle changes, even if their LDL level alone doesn't warrant it. You have the metabolic syndrome if you have three or more of these risk factors: HDL under 40 in men, 50 in women; systolic blood pressure of 130 or more or diastolic pressure of 85 or more; fasting glucose level of 110 to 125; triglyceride level of 150 or more; and waist circumference over 40 inches in men, 35 inches in women. People with the syndrome should limit their carbohydrate intake, get up to 30 to 35 percent of their calories from total fat (more than usually recommended), and make the other lifestyle changes, including restriction of saturated fat.
2. The major coronary risk factors are cigarette smoking; coronary disease in a father or brother before age 55 or a mother or sister before age 65; systolic blood pressure of 140 or more, a diastolic pressure of 90 or more, or being on drugs for hypertension; and an HDL level under 40. If your HDL is 60 or more, subtract one risk factor. (High LDL is a major factor, of course, but it's already figured into the table.)
3 While the goal is to get LDL under 130, the use of drugs in these people usually isn't worthwhile, even if lifestyle steps fail to achieve that goal.
4. People in this group usually have less than 10 percent 10-year risk. Those who have higher risk should ask their doctor whether they need more aggressive treatment than shown here.

Understanding Your CVD Risk

NAME _____ DATE _____

Each of us has a unique level of risk for various diseases. Some of these risks are things you can take action to change; others are risks that you need to consider as you plan a lifelong strategy for overall risk reduction. Complete each of the following questions and total your points in each section. If you score between 1 and 5 in any section, consider your risk. The higher the number, the greater your risk. If you answered "don't know" for any question, talk to your parents or other family members as soon as possible to find out if you have any unknown risks.

PART I: ASSESS YOUR FAMILY RISK FOR CVD

1. Do any of your primary relatives (mother, father, grandparents, siblings) have a history of heart disease or stroke?

   YES _____ (1 point)   NO _____ (0 points)   Don't Know _____

2. Do any of your primary relatives (mother, father, grandparents, siblings) have diabetes?

   YES _____ (1 point)   NO _____ (0 points)   Don't Know _____

3. Do any of your primary relatives (mother, father, grandparents, siblings) have high blood pressure?

   YES _____ (1 point)   NO _____ (0 points)   Don't Know _____

4. Do any of your primary relatives (mother, father, grandparents, siblings) have a history of high cholesterol?

   YES _____ (1 point)   NO _____ (0 points)   Don't Know _____

5. Would you say that your family consumed a high fat diet (lots of red meat, dairy, butter/margarine) during your time spent at home?

   YES _____ (1 point)   NO _____ (0 points)   Don't Know _____

Total Points _____

PART II: ASSESS YOUR LIFESTYLE RISK FOR CVD

1. Is your total cholesterol level higher than it should be?

   YES _____ (1 point)   NO _____ (0 points)   Don't Know _____

2. Do you have high blood pressure?

   YES _____ (1 point)   NO _____ (0 points)   Don't Know _____

3. Have you been diagnosed as prediabetic or diabetic?

   YES _____ (1 point)   NO _____ (0 points)   Don't Know _____

(continued on next page)

4. Do you smoke?

   YES _____ (1 point)   NO _____ (0 points)   Don't Know _____

5. Would you describe your life as being highly stressful?

   YES _____ (1 point)   NO _____ (0 points)   Don't Know _____

Total Points _____

PART III: ASSESS YOUR ADDITIONAL RISKS FOR CVD

1. How would you best describe your current weight?

   a. Lower than what it should be for my height and weight (0 points)

   b. About what it should be for my height and weight (0 points)

   c. Higher than it should be for my height and weight (1 point)

2. How would you describe the level of exercise that you get each day?

   a. Less than what I should be exercising each day (1 point)

   b. About what I should be exercising each day (0 points)

   c. More than what I should be each day (0 points)

3. How would you describe your dietary behaviors?

   a. Eating only the recommended number of calories/day (0 points)

   b. Eating less than the recommended number of calories each day (0 points)

   c. Eating more than the recommended number of calories each day (1 point)

4. Which of the following best describes your typical dietary behavior?

   a. I eat from the major food groups, trying hard to get the recommended fruits and vegetables (0 points)

   b. I eat too much red meat and consume much saturated fat from meats and dairy products each day (1 point)

   c. Whenever possible, I try to substitute olive oil or canola oil for other forms of dietary fat. (0 points)

5. Which of the following best describes you?

   a. I watch my sodium intake and try to reduce stress in my life (0 points)

   b. I have a history of *Chlamydia* infection (1 point)

   c. I try to eat 5 to 10 milligrams of soluble fiber each day and to substitute a soy product for an animal product in my diet at least once each week. (0 points)

Total Points _____

Assessing Your Genetic Predisposition for Cardiovascular Disease

NAME —————————————————————— DATE ——————————————————————

The following is a family tree that allows you to fill in risk factors and conditions for heart disease in your family members. Remember that heart disease has a genetic contribution, so examining your relatives' health and lifestyles will provide insight into your future susceptibility to heart disease. Write in risk factors directly related to heart disease. Examples include: hypertension, high blood cholesterol, diabetes, stroke, obesity, heart attack.

Your Family History of Heart Disease

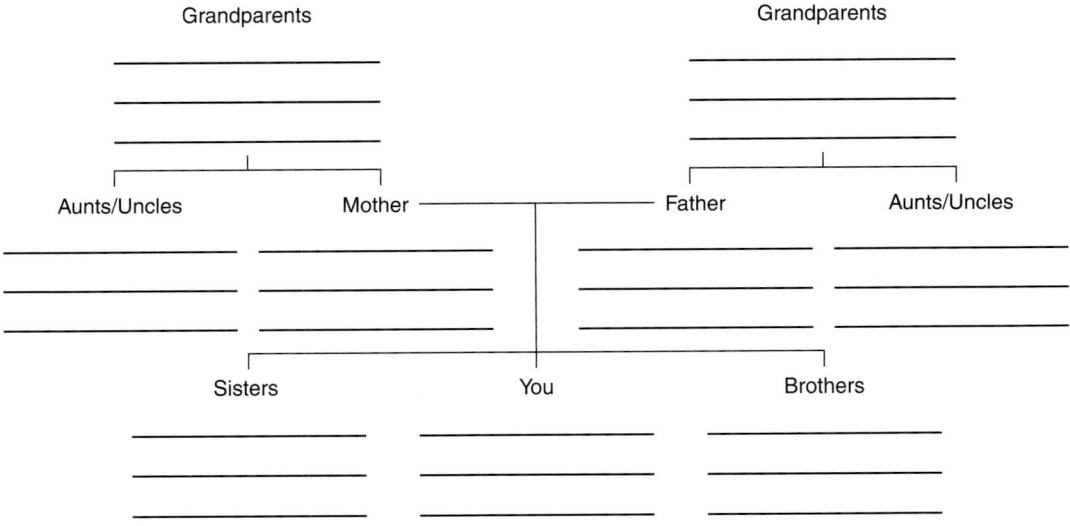

Note: This family tree can be copied and used for other diseases with an inheritable component, such as cancer.

(continued on next page)

In the space below, list any diet, behavior, or lifestyle risks in your life that may contribute to heart disease. Examples include high stress level, high fat diet, physical inactivity, high sodium intake.

_____

_____

_____

_____

INTERPRETATION

Inherited traits can increase your risk of cardiovascular disease. The good news is that you are not destined to develop heart disease or any of the conditions present in your relatives. Lifestyle changes that include moderate exercise and proper diet can reduce your risk of developing cardio-vascular diseases. Being aware of health concerns and problems within your family that may be passed on genetically will make you a more informed, health-conscious individual.

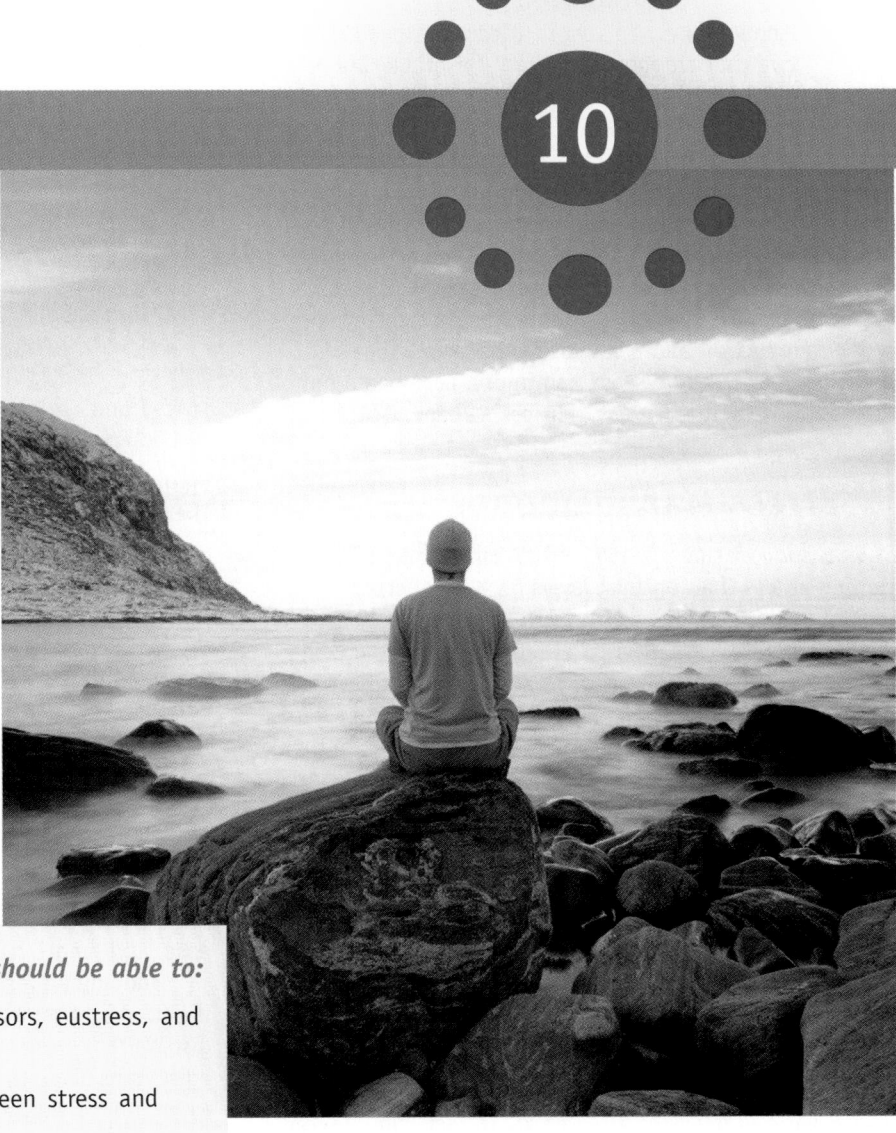

10

After studying this chapter, you should be able to:

1. Discuss the terms stress, stressors, eustress, and distress.

2. Describe the relationship between stress and disease.

3. Discuss physical responses to stress.

4. List common sources of stress.

5. Outline the steps involved in stress management.

6. List two relaxation techniques that will help lower stress.

7. Discuss the Health Belief Model and how it relates to behavior change.

8. Provide an example of how behavior modification can be used to modify unhealthy behavior.

9. Identify the most common types of accidents.

10. Outline steps to reduce your risk of accidents.

Stress Management and Modifying Unhealthy Behavior

Although many behaviors affect your health, the five that are most important for promotion of good health (1–5) are regular exercise, good nutrition, weight control, stress management, and modification of unhealthful behaviors that increase your risk of getting a disease or becoming injured. Earlier chapters have focused on improving health through physical fitness, proper diet/weight control, and actively reducing the risk of cancer and heart disease. This chapter expands on these strategies by introducing the concepts of stress reduction and behavior modification aimed at reducing your risk of disease and injury. Let's begin our discussion with an overview of stress management.

☀ Stress Management

Studies suggest that 10–15% of U.S. adults may be functioning at less than optimal levels because of stress-related anxiety and depression (5). Approximately 75–90% of all physician visits are for stress-related complaints resulting in millions of people taking medication for stress-related illnesses (6). Stress-related problems result in an annual loss of billions of dollars to both businesses and government due to employee absenteeism and health care costs. Therefore, stress is a major health problem in the United States that affects individual lives and the economy as a whole. In the following sections we discuss several key aspects of stress management.

STRESS: AN OVERVIEW

As described in Chapter 1, wellness focuses on balanced interactions among the wellness components. An imbalance between these areas of life will cause individuals to feel varying levels of discomfort. In fact, the greater the imbalance the more discomfort the individual experiences.

Stress is a physiological and mental response to forces and pressures of modern life that cause us to become uncomfortable. Any factor that produces stress is called a **stressor.** Stressors can be physical in nature (such as an injury) or mental (such as emotional distress resulting from a personal relationship). Regardless of the nature of the stressor, the physiological and mental responses to stress usually include the feelings of strain, tension, and anxiety.

There are many sources of stress in everyday life. Driving in heavy traffic, being involved in a motor ve-

stress A physiological and mental response to something in the environment that causes people to become uncomfortable.
stressor A factor that produces stress.

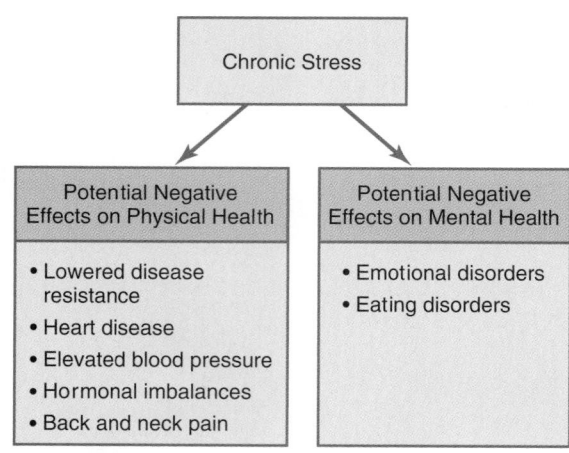

FIGURE 10.1
The health effects of chronic stress.

hicle crash, encountering emotional conflicts at work or school, and experiencing personal financial problems are just a few. Let's continue our discussion of stress by examining the link between stress and disease.

STRESS AND DISEASE

From a medical standpoint, stress can affect both emotional and physical health. Chronic (persistent) stress has been linked to elevated blood pressure, heart disease, hormonal imbalances, reduced resistance to disease, and emotional disorders (1–5) (Figure 10.1).

The human response to stress, known as the "fight or flight" response, was first discovered by Harvard physiologist Walter Canon (7) and later elaborated on by the biologist Hans Selye (8). Canon described the stress response as an inborn, automatic, and primitive response designed to prepare individuals to face (fight) or run away (flight) from any type of perceived harm or threat to survival. According to Canon, once a person perceives a threat, the brain initiates a sequence of physiological and physical changes that ready the body for action.

Imagine you are a caveman looking for some berries to eat and suddenly you sense something is behind you. You look around and see a hungry saber-tooth tiger closely stalking you. You know you are in danger. Do you run or use your spear to protect yourself? No matter what you decide your brain has activated your fight or flight response. Now, imagine you are at home and the telephone awakens you from a sound sleep. You answer the phone and hear your professor's voice asking why you missed the final exam. You look at your clock and realize you overslept and missed class! Suddenly you notice your heart is racing, perspiration is pouring, blood pressure is up, and your hands are cold and clammy. Do you try to explain the situation to your professor (fight) or quickly hang up and never return to school again (flight)? The fight or

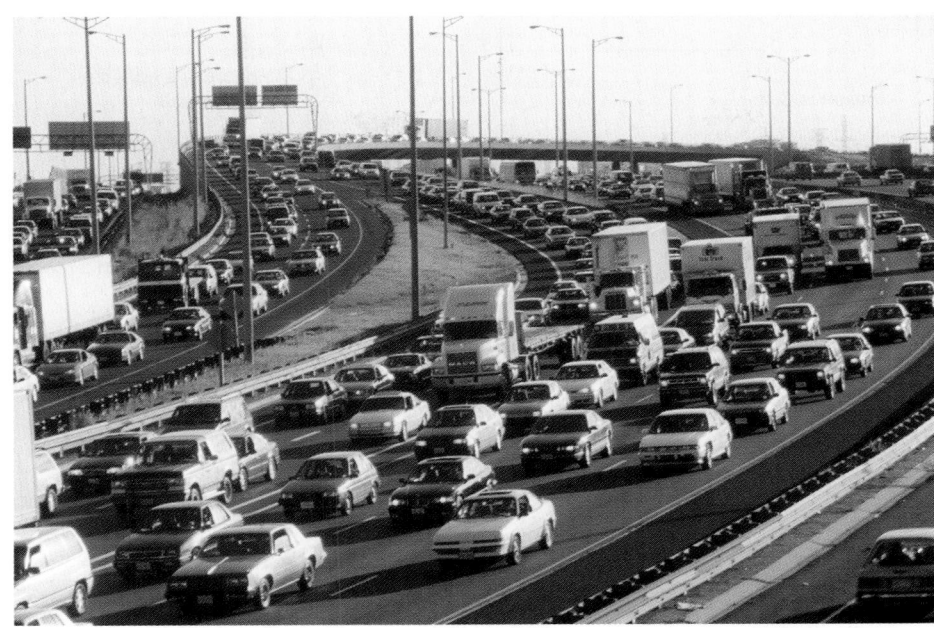

Traffic jams are one of many sources of stress in today's society.

flight response is called a "primitive response" because it has not changed from the early beginnings of humankind. Regardless of whether a saber-tooth tiger or an angry professor is stalking you, the perceived threat brings about the same bodily response (8).

The body's responses to stress are mediated by an area in the brain called the hypothalamus and initiated when the hormones **epinephrine, norepinephrine,** and **cortisol** are released into the bloodstream. The hormones cause a number of physiological changes to occur (Figure 10.2), including an increased rate of breathing and enlargement (dilation) of the pupils of the eyes. In addition, blood is directed away from the digestive tract and redirected into the muscles to provide extra energy for fighting or fleeing. During this time individuals have an increased awareness of their surroundings, quickened impulses, diminished pain perception, and a heightened immune response. In other words, the body is prepared physically and mentally for battle, and as long as the person perceives the threat, the body will stay in this aroused state. Once the threat is eliminated, the body returns to its normal state of balance.

As you can see during the fight or flight response people are in an "attack mode" and focused on short-term survival; fear is heightened and body systems are distorted. While primitive people were required to exert physical activity while fighting or fleeing from wild animals, modern stressors such as congested roads, too few parking spaces, missing an exam, bouncing a check, or having an argument with your significant other do not typically require physical exertion. In primitive times, the physical exertion related to the act of fighting or fleeing would rid the body of excess levels of stress hormones and allow it to return to its prearoused state of balance and calm. Today, people

living highly stressful lives remain in a state of heightened alarm (chronic stress), and often have no release from these stressors in the form of physical exertion; over time the stress hormones accumulate in the body, causing illness and chronic disease.

Hans Selye developed a scientific theory to explain the relationship between stress and disease. Selye proposed that humans adapt to stress in a response he termed the **general adaptation syndrome,** which involves three stages: an alarm stage, a resistance stage, and an exhaustion stage (8).

During the alarm stage, the release of the stress hormones and their effects on the body (8) can cause individuals to experience generalized anxiety, headaches, and disrupted patterns of sleeping and eating. During this phase, the body becomes susceptible to disease and more prone to injury.

With continued exposure to stress, the individual reaches the resistance stage, during which the body's resistance to stress is higher than normal and mechanisms are activated that allow it to resist disease effectively.

Epinephrine A hormone secreted by the inner core (medulla) of the adrenal gland; also called adrenaline.

Norepinephrine A hormone secreted by the inner core (medulla) of the adrenal gland

Cortisol A hormone secreted by the outer layer (cortex) of the adrenal gland.

general adaptation syndrome A pattern of responses to stress that consists of an alarm stage, a resistance stage, and an exhaustion stage.

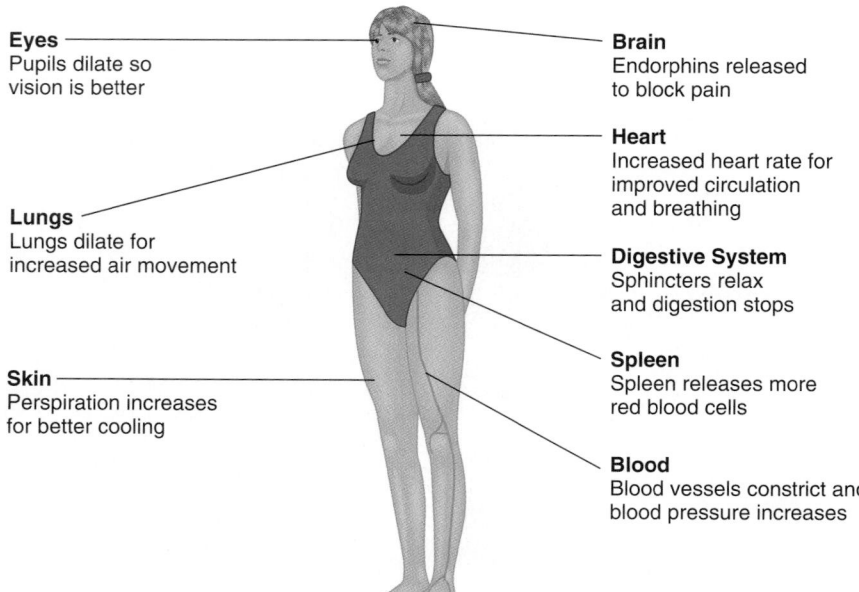

Eyes
Pupils dilate so
vision is better

Lungs
Lungs dilate for
increased air movement

Skin
Perspiration increases
for better cooling

Brain
Endorphins released
to block pain

Heart
Increased heart rate for
improved circulation
and breathing

Digestive System
Sphincters relax
and digestion stops

Spleen
Spleen releases more
red blood cells

Blood
Blood vessels constrict and
blood pressure increases

FIGURE 10.2
**The body's physiological response to
stress.**

In short, the resistance stage represents an improved ability to cope with stress (8).

If the stress persists, however, the individual reaches the exhaustion stage. (Note that "exhaustion" in this sense is a life-threatening type of physical and psychological depletion that occurs due to days or weeks of exposure to constant stress.) Selye suggests that the body is vulnerable to disease during this stage because the resources needed for the stress response have been depleted. During this phase, physical symptoms that appeared in the alarm stage can reappear, but now are more serious and can sometimes lead to death.

Although Selye's model of adaptation to stress is still viewed as an important contribution to our understanding of the stress response, newer research findings have improved our understanding of the relationship between stress and disease. For example, today we know that the underlying cause of many stress-related diseases is not the body's inability to respond to stress because of depleted resources, but the prolonged response to stress brought about by the relationship between the nervous, endocrine (produces hormones), and immune (protects against disease) systems, which results in the continual release of stress hormones, including cortisol. One's risk of developing a stress-related illness increases because, over time, high levels of cortisol in the blood impair the immune system's ability to fight infections (9–11). As you have realized

by now, prolonged stress places an individual at greater risk for illness and other associated problems. As a result, knowledge of stress management skills is an important tool for maintaining a high level of wellness. Before we discuss stress management skills, let's begin with a discussion of how to assess your own level of stress.

ASSESSMENT OF STRESS

Stressors can be acute (such as the death of a loved one), cumulative (such as a series of events leading to a divorce), or chronic (such as daily job- or school-related pressures). Although it is clear that chronic or extreme stress is unhealthy, some degree of stress is required to maximize performance. Indeed, for any type of "performance" activity there is an optimal level of stress. This optimal level of stress pushes us to perform and excel, while experiencing positive health effects. For instance, athletes and business professionals often perform better when faced with mild-to-moderate stress. A stress level that results in improved performance is called **eustress** or positive stress. This type of stress is exhilarating and energizing. Although some level of stress is desirable, each of us has a breaking point in terms of stress. This idea is illustrated in Figure 10.3. When we surpass the stress level needed to optimize performance (optimal stress), we reach our stress "break point," and distress (negative stress) results. For example, regular exercise can be described as positive stress. However, regular exercise at too high a frequency or intensity turns into overtraining which is negative stress. As a result, the chronic stress promotes a decline in performance, and increases the individual's risk of injury and illness.

eustress A stress level that results in improved performance.

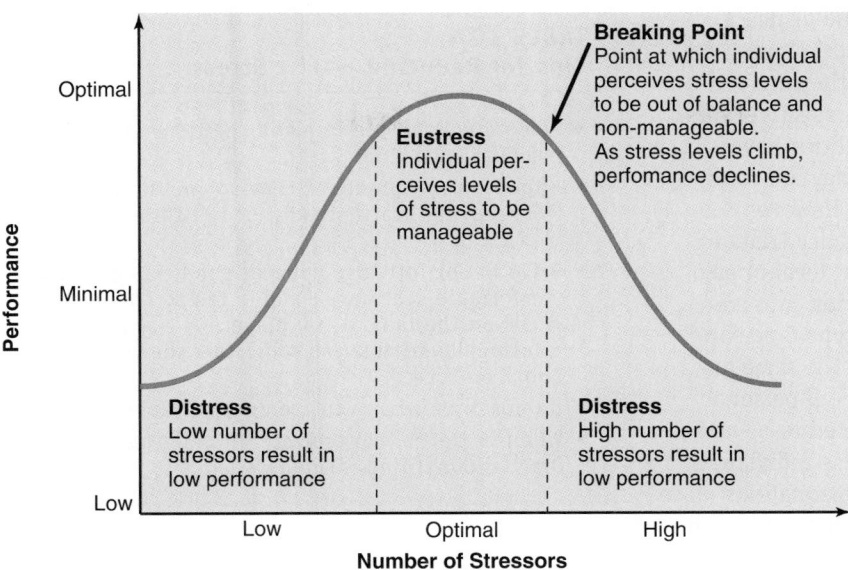

FIGURE 10.3
The concepts of eustress and distress.

People may react differently to the same stressful situation; for example, arriving late for class may evoke strong feelings of anxiety in one student and no emotion at all in another. This difference in "stress perception" is due to personality differences.

There are many different ways to describe personalities. An Internet search for "personality types" will result in thousands of sites and tools that can be used to determine personality type. For instance, the Myers Briggs Temperament Indicator (MBTI) is a widely used personality test that describes 16 distinct temperament (personality) types, each of which reacts differently to stress. Readers should note that while there is not one specific (or completely reliable) way of identifying stress-prone personalities, one of the most

common, and easily interpreted, classification groupings describe individuals as belonging to one of four personality categories: type A, type B, type C, and type D (Figure 10.4). This method of identifying a stress-prone personality was developed in the 1970s by two cardiologists, Drs. Friedman and Rosenman, who were interested in the relationship between heart attacks and stress. The physicians described each of the four most common personality types as follows. Type A individuals are highly motivated, time-conscious, hard driving, impatient, and sometimes hostile. They have a heightened response to stress and their hostility places them at a greater risk for heart disease (5). In contrast, type B individuals are easygoing, nonaggressive, patient, and are not prone to hostile episodes as type

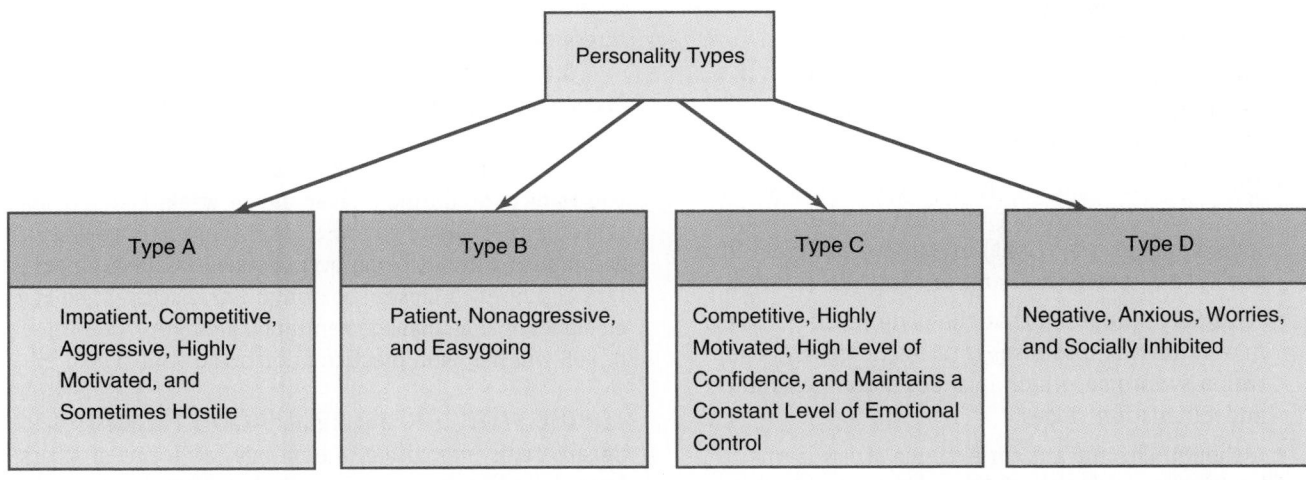

FIGURE 10.4
Personality types and their risks for heart disease.

As are. Type B personalities are relaxed and at peace with themselves. Their sense of inner peace allows them to cope with stress effectively; therefore they are considered to be at low risk (from a stress perspective) for heart disease. People with type C personalities have many of the qualities of type A people. They are confident, highly motivated, and competitive. However, these unique individuals use their personality traits to their advantage by maintaining a constant level of emotional control and channeling their ambition into creative directions. Interestingly, although type C personalities are highly driven, they experience the same low stress-related risk for heart disease as type B personalities. Type D personalities are also considered to be at greater risk for stress-related disease. These individuals are prone to worry and anxiety. Type D personalities are socially inhibited and uneasy when interacting with others. Their social clumsiness results in a chronic state of anxiety, which places them at greater risk for heart disease (12, 13).

While discovering aspects of one's personality can be interesting and entertaining, we must keep in mind that ultimately, it is our perception of the stressor and the way we respond to it that will determine any resulting health effects. Regardless of your personality type, you can learn ways to deal with the stress in your life, and the first step in this is to examine your stress level.

The most convenient way to do this is to complete a questionnaire designed to evaluate your stress level. Laboratory 10.1 on p. 301 is designed to accomplish this goal. If the results suggest that you are under stress, you should begin implementing stress reduction techniques.

☀ IN SUMMARY

- Stress is a physiological and mental response to things in our environment (stressors) that cause us to be uncomfortable.
- Studies suggest that 10–15% of U.S. adults may be functioning at below optimal levels due to stress-related anxiety and/or depression.
- The "fight or flight" response is an inborn, automatic, and primitive response designed to prepare individuals to face (fight) or run away (flight) from any type of perceived harm or threat to survival.
- Hans Selye proposed that the body reacts to stress in a pattern of responses termed the general adaptation syndrome, which includes alarm, resistance, and exhaustion stages.
- Although chronic and/or extreme stress is unhealthy, some degree of stress is required to maximize performance. A stress level that results in improved performance is called eustress.

TABLE 10.1
Tips for Reducing Traffic Stress

- Alter your schedule to avoid the times of heaviest congestion.
- Allow yourself plenty of time so you do not have to speed, run traffic lights, or roll through stop signs.
- Drive in comfort. Use your air conditioner, get a comfortable seat cover, and listen to classical music on the radio or CD player. Do not listen to emotionally stimulating radio talk shows. Enjoy books on tape.
- Do not drive when you are angry or upset.
- When in traffic, concentrate on being relaxed. Practice breathing for relaxation.

STEPS IN STRESS MANAGEMENT

Now that you have identified your stress level, it is time to deal with stress by using techniques known collectively as "stress management." Although there are no magic formulas or nutritional supplements capable of eliminating stress, there are two general steps to managing stress (5, 14): Reduce the amount of stress in your life, and learn to cope with stress by improving your ability to relax. Laboratory 10.2 on p. 303 is designed to help you analyze your sources of stress and your responses to them. Let's discuss each of these steps individually.

STRESS REDUCTION Reducing sources of stress is the ideal means of lowering the impact of stress on your life. The first step in stress reduction is to recognize those factors that promote daily stress. After identifying these factors, you should eliminate activities that result in daily stress. While it may not be possible to avoid all sources of stress, many "unnecessary" forms of stress can be eliminated.

A classic example of stress that can often be avoided is overcommitment, a frequent cause of stress in college students. Plan your time carefully and prioritize your activities. It may not be possible to do everything that you want to do during a given day or week. Plan a daily schedule that allows you to do the things you need to accomplish without being overwhelmed with less important activities. A Closer Look on p. 287 discusses the key elements of time management and Laboratory 10.3 on p. 305 will help you practice prioritizing your time.

COPING WITH STRESS: RELAXATION TECHNIQUES
Because it is impossible to eliminate all forms of stress from daily life, it is necessary to use stress management

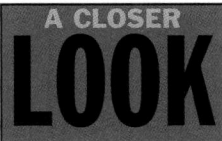

Time Management Guidelines

Use the following guidelines to improve your time management skills and increase productivity:

Establish goals. Establish a list of goals you plan to accomplish. Identify short- and long-term goals, and rank the goals according to priority. Focus your efforts on the goals that are most important to you.

Plan ahead. Planning is an essential component of time management. You can plan your day by using a daily planner or prioritized task lists. No matter what you prefer make sure you spend as much time as you need each day planning how you will use your time. Remember, it is not enough to plan your schedule; you must be able to implement it. This means allowing time for unscheduled events and delays.

Schedule time for you. Find time each day to relax and do something you enjoy. Also, to improve your overall productivity and energy level make sure you take regular breaks during your workday. Plan your whole life: work and leisure time. Regularly evaluate your ratio of work to home and leisure time; remember the key to effective stress management is balance.

Under-promise and over-deliver. Schedule task due dates that you can accomplish on time, even if something unforeseen occurs. Overestimate the time you think it will take you to accomplish a task. Stress levels associated with homework and other tasks will be much lower and you will delight your professors by turning your assignments in on time or even early!

Baby steps. Tasks that seem too big to accomplish usually are not. Break a big task into several smaller, more manageable ones, and develop a reasonable time schedule for completion.

Delegate responsibility. Many people feel they lose control of a project by delegating tasks. Can you delegate or do you hear yourself saying things like, "It takes too long to explain it to someone else" or "Nobody ever does it like I like it"? If so, you may need to practice delegating tasks. Start with small ones and work up to the larger ones. Once you become comfortable delegating tasks it is easier to ask for help when working on group projects or when you feel the stress of work overload. Delegating responsibility to others is an easy way to reduce your workload and lower stress while teaching others beneficial skills.

Learn to say "no" to those activities that prevent you from achieving your goals. Saying "no" is often difficult, but it is critical for effective time management. Before accepting a new responsibility, complete your current task or eliminate an unnecessary project. Adding tasks to an already full schedule causes you to work longer hours and upsets the work-to-leisure time ratio that is so critical for your health and well-being.

Learn to prioritize. Develop and follow your list of priorities. High priority tasks are very important; medium-priority ones are less important; and low-priority tasks are those tasks that would be nice to accomplish, but only when there is time. Establish a daily goal of accomplishing the three most important tasks on your priority list.

Reward yourself when you complete a goal. One of the simple pleasures in life is to reward yourself after you complete a goal. The reward can come in many forms: a new pair of shoes, a movie, a few days of relaxation, and so on. People perform better when rewarded for a job well done, and a reward is an excellent way to provide encouragement and reinforcement for future good behavior.

---

techniques to reduce the potentially harmful effects of stress. Most of these techniques are designed to produce relaxation, which reduces the stress level. When trying to relax, individuals should ask themselves two questions: (1) What am I doing that prevents me from relaxing? And (2) What am I not doing that could help me relax? (3) Your answers can help you determine where to focus your stress reduction efforts. Lowering your levels of stress and practicing effective stress management techniques will increase your overall level of

wellness (14). The following are some of the more common approaches used in stress management.

PROGRESSIVE RELAXATION   Progressive relaxation is a stress reduction technique for reducing muscular tension using exercises designed to promote relaxation. In essence, the technique is practiced as follows. While sitting quietly or lying down, contract and then relax various muscle groups one at a time, beginning with your feet and then moving up the body to the hands

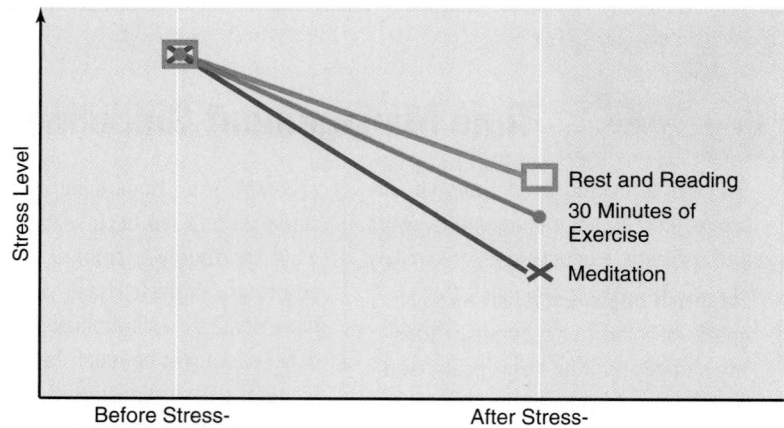

Rest and Reading

30 Minutes of Exercise

Meditation

Before Stress-
Reduction Technique

After Stress-
Reduction Technique

FIGURE 10.5
The effects of exercise and other activities on stress reduction.

and neck, until a complete state of muscle relaxation is achieved. The details of this technique are outlined in A Closer Look, p. 289.

The proponents of progressive relaxation techniques for reducing stress argue that relaxing the muscles in this manner will also relax the mind and therefore relieve stress. The theory behind this concept is that an anxious (stressed) mind cannot exist in a relaxed body.

BREATHING EXERCISES A simple way of achieving relaxation is by performing **breathing exercises.** A sample breathing exercise designed to reduce stress is performed as follows (5):

1. Assume a comfortable position, sitting or lying down, with eyes closed.

2. Begin inhaling and exhaling slowly. Count from one to three during each inhalation and each exhalation to maintain a slow and regular breathing pattern.

3. Now combine stretching and breathing to provide greater relaxation and stress reduction. For example, stretch your arms toward the ceiling as you inhale, then lower your arms during exhalation.

Try this exercise for 5 to 15 minutes in a quiet room. Although breathing exercises may not reduce all stress, they have been shown to be a simple means of stress reduction.

REST AND SLEEP One of the most effective means of reducing stress and tension is to get an adequate amount of rest and sleep. How much sleep do you need? It appears that individual needs vary greatly;

however, a good rule of thumb is 7 to 9 hours of restful sleep per night (A Closer Look, p. 290). Further, because of the body's natural hormonal rhythms, it is recommended that you go to bed at approximately the same time every night.

In addition to a good night's sleep, 15 to 30 minutes of rest per day is useful in stress reduction. This can be achieved as simply as putting your feet up on a desk or table and closing your eyes. A well-rested body is the best protection against stress and fatigue.

EXERCISE Although prolonged or high-intensity exercise can impose both mental and physical stress, research has shown that light-to-moderate exercise can reduce many types of stress. The recommended types of exercise for optimal stress reduction are low- to moderate-intensity aerobic exercises such as running, swimming, and cycling. The guidelines for this type of exercise prescription are presented in Chapter 4. Other popular types of exercise for reducing stress and achieving relaxation are yoga, tai-chi, and Pilates. Many gyms and health clubs offer classes in these forms of exercise.

How good is exercise at reducing stress? Studies have shown that exercise is a very effective form of stress reduction (15–17). Figure 10.5 compares the effects of a 30-minute session of light-to-moderate exercise (running) to three other common forms of stress reduction: rest, reading, and meditation. In this study, meditation provided the greatest stress reduction, with exercise finishing a close second (17).

Why does regular exercise reduce stress? Several possibilities exist. One theory is that exercise causes the brain to release several naturally produced tranquilizers, called *endorphins,* which reduce stress levels (18). Endorphins work by blocking the effects of stress-related chemicals in the brain. Another theory is that exercise may be a diversion that frees your mind from worry or other stressful thoughts. Another possibility is that regular exercise results in an improvement in

breathing exercises A simple way of achieving relaxation.

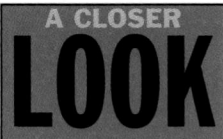

A CLOSER LOOK

Progressive Relaxation Training

There are many types of progressive relaxation training methods, and over 200 different exercises have been described. In essence, the technique involves contracting and relaxing muscle groups, starting in your lower body and moving toward your upper body. The following technique is one of the many forms that you can use:

1. Find a quiet, comfortable, and private place. Remove your shoes and loosen any tight clothing. At first, expect emerging thoughts and emotions to distract your attempts to relax. It helps to play soothing music during your relaxation sessions. There are many commercial relaxation musical CDs available. You may also read the instructions into a tape recorder and use them to guide you through your relaxation session; this will avoid your having to remember the steps involved.

2. Assume a relaxed position (either sitting or lying down). Close your eyes. Begin by focusing on your breathing; just become aware of how it feels to breathe in and breathe out. While breathing deeply and slowly through your nose, imagine breathing in good healing air and breathing out stress and muscle tension. While developing your breathing you may find it useful to breathe in to a count of seven, 1-2-3-4-5-6-7, and out to the same count. Breathe this way several minutes before starting your progressive relaxation exercise.

3. Without speaking, successively focus on telling each of the following parts of your body to relax. Do not move on to the next area until you have relaxed the part you are focusing on. Begin by relaxing:

   a. Toes of left foot
   b. Toes of right foot
   c. Left root
   d. Right foot
   e. Left ankle
   f. Right ankle
   g. Lower left leg
   h. Lower right leg
   i. Left thigh
   j. Right thigh
   k. Buttocks
   l. Abdomen
   m. Chest
   n. Left shoulder
   o. Right shoulder
   p. Right arm
   q. Right hand
   r. Right fingers
   s. Left arm
   t. Left hand
   u. Left fingers
   v. Neck
   w. Face

4. Now you should be completely relaxed. Take a few minutes to continue breathing. Try not to let your mind wander—remain in this relaxed state.

5. At the end of your session take a deep breath and slowly bring yourself out of your relaxed state. Stand up and stretch. You should feel renewed and refreshed.

physical fitness and self-image, which increases your resistance to stress. A final possibility is that all of these factors may be involved in the beneficial effects of exercise on stress management. The next time you feel stressed, try exercising; you will feel and look better as a result.

MEDITATION   **Meditation** has been practiced for ages in an effort to produce relaxation and achieve inner peace. There are many types of meditation, and there is no scientific evidence that one form is superior to another. Most types of meditation have the same common elements: sitting quietly for 15 to 20 minutes twice a day, concentrating on a single word or image, and breathing slowly and regularly. The goal of meditation is to reduce stress by achieving a complete state of physical and mental relaxation. Although beginning a successful program of meditation

meditation A method of relaxation that has been practiced for ages in an effort to produce relaxation and achieve inner peace. No scientific evidence indicates that one form of meditation is superior to another.

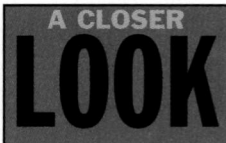

How Much Sleep Is Enough?

Adolescents and young adults need approximately nine hours of sleep each night. If you are falling asleep in class, have difficulty waking up in the morning, or have difficulty concentrating, you are exhibiting signs of sleep deprivation. Making sure that you are getting enough sleep will help you effectively deal with your daily stressors and it may also help improve your grades. So how do you know if you are getting enough sleep? One way is to figure out how long it takes you to fall asleep. Set your alarm clock to go off 10 minutes after you go to bed. If you are still awake when it goes off then you are probably getting enough sleep. Experts say that it should take you at least 15 minutes to fall asleep once you are in bed. If you are asleep in less than 10 minutes then you may not be getting enough sleep. The following tips can help you get more sleep:

- Don't drink beverages containing caffeine after 4 P.M.
- Avoid stimulating reading or television/movies in the evening.
- Do not nap more than 30 minutes during the day.
- Avoid disrupting your sleep patterns by staying up all night before an exam.
- Don't exercise close to bedtime. Instead, try meditating, reading, or soothing music to help you unwind and relax.
- Go to bed and get up at the same time each day. Avoid disrupting your regular sleep pattern by using the weekend to play "catch up" on sleep missed during the week.
- Use bright light in the morning to help you wake up.

may require initial instruction from an experienced individual, the following is a brief overview of how meditation is practiced (5):

1. First, you must choose a word or sound, called a *mantra,* to be repeated during the meditation. The idea of using a mantra is that this word or sound should become your symbol of complete relaxation. Choose a mantra that has little emotional significance for you, such as the word *red.*

2. To begin meditation, find a quiet area and sit comfortably with your eyes closed. Take several deep breaths and concentrate on relaxation; let your body go limp.

3. Concentrate on your mantra. This means that you should not hear or think about anything but your mantra. Repeat your mantra over and over again in your mind and relax. Avoid distracting thoughts and focus only on the mantra.

4. After 15 to 20 minutes of concentration on the mantra, open your eyes and begin to move your thoughts away from the mantra. End the session by making a fist with both hands and saying to yourself that you are alert and refreshed.

VISUALIZATION **Visualization** (sometimes called imagery) uses mental pictures to reduce stress. The idea is to create an appealing mental image (such as a quiet mountain setting) that promotes relaxation and reduces stress. Visualization is similar to meditation except that instead of using a mantra, you substitute a relaxing scene.

To practice visualization, simply follow the instructions presented for meditation, substituting your relaxing scene for the mantra. If you fail to reach a complete state of relaxation after your first several sessions, don't be discouraged. Achieving complete relaxation with this technique may require numerous practice sessions.

In summary, there are many ways to successfully manage stress. The key is to find the technique that is best for you and stick with it. Regular exercise may be the only type of stress management you require. However, if exercise alone is not sufficient, try one of the other forms of stress management as well. Remember, regardless of your personality type or your lifestyle, you can successfully manage stress by applying one or more of the previously discussed techniques.

visualization A relaxation technique that uses appealing mental images to promote relaxation and reduce stress; also called *imagery.*

STRESS MANAGEMENT: CLOSING REMARKS

If you are one of the millions of Americans who suffer from one or more stress-related disorders, the first step in preventing or treating stress-related problems is recognizing that a problem exists. The way to begin is to assess your level of stress using an appropriate stress identification questionnaire such as the one in Laboratory 10.1 on p. 301. Next, practice prioritizing your tasks and effective time management, using strategies offered in Laboratories 10.2 and 10.3. Then, select a stress management technique that is right for you—one that you enjoy, and, perhaps most importantly, one that you will practice regularly. And lastly, keep in mind that your stress response is determined not by the actual stressor, but by your perception of the stressor. Therefore, the way you frame the stressors in life will determine how positively or negatively they impact you and ultimately your health. Remember, "stressed" spelled backward is "desserts"; it's all in the way you look at it! To learn more about the effects of stress, see A Closer Look on p. 294.

⚙ IN SUMMARY

- The two general steps involved in stress management are reducing the sources of stress and using relaxation techniques to help you learn to cope with stress.
- The ideal way to lessen the effects of stress on your life is to reduce the sources of stress.
- Among the many relaxation techniques that can help you cope with stress are progressive relaxation, breathing exercises, getting more rest and sleep, exercise, meditation, and visualization.

⚙ Modifying Unhealthy Behavior

A healthy lifestyle sometimes requires behavior change, or eliminating unhealthy behaviors and replacing them with behaviors that will contribute positively to our overall level of wellness. Changing behavior is not easy. For example, many people with high blood pressure are aware that maintaining a healthy weight and exercising regularly will lower their risk of stroke and heart disease. Even so, some continue to neglect their diets and exercise. In order to gain insight into the complexity of behavior change it is important to discuss two widely used health behavior change theories, namely the Health Belief Model and the Transtheoretical Model.

Theory is defined as a "systematic arrangement of fundamental principles that provide a basis for explaining certain happenings of life" (22–23). In other words,

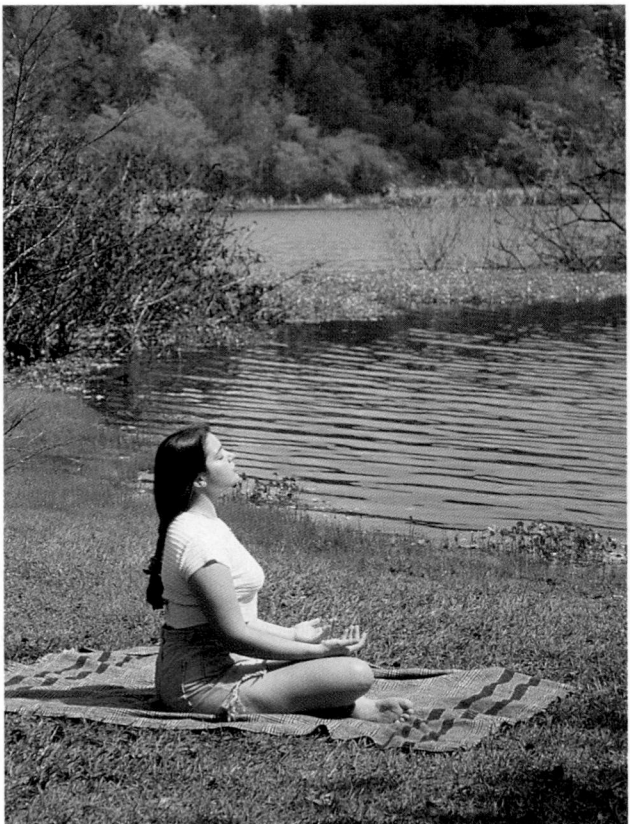

Assuming a relaxed position is important in progressive relaxation techniques.

a theory helps us to explain why people do or do not practice healthy behaviors and suggests ways to achieve behavior change. Theories are composed of **concepts** or **constructs**. Imagine a theory as a pearl necklace; each individual pearl is a concept, but once they are strung together they become constructs. For our purposes we will not distinguish between concepts and constructs. Rather, we'll focus on the concepts that come together to form a theory that allows us to explain why some things happen and others do not. Trying to understand behavior change without the use of theory is like getting into a car without a map and any knowledge of

---

Concepts the primary elements or major components of a theory
Construct a concept that has been developed or adopted for use within a specific theory
Theory a systematic arrangement of fundamental principles that provide a basis for explaining why certain things happen.

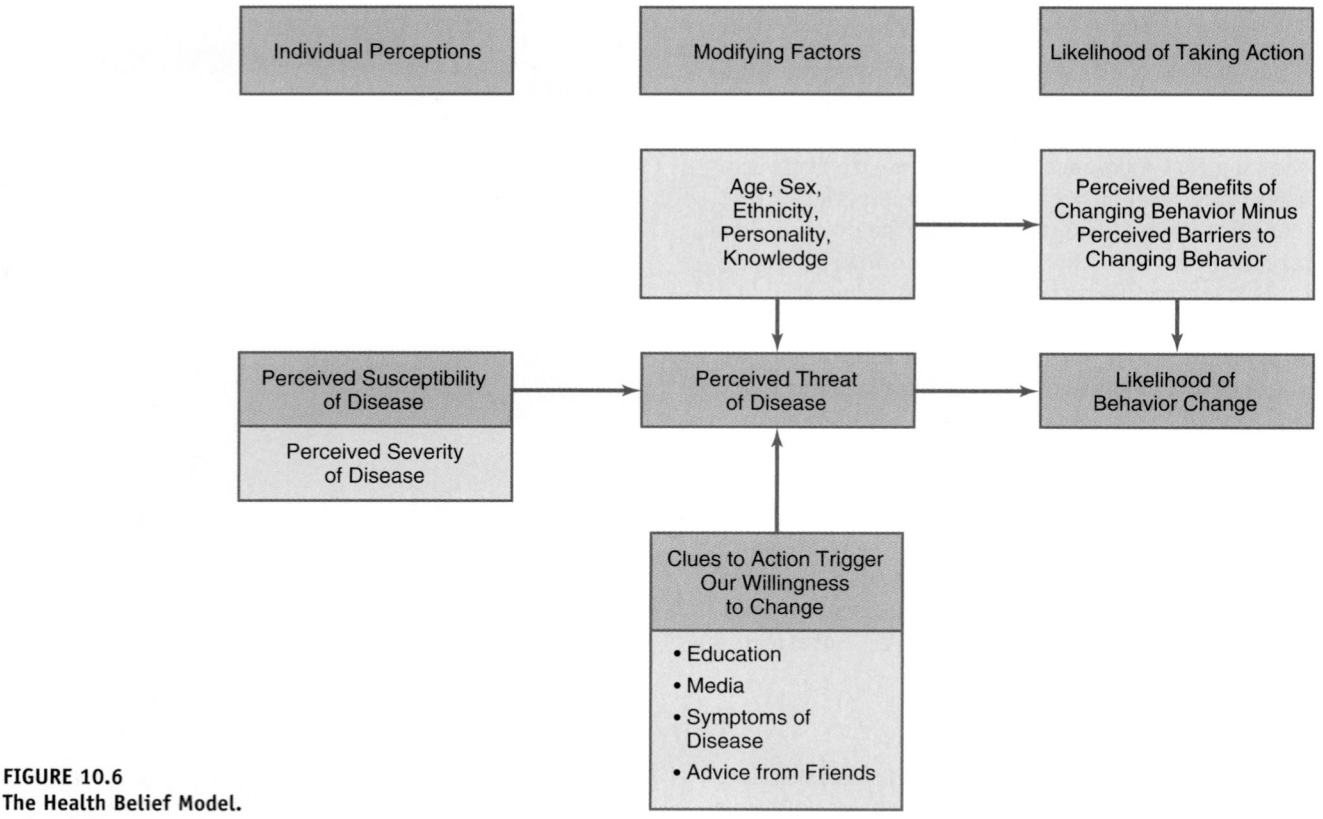

FIGURE 10.6
The Health Belief Model.

where you are going; you may arrive somewhere but you may not know where you are and you certainly won't be able to explain how you got there. In other words, theory provides direction.

A theoretical **model** attempts to explain behavior by borrowing ideas from more than one theory. The Health Belief Model (HBM) was developed in the 1950s by a group of psychologists who wanted to understand why people would or would not use health services available to them (22). Since that time the HBM has been used extensively to study behavior. Based on past research we now believe that people will take action to prevent, change, or control health behaviors if they believe they are susceptible to the disease or condition (perceived susceptibility), if they believe the disease or condition has the potential to cause serious consequences (perceived severity), if they believe the suggested behavior change will benefit them (perceived benefits), and if they believe the benefits associated with the behavior change outweigh the associated costs (perceived barriers). In addition, there must be some event that gets one thinking about making the change;

Model a subclass of theory

this is called a cue to action. For example, a student sees a news report discussing the relationship between stress and disease. The following day a free stress management workshop is offered on campus. What is the likelihood he will decide to attend? Based on the HBM if he believes he is susceptible to illness when overstressed and will become ill and have to miss class which may affect his grade, and the benefits of attending the workshop outweigh the barriers, he will most likely attend. Figure 10.6 offers a graphic representation of the HBM.

The Transtheoretical Model (TTM) is a framework for understanding how individuals move toward adopting and maintaining health behavior change. The TTM suggests that there are a series of six stages to behavior change: precontemplation, contemplation, preparation, action, maintenance, and termination. Individuals in the *precontemplation* stage of behavior change do not realize their need to change. They do not read, talk, or think about their negative behavior. In the *contemplation* stage a person is aware of their need to change and intends to do so within the next six months. During the *preparation* stage the person is getting ready to make the change within the next 30 days. This would be the time a person may buy a daily planner and practice listing and prioritizing their daily tasks. The next stage is described as the *action* stage because the

FITNESS-WELLNESS
CONSUMER

Can Nutritional Supplements Reduce Emotional Stress?

Currently, no scientific evidence exists that any specific nutritional supplement will reduce emotional stress. Because vitamins are good for us, many people mistakenly believe that the more they take, the better they will feel. As a result, many manufacturers have taken advantage of this belief by marketing products they advertise as "magic bullets" for reducing stress. According to researchers at the University of Texas Southwestern Medical Center at Dallas, most "stress formulas" contain B vitamins, such as niacin and riboflavin, which are meant for aiding in recovery from physical stress, not emotional stress. The B vitamins are important for injury recovery (physical stress) and are sometimes used to supplement the diets of people recovering from surgery. However, emotional stress does not increase the body's energy or nutrient needs so taking vitamins will not calm us down. Getting plenty of rest and regular exercise combined with a healthy diet are the best ways to deal with emotional stress. Combining healthy lifestyle practices with stress management techniques such as those offered in this chapter can aid in dealing with life's stressors. Unfortunately, while everyone would like to find a simple and effective means for reducing life's stressors, there are no "magic bullets." For a complete review of vitamins and minerals see reference 19. For readers wishing information on dietary supplements, two excellent online resources are the National Institutes of Health (NIH) Office of Dietary Supplements (http://ods.od.nih.gov) or Memorial Sloan-Kettering Cancer Center (http://www.mskcc.org/mskcc/html/11570.cfm).

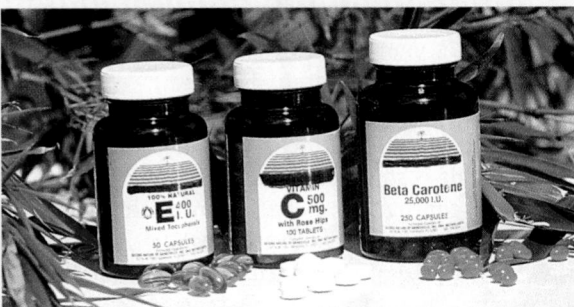

Although the advertisements for numerous nutritional products claim the products reduce stress, none of these products have been proven effective for stress reduction

TABLE 10.2
General Steps in Behavior Modification

Step No.	Action
1	Identify the problem.
2	Desire change.
3	Analyze the past and current history of the problem.
4	Establish short-term written goals.
5	Establish long-term written goals.
6	Sign a contract (with friends).
7	Develop a strategy for change.
8	Implement the strategy and learn new coping skills to deal with the problem.
9	Evaluate your progress in making behavioral changes. Provide friends with progress reports.
10	Plan a long-term strategy for maintaining behavior changes.

behavior change has occurred, but for less than six months. Once the behavior change has been sustained for six months, the person enters the *maintenance* stage. During this stage the behavior change is more of a habit and requires less conscious effort. As this stage progresses, the temptation to resume old habits becomes less and less. Individuals are said to be in the *termination* stage when they have maintained the behavior change for at least six months and have no temptation to return to their old behavior. The length of time that one spends in each stage is highly individual and progression from stage-to-stage is not usually linear. Often, people move back and forth among the stages many times before they are able to make the behavior change permanent. In the next two sections we discuss how to change behavior and provide specific examples of how unhealthy behavior can be eliminated.

MODEL FOR CHANGING BEHAVIOR

The key element in any behavior modification plan is the desire to change. Without a genuine desire to make lifestyle changes, the best behavior modification plan is doomed to fail. In the previous section we presented two widely used behavior change models. Remember that concepts from various models and theories can be combined to create other behavior change models. This section illustrates how concepts from the HBM and TTM can be used with other behavior modification techniques to achieve behavior change. The general plan for modifying behavior is similar for all types of behavior modification (Table 10.2). A logical starting point in eliminating unhealthful behavior is to analyze your

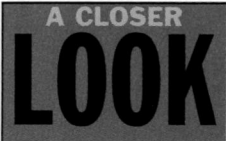

A CLOSER LOOK

How Much Stress Is Too Much?

While the number of stressors that each person can deal with, as well as our reaction to the stressors is very individual, there are some common signs of being overstressed. People who remain in extreme states of stress and its associated feelings of anxiety can become what is called "burned out." Burnout is a term used to describe the loss of physical, emotional, and mental energy which, if ignored, can lead to emotional exhaustion and withdrawal (21). If you are experiencing any of the following warning signals of burnout, begin practicing the stress management techniques offered in this chapter.

1. **Changes in sleeping patterns.** You may sleep too much or too little. Also, you may have trouble falling asleep and/or awaken during the night and not be able to fall back asleep. Usually when you awaken you find yourself thinking about events or activities that are causing you stress.

2. **Changes in eating habits.** You either over eat or under eat. During stressful times some people gain weight, especially in the abdominal area, while others lose pounds. Once again, this response is highly individual.

3. **Greater susceptibility to illness.** You begin to notice more frequent headaches (migraines), stomachaches, muscle tension, and other aches or pains. Over time you may be more susceptible to colds or other viral and bacterial infections. In addition, you don't recover as quickly as you once did.

4. **Intense cravings.** Depending on your personal preferences and behaviors these can include coffee (caffeine), cigarettes, alcohol, and special "comfort" foods such as chocolate, ice cream, and other high-fat, high-calorie foods. Most people find that it takes larger quantities of these substances to alleviate their anxiety, and sometimes the cravings do not relieve the negative feelings caused by their high levels of stress.

5. **Increased feelings of hopelessness and exhaustion.** Over time the lack of sleep, coupled with the ever-increasing unhealthy lifestyle and its negative consequences, causes you to want to "give up." At this point you may find yourself thinking about dropping a class, quitting your job or school, leaving your mate, moving, or doing anything that may relieve some of the stress in your life.

---

current behavior and identify problem areas. Laboratory 10.1 on p. 301 is designed to assist you. While you are completing the exercise think about the HBM concepts from the previous section. For instance, how susceptible do you feel to the health effects related to the behavior you wish to change? Can you identify where you are in the TTM stages of change? Do you need to gather more information before you initiate your behavior change plan? Remember, for behavior change to be successful you must be ready physically and mentally.

The desire to change is the key point in any behavior modification plan. Without a genuine desire to make lifestyle changes, any behavior modification plan is doomed to fail.

After identifying the problem and establishing a desire to change a specific behavior, the next move is to analyze the history of the problem. The objective here is to learn what factors contribute to the development of the behavior to be modified. Learning the cause is useful when developing a strategy for change.

The next two steps in the behavior modification plan (steps 4 and 5 in Table 10.2) are the development of both short- and long-term goals for behavior change. Short-term goals establish the need for a rapid change in behavior. Long-term goals provide the incentive required to maintain behavior changes. The importance of goal setting in behavior modification cannot be overemphasized. A behavior modification plan without goals is like a race without a finish line. Remember the stages of change and the time required to pass through each stage. If you try to move into the maintenance stage too soon, your behavior modification efforts may be compromised or ultimately defeated.

The sixth stage in the behavior modification plan is to sign a behavior modification contract in the presence of friends (Laboratory 10.2). The purpose of signing a formal contract is to confirm in writing your commitment to a behavior change. Having friends present during the signing of the contract is important. They provide moral support and encouragement during the difficult early periods of behavior change.

The final four steps (steps 7–10) incorporate the development of a strategy for behavior change, the learning of new coping skills, evaluation of your

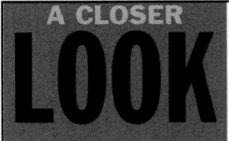

A CLOSER LOOK

Stress and College Students

How does stress affect college students? Here are some facts relating to academic performance revealed by Michigan State University's 2002 National Collegiate Health Assessment survey:

- Nearly 8 out of 10 students who responded (respondents) reported having a cold, flu, or sore throat, or experiencing stress during the last school year.

- 27% of the respondents said they experienced stress to the point that their academic performance was negatively affected; while 19.4% said their academic performance was negatively impacted by a cold, flu, or sore throat.

- Approximately 23% said their academic performance was impaired by sleep difficulties, 15.7% by relationship difficulties, and 14.6% by concerns for a troubled friend or family member.

- Approximately 9% of respondents said their academic performance was negatively affected by alcohol use; 10.9% by depression, an anxiety disorder, or seasonal affective disorder; and 7.7% by a sinus/ear infection, bronchitis, or strep throat.

- Almost 13% said their academic performance had been impaired due to problems they experienced because of Internet use or computer games.

---

progress, and the planning of long-term maintenance for behavior change.

Many people who have had previous difficulty in changing behavior develop the attitude that some bad habits cannot be changed. This is not true! It takes the proper tools to successfully modify behaviors—possibly your previous efforts did not succeed because you were missing the proper skills or didn't have some vital information. Unhealthful behaviors are learned; therefore, they can be unlearned. You now have the tools you need to begin modifying your behavior.

SPECIFIC BEHAVIOR MODIFICATION GOALS

Let's fill in the details of our behavior modification model by illustrating how these plans can be applied specifically to smoking cessation and weight loss.

SMOKING CESSATION   As previously mentioned, cigarette smoking is a serious health risk that increases the risk of cancer and heart disease. Research shows that smoking is the largest avoidable cause of death in the United States (24). Although millions of people have quit smoking, the number of smokers has increased since the late 1960s because of an increase in young smokers, particularly young women.

The first step in smoking cessation is having the desire to stop. The desire to stop smoking can be influenced by your belief that you are susceptible to the negative health effects from smoking, by having important people in your life who want you to quit, and perceiving that there are few benefits to smoking. After expressing this desire and analyzing smoking be-

havior, each individual can develop a three-phase plan to stop smoking that incorporates steps 4 through 10 of the general steps of the behavior modification model. Phase one is often termed the *preparation phase.* In this phase, smokers develop the confidence to stop smoking by establishing both short-term and long-term goals, signing a written contract, and developing a plan to stop smoking.

The second phase of smoking cessation is commonly termed *cessation.* On the cessation date established in the *stop smoking contract,* the individual stops smoking. Quitting smoking "cold turkey" has been shown to be more effective than a gradual slowdown (2). After a smoking cessation program has begun, it is important that the individual get strong peer support, especially during the first few days and weeks. The "action" stage of change requires that you remain smoke free while in this stage. If you smoke even one cigarette during this stage, you move from the action stage back into the preparation or possibly the contemplation stage.

The final phase of smoking cessation is termed the *maintenance phase.* The obvious objective of the maintenance phase is to ensure that the individual does not start smoking again. Several strategies can assist in this process. Continued peer and family support for the individual's decision to stop smoking is critical, and its importance cannot be overemphasized. A second strategy is to avoid social circumstances that accept or encourage smoking. For example, if going to a bar encourages smoking, then the individual should avoid bars. Finally, self-education about the health hazards of smoking provides a continual incentive to maintain a

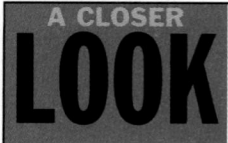

A CLOSER LOOK

Road Rage

What is road rage?

The term originated during the late 1980s in the United States and refers to extreme acts of aggression directly resulting from disagreements between drivers. Typical acts of aggression include tailgating, headlight flashing, obscene gestures, deliberately blocking other vehicles, verbal abuse, and its most extreme form—physical assault. According to estimates aggressive driving injures or kills at least 1,500 people each year. Road rage is a serious problem and a criminal offense.

What causes road rage?

For many of us, driving is our most stressful daily activity. Roadways are crowded and we must deal with drivers who make driving errors. Many instances of road rage start out as a misunderstanding between drivers and escalate into more serious events. Usually, the driving incident is not the immediate cause of anger. For some, mounting professional and/or personal troubles, plus frustration over another driver's "stupid" mistakes, is enough to cause them to erupt in anger. Drivers in

a "bad mood" before they get behind the wheel are more likely to become upset by the actions of other drivers. Researchers believe that some personalities are more prone to aggressive driving. If you drive aggressively use the tips provided in Table 10.1 to reduce your traffic stress. For more information visit the American Automobile Association's (AAA) website at http://www.aaafoundation.org.

---

smokeless life. Remember, you must remain in this stage for at least six months. For some, the temptation to smoke will linger longer than six months. If this applies to you remember to stay away from situations that may tempt you to begin smoking. Keep in mind the HBM concepts and review the benefits of remaining smoke free.

WEIGHT CONTROL In Chapter 8 we discussed the general principles of losing weight. Unfortunately, losing weight and maintaining weight loss are difficult for many people. Clearly, the application of behavior modification principles and the use of behavior change models is essential in the weight loss process. Although no single weight loss program works for all people, the following eight components are common ingredients of most successful efforts:

1. The individual desires to lose weight.
2. The program begins with a 2-week dietary diary that includes the kind and amount of food eaten and the environmental and social circumstances involved.
3. Short- and long-term weight loss goals are established.
4. The individual signs a weight loss contract with friends.
5. The new dietary plan includes a balanced diet that results in a negative caloric balance and a fat deficit so that a loss of fat will result. Further, the addition of a regular exercise program is a key factor in any successful weight loss plan. (See Chapter 8 for details.)

6. New coping skills for overeating include avoiding those environments or social settings (such as parties) that promote it.
7. The individual evaluates weight loss progress on a weekly basis and gets positive feedback from a support group (such as a spouse, friends, or relatives).
8. After establishing weight loss goals, the individual makes a plan for long-term behavioral changes that maintain the desired weight.

In summary, weight control is a specific application of general behavior modification principles. Indeed, these eight components incorporate most of the general behavior modification principles outlined in Table 10.2. Remember: the key elements in a weight control program are the desire to lose weight, establishment of goals, development of a plan, and positive feedback from peer/family support. As you develop your plan, assess your readiness for change as well as the benefits, barriers, and other factors that will contribute to your success!

INJURY PREVENTION

In the United States, **unintentional injuries** are the number one killer of people ages 1 to 34 years (25). Each year, unintentional injuries claim the lives of more than 5,600 children, or about 15 per day (26). In addition, for children under the age of 14 years, unintentional injuries cause the need for about 11.8 million medical visits each year with more than 16% resulting in permanent disability (26). Although unintentional injuries can result from many causes, the most common types are motor vehicle crashes,

TABLE 10.3
Five Leading Causes of Injury or Death for Young Adults

	Age Groups	
Rank	15–24	25–34
1	**Unintentional Injury**	**Unintentional Injury**
	Motor Vehicle Crash (73%)	Motor Vehicle Crash (57.1%)
	Poisoning (9.5%)	Poisoning (21.2%)
	Drowning (4.1%)	Drowning (3.2%)
	Other (13.4%)	Other (18.5%)
2	Homicide Firearm	Homicide Firearm
3	Suicide Firearm	Suicide Firearm
4	Unintentional Poisoning	Unintentional Poisoning
5	Suicide Suffocation	Suicide Suffocation

Adapted from the Centers for Disease Control and Prevention http://www.cdc.gov/ncipc/osp/charts.html

falls, poisonings, drowning, and fires. While most unintentional injury events may seem to be a matter of chance or "accidents," this is not the case. In fact, public health officials prefer using the term "unintentional injury" instead of **"accident"** since the latter implies random events, bad luck, and an inability to change the outcome through modifying events or behavior (27). Throughout this section, the terms unintentional injury and accident are used interchangeably. Keep in mind that accident refers to the sequence of events that lead up to the injury, while the injury is the health consequence of the accident. By using behavior modification, you can reduce your risk of injury by gaining control over many risk factors. Let's examine the most common risk factors for accidents.

RISK FACTORS FOR INJURY   One of the most important injury risk factors is an unsafe attitude, which promotes risk-taking behaviors. For example, people who are overly confident in their driving skills may speed on a winding or wet road and increase their risk of being in a motor vehicle crash. Similarly, people who are overconfident in their job skills may take unnecessary risks at work.

Some people crave excitement or the sensation of danger (2). This type of thrill-seeking attitude increases the risk of accidents. These people often engage in high-risk physical activities such as skydiving, auto racing, or rock climbing, which increase their risk of injury due to accidents.

Stress also increases your risk of accidents (1, 2). During periods of emotional or physical stress, people tend to be less careful. If you find yourself having a series of small mishaps or "near misses" when performing routine activities such as yardwork, house cleaning, or sports activities, this may be an indication that you

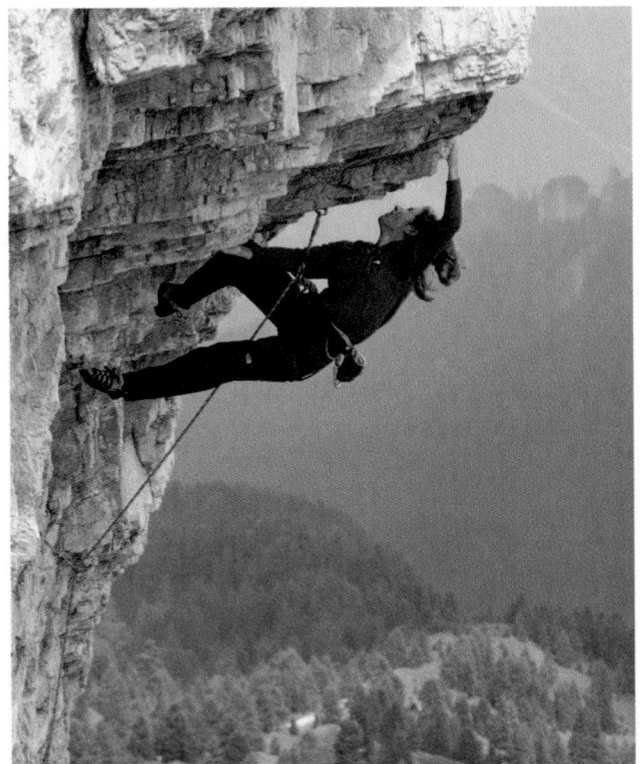

Rock climbing is a high-risk activity.

Unintentional injury injury resulting from unplanned actions; preferred term for accidental injury.
Accident sequence of events producing unintended injury, death, or property damage; refers to the event and not the consequences of the event.

TABLE 10.4
Reducing Your Risk of Injury

Bicycle or motorcycle accidents
- Always wear a helmet and use reflectors and protective clothing when riding.
- Ride with the traffic or use bike paths when available.
- Obey the rules of the road (e.g., use turn signals) and ride defensively.

Motor vehicle crashes
- Never drive while or after using drugs or alcohol.
- Do not drive when you are overly tired or sleepy.
- Maintain your motor vehicle in good mechanical condition.
- Obey the rules of the road and drive defensively.
- If you need assistance, stay in your car and wait for help.
- Always wear your seat belt.
- Always drive within the legal speed limit.
- Do not drive when emotionally upset.
- Do not respond to aggressive drivers.

Falls
- Use handrails when going up and down stairs.
- Do not attempt to climb ladders or stairs when ill or physically impaired due to drug use.
- Maintain ladders and steps in good working condition.
- Never run up or down stairs.
- Make sure stairways are well lit.
- Use skidproof backing on rugs that are not attached to floor.
- Use handrails or non-slip mats in the bathtub and shower.

Poisoning
- Properly label all drugs.
- Never take more of any drug than is recommended.

- Keep all drugs out of the reach of children.
- Use only nontoxic cleaning materials.
- Increase your knowledge of poisons.
- Do not take medication in the dark.
- Discard old or expired prescriptions.
- Do not combine drugs.
- Keep the poison control center's telephone number near your phone.
- Store all drugs and chemicals in their proper containers.

Fire
- Reduce the risk of fire in your home or workplace by storing combustible materials in a safe place.
- Maintain smoke detectors, fire extinguishers, and sprinkler systems in proper working condition.
- Know how to use a fire extinguisher properly.
- Practice safe evacuation procedures from your home and workplace.
- Never smoke in bed.
- Never leave portable heaters unattended.
- Do not overload electrical outlets.

Drowning
- Never allow children to swim unsupervised.
- Learn to swim, and learn proper water safety procedures.
- Do not swim alone or in the dark.
- Dive only in designated areas.
- Do not swim immediately after eating or when tired.
- Do not swim when using drugs of any kind.
- Avoid swimming in dangerous waters, such as rivers with strong currents.
- Learn cardiopulmonary resuscitation.
- Make sure residential pools are fenced.

---

should reduce your stress level by resting and using stress management techniques.

Alcohol and other drugs are other factors that increase your risk of accidents. Drug use does this by altering your judgment and by decreasing both reaction speed and motor coordination. In the United States, every 33 minutes someone dies in an alcohol-related motor vehicle crash and every two minutes someone is non-fatally injured (25). If your class is one hour long, 30 people have been injured and at least one person has died while you have been learning about wellness. Alcohol use is also involved in about 25–50% of adolescent and adult water recreation deaths (24), and among adolescent males, alcohol is a contributing factor in 50% of drowning deaths (25). The effects of alcohol on balance, coordination, and judgment are increased by sun exposure and heat. Similarly, cocaine and marijuana use are

associated with a wide range of accidents, including falls, drownings, fires, and automobile accidents.

A number of environmental factors can increase your risk of accident. For example, storing combustible materials close to a heater and failing to have properly operating smoke detectors both increase your risk of injury due to fire. Other factors, such as failing to properly maintain ladders or steps around your home or workplace, may also increase your risk of accidental injury.

REDUCING YOUR RISK OF ACCIDENTS   You can take a number of steps to reduce your risk of injury. The key is to increase your awareness of the risk factors. Table 10.4 summarizes key steps that can reduce your risk of injury due to vehicular accidents, fire, falls, drowning, and poisoning. Study each of these recommendations and alter your lifestyle to reduce your injury risk.

☀ **IN SUMMARY**

- A healthy lifestyle can be achieved by eliminating unhealthful behaviors.
- Theory helps us predict and explain behavior change.

- Behavior modification is the process of changing an undesirable behavior to a more desirable behavior.
- The 10 general steps of behavior modification begin with the identification of a problem and the desire to change. The process concludes with a long-term plan for maintaining the desired behavior change.

Summary

1. The five key behaviors that promote a healthy lifestyle are health-related physical fitness, good nutrition, weight control, stress management, and modification of unhealthful behaviors.

2. *Stress* is defined as a physiological and mental response to things in our environment that make us feel uncomfortable. Any factor that produces stress is called a *stressor*.

3. Two steps in stress management are to reduce stressors in your life and to learn to cope with stress by improving your ability to relax.

4. Common relaxation techniques to reduce stress include progressive relaxation, visualization, meditation, breathing exercises, rest and sleep, and exercise.

5. Behavior modification is the process of changing an undesirable behavior to a more desirable behavior. The general model of behavior modification can be applied to achieve any desired health-related behavior.

6. The five most common types of unintentional injuries are motor vehicle crashes, fires, drownings, poisonings, and falls.

7. Risk factors for accidents and injuries include unsafe attitudes, stress, drug use, and an unsafe environment.

Study Questions

1. Define *stress*. What is a *stressor*?

2. Why is stress management important to health?

3. List the steps in stress management. Identify some common stress management (relaxation) techniques.

4. Define *behavior modification*. What are the steps involved in behavior modification?

5. Outline a plan to use behavior modification to eliminate a specific unhealthful behavior.

6. Discuss the concept of eustress.

7. Explain how exercise is useful in reducing stress.

8. List the key guidelines for the development of a time management program.

9. Discuss the five stages of change.

10. Discuss the difference between the terms "accident" and "unintentional injury."

11. List the steps to reduce your risks of injury due to motor vehicle crashes, falls, fires, water-related incidents, and poisonings.

Suggested Reading

Barrett, S., W. Jarvis, M. Kroeger, and W. London. *Consumer Health: A Guide to Intelligent Decisions,* 7th ed. New York: McGraw-Hill, 2002.

Benson, H. *The Relaxation Response.* New York: Avon, Wholecare, 2000.

Cowley, G. Stress-busters: What works. *Newsweek,* June 14, 1999, pp. 60–62.

Daniel, E. (ed.). *Annual Editions: Health,* 25th ed. Guilford, CT: McGraw Hill, 2004.

Donatelle, R. *Health: The Basics,* 6th ed. San Francisco, CA: Benjamin Cummings, 2005.

Donatelle, R., *Access to Health*, 8th ed. San Francisco, CA: Benjamin Cummings, 2004.

Donatelle, R., and L. Davis. *Access to Health.* Needham Heights, MA: Allyn & Bacon, 2000.

Edlin, G., E. Golanty, and K. M. Brown. *Essentials for Health and Wellness,* 4th ed. Boston, MA: Jones and Bartlett, 2000.

Greenberg, J. *Comprehensive Stress Management,* 6th ed. Dubuque, IA: Brown and Benchmark, 1999.

Spera, S., and L. Lanto. *Beat Stress with Strength.* Indianapolis: Park Avenue Productions, 1997.

For links to the web sites below visit The Total Fitness and Wellness Website at www.aw-bc.com/powers.

American Automobile Association

Contains information and resources relating to traffic safety.

American College Counseling Association

Offers information related to counseling and college students.

American College Health Association (ACHA)

Offers health related information for college students.

Centers for Disease Control and Prevention

National Center for Injury Prevention and Control

Information relating to injury prevention including specific injury prevention fact sheets.

National Institute of Mental Health

Working to improve mental health through biomedical research on mind, brain, and behavior.

Weil Lifestyle

Provides a wide range of wellness information.

Mayo Clinic Health

Contains wide-ranging information about stress, diet, fitness, and mental health.

American Medical Association

Includes many sources of information about a wide variety of medical problems, including stress-related disorders.

WebMD

Contains information about a wide variety of diseases and medical problems, including stress-related disorders.

American Psychological Association

Provides information on stress management and psychological disorders.

References

1. Donatelle, R., *Access to Health,* 8th ed. San Francisco, CA: Benjamin Cummings, 2004.

2. Hales, D. *An Invitation to Health,* 8th ed. San Francisco, CA: Benjamin Cummings, 1998.

3. Weil, Andrew. *Stress and Relaxation: An Introduction.* http://www.drweil.com/app/cda/drwCDAArticlePreview.html-articleId=129

4. Margen, S., et al., eds. *The Wellness Encyclopedia.* Boston: Houghton Mifflin, 1992.

5. Williams, M. *Lifetime Fitness and Wellness.* Dubuque, IA: Wm. C. Brown, 1996.

6. American Psychological Association HelpCenter: How does stress affect us? http://www.helping.apa.org/work/stress2.html

7. Canon, W. *The Wisdom of the Body.* New York: Norton Publishing, 1932.

8. Selye, H. *The Stress of Life,* revised edition. New York: McGraw-Hill, 1978.

9. Abercrombie, H., et. al. Flattened cortisol rhythms in metastatic breast cancer patients. *Psychoneuroendocrinology* 29(8):1082–1092, 2004.

10. Holroyd, K. A., et al. Management of chronic tension-type headache with tricyclic antidepressant medication, stress management therapy, and their combination: A randomized trial. *Journal of the American Medical Association* 285(17):2208–2215, 2001.

11. Sewitch, M., et al. Psychological distress, social support, and disease activity in patients with inflammatory bowel disease. *American Journal of Gastroenterology* 96(5):1470–1479, 2001.

12. DeFruyt, F., and J. Denollet. Type D personality: A five factor model perspective. *Psychology and Health* 17(5): 671–683, 2002.

13. Albus, C., J. Jordan, and C. Herrmann-Lingen. Screening for psychosocial risk factors in patients with coronary heart disease—recommendations for clinical practice. *European Journal of Cardiovascular Rehabilitation* 11(1): 75–79, 2004.

14. Howley, E., and B. D. Franks. *Health Fitness: Instructors Handbook.* Champaign, IL: Human Kinetics, 1997.

15. Tsai, J.C., et al. The beneficial effects of Tai Chi Chuan on blood pressure and lipid profile and anxiety status in a randomized controlled trial. *Journal of Alternative Complementary Medicine* 9(5):747–754, 2003.

16. Berger, B., and D. Owen. Stress reduction and mood enhancement in four exercise modes: Swimming, body conditioning, hatha yoga, and fencing. *Research Quarterly for Exercise and Sport* 59:148–159, 1988.

17. Oliver, S., and D. Alfermann. Effects of physical exercise on resources evaluation, body self-concept and well-being among older adults. *Anxiety, Stress, and Coping* 15(3): 311–320, 2002.

18. Farrell, P. Enkephalins, catecholamines, and psychological mood alterations: Effects of prolonged exercise. *Medicine and Science in Sports and Exercise* 19:347–353, 1987.

19. Clarkson, P. Vitamins and trace minerals. In *Ergonomics,* D. Lamb and M. Williams, eds. Madison, WI: Brown and Benchmark, 1991, 123–175.

20. Ystgaard, M. Life stress, social support, and psychological distress in late adolescence. *Social Psychiatry and Psychiatric Epidemiology* 32:277–283, 1997.

21. Musick, J. How close are you to burnout? Family Practice Management 4(4): http://www.aafp.org/fpm/970400fm/lead.html

22. McKenzie, J., and J. Smeltzer. *Planning, Implementing, and Evaluating Health Promotion Programs: A Primer,* 3rd ed. Boston, MA: Allyn and Bacon, 2001.

23. Glanz, K., et al. (eds.). *Health Behavior and Health Education,* 3rd ed. San Francisco: Jossey-Bass, 2002.

24. Edwards, R. ABC of smoking cessation: The problem of smoking. *BMJ: British Medical Journal* 328(7433): 217–219, 2004.

25. National Center for Injury Prevention and Control. Injury Fact Book 2001–2002. Atlanta, GA: Centers for Disease Control and Prevention, 2001.

26. National SAFE KIDS Campaign. Report to the Nation: Trends in Unintentional Childhood Injury Mortality, 1987–2000. 2003.

27. Institute of Medicine. *Reducing the Burden of Injury: Advancing Prevention and Treatment.* Washington, DC: National Academies Press, 1999.

Stress Index Questionnaire

NAME _____ DATE _____

DIRECTIONS

The purpose of this stress index questionnaire is to increase your awareness of stress in your life. Circle either "yes" or "no" to answer each of the following questions.

Yes	No	1.	I have frequent arguments.
Yes	No	2.	I often get upset at work.
Yes	No	3.	I often have neck and/or shoulder pains due to anxiety/stress.
Yes	No	4.	I often get upset when I stand in long lines.
Yes	No	5.	I often get angry when I listen to the local, national, or world news or read the newspaper.
Yes	No	6.	I do not have a sufficient amount of money for my needs.
Yes	No	7.	I often get upset when driving.
Yes	No	8.	At the end of a workday I often feel stress-related fatigue.
Yes	No	9.	I have at least one constant source of stress/anxiety in my life (e.g., conflict with boss, neighbor, mother-in-law, etc.).
Yes	No	10.	I often have stress-related headaches.
Yes	No	11.	I do not practice stress management techniques.
Yes	No	12.	I rarely take time for myself.
Yes	No	13.	I have difficulty in keeping my feelings of anger and hostility under control.
Yes	No	14.	I have difficulty in managing time wisely.
Yes	No	15.	I often have difficulty sleeping.
Yes	No	16.	I am generally in a hurry.
Yes	No	17.	I usually feel that there is not enough time in the day to accomplish what I need to do.
Yes	No	18.	I often feel that I am being mistreated by friends or associates.
Yes	No	19.	I do not regularly perform physical activity.
Yes	No	20.	I rarely get 7 to 9 hours of sleep per night.

SCORING AND INTERPRETATION

Answering "yes" to any of the questions means that you need to use some form of stress management techniques (see the text for details). Total your "yes" answers and use the following scale to evaluate the level of stress in your life.

Number of "Yes" Answers	Stress Category
6–20	High stress
3–5	Average stress
0–2	Low stress

Keeping a Stress Diary

DIRECTIONS

For this exercise you will need seven copies of this worksheet. Keep a daily stress diary for one week. Indicate the time of day the stressor occurred, as well as your perceived level of stress (10 is the worst stress you have ever felt), any symptoms you experienced, and your response to the symptoms. A response can include things like practicing a relaxation technique, getting angry, or doing nothing. At the end of seven days analyze your stress diary to determine the greatest sources of stress and the times that they occur. Once you have done this you will be ready to practice effective stress management techniques.

DATE				
Time	Level of Perceived Stress 0 to 10	Cause of Stress	Symptoms of Stress	Your Response
7:00				
8:00				
9:00				
10:00				
11:00				
12:00				
1:00				
2:00				
3:00				
4:00				
5:00				
6:00				
7:00				
8:00				

Time Management and Establishing Priorities

NAME _____ DATE _____

Often people feel that that there are not enough hours in the day. They feel that at some future point, like "when I graduate," they will have more time to focus on priorities. Often, delaying things until the future results in lack of completion. Use the following time management tool to help you budget your time and organize your priorities.

STEP 1. ESTABLISHING PRIORITIES

Rank each priority that applies to you in the list below. Use a 1 for the highest priority, 2 for the second highest, and so on. You may add priorities as necessary.

	Rank		Rank
More time with family	_____	More time for physical fitness	_____
More time for leisure	_____	More time to relax	_____
More time for work success	_____	More time to study	_____
More time for other recreation	_____	More time to improve myself	_____
More time with boyfriend/girlfriend	_____	Other _____	_____
More time with spouse	_____	Other _____	_____

STEP 2. MONITOR YOUR CURRENT TIME USE

Pick one day of the week and keep track of daily time expenditure. Write in exactly what you did for each time block.

Time	Activity
5:00am	
6:00	
7:00	
8:00	
9:00	
10:00	
11:00	
12:00 pm	
1:00	
2:00	
3:00	
4:00	

(continued on next page)

Time	Activity
5:00	
6:00	
7:00	
8:00	
9:00	
10:00	
11:00	
12:00am	

STEP 3. ANALYZE YOUR CURRENT TIME USE

1. In what activity can you spend less time? For example, did you watch TV for three hours?

2. What can you do to spend less time in these activities?

3. Where can you spend time doing activities that are important to you?

(continued on next page)

STEP 4. MAKE A SCHEDULE

Write in your planned activities for the next day and try to stick closely to this schedule.

Time	Activity
5:00am	
6:00	
7:00	
8:00	
9:00	
10:00	
11:00	
12:00pm	
1:00	
2:00	
3:00	
4:00	
5:00	
6:00	
7:00	
8:00	
9:00	
10:00	
11:00	
12:00am	

Were you able to modify your schedule to find time for your priorities?

Task Management

DIRECTIONS

Keep a running list of tasks you want to accomplish. Next to each task indicate when the task should be accomplished. Those tasks that should be completed by the end of the day are given an "A" priority. Tasks that can be completed within the next 24 hours are assigned a "B" priority. Level "C" tasks can be accomplished at a later date. This exercise will help you better plan your daily activities. Remember you should not have a schedule that does not allow for daily exercise and adequate rest.

Priority	Time	To Do List	Completed

Assessing Your Personality Type

NAME _____ DATE _____

Where do you fall on the continuum? Circle the position that you feel best reflects your typical behavior in the situations described. Behaviors exhibited by extreme Type A personalities fall to the left and those exhibited by extreme Type B personalities fall to the right.

Extreme Type A						Extreme Type B
Fast at doing things	1	2	3	4	5	Slow at doing things (eating, talking, walking)
Unable to wait patiently	1	2	3	4	5	Able to wait patiently
Never late	1	2	3	4	5	I don't worry about being on time
Very competitive	1	2	3	4	5	Not competitive
Poor listener (I finish other people's sentences for them)	1	2	3	4	5	Good listener
Always in a hurry	1	2	3	4	5	Never in a hurry
Always do two or more things at once	1	2	3	4	5	I take one thing at a time
Speak quickly and forcefully	1	2	3	4	5	Speak slowly and deliberately
Need recognition from others	1	2	3	4	5	Don't worry about what others think
Push yourself (and others) hard	1	2	3	4	5	Easy going
Don't express feelings	1	2	3	4	5	Good at expressing feelings
Few interests outside school or work	1	2	3	4	5	Many hobbies and interests
Very ambitious	1	2	3	4	5	Not ambitious
Eager to get things done	1	2	3	4	5	Deadlines don't bother me

(continued on next page)

Extreme Type A = The majority of your responses are 1. This personality type is described as extremely competitive, highly committed to work with an extreme sense of time urgency. Extremely goal-oriented with a tendency to become hostile if someone gets between them and a goal they have established.

Type A = The majority of your responses are 2s with a few 1s. Type A personalities have the traits listed for Extreme Type A but they are moderated somewhat. This personality type is ambitious, time urgent, competitive, and goal-oriented.

If your responses are a mixture of the personality types, you are described as a "balanced personality." The Balanced Personality gets things done, but not at all costs. They can compete, but do not have too. They are more laid back and give people the benefit of the doubt. Leisure time and work time are balanced.

Type B = The majority of your responses are 4s with some 5s. Type Bs are easy going and lack a strong sense of time urgency. They don't like to compete and won't let deadlines interfere with vacation or leisure time. It is not that they are less ambitious than Type As, just more relaxed.

Extreme Type B = The majority of your responses are 5. This personality type is very relaxed with no sense of time urgency. In fact, extreme Type Bs typically don't wear a watch. They try to avoid competition at all costs and never mix leisure time and work time.

Remember: This inventory is only one aspect of your personality type. If your responses indicate Type A tendencies you may want to assess your lifestyle and address some of the more stressful areas.

Assessing Your Risk of Stress-Related Illness

NAME _____ **DATE** _____

In 1967, Drs. Holmes and Rahe developed a scale of life-change events to study the relationship between stress and illness. These events have been updated through the years to better reflect the amount of stress that life changes can bring about. This list of life events has been adapted to better reflect stressful events in the lives of young adults. To learn the level of stress in your life, circle each of the following Life Change Events that you have experienced during the past 12 months. Add the assigned LCU values to determine your total LCU score. Refer to the scoring chart below the table to determine your risk of developing a stress-related illness.

Life Event	Life Change Units (LCU)
Death of spouse, parent, boyfriend/girlfriend	100
Divorce (yourself or your parents)	65
Pregnancy (or causing pregnancy)	65
Marital separation or breakup with boyfriend/girlfriend	60
Jail term or probation	60
Death of other family member (other than spouse, parent, boyfriend/girlfriend)	60
Broken engagement	55
Engagement	50
Serious personal injury or illness	45
Marriage	45
Entering college or beginning next level of school	45
Change in independence or responsibility	45
Any drug or alcohol use	45
Fired at work or expelled from school	45
Change in alcohol or drug use	45
Reconciliation with spouse or significant other	40
Trouble at school	40
Serious health problem of a family member	40
Working while attending school	35
Working more than 40 hours per week	35
Changing course of study	35
Change in frequency of dating	35

(continued on next page)

Life Event	Life Change Units (LCU)
Sexual adjustment problems (confusion of sexual identity)	35
Gain new family member (new baby born or parent remarries)	35
Change in work responsibilities	35
Change in financial state	30
Death of a close friend (not family member)	30
Change to a different kind of work	30
Change in number of arguments with spouse, significant other, family, or friends	30
Sleeping less than 8 hours per night	25
Trouble with in-laws or family of significant other	25
Outstanding personal achievement (awards, grades, etc.)	25
Significant other or parents start or stop working	20
Begin or end school	20
Change in living conditions (visitors in home, change in roommates, etc.)	20
Change in personal habits (start or stop a habit like smoking or dieting)	20
Chronic allergies	20
Trouble with boss	20
Change in work hours	15
Change in residence	15
Change to a new school (other than graduation)	10
Change in religious activity	15
Going in debt (you or your family)	10
Change in frequency of family gatherings	10
Vacation	10
Presently in winter holiday season	10
Minor violation of the law	5
Total Life Change Events	

LCU for Young Adults retrieved from http://www.markhenri.com/health/stress.html

(continued on next page)

SCORING:

- Less than 150 LCU   37% chance of developing a stress-related illness.
- 150–299 LCU   51% chance of developing a stress-related illness.
- Over 300 LCU   80% chance of developing a stress-related illness.

Remember: This score indicates your *probability* or risk of developing a stress-related illness. It does not *guarantee* that you will develop a stress-related illness. Persons with a low stress tolerance may develop a stress-related illness with less than 150 LCUs and others remain healthy in spite of high numbers of LCUs. It is your perception of the stressors, as well as your ability to effectively manage them, that influences your chance of developing a stress-related illness. Developing a realistic perception of the stressor(s), plus employing effective coping strategies such as those presented in this chapter will lessen your chances of becoming ill. After evaluating the level of stress in your life, if you would like to learn more about stress management or contact a professional for help in this area, refer to the websites listed at the end of this chapter.

Are You An Aggressive Driver?

Direct your web browser to http://www.aaafoundation.org/quizzes/index.cfm?button=aggressive

You will be directed to a Web-based Driver Stress Profile. After responding to the questions you will receive your Driver Stress Profile results. The results will include tips on how to lower your levels of driving stress.

Record your profile results below and answer the following questions.

Category	Rating	Score	Rating	Score
Anger	_____	_____	_____	_____
Impatience	_____	_____	_____	_____
Competing	_____	_____	_____	_____
Punishing	_____	_____	_____	_____

What have you learned about your driving style as a result of this quiz?

_____

_____

_____

_____

_____

_____

What can you do to lower your levels of traffic-related stress?

_____

_____

_____

_____

_____

_____

For the next two weeks implement the suggested changes. Then retake the profile and indicate your score above.

(continued on next page)

What changes did you make? How did it affect your level of driving stress?

_____

_____

_____

_____

_____

_____

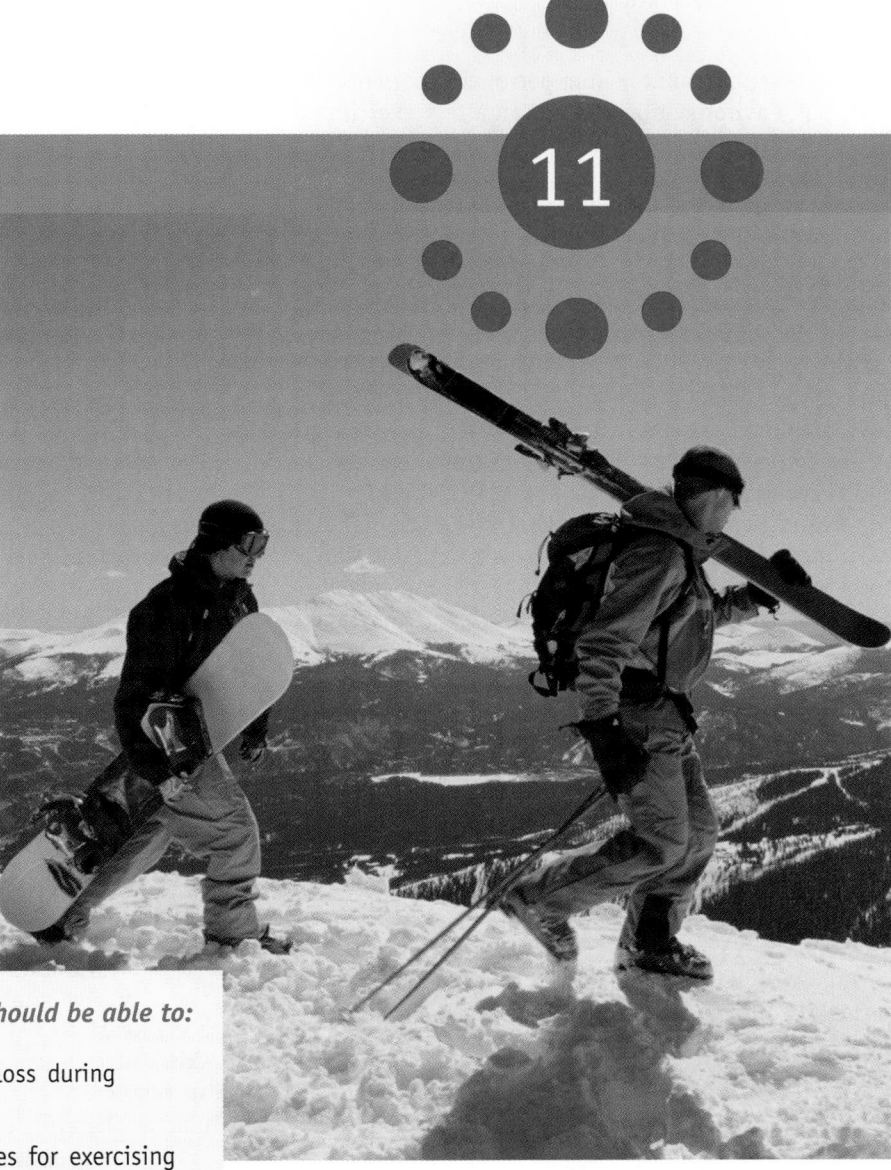

Exercise and the Environment

After studying this chapter, you should be able to:

1. Describe how to prevent heat loss during exercise.

2. List several important guidelines for exercising in a hot environment.

3. Describe the appropriate exercise clothing for exercising in the heat.

4. Differentiate among the various types of heat injury.

5. Discuss how heat acclimatization reduces the risk of heat injury.

6. Describe the appropriate clothing for exercise in a cold environment.

7. Explain why exercise at high altitude results in higher heart rate and increased ventilation.

8. List two major forms of air pollution that affect exercise performance.

9. Outline an exercise strategy for coping with air pollution.

Most of us know from personal experience that environmental factors can affect exercise performance. For example, hot environments, high altitude, and air pollution can elevate exercise heart rates, promote labored breathing, and impair exercise tolerance. A general understanding of how environmental factors can influence exercise performance is important for the physically active individual. In this chapter we discuss common environmental hazards that should be considered when planning workouts or strenuous outdoor activities and outline ways to cope with environmental stress. In particular, we focus on the following environmental concerns: heat and humidity, cold, altitude, and air pollution.

Before we turn to a discussion of exercise in a hot environment, it's important to know a little bit about body temperature regulation in humans. Humans are **homeotherms** (*homeo*, "same," and *therm* "temperature"), which means our body temperature is regulated to remain close to a set point—in our case, 98.6°F or 37°C. If body temperature falls too far below or rises too far above this "normal" temperature, serious bodily injury can result (Figure 11.1), so the body must maintain precise control over its temperature to avoid a life-threatening situation.

☀ Exercise in the Heat

During exercise, heat is produced as a by-product of muscular contractions. High-intensity exercise using large muscle groups produces more body heat than low-intensity exercise involving small muscle groups. Thus, when large muscle groups are vigorously exercised under hot conditions, the body must eliminate excess heat in order to prevent a dangerous rise in body temperature. If the body cannot eliminate enough heat to keep body temperature from exceeding 105°F (41°C), then heat injury can ensue (1). The signs of impending heat injury are cramps; dizziness; nausea; lack of sweat production; and dry, hot skin.

In the next several paragraphs we discuss the ways by which heat is lost from the body during exercise, and we outline key factors to consider when exercising in a hot environment.

HEAT LOSS DURING EXERCISE

The primary means of heat loss during exercise are convection and evaporation. **Convection** is heat loss by the movement of air (or water) around the body. During **evaporation,** heat loss occurs due to the conversion of sweat (water) to a gas (water vapor). Let's discuss each of these methods individually.

Convective heat loss occurs only when the air or water molecules moving over the surface of the body are cooler than skin temperature; the faster the flow of cool air or water around the body, the greater the heat loss. Minimal convective cooling occurs during exercise in a hot environment where there is limited air movement (riding a stationary exercise bicycle, for example). In contrast, bicycling outdoors on a cold day or swimming in cool water results in a large amount of convective cooling.

On a warm day with limited air movement around the body, evaporation is the most important means of body heat loss (1). The evaporation of sweat on the skin's surface removes heat from the body, even if the air temperature is higher than body temperature, as long as the air is dry. However, if the air temperature is high and the **humidity** is also high (i.e., the air is relatively saturated with water), then evaporation is retarded and body heat loss is drastically decreased. Under these conditions, heat produced by the contracting muscles is retained, and body temperature increases gradually throughout the exercise session. Prolonged exercise in a hot and humid environment can result in a dangerously high increase in body temperature. Figure 11.2 illustrates the differences in body temperature rise during exercise in a high-temperature/high-humidity environment, a high-temperature/low-humidity environment, and a low-temperature/low-humidity environment.

GUIDELINES FOR EXERCISE IN THE HEAT

Short-term exposure (30–60 min) to an extremely hot environment is sufficient heat stress to cause heat injury in some people (2), especially those at high risk for heat injury. (The elderly and those with low

---

homeotherms Animals that regulate their body temperature to remain close to a set point. Humans regulate their body temperature around the set point of 98.6° or 37°C.

convection Heat loss by the movement of air (or water) over the surface of the body.

evaporation The conversion of water (or sweat) to a gas (water vapor); the most important means of removing heat from the body during exercise.

humidity The amount of water vapor in the air. If the relative humidity is high (meaning the air is relatively saturated with water) while the air temperature is also high, evaporation is retarded and body heat loss is drastically decreased.

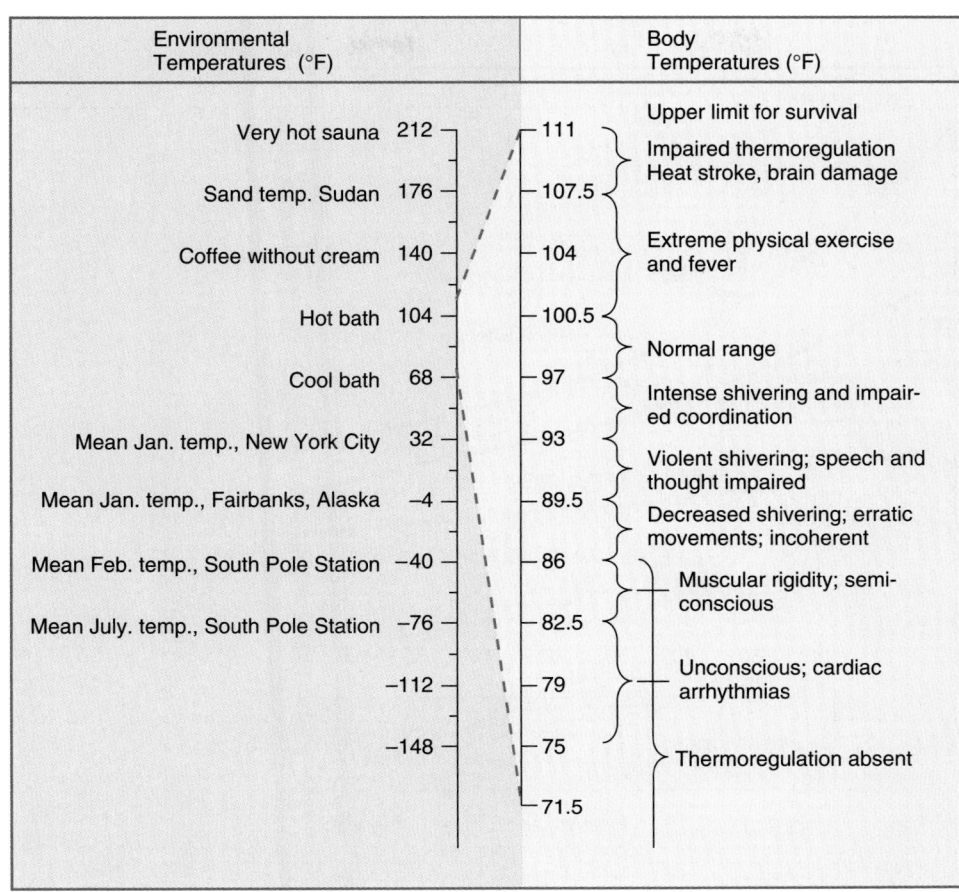

FIGURE 11.1
A comparison of temperature extremes: the environment (at left) and the body (at right). Note that even the relatively small changes in body temperature can have serious consequences.
Source: Adapted from Brooks, G., T. Fahey, K. Baldwin and T. White. *Exercise Physiology: Human Bioenergetics and Its Application.* New York: Macmillan, 2000.

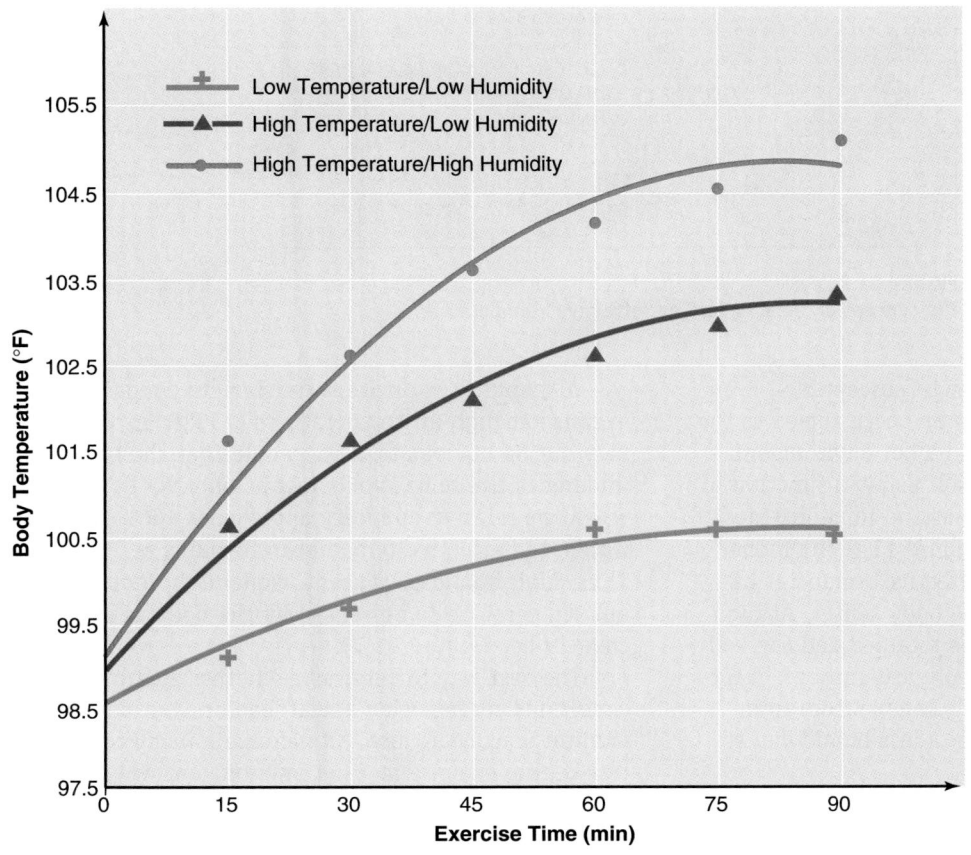

FIGURE 11.2
Body temperature responses to prolonged exercise in a high-temperature/high-humidity environment, a high-temperature/low-humidity environment, and a low-temperature/low-humidity environment.
Source: Donatelle, R. J. *Access to Health,* San Francisco, Benjamin Cummings, 2004.

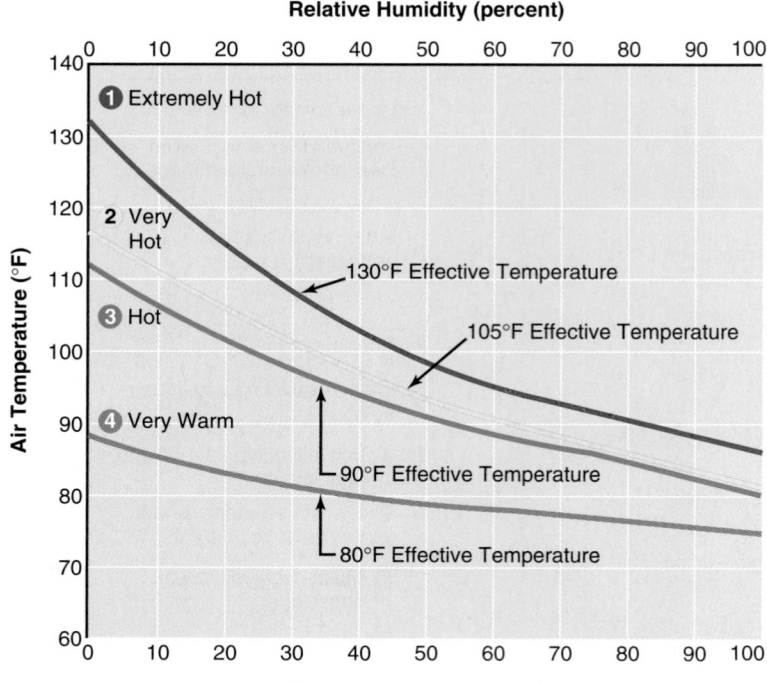

FIGURE 11.3
The concept of "heat index" or "effective" temperature.

Category	Heat Index	General Effect of Heat Index on People in Higher Risk Groups
❶	130° or higher	Heat/sunstroke highly likely with continued exposure
2	105°–130°	Sunstroke, heat cramps, or heat exhaustion likely and heatstroke possible with prolonged exposure and/or physical activity
❸	90°–105°	Sunstroke, heat cramps, and heat exhaustion possible with prolonged exposure and/or physical activity
❹	80°–90°	Fatigue possible with prolonged exposure and/or physical activity

cardiovascular fitness levels are most susceptible.) Even individuals who are physically fit and accustomed to the heat are at risk if they exercise in a hot environment.

Heat stress on the body is not simply a function of the air temperature; both the heat and humidity must be considered. As indicated in Figure 11.3, the higher the humidity, the higher the "effective" temperature—that is, the temperature that the body senses. At high levels of humidity, evaporation is retarded and the body cannot get rid of the heat normally lost through evaporative processes. This causes body temperature to increase above what it would be on a less humid day at the same ambient temperature.

Although it is obviously extremely dangerous to exercise at high air temperatures (130°F, 55°C), it may not be obvious to most people that the body undergoes the same heat stress at only 90°F (29°C) when the relative humidity approaches 100%. In other words, the effective temperature remains at 130°F. Thus, high humidity causes a moderately high ambient temperature to be sensed by the body as extremely hot (Figure 11.3).

The best way to determine whether environmental conditions are imposing a heat load on your body is to monitor your heart rate. An increase in body temperature during exercise in a hot environment will result

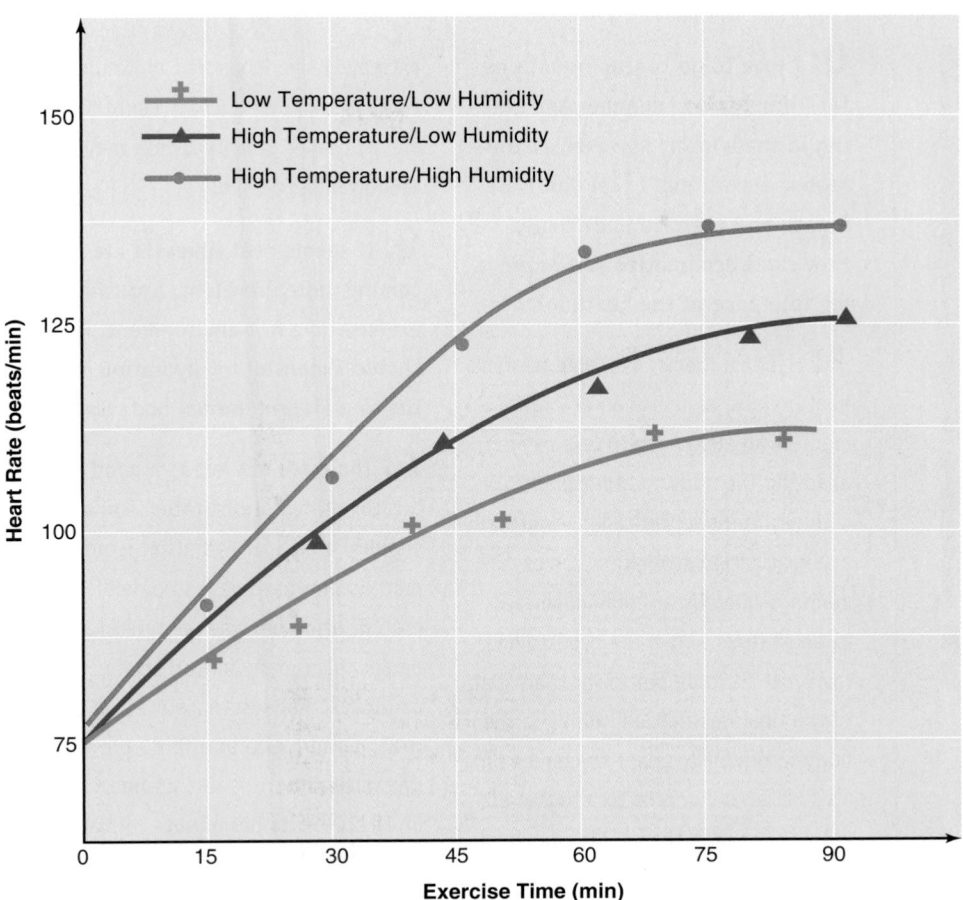

FIGURE 11.4
Changes in heart rate during prolonged exercise under three different environmental conditions.

in large increases in heart rate compared with exercise in a cooler environment. This point is illustrated in Figure 11.4, which shows the large differences in exercise heart rates in responses to three different conditions. A temperature-induced increase in exercise heart rate is significant because it increases the difficulty of staying within your target heart rate zone (Chapter 4).

EXERCISE CLOTHING FOR HOT ENVIRONMENTS

Although it may be impossible to prevent body heat gain during physical exertion in a hot environment, there are ways to reduce the risks of heat injury. Wearing the proper clothing is essential to minimizing the possibility of overheating (3). Clothing should be minimal to maximize the body surface area exposed for evaporation. It should be lightweight and made from materials that readily absorb moisture and allow air to move through them freely, features that promote evaporative and convective cooling. Cottons and linens are best for these purposes. Because dry clothing retards heat exchange compared to the same clothing when wet, switching to dry clothing when your clothes

become saturated with sweat delays the resumption of evaporative cooling, and thus makes little sense when you want to stay cool. Heavy clothing and clothing made of rubber or plastic retard evaporative heat loss by trapping humid air next to the skin. In addition, because dark colors absorb radiant heat from the sun, light-colored clothing should be worn during outdoor exercise.

HEAT ACCLIMATIZATION

Exercise in a hot, or even a moderately hot, environment will cause the body to adapt or *acclimatize* to this condition. **Acclimatization** refers to the physiological adaptations that occur to assist the body in adjusting

---

acclimatization Refers to the physiological adaptations that occur to assist the body in adjusting to environmental extremes. Exercise in a hot or even moderately hot environment will cause the body to acclimatize to these conditions.

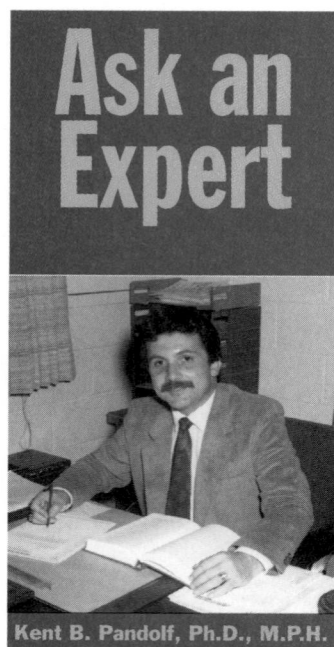

Kent B. Pandolf, Ph.D., M.P.H.

Exercising in Extreme Conditions

Dr. Pandolf is an internationally known researcher at the U.S. Army Research Institute of Environmental Medicine in Natick, Massachusetts. His work describes the body's response and adaptations to environmental extremes and exercise. He has published scientific papers, books, and book chapters related to exercise in the extremes of cold, heat, and altitude and is currently the Editor-in-Chief of Medicine & Science in Sports & Exercise, *the flagship journal of the American College of Sports Medicine. In the following interview, Dr. Pandolf addresses several hot topic questions related to exercise and the environment.*

Q: I love to go to the mountains for hiking in the summer and skiing in the winter; however, at the higher elevations, I feel short of breath and exercise is difficult. How can I acclimatize and improve my tolerance of the altitude?

A: Hypoxia rooms, available in some health clubs, simulate an environment at an altitude with less oxygen, adapting the body to atmosphere changes in higher altitudes. Another acclimatization strategy involves staging, whereby an individual goes to an altitude above the accustomed residence altitude but lower than that of the final destination, allowing the body to gradually adapt to changes in altitude before accent to a higher elevation. The prescription drug acetazolamide helps prevent some of the altitude-associated illnesses referred to as acute mountain sickness.

Q: I exercise regularly, sometimes in a hot environment. I hear a great deal of discussion about the best drink (water, electrolyte drink, glucose drink) for replenishment of fluid lost through sweating. What drink do you advise for the replenishment of fluid when exercising?

A: The best fluid for replenishment depends on the weather and the intensity and duration of exercise. In general, water is the best fluid to be used in most exercise conditions to maintain proper hydration and avoid dehydration. Absorption of fluids in the gut, which is the most important step in fluid replenishment, is best accomplished with cold water. For extremely strenuous and prolonged types of exercise such as marathons, electrolyte or glucose drinks may be appropriate.

Q: It seems heat illnesses are becoming more prevalent. I routinely exercise in a hot environment. How should I monitor my hydration status to maintain normal body water?

A: The color of urine is a good indicator of hydration status. Urine should be clear if hydration is normal. As one becomes more dehydrated, urine becomes progressively darker. Also, dehydration strains the cardiovascular system, elevating the resting heart rate in a fairly predictable fashion. A resting heart rate of 10–20 beats per minute higher than normal after exercise indicates significant dehydration.

Q: Quite often I hear press reports warning about the dangers of exercising in the heat. Is it not just as dangerous to exercise in extremely cold weather?

A: The dangers of exercising in a cold versus a hot environment are completely different. In a hot environment, you must get rid of heat produced during exercise. In a cold environment, you must retain some of the heat produced during exercise. Thus, if you are adequately clothed, the risks of injury or illness in extremely cold weather can be minimized. Hypothermia in extremely cold weather will only become a problem during very lengthy exposures or if you remain at rest rather than exercising.

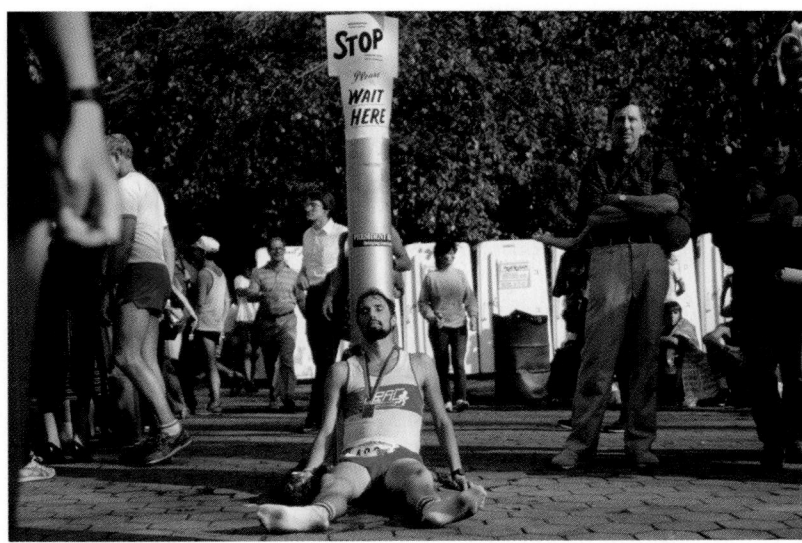

Be aware of the signs of heat injury. Distance runners and athletes who wear heavy equipment in hot conditions are especially prone to the serious effects of heat injury.

to environmental extremes. When the body needs to dissipate heat, these changes include an earlier onset of sweating, a higher exercise sweat rate (i.e., more evaporative cooling), and an increase in blood volume (3). Interestingly, heat acclimatization occurs rapidly. Within 10 to 12 days of heat exposure, the physiological responses to exercise in the heat are drastically altered (3). The end result is that heat acclimatization promotes a decreased exercise heart rate and lower body temperature. A key point here is that heat acclimatization decreases the likelihood of experiencing heat injury during exercise.

Heat injury can occur when the exercise heat load exceeds the body's ability to regulate body temperature. It is a serious condition and can result in damage to the nervous system, and in extreme cases, death. The following are the most common types of heat injury.

Heat Cramps: Heat cramps are characterized by muscle spasms or twitching of limbs. This usually occurs in people who are unacclimatized to the heat. Anyone with these symptoms should be moved to a cool place, laid down, and given 1 to 2 glasses of water with 1/2 teaspoon of salt added to each glass.

Heat Exhaustion: Heat exhaustion results in general weakness, fatigue, a possible drop in blood pressure, blurred vision, occasionally a loss of consciousness, and profuse sweating from pale, clammy skin. Heat exhaustion can occur in an acclimatized individual. First aid should consist of moving the victim to a cool place, removing the clothing, applying cold water or ice, and administering 1 cup of water containing 1/2 teaspoon of salt every 15 minutes for 1 hour.

Heat Stroke: Heat stroke is a life-threatening emergency. A person experiencing heat stroke stops sweating, and the skin is hot and red. Muscles are limp. There is involuntary limb movement,

seizures, diarrhea, vomiting, and a rapid, strong heart beat. The individual may hallucinate and eventually lapse into a coma. Any of these signs should be taken very seriously. Seek emergency medical assistance immediately, and administer first aid by moving the victim to a cool place, removing clothing, and lowering body temperature as rapidly as possible (by giving soft drinks, immersing in water or ice, and/or fanning).

Each of these conditions has several similarities: They are initiated by heat exposure; they involve significant loss of water and electrolytes; and the body undergoes an increase in heat storage, as indicated by a high core temperature. The most important of these is the loss of water, a factor that can be prevented by drinking plenty of fluids whenever it's hot. Inattention to any of the signs of heat injury can lead to heat stroke and finally to death. Do not take these symptoms lightly!

Given the dangers of combined high heat and humidity, should you even consider exercising under these conditions? The answer is "yes," but when exercising in the heat, keep the following in mind:

- Start exercising slowly, and keep your exercise session relatively short (15 to 20 minutes).
- Monitor your exercise heart rate often, and keep your exercise intensity low so that you stay within your target heart rate zone.

---

heat injury Bodily injury that can occur when the heat load exceeds the body's ability to regulate body temperature. This serious condition can result in damage to the nervous system and, in extreme cases, death. Also called *heat illness.*

Nutritional Links

Guidelines for Fluid Intake During Exercise in a Hot Environment

Because the sweat you lose during exercise is replaced with water from the blood, the ultimate danger during prolonged exercise in the heat is the loss of blood volume. The best strategy for preventing a decrease in blood volume is maintaining a regular schedule of fluid intake during exercise. However, thirst for fluid lags behind fluid loss, because your body does not recognize a need for fluid until the composition of the blood has changed. Therefore, you should begin to drink within 10 to 20 minutes after beginning exercise, before a fluid deficit accumulates (4). The following fluid replacement schedule will help in meeting your body's need for water:

CONTENTS OF FLUID
The drink should:

- be low in sugar (generally less than 8 grams per 100 ml of water)

- be low in electrolytes (sodium and potassium)
- be cold (approximately 45–55°F, or 8–13°C)

FLUID INTAKE BEFORE WORKOUT
Drink approximately 200 ml (6 oz) of the fluid 20 to 30 minutes prior to the workout.

FLUID INTAKE DURING WORKOUT
Thirst is a poor gauge of the amount of fluid needed. Drink approximately 100 to 200 ml (3–6.6 oz) every 10 to 20 minutes during exercise, regardless of whether you feel thirsty.

FLUID REPLACEMENT AFTER WORKOUT
In general, you should consume 30 ml (~1 oz) of fluid for every minute of exercise performed. Another means of estimating how much fluid you need is to weigh yourself before exercising and immediately after your cool-down period. The difference in body weight is a measure of how much fluid was lost via sweating, and more than that amount should be replaced. In fact, each ounce of body weight lost due to sweating is equivalent to 1 fluid ounce. For example, a pre/postexercise body weight difference of 1 pound indicates that 16 ounces of sweat were lost during exercise. Therefore, consumption of more than 16 fluid ounces (~475 ml) of fluid is required to replenish body fluid stores.

- Wear appropriate clothing. (See the section on exercise clothing on p. 323.)
- Drink plenty of cold fluids before, during, and after the exercise session (Nutritional Links to Health and Fitness, above).
- Do not use salt tablets. Although people involved in athletics once thought that salt tablets replace the salt lost from the body in sweat during exercise, recent research indicates that no supplemental salt is necessary. As discussed in Chapter 7, many people consume too much salt in their diets, and supplemental salt is actually counterproductive to coping with heat stress. The crucial element in staying hydrated is not taking supplemental salt, but instead replacing lost body water. See A Closer Look on p. 327 for a brief discussion of the adverse effects of dehydration.
- Exercise in the coolest part of the day. Mornings are best because much of the radiant heat from the ground has been lost overnight and the air temperature is most likely the lowest of the day. After sunset would be the second best time because the radiant heat from the sun will not be a factor. If you must exercise during the heat of the day, try to find a shaded area. This might mean exercising indoors or hiking/jogging in a wooded area.

☀ IN SUMMARY

- Evaporation is the most important means of heat loss when exercising in a hot environment.
- It is generally safe to exercise in a hot environment, but the following guidelines should be observed: Start slow and reduce your total exercise time; adjust your exercise intensity to avoid exceeding your target heart rate; wear loose, light-colored clothing; and drink plenty of fluids before, during, and after the exercise session.
- Heat acclimatization occurs after several days of exposure to a hot environment. It results in a greater ability to lose body heat and thus reduces the likelihood of heat injury.

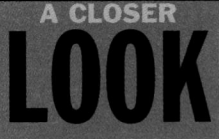

A CLOSER LOOK

Adverse Effects of Dehydration

Exercise in the heat can be extremely dangerous depending on exercise intensity, ambient temperature, relative humidity, clothing, and state of hydration (water content of the body). Although some forms of heat injury can occur prior to significant weight loss due to sweating, the table in this box shows how weight loss during exercise can be a predictor of some of the dangers associated with exercise in the heat. The loss of body weight during exercise in the heat is simply due to water loss through sweating. Thus, prolonged, profuse sweating is the first warning signal of impending dehydration.

% Body Weight Loss	Symptoms	% Body Weight Loss	Symptoms
0.5	Thirst	6.0	Impaired temperature regulation, increased heart rate
2.0	Stronger thirst, vague discomfort, loss of appetite	8.0	Dizziness, labored breathing during exercise, confusion
3.0	Concentrated blood, dry mouth, reduced urine output	10.0	Spastic muscles, loss of balance, delirium
4.0	Increased effort required during exercise, flushed skin, apathy	11.0	Circulatory insufficiency, decreased blood volume, kidney failure
5.0	Difficulty in concentrating		

☀ Exercise in the Cold

Exercising below an effective temperature of about 80°F (Figure 11.3) increases your ability to lose heat and therefore greatly reduces the opportunity for heat injury. However, exercising at ambient temperatures below about 60°F dictates that some combination of warm clothing and production of muscle heat is required to prevent too much body heat loss. Failure to adequately combine warm clothing with muscle heat in extremely cold temperatures increases the likelihood of experiencing a large decline in body temperature (hypothermia), which can be life threatening (1). Indeed, exercise in the cold for long periods (e.g., 1–4 hours) or swimming in cold water may overwhelm the body's ability to prevent heat loss, resulting in hypothermia. Severe hypothermia can result in a loss of judgment, which increases the risk of further cold injury. Hypothermia can be avoided by limiting the duration of exercise in a cold environment, dressing appropriately, and avoiding cold water (water can be considered too cold if it makes you start to shiver).

A question that is often asked is, "Can you damage your lungs by breathing cold air during exercise?" Research suggests that exercise when the temperature is between 15°F and 32°F (−10–0°C) does not present a major risk to lung tissues (6). Indeed, inhaled cold air is rapidly warmed by the nasal passages and airways, so that by the time the gas reaches the lungs, it is close to body temperature.

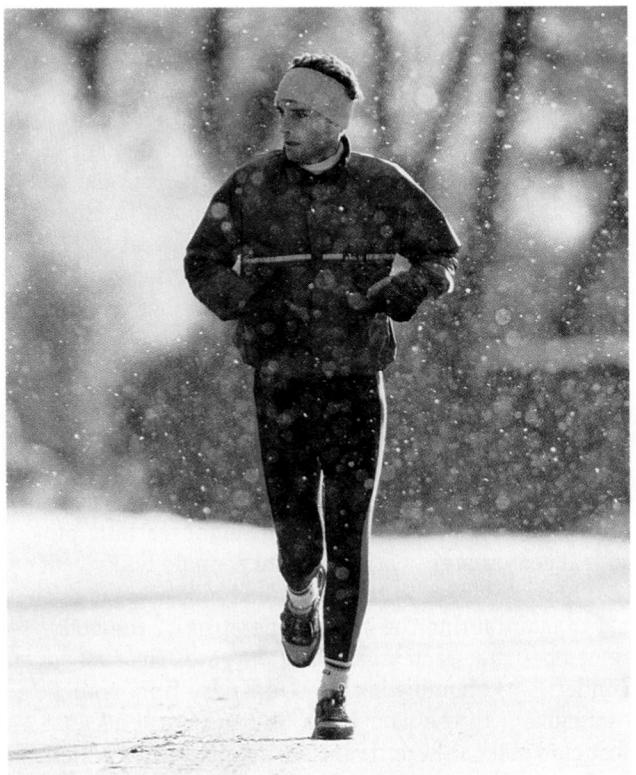

Exercise in the cold can be enjoyable if the proper clothing is worn.

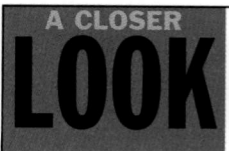

Exercise in the Cold— But Don't Get Wet!

Exercise in a cool or cold environment can be safe as well as pleasurable if the proper clothing is worn. If the intensity of the exercise causes a person to sweat or if a person gets wet in the rain, a dangerous condition could occur. One study (5) examined the effects of cold, rain, and wind on exercise tolerance and hypothermia. Subjects were asked to attempt a 5-hour walk at 5°C (41°F) at a brisk pace. At the end of 1 hour the subjects were exposed to constant rain and wind in addition to the cold. These conditions were severe enough that only 5 of 16 subjects could complete the 5-hour walk.

During the first hour of walking, body temperature actually rose 1 degree! However, with the onset of wind and rain, body temperature started to decrease, even when some subjects began shivering. The shivering produced weakness and loss of manual dexterity. Over the last 2 hours, body temperature was variable in those completing the walk. Of the five subjects that completed the walk, two experienced a severe decrease in body temperature because they were not able to maintain the walking pace due to fatigue from shivering.

This study illustrates the important air temperature, wind, and water interaction. If clothing gets wet, it conducts heat from the body so fast that heat production during exercise may not be sufficient to maintain body temperature. It is important to note that the subjects in this study were not wearing protective rainwear. Any type of waterproof clothing would have given them significant additional time to exercise in the wind and rain. In contrast, a very fit individual who was capable of increasing exercise intensity in the conditions of this study may have been able to complete the 5 hours without rainwear.

EXERCISE CLOTHING FOR COLD ENVIRONMENTS

The key to exercising in the cold is wearing the proper clothing—that is, clothing that traps just enough of the heat produced during exercise so that normal body temperature is maintained, but not enough to produce overheating. The ideal clothing permits sweat to be transferred from the skin to the outer surface of the clothing, so that it does not evaporate from your skin and cause too much heat loss.

Trapping heat is best accomplished by **layering**—wearing multiple layers of clothing so that air, an excellent insulator, is trapped between the layers. The thicker the zone of trapped air between the body and the outside of the clothing, the more effective the insulation; thus several layers of lightweight clothing provide much greater insulation than a single bulky coat.

Because dressing the upper body in layers is critical to maintaining the core temperature of the body, remember that each layer has a purpose. The *base layer* (underwear) should wick moisture away from your skin and move it to the next layer. This is critical because wet clothing can lose its insulating properties which facilitates the loss of body heat (see A Closer Look, above). Try to wear a CoolMax type of shirt (see Fitness-Wellness Consumer box on p. 329). At all costs, avoid cotton! Cotton will get wet when you perspire and then stay wet, chilling you to the bone. The primary purpose of the *middle layer* is to further insulate the body while still wicking moisture outward. Middle layers are often a bit heavier than the base layer. They should only be used in very cold conditions and should fit loosely over the base layer. The middle layer should be easy to remove for changing environmental conditions. Suggested fabrics include Polartec, Thermax, and fleece. The *outer layer* should protect you from wind and water. The wind makes the "effective" temperature colder than the actual air temperature (called the wind-chill effect). Water causes virtually the same effect by conducting heat away from the body more rapidly than air. Thus, the outer layer should be a lightweight, micro fiber, well-ventilated, windproof jacket. This type of material will protect you against cold, wind, rain, or snow while still allowing perspiration to evaporate.

The proper amount of clothing to provide comfort during exercise varies with the temperature, the wind speed, and the intensity and duration of exercise. Wearing too little clothing obviously allows the loss of too much heat. It's often important to cover your head, because 30–40% of body heat is lost through the head. Too much clothing, in contrast, can limit your freedom of movement, but more importantly it can cause a gain

layering Dressing for exercise in the cold by using layers of clothes to trap air.

CONSUMER

Advances in Cold-Weather Clothing

Even though wearing several layers of clothing is beneficial while exercising in the cold (because the air trapped between layers provides great insulation), exercising in the cold can be extremely dangerous if the clothing gets wet from perspiration. Thus materials that help remove moisture from the skin (a process called "wicking") are better when worn next to the skin than are materials that absorb moisture, such as cotton.

Dupont has designed a fabric called CoolMax®, that according to comparison tests "wicks" moisture away from the skin better than wool, polypropylene, cotton, and other fibers. CoolMax® contains specially engineered fibers that transport perspiration away from the body and to the surface of the garment, where it can evaporate quickly, while providing great breathability, even when wet.

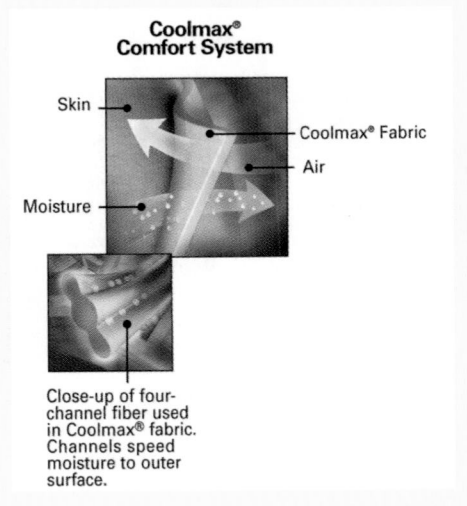

Coolmax® Comfort System

Skin
Coolmax® Fabric
Air
Moisture

Close-up of four-channel fiber used in Coolmax® fabric. Channels speed moisture to outer surface.

in body heat and sweating. During extreme cold, the loss of body heat that results from sweating can lead to hypothermia, which can be fatal (3).

☀ IN SUMMARY

- Exercise in the cold can be safe and enjoyable, provided that exercisers take the necessary precautions to maintain heat balance and avoid hypothermia, limit the duration of exercise, avoid cold water, and dress in layers consisting of the appropriate amounts and types of clothing.

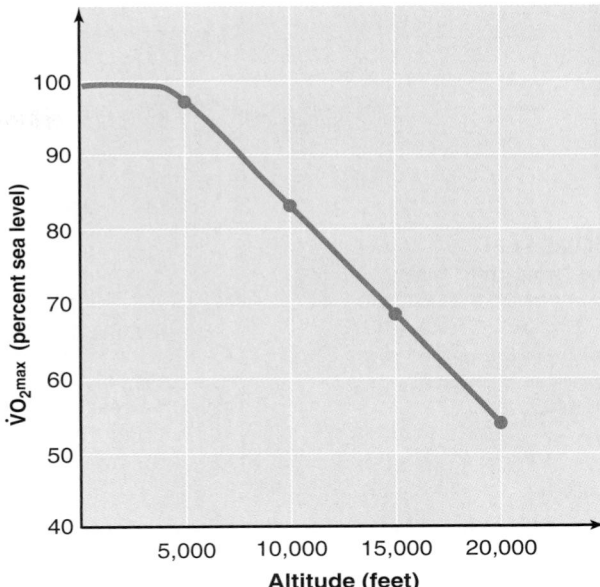

FIGURE 11.5
The effects of altitude on maximal exercise capacity.

☀ Exercise and Altitude

Each year, more and more people go to high altitudes to participate in recreational activities such as skiing, hiking, and camping. How does the body respond to exercise at high altitudes, and how can you adjust your exercise prescription?

The primary concern with exercise at high altitude (i.e., altitudes above 5000 feet) is that the lower barometric pressure limits the amount of oxygen transported in arterial blood (1). This results in a reduction in oxygen transport to the exercising muscles, and therefore both exercise tolerance and $\dot{V}O_{2max}$ are reduced. As shown in Figure 11.5, at altitudes above about 5000 feet (which is the approximate elevation of Denver, Colorado), the reduction increases as a function of increasing altitude: The higher the altitude, the greater the reduction in $\dot{V}O_{2max}$ and exercise tolerance.

To cope with this lowered oxygen delivery to the exercising muscles, the body makes several physiological adjustments (Figure 11.7, p. 330). Breathing becomes deeper and faster in an attempt to maximize oxygen transfer from the lungs to the blood. Exercise heart rate rises to increase blood flow and oxygen delivery to the exercising muscles. To stay within your target heart rate zone during exercise at high altitude, it is necessary to lower your exercise intensity to a level below your normal intensity. In general, there is little need to alter your duration or frequency of training during a brief stay at high altitude. However, the air is very dry at high altitudes, which results in increased water loss during breathing (1). In addition,

FIGURE 11.6
The "wind-chill" index.

Source: McArdle, W. D., F. I. Katch, and V. L. Katch. *Exercise Physiology: Essentials of Exercise Physiology,* 2nd ed. Lippincott Williams and Wilkins, 2000.

	Ambient Temperature, °F*														
	40	35	30	25	20	15	10	5	0	−5	−10	−15	−20	−25	−30
Wind Speed, mph	**Effective Temperature, °F***														
Calm	40	35	30	25	20	15	10	5	0	−5	−10	−15	−20	−25	−30
5	37	33	27	21	16	12	6	1	−5	−11	−15	−20	−26	−31	−35
10	28	21	16	9	4	−2	−9	−15	−21	−27	−33	−38	−46	−52	−58
15	22	16	11	1	−5	−11	−18	−25	−36	−40	−45	−51	−58	−65	−70
20	18	12	3	−4	−10	−17	−25	−32	−39	−46	−53	−60	−67	−76	−81
25	16	7	0	−7	−15	−22	−29	−37	−44	−52	−59	−67	−74	−83	−89
30	13	5	−2	−11	−18	−26	−33	−41	−48	−56	−63	−70	−79	−87	−94
35	11	3	−4	−13	−20	−27	−35	−43	−49	−60	−67	−72	−82	−90	−98
40	10	1	−6	−15	−21	−29	−37	−45	−53	−62	−69	−76	−85	−94	−101

Little Danger **Danger** **Great Danger**

*°C = 0.556 (°F −32)
Convective heat loss at wind speeds above 40 mph have little additional effect on body cooling.

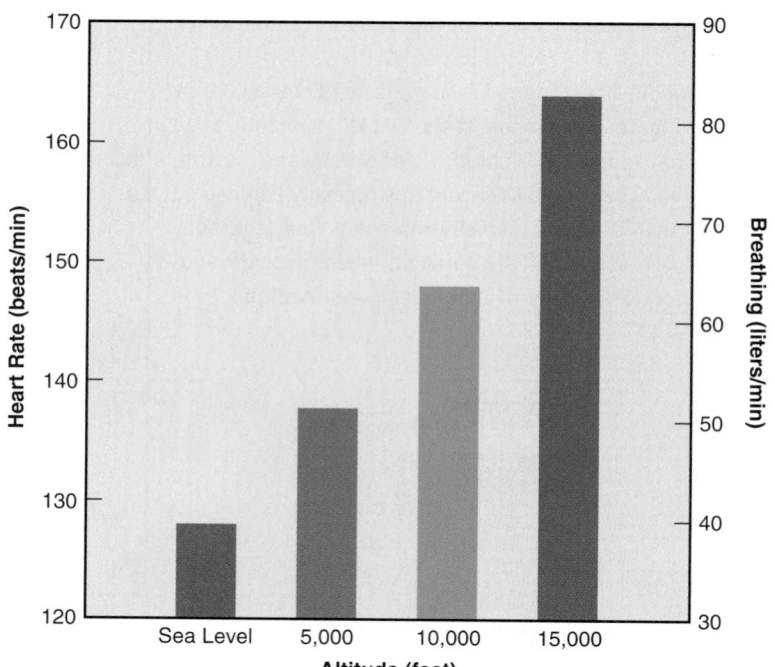

FIGURE 11.7
The effect of elevation on heart rate and ventilation during moderate exercise. Exercise workload is constant at each altitude.

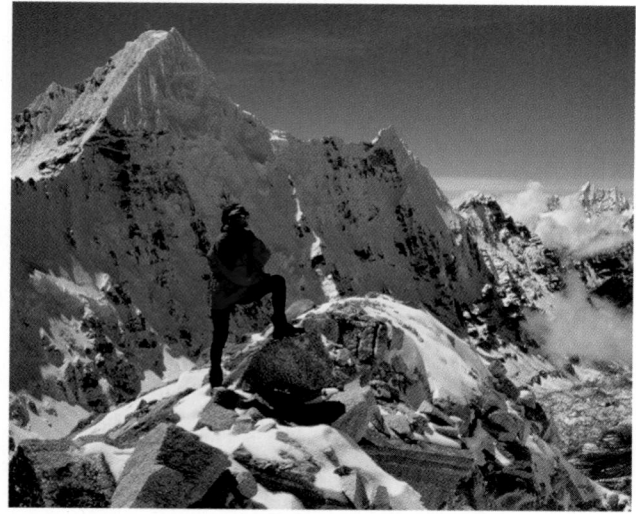

Altitude presents a significant challenge to the body.

the body decreases its water content as a way of coping with the stress of altitude exposure. Be sure to drink plenty of fluids during and after exercise.

☀ IN SUMMARY

- Exercise at high altitude results in a reduced amount of oxygen in the arterial blood, which reduces oxygen transport to the working muscles and lowers both $\dot{V}O_{2max}$ and exercise tolerance.

- At altitude, it is necessary to reduce the intensity of exercise below normal in order to stay within your target heart rate range. However, there is little need to reduce your duration or frequency of exercise training during brief stays at altitude.

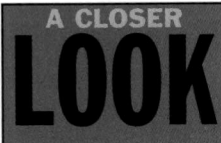

A CLOSER LOOK

Be Cautious of High Altitudes!

The numbers of people going to high altitudes for hiking, skiing, camping, mountain climbing, and other activities is growing yearly. In fact, according to the National Ski Area Association, over 52 million visits are made to ski slopes alone each year. One of the problems associated with recreation at high altitude (above ~8000 ft.) is Acute Mountain Sickness (AMS). This occurs in ~20% of people going above this altitude and may occur in as many as 80% of those who fly in to 12,000 feet elevations. AMS is characterized by severe headaches, nausea, weakness, and dizziness which, if not corrected, can lead to a life-threatening condition of fluid collecting in the brain or lungs.

There are no specific factors that correlate with your susceptibility to AMS (i.e., age, sex, fitness level). The major cause of AMS is going too high, too fast so that your body doesn't have time to adjust the rate and depth of breathing, to increase the number of red blood cells, etc. If you know you get AMS, or if you want to reduce your chance on your first trip, try the strategies listed below before your next trip to the mountains;

- Ascend slowly. (Hiking is best; if you drive, try to spread the trip over several days; if you fly, remain at that altitude for at least 24 hours)
- If you go above 10,000 feet increase your altitude by no more than 1000 feet per day.

- Sleep at the lowest elevation possible.
- If you feel the onset of AMS, don't go higher—if symptoms get worse, get off of the mountain.
- Drink plenty of water. Mountain air is typically dry and you can dehydrate without sweating (make sure urine output is normal and clear).
- Avoid tobacco, alcohol, and other depressants because they decrease your rate of respiration, or breathing.
- Eat a high carbohydrate diet.
- If you know you get AMS, see your doctor, there are medications that can help with acclimatization.

☀ Exercise and Air Pollution

Air pollution is a growing problem in many parts of the world. In this section we examine the effects of air pollution on exercise performance and establish guidelines for minimizing its effects.

MAJOR FORMS OF AIR POLLUTION

Two major pollutants that affect exercise performance are ozone and carbon monoxide (7, 8). **Ozone** is a gas produced primarily by a chemical reaction between sunlight and the hydrocarbons emitted from car exhausts. This form of pollution is extremely irritating to the lungs and airways. It causes tightness in the chest, coughing, headaches, nausea, throat and eye irritation, and, worst of all, bronchoconstriction (8). In fact, exposure to ozone can trigger an asthma attack.

In an effort to protect citizens from air pollution, many cities monitor air quality and issue health alerts when it is poor. Stage 1 health alerts are issued when ozone reaches 0.2 ppm (parts per million), and stage 2 alerts are issued at 0.35 ppm. These alerts suggest that anyone with lung problems, such as asthma, should not exercise outdoors.

Many large metropolitan areas now have stage 1 alerts on more than 100 days out of the year. Although the long-term effects of ozone exposure are not clear, recent research suggests that chronic exposure to ozone results in diminished lung function (8).

Carbon monoxide is a gas produced during the burning of fossil fuels, such as gasoline and coal, and it is also present in cigarette smoke. This pollutant binds to hemoglobin in the blood and reduces the blood's oxygen-carrying capacity. High levels of carbon monoxide can impair exercise performance by reducing oxygen

---

ozone A gas produced by a chemical reaction between sunlight and the hydrocarbons emitted from car exhausts. This form of pollution is extremely irritating to the lung and airways. It causes tightness in the chest, coughing, headaches, nausea, throat and eye irritation, and, worst of all, bronchoconstriction.
carbon monoxide A gas produced during the burning of fossil fuels such as gasoline and coal; also present in cigarette smoke. This pollutant binds to hemoglobin in the blood and reduces the blood's oxygen-carrying capacity.

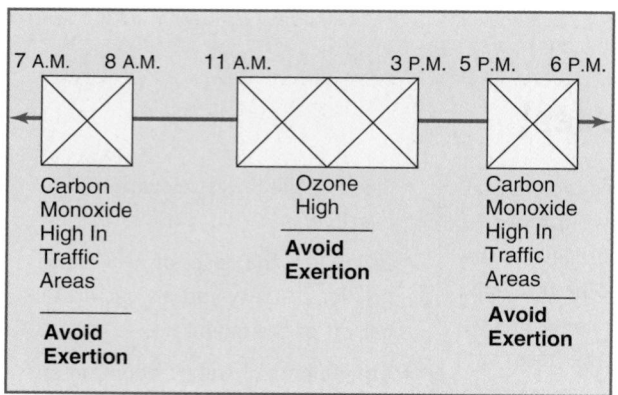

FIGURE 11.8
Times of day to avoid exercise due to high levels of ozone and carbon monoxide.

delivery to the exercising muscles (8). In cities where traffic is heavy and congested, carbon monoxide can be a serious deterrent to exercise. For example, research suggests that runners in large metropolitan areas exhibit carbon monoxide levels in the blood that are twice the level necessary to negatively affect exercise performance (9).

COPING WITH AIR POLLUTION

The best way to minimize the effects of air pollution during exercise is to avoid exercising when ozone or carbon monoxide levels are highest (Figure 11.8). On hot summer days, ozone levels are highest during midday (11 A.M. to 3 P.M.) when the sun's ultraviolet rays are strongest. Avoid exercising during this time and also when automobile traffic is heavy. Carbon monoxide levels reach approximately 35 ppm in moving traffic and can exceed 100 ppm in slow and congested conditions (8).

Because these levels can extend 20 to 30 yards away from traffic, exercisers should avoid heavily traveled roads and/or stay at least 30 yards away from the road if possible. Exposure to carbon monoxide (from sitting in traffic with the windows down or being in a smoke-filled room) can be detrimental before exercise, too, because carbon monoxide leaves the blood so slowly. In fact, the body may require over 6 hours to remove significant amounts of carbon monoxide from the blood (8).

Remember: Air pollution is not always visible. Therefore, you must be aware of the times of day at which various pollutants are in highest concentrations and avoid exercising then. Pollutants not only affect exercise performance; chronic exposure to them is also hazardous to your health. So, don't simply try to avoid pollution; do what you can to reduce pollution in order to have a cleaner environment in which to exercise. Walk or take the bus when possible, recycle waste, don't burn leaves or garbage; these are just a few things that we can do to make a better environment in which to live and exercise.

☀ IN SUMMARY

- Ozone is produced by a chemical reaction between sunlight and automobile exhaust. Carbon monoxide is produced by the burning of fossil fuels. Both forms of air pollution can impair exercise tolerance.

- The best way to minimize the effects of air pollution during exercise is to avoid exercising when ozone or carbon monoxide levels are highest. Ozone levels are highest during midday on hot summer days. Carbon monoxide levels are highest when automobile traffic is heavy.

Summary

1. Evaporation is the most important means of heat loss during exercise in a hot environment.

2. Although it is generally safe to exercise in a hot environment, these guidelines need consideration:
   - Start slowly and reduce your total exercise time.
   - Adjust your exercise intensity to avoid exceeding your target heart rate.
   - Wear loose, light-colored clothing.
   - Drink plenty of fluids before, during, and after the exercise session.

3. Heat acclimatization occurs after several days of exposure to a hot environment. It results in a greater ability to lose body heat and reduces the likelihood of heat injury.

4. Although long-term exercise in a cold environment could result in hypothermia, short-term exercise in a cold environment does not generally pose a serious threat to heat balance.

5. Exercise at high altitude results in a reduced amount of oxygen in the arterial blood, which reduces oxygen transport to the working muscles and lowers both $\dot{V}O_{2max}$ and exercise tolerance.

6. At high altitude, it is necessary to reduce the intensity of exercise below normal in order to stay within your target heart rate range. However, there is little need to reduce your duration or frequency of exercise training during brief stays at moderate altitudes.

7. Ozone is produced by a chemical reaction between sunlight and automobile exhaust. Carbon monoxide is produced by the burning of fossil fuels. Both forms of air pollution can impair exercise tolerance.

8. The best way to minimize the effects of air pollution during exercise is to avoid exercising when ozone or carbon monoxide levels are highest. Ozone levels are highest during hot summer days. Carbon monoxide levels are highest when automobile traffic is heavy.

Study Questions

1. Define the term *homeotherm*.

2. How is body heat lost during swimming?

3. What is the most important means of heat loss during exercise in a hot environment?

4. List key guidelines for exercising in the heat.

5. List guidelines for fluid intake during and after exercise in hot environments.

6. Describe the appropriate clothing for exercising in hot and cold environments.

7. Outline the major types of heat injury, and list the symptoms of each.

8. Why does exercise at high altitude result in higher heart rates and increased ventilation compared to the same exercise performed at sea level?

9. Discuss the effects of air pollution on exercise tolerance.

10. What guidelines should you follow to minimize your exposure to air pollution?

11. Define the term *acclimatize*.

12. Distinguish between the terms *ozone* and *carbon monoxide*.

13. Describe the difference between *convection* and *evaporation*.

Suggested Readings

Burke, L. M. Nutritional needs for exercise in the heat. *Comparative Biochemistry and Physiology* 128(4): 735–748, 2001.

"Exercise and Fluid Replacement." American College of Sports Medicine, Position Stand, MSSE 28:1, 1996.

"Heat and Cold Illnesses During Long Distance Running." American College of Sports Medicine, Position Stand, MSSE 28:12, 1996.

Holden, C. Peering under the hood of Africa's runners. *Science* 305(5684):637–639, 2004.

Nieman, D. C. Current perspective on exercise immunology. *Current Sports Medicine Reports* 2(5):239–242, 2003.

Noakes, T. D. Exercise and the cold. *Ergonomics* 43(10):1461–1479, 2000.

Powers, S. K., and E. T. Howley. *Exercise Physiology: Theory and Application to Fitness and Performance,* 4th ed. Dubuque, IA: McGraw Hill, 2004.

Reilly, T., Dowzer, C. N., and Cable, N. T. The physiology of deep-water running. *Journal of Sports Science* 21(12): 959–972, 2003.

Sawka, M. N., and S. J. Montain. Fluid and electrolyte supplementation for exercise heat stress. *American Journal of Clinical Nutrition* 72(Suppl):564S–572S, 2000.

Stocks, J. M., Taylor, N. A., Tipton, M. J., and Greenlead, J. E. Human physiological responses to cold exposure. *Aviation, Space, and Environmental Medicine* 75(5):444–457, 2004.

For links to the web sites below visit The Total Fitness and Wellness Website at www.aw-bc.com/powers.

About.com

Exercising in Extreme Conditions (Temperature, Air Pollution, and Altitude) Information from heat stroke to ozone to hypothermia. How the environment affects athletic performance.

DestinationOutdoors.com

Outdoor tips and information. From insect repellant to first aid.

Gatorade Sports Science Institute

Contains many articles related to fluid replacement during exercise; enables visitors to add their names to a mailing list and receive new articles.

Northern Outfitters

Contains the sites for several cold-weather clothing outfitters.

References

1. Brooks, G., T. Fahey, T. White, K. Baldwin, and T. Fahey. *Exercise Physiology: Human Bioenergetics and Its Applications,* 5th ed., New York: Macmillan, 2000.

2. Coris, E., Ramirez, A., and Van Durme, D. Heat illness in athletes: The dangerous combination of heat, humidity and exercise. *Sports Medicine* 34(1):9–16, 2004.

3. McArdle, W. D., F. I. Katch, and V. L. Katch. *Exercise Physiology: Energy, Nutrition, and Human Performance,* 5th ed. Lippincott Williams and Wilkins, 2001.

4. Von Duvillard, S., Braun, W., Markofski, M., Beneke, R., and Leithauser, R. Fluids and hydration in prolonged endurance performance. *Nutrition* 20(7–8):651–656, 2004.

5. Thompson, R. L., and J. S. Hayward. Wet-cold exposure and hypothermia: Thermal and metabolic responses to prolonged exercise in the rain. *Journal of Applied Physiology* 81(3):1128–1137, 1996.

6. Irlbeck, D. Normal mechanisms of heat and moisture exchange in the respiratory tract. *Respiratory Care Clinics of North America* 4(2):189–198, 1998.

7. Carlisle, A. J., and N. C. Sharp. Exercise and outdoor ambient air pollution. *British Journal of Sports Medicine* 35(4): 214–222, 2001.

8. Carlisle, A. J., and Sharp, N. C. Exercise and outdoor ambient air pollution. *British Journal of Sports Medicine* 35(4): 214–222, 2001.

9. Tikuisis, P., D. M. Kane, T. M. McLellan, F. Buick, and S. M. Fairburn. Rate of formation of carboxyhemoglobin in exercising humans exposed to carbon monoxide. *Journal of Applied Physiology* 72(4):1311–1319, 1992.

Exercising in Harsh Environments

NAME _____ DATE _____

Answer the following true or false questions related to exercise and the environment. If a statement is false, change it to make it true. You can check your answers against those provided on the next page.

TRUE/FALSE

_____ 1. Evaporation is the primary means of heat loss during exercise in a hot environment.

_____ 2. When exercising in a hot, humid environment, you should wear loose, dark-colored clothing.

_____ 3. Exercise at high altitude results in an increased amount of oxygen in the arterial blood.

_____ 4. At high altitude, it is necessary to reduce the intensity of exercise to stay within your target heart rate range.

_____ 5. Ozone levels are highest during cool, winter days.

_____ 6. Humans regulate their body temperature around the set point of 37°C.

_____ 7. Low-intensity exercise using small muscle groups produces more body heat than high-intensity exercise incorporating large muscle groups.

_____ 8. An increase in body temperature during exercise in a hot environment will result in large increases in heart rate compared with exercise in a cool environment.

_____ 9. The strategy for exercising in the cold is to wear enough clothing necessary to trap just enough heat to maintain body temperature but not overheat.

_____ 10. Heat injuries are nonfatal conditions that result in cramps and fatigue.

(continued on next page)

ANSWERS

1. True

2. False: When exercising in a hot, humid environment, you should wear loose, *light-colored* clothing.

3. False: Exercise at high altitude results in a *reduced* amount of oxygen in the arterial blood.

4. True

5. False: Ozone levels are highest during *hot, summer* days.

6. True

7. False: *High-intensity exercise using large muscle groups produces more body heat than low-intensity exercise incorporating small muscle groups.*

8. True

9. True

10. False: Heat injuries are *serious and can result in damage to the nervous system and, in extreme cases, death.*

1. If your friend planned to exercise in a warm, high humidity environment, what advice would you give to him/her to remain safe?

_____

_____

_____

_____

2. What advice would you give to a friend exercising in a cold climate?

_____

_____

_____

_____

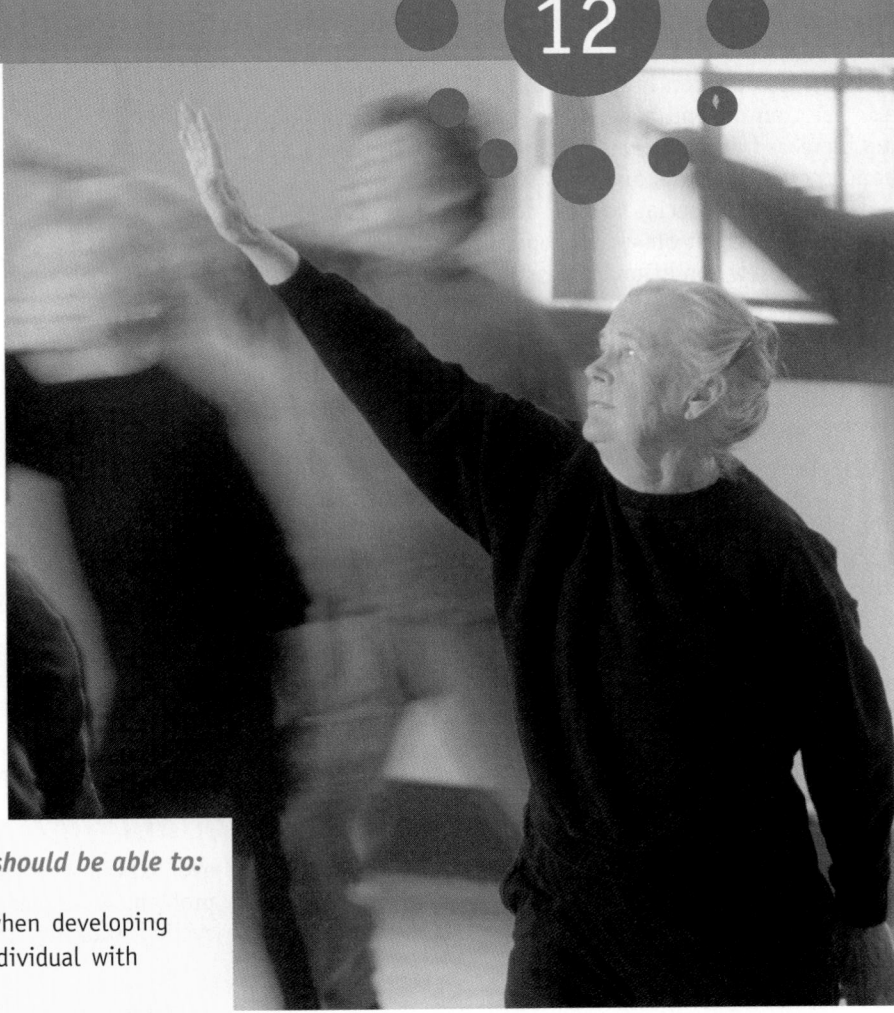

12

After studying this chapter, you should be able to:

1. Describe factors to consider when developing an exercise program for an individual with orthopedic problems.

2. Outline the exercise guidelines for an obese individual.

3. Discuss exercise training programs for type I and type II diabetics.

4. Discuss the benefits of exercise for asthmatics.

5. Outline the considerations for beginning or continuing an exercise program during pregnancy.

6. Discuss the physiological changes that accompany aging, and list the general guidelines for maintaining an exercise program throughout life.

Exercise for Special Populations

Many people with special medical concerns want and need to participate in an exercise program. For most of these individuals, it is both safe and healthy to exercise. Although the exercise program may or may not have a direct benefit on the condition in question, in almost all cases exercise training will benefit the individual by providing increased energy levels, increased stamina, enhanced quality of life, and overall wellness.

People with special medical concerns may need to use certain precautions when beginning an exercise program. A few conditions necessitate medical supervision during exercise, and in some conditions exercise may be ill advised. In most instances, the decision to start an exercise program should be made in consultation with a physician.

For example, people with serious heart problems are likely to need medical supervision while exercising. Usually, exercise is performed under the direct supervision of nurses and exercise specialists in a hospital or other institutional setting. In contrast, after consulting with their physician, individuals with an orthopedic problem (e.g., joint problems) or diabetes often need only modify the "standard" exercise prescription (discussed in Chapter 4).

In this chapter we provide exercise guidelines for individuals with some of the more common health concerns that do not require medical supervision. Certainly, a huge variety of special concerns may dictate modification of an exercise program. If you have special health concerns that are not discussed here, consult your physician before beginning an exercise program.

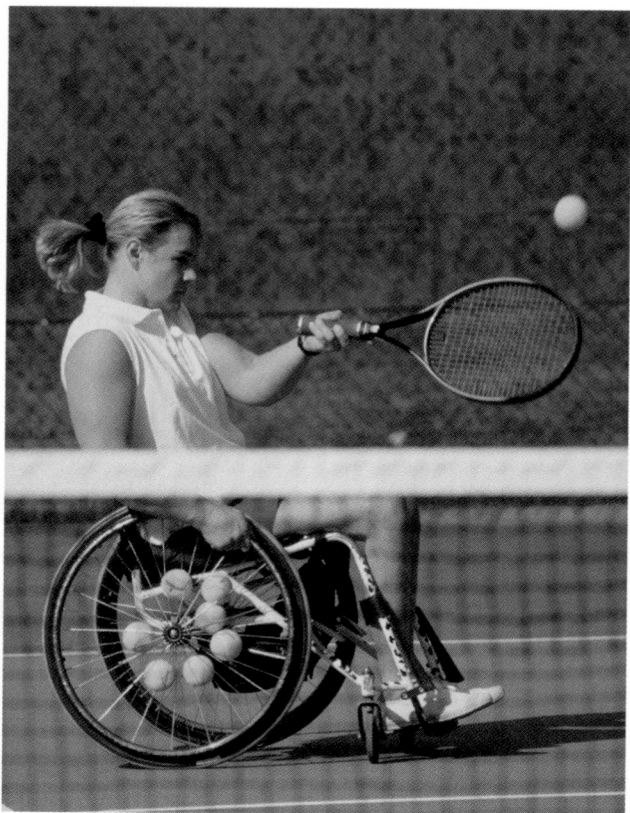

By using alternate modes of exercise, fitness levels can be maintained even when injury or disability makes exercise difficult.

Orthopedic Problems

Individuals with orthopedic problems, such as bone or joint disorders, often need to take special care when designing an exercise program. The objective of the exercise prescription is to find an exercise mode that uses large muscle groups that are not associated with the problem area. For example, if the orthopedic problem is in the lower leg, this would mean undertaking exercise other than running, walking, or any other weight-bearing activity. Riding a stationary exercise bicycle, swimming, and using a rowing machine are non–weight-bearing exercises that use large muscle groups and are considered excellent for developing aerobic fitness. In addition, the muscles of the upper body and the uninjured leg could undergo resistance training exercises.

The exercise prescription is made somewhat easier if the problem is in the arm. In this instance, the individual could exercise using the legs as well as the uninjured arm. Because arm movement provides balance in many whole-body exercises, it would be wise to select

exercises in which maintenance of balance is not a problem. Examples of these exercises are stationary cycling, walking, and stair-climbing.

Obesity

Although it is well established that exercise is an important factor in promoting weight loss (Chapter 8), exercise prescriptions for obese individuals require special attention. For example, in obese individuals, exercise limitations are produced by the following conditions: heat intolerance, shortness of breath during heavy exercise, lack of flexibility, frequent musculoskeletal injuries, and a lack of balance during weight-bearing activities such as walking or running (1, 2).

Exercise programs for obese individuals should emphasize activities that can be sustained for long periods of time (30+ minutes), such as walking, swimming, or bicycling. Further, obese people should avoid exercise in a hot or humid environment. The initial goal of the exercise program should not be to improve cardiovascular fitness but rather to increase voluntary energy expenditure and to establish a regular exercise routine. Therefore, the beginning exercise intensity should be below the typical target heart rate range for improving cardiorespiratory

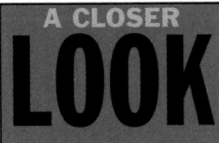

Use Exercise Accessories to Help with Special Conditions

For the elderly, obese individuals, or people with orthopedic problems, stability and weight support may be insurmountable problems when considering an exercise program. One solution may be the use of exercise accessories that are typically used in rehabilitation clinics. *Exercise balls* are large, inflatable heavy-duty balls made of rubber or vinyl that come in various sizes to accommodate various movements and body sizes. They are helpful in stabilizing or balancing body weight in different exercises. These balls, first used in physical therapy clinics, are relatively inexpensive and now found in many fitness centers. The photo shows an example of how they can be used.

Also inexpensive and found in many fitness centers are rubber tubes or bands that come in various thick-

nesses (to vary the resistance to stretch) and are useful for those individuals who might not have the mo-

bility to use weights or weight machines.

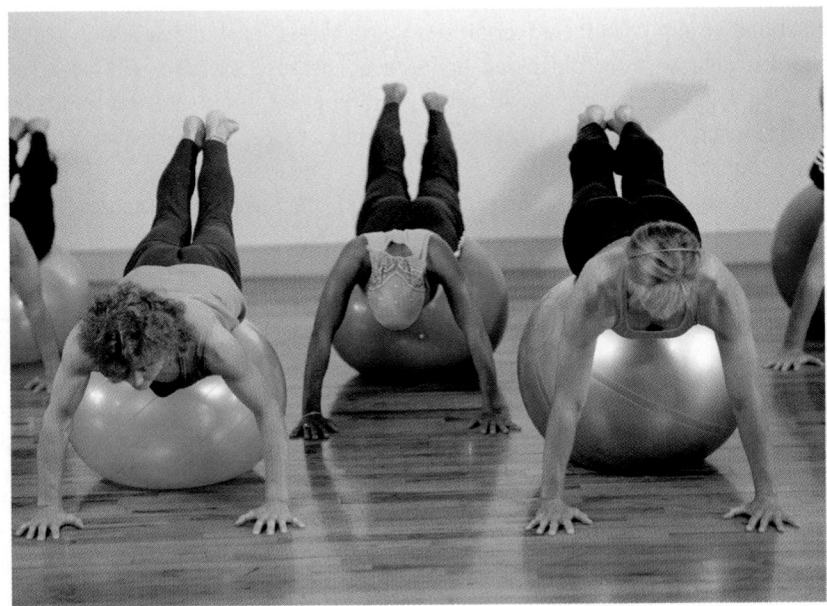

fitness, and the initial duration of exercise should be short (about 5–10 min/day) to reduce the risk of soreness and injury (3). The duration can be gradually increased in 1-minute increments to achieve an energy expenditure of approximately 300 kcals per workout. As the musculoskeletal system adapts to the exercise regimen, the intensity, too, can gradually be increased.

Diabetes

Diabetes is a metabolic disorder affecting over 18 million people and is characterized by high blood glucose levels. Chronic elevation of blood glucose is associated with increased incidence of heart disease, kidney disease, nerve dysfunction, and eye damage (4). In fact, diabetes is one of the leading causes of death in the United States, and its incidence is increasing (4).

There are two types of diabetes. Type I diabetes usually occurs in the young and is due to abnormally low levels of the hormone insulin; it is often called *insulin-dependent diabetes.* The cause of this type of diabetes is now thought to be the immune system's de-

struction of the cells in the pancreas that produce insulin. Type II diabetes often occurs in overweight, middle-aged adults due to a reduction in the ability of insulin to transport glucose from the blood into cells. This form of diabetes generally is due to the lack of sensitivity of the cells to the action of insulin. Although the specific cause of the problem is not known, it is clear that obesity increases the severity of the disease (5). Because type II diabetics generally do not have a problem producing insulin, they generally do not require insulin treatment, and their condition is referred to as *non–insulin-dependent diabetes.*

The three most important tools for managing diabetes are diet, exercise, and insulin (5, 6). Although about three-fourths of known diabetics are taking insulin, it is estimated that 90% of non–insulin-dependent diabetes cases can be prevented with proper diet and exercise regimens (6, 7). There is great motivation to use diet and exercise to control blood glucose because of the considerable trouble, expense, and even danger associated with taking insulin. The danger is associated with the possibility of taking too much, which could result in a coma. Moreover, diabetics who take

Nutritional Links

The Roles of Diet and Exercise in Controlling Blood Glucose

The interaction between the types and amounts of macronutrients in the diet, and the type and amount of exercise, greatly influences the level of glucose in the blood. Both exercise and the hormone insulin have the effect of removing glucose from the blood and getting it into exercising muscle cells.

Whereas nondiabetic individuals on a normal diet need not be concerned about blood glucose levels during a normal exercise training session, diabetics who are about to begin an exercise training session must be concerned with the amount and type of micronutrients they have taken in. Among the three major macronutrients, carbohydrates affect blood glucose levels most dramatically. Moreover, because exercise reinforces the action of insulin in clearing the blood of glucose (6), diabetics must learn how different types of exercise affect blood glucose levels. Diabetics who fail to recognize the effects of various types of exercise on their blood glucose levels run the risk of lowering those levels so much that they become lethargic and disoriented and appear to be drunk. Thus, the primary goal in beginning an exercise program for the person with diabetes is to try different types of exercise and determine the effects on blood glucose. In this way, the individual can learn to manage blood glucose levels and keep blood glucose in a safe range.

oral medication to control blood glucose are at increased risk of cardiovascular disease (8).

Exercise training can benefit diabetics in four major ways. First, exercise training may help control blood glucose in non–insulin-dependent diabetics by improving the transport of glucose into cells, which also reduces insulin requirements. Although this effect has been thought to last only a short time after an exercise session, mounting evidence suggests that the effect may be long lasting for non–insulin-dependent diabetics (9). Simply learning to control blood glucose levels for the duration of each exercise session may be motivation enough to make exercise beneficial. The roles of diet and exercise in controlling blood glucose are briefly discussed in Nutritional Links to Health and Fitness above.

Second, the greatest benefit of exercise to diabetics may be that it helps in controlling body weight (5, 7). One of the single most important objectives for individuals with diabetes is not to become overweight, because this leads to higher blood glucose levels, increased blood lipids, and elevated blood pressure. If an overweight person with diabetes loses weight, glucose levels may return to normal without taking insulin or oral hypoglycemic drugs (5). Obviously, exercise can play an important role in weight management for diabetics.

Third, diabetics are at high risk for heart disease. As we have seen, a lack of exercise is now considered a primary risk factor for heart disease. Because exercise leads to reduced blood pressure, total cholesterol, LDLs, and triglycerides, and to increased HDLs in overweight diabetic individuals (10), the importance of exercise in lowering their risk of heart disease cannot be overlooked.

Last, but certainly not least, regular exercise results in many psychological and social benefits that act to enhance the daily lives of individuals with diabetes (11). Improvements in self-confidence, self-control, self-esteem, vigor, and wellness in general are especially important.

Because the guidelines for developing exercise prescriptions differ for the two categories of diabetes, we next examine each separately.

EXERCISE FOR TYPE I DIABETICS

Before beginning an exercise program, insulin-dependent diabetics must work with a personal physician to learn to manage resting blood glucose levels. This is important because exercise, like insulin, acts to lower blood glucose (9). Indeed, the combination of exercise and insulin can produce low blood glucose levels, which can lead to seizures or loss of consciousness.

Generally, type I diabetics can participate in the same activities as nondiabetics. The recommended training intensity for type I diabetics is identical to the recommended values for healthy individuals (Chapters 4–6). However, exercise should be performed daily so that a regular pattern can be established for glucose control, and the daily exercise duration should be only 20 to 30 minutes. Insulin-dependent diabetics should adopt the following guidelines when beginning an exercise training program:

- Get a thorough medical examination, and tell your physician about your plans to begin an exercise program.

- Do not exercise alone.

- Use footwear designed for the planned activity, and maintain good foot hygiene.
- Consume a meal 1 to 3 hours prior to exercise.
- Consume a snack composed of complex carbohydrates after exercise.
- If so advised by your physician, reduce your insulin dose before the exercise session. (The amount will depend on the type of insulin you take and the amount of exercise you do.)
- Avoid exercising the muscle in which a short-acting insulin injection is given.
- Avoid late-evening exercise, because while you are asleep you cannot monitor any exercise-induced changes in blood glucose.
- Monitor blood glucose before, during, and after exercise.
- Carefully monitor how your blood glucose responds to different forms of exercise.

EXERCISE FOR TYPE II DIABETICS

The most important factor for type II diabetics is exercise duration. Because one of the major objectives of exercise for type II diabetics is assisting in the reduction of body fat, the recommended exercise duration is longer than that for type I diabetics. It is generally short initially (5–10 min/day) and is gradually increased over a period of weeks, reaching a total workout time of 40 to 60 minutes/session. The frequency of exercise should be increased gradually from 3 days per week to 5 in an effort to maximize energy expenditure and promote weight loss. Because of the long duration and relatively high frequency of exercise, type II diabetics should maintain an exercise intensity near the lower end of the target range (40–60% of aerobic capacity) to reduce the risk of injury (7, 8).

☀ IN SUMMARY

- Designing an exercise program for individuals with orthopedic problems often requires special considerations. The objective of the exercise prescription is to find an exercise mode that increases physical fitness without aggravating the existing orthopedic condition.
- Obese individuals should emphasize the use of non–weight-bearing activities (swimming, cycling, and so on). In addition, exercise should be of lower-than-normal intensity.
- Diabetes results from a deficiency in the amount or effectiveness of the hormone insulin, which acts to transfer glucose from the blood and into cells.

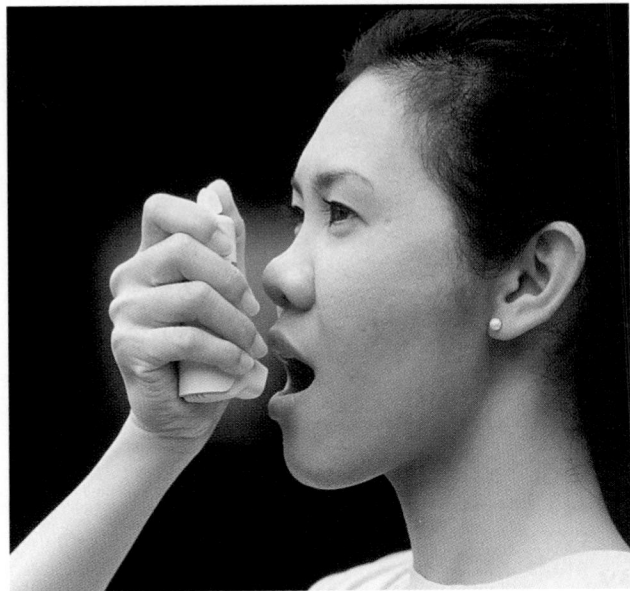

Exercise can be both safe and healthy for individuals with asthma who take the proper precautions.

- The key to developing a sound exercise program for type I diabetics is learning how to manage blood glucose levels during exercise. If blood glucose can be managed, type I diabetics can participate in the same activities as nondiabetics.
- Only minor differences exist in the exercise guidelines for type I and type II diabetics. The most important difference is that type II diabetics can generally participate in longer exercise sessions.

☀ Asthma

Asthma is a condition that reduces the size of the airways leading to the lungs, and it can result in a sudden difficulty in breathing. It is triggered by a number of factors, including air pollution, pollen, and exercise. Unfortunately, the incidence of asthma is on the rise (especially in children). Although solid evidence is lacking, this increased incidence may result from the presence of molds, mildew, and pollutants in indoor air. Fortunately, asthma can be controlled by proper medication.

It is generally agreed that asthmatics can safely participate in all types of exercise training. However, a prerequisite for exercise programs for asthmatics is that

---

asthma A condition that reduces the size of the airways leading to the lungs; it can result in a sudden difficulty in breathing. It is triggered by a number of factors, including air pollution, pollen, and exercise.

they have the proper medication program to control the asthma (12). Once the asthma is under control, the exercise prescription is identical to those for individuals without asthma. However, a wise precaution is to exercise with others and keep an inhaler of asthma medication handy during training in case of a sudden asthma attack.

The following guidelines should be followed by asthmatics who are beginning an exercise training program.

- Work with your personal physician to develop the proper medical protocol to control your asthma.
- Never exercise alone.
- Avoid exercising in cold weather.
- Carry your inhaler while you exercise.
- Avoid exercising in polluted environments; properly filtered indoor air may be preferable to outdoor air.

☀ Pregnancy

Can women continue an exercise program safely during a normal pregnancy? The answer is generally "yes," but the decision to exercise during pregnancy must be made by each woman after consultation with her physician. To date, most of the evidence suggests that short-duration, low-to-moderate intensity exercise does not pose a serious risk to the health of the fetus or the mother (13). However, prolonged or high-intensity exercise may impair fetal development. The best evidence suggests that intense exercise during pregnancy results in reduced birth weights (13). The reason is unknown but may be related to decreased blood flow to the fetus or an elevation in body temperature during exercise (13). It is recommended that pregnant women choosing to exercise perform low-intensity, short-duration exercise (10 to 20 minutes).

The following guidelines should be followed while performing exercise during pregnancy.

- Consult your physician about your exercise plan.
- Do not increase the amount of exercise you typically performed before your pregnancy.
- Do not participate in sports that have a high risk of injury (e.g., contact sports).
- Do not use exercises that require lying on the back for more than 5 minutes. The weight of the fetus may reduce blood flow through vessels supplying blood to the lower extremities.
- In the final 3 months of the pregnancy, avoid exercises that use quick, jerking movements because they may cause joint strains.

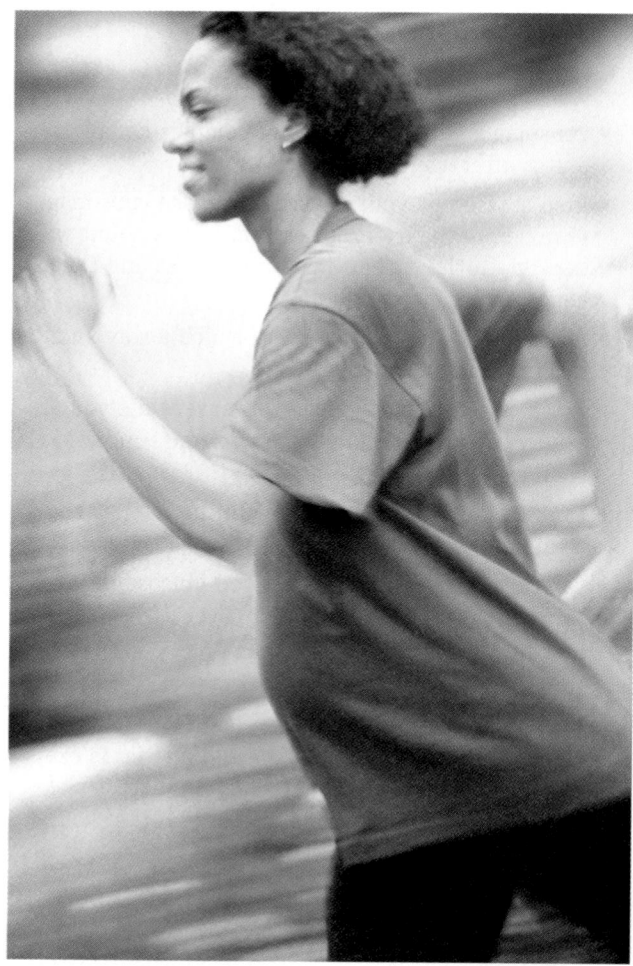

Short-duration, low-to-moderately intense exercise can be beneficial for the mother while posing little risk for the fetus.

- Wear good supportive footwear and adequate breast support.
- Avoid exercise in the heat. Remember: The primary dangers of exercise during pregnancy are elevated body temperature and lack of blood flow to the baby. Because water removes heat from the body better than does air, aquatic exercise is an excellent means of preventing large gains of body heat.
- Monitor your pulse and stay at the low end of your target heart rate zone. Don't exceed 140 beats/minute.
- Concentrate on non–weight-bearing exercises such as cycling or swimming.
- Drink plenty of fluids.
- Stop exercising immediately and call your doctor if you experience any of the following: shortness of breath, dizziness, numbness, tingling, abdominal pain, or vaginal bleeding.

☀ Aging

Throughout this text we have focused on young individuals (about 18 to 25 years of age). In this section we shift our focus to consider exercise for older individuals. Who are the elderly? Usually, the defining age for elderly is considered to be 65 because this is the age when retirement and Social Security benefits begin. However, when considering exercise capacity, we cannot equate ability with age. Many individuals above 65 years of age have the exercise capacity of people one-third their age, and their number is growing.

Everyone experiences a significant decline in $\dot{V}O_{2max}$ with age (Figure 12.1). However, recent research has shown that older individuals engaging in a regular program of vigorous physical activity can maintain the aerobic capacity of someone one-third their age (14). Note in Figure 12.1 that a 75-year-old individual may have the aerobic capacity of a 25-year-old!

Although this may seem like a new idea, the adaptability of the human body has been known for centuries. About 400 B.C., Hippocrates said,

All parts of the body which have a function, if used in moderation and exercised in labors in which each is accustomed, become thereby healthy, well-developed and age more slowly, but if unused and left idle they become liable to disease, defective in growth, and age quickly.

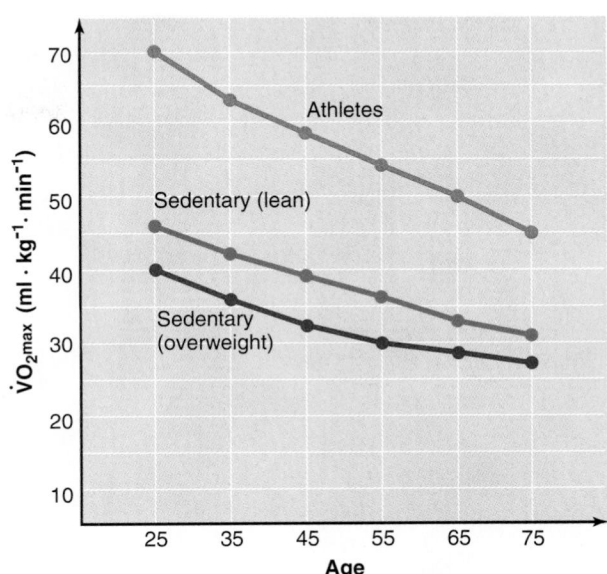

FIGURE 12.1
Changes in $\dot{V}O_{2max}$ with advancing age. A decline of approximately 10% per decade occurs after age 25.
Source: Neiman, D. *Exercise Testing Prescription: A health related approach.* Copyright 1995. Reprinted by permission of McGraw Hill.

Obviously, the normal biological changes that take place during aging are inevitable. However, recent scientific evidence suggests that an active lifestyle can delay the aging process and result in a longer, healthier, and happier life (15).

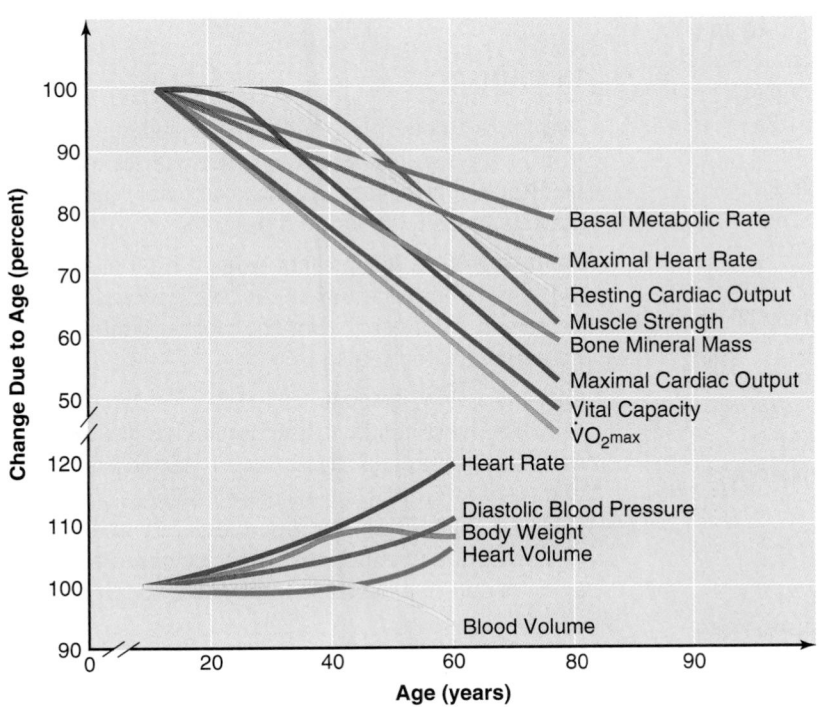

FIGURE 12.2
Physiological changes that accompany aging.
Source: Neiman, D. *Exercise Testing Prescription: A health related approach.* Copyright 1995. Reprinted by permission of McGraw Hill.

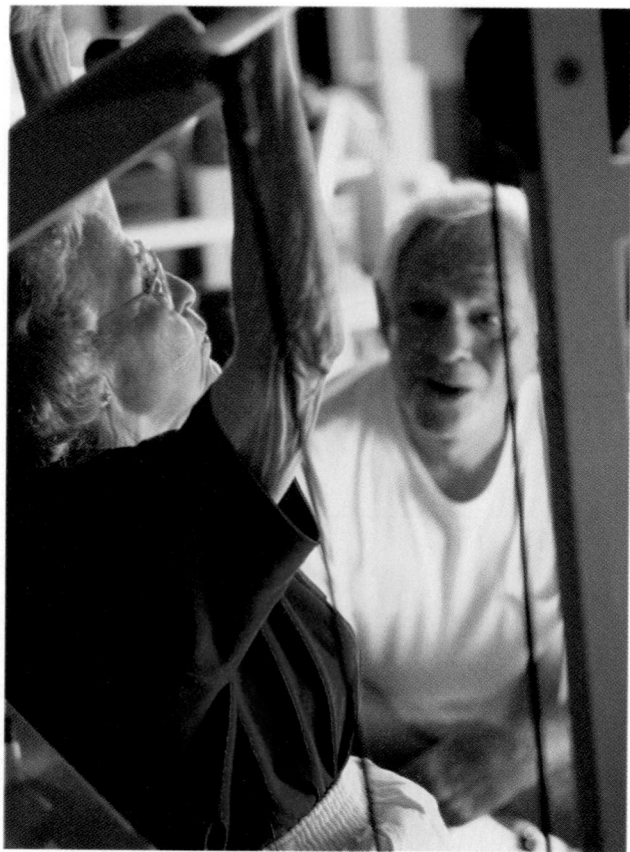

Chronological age and physiological age are not necessarily equivalent.

PHYSIOLOGICAL CHANGES WITH AGING

Aging results in a gradual decline in biological function. Many of the age-related changes in the body begin to appear between the ages of 30 and 40 (15). As illustrated in Figure 12.2, the physiological changes that accompany aging are similar to those seen with inactivity or the prolonged weightlessness experienced by astronauts.

The most common functional changes with aging are decreased cardiorespiratory function, increased body fat, and musculoskeletal fragility (15). What causes these age-related changes? Interestingly, approximately one-half of the decline in functional capacity is due to a decrease *in physical activity* (15). Therefore, regular exercise may improve cardiorespiratory function, assist in maintaining a satisfactory percent body fat, and maintain the mineral content of bone during the aging process. For more on the changes your body undergoes as you age, see Chapter 17.

GUIDELINES FOR EXERCISE

It is important for everyone to remain physically active. However, older individuals should both seek exercise advice from their physicians and avoid physical activities that present a high risk of causing orthopedic problems. Activities such as walking, cycling, swimming, and light weight training are generally recommended. When designing an exercise prescription for older individuals, the basic principles for the development of fitness apply (Chapter 3). The following guidelines outline some specific considerations for exercise after age 40 for men and after age 50 for women.

- Due to the risks of heart disease associated with age, it is wise for men over 40 and women over 50 to perform a physician-supervised, graded exercise stress test before engaging in any vigorous physical fitness program.

- Non–weight-bearing exercises are recommended to reduce the risk of musculoskeletal problems. Weight-bearing exercises are beneficial but should be performed with balance support to avoid falls.

- Exercise intensity should be at the lower end of the target heart rate range.

- Exercise frequency should be limited to 3 to 4 days per week to reduce the risk of injury.

- Exercise duration should be modified to meet the needs (and abilities) of each individual. For example, in the beginning stages of the exercise program, it is likely that many unconditioned elderly individuals cannot exercise for more than 5 to 10 minutes per exercise session. In this case, individuals may exercise several times per day for short durations (three 10-minute sessions/day). As the program progresses, individuals can slowly increase the duration of each session and begin to have fewer daily sessions (two 15-minute sessions/day).

☀ IN SUMMARY

- Asthma is a condition that causes a sudden reduction in the size of the airways. Asthmatics who can medically control their asthma can safely participate in an exercise training program.

- Pregnancy need not prevent women from exercising. Short-duration, low-to-moderate intensity exercise can be beneficial for the mother while posing little risk for the fetus.

- Aging is a slow, gradual decline in biological function. The most common functional changes seen with both aging and inactivity are decreased cardiorespiratory function, increased body fat, and musculoskeletal fragility. Approximately one-half of the decline in functional capacity observed with aging is due to a decrease in physical activity.

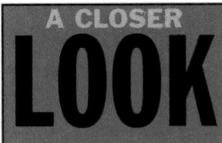

Find a Sport for Your Disability

Can people with disabilities benefit from participation in sports? What precautions need to be taken? What benefits are obtained? These are important questions and bring up many issues concerning the involvement of disabled people in organized sports. People with disabilities are more visible in today's society compared to that of 50 years ago. This wide involvement illustrates the desire disabled people have and demonstrates that they can be active participants, despite their disability.

With participation in sports, precautions need to be taken to ensure safety. These precautions include the following:

- environment (field, court, etc.)
- equipment
- knowledge of the rules
- knowledge about their disability and their limitations

Benefits for the disabled athlete are very much like those of the able-bodied person. These benefits include:

- improved physical health
- improved psychological health, including the cognitive, social, and affective aspects
- improved self-concept, self-esteem, and self-confidence

Numerous organizations have been developed for athletic participation of disabled persons. Some of these include Special Olympics, International Sports Organization for the Disabled, International Committee of Sports for the Deaf, and International Paralympic Committee. This list is a small representation of the organizations that are available for the disabled. A more detailed list (with addresses and phone numbers) can be obtained from the Web site "Sports: National Disabled Sports Organizations" listed at the end of this chapter.

Summary

1. Exercise programs for individuals with orthopedic problems often require special considerations. The objective of the exercise prescription is to find an exercise mode that increases physical fitness but does not aggravate the existing orthopedic condition.

2. Obese individuals should emphasize the use of non–weight-bearing activities (e.g., swimming, cycling). In addition, the exercise should be of lower-than-normal intensity.

3. Diabetes results from a deficiency in the amount or effectiveness of the hormone insulin, which acts to transfer glucose from the blood and into cells.

4. The key to developing a sound exercise program for type I diabetics is learning how to manage blood glucose levels during exercise. If blood glucose can be managed, diabetics can participate in the same activities as nondiabetic individuals.

5. Only minor differences exist between the exercise guidelines for type I and type II diabetics. The most important difference is that type II diabetics can generally participate in longer exercise sessions.

6. Asthma is a condition that results in a sudden reduction in the size of the airways. Asthmatics who can control their asthma medically can safely participate in an exercise training program.

7. Aging is a slow, gradual decline in biological function. The most common functional changes seen with both aging and inactivity are decreased cardiorespiratory function, increased body fat, and musculoskeletal fragility. Approximately one-half of the decline in functional capacity observed with aging is due to a decrease in physical activity.

8. Pregnancy need not prevent women from exercising. Short-duration, low-to-moderate intensity exercise can be beneficial for the mother while posing little risk for the fetus.

Study Questions

1. What exercises may be prescribed for an individual with an orthopedic problem in the lower extremity? The upper extremities? The back?

2. List the problems likely to be encountered by an obese individual who is beginning an exercise program.

3. Distinguish between type I and type II diabetes.

4. Contrast the special guidelines to be followed by type I and type II diabetics who wish to start an exercise program.

5. What physiological changes occur during exercise that may have detrimental effects on the fetus?

6. List the guidelines to be followed for starting or maintaining an exercise program during pregnancy.

7. List the primary physiological changes seen with aging.

8. List the guidelines for establishing a fitness program for an older individual.

9. What special considerations should be taken by an individual with asthma who is starting an exercise program?

10. What is the purpose of the hormone insulin?

Suggested Reading

American College of Sports Medicine. Position stand: Exercise and physical activity for older adults. *Medicine and Science in Sports and Exercise* 30(6):992–1008, 1998.

Bouchard, C. *Physical Activity and Obesity.* Champaign, IL: Human Kinetics, 2000.

Clapp, J. F. Exercise during pregnancy: A clinical update. *Clinics in Sports Medicine* 19(2):273–286, 2000.

Clark, C. J., and L. M. Cochrane. Physical activity and asthma. *Current Opinion in Pulmonary Medicine* 5(1):68–75, 1999.

Fransen, M. Dietary weight loss and exercise for obese adults with knee osteoarthritis: Modest weight loss targets, mild exercise, modest effects. *Arthritis and Rheumatology* 50(5):1366–1369, 2004.

Hawkins, S. A., Wiswell, R. A., and Marcell, T. J. Exercise and the master athlete—a model of successful aging? *Journal of Gerontology* 58(11):1009–1011, 2003.

Hurley, B. F., and S. M. Roth. Strength training in the elderly: Effects on risk factors for age-related diseases. *Sports Medicine* 30(4):249–268, 2000.

Mador, M. J., Bozkanat, E., Aggarwal, A., Shaffer, M., Kufel, T. J. Endurance and strength training in patients with COPD. *Chest* 125(6):2036–2045, 2004.

Powers, S. K., and E. T. Howley. *Exercise Physiology: Theory and Application to Fitness and Performance,* 4th ed. Dubuque, IA: Brown and Benchmark, 2001.

Ryan, D. H. Diabetes Prevention Program Research Group. Diet and exercise in the prevention of diabetes. *International Journal of Clinical Practice: A Supplement* 134:28–35, 2003.

Sato, Y. Diabetes and life-styles: Role of physical exercise for primary prevention. *British Journal of Nutrition* 84(Suppl 2):S187–S190, 2000.

Soultanakis-Aligianni, H. N. Thermoregulation during exercise in pregnancy. *Clinical Obstetrics and Gynecology* 46(2):442–455, 2003.

Spirduso, W. W., and D. L. Cronin. Exercise dose-response effects on quality of life and independent living in older adults. *Medicine and Science in Sports and Exercise* 33 (6 Suppl):S598–S608, 2001.

For links to the web sites below visit The Total Fitness and Wellness Website at www.aw-bc.com/powers.

About.com

Provides information about many aspects of fitness, health benefits of exercise, and wellness concepts for special populations.

American Lung Association

Exercise guidelines for exercise and asthma

Sports: National Disabled Sports Organizations

National Disabled Sports Organizations (DSOs) are members of the U.S. Olympic Committee responsible for providing disability specific sports opportunities. Lists contact information for most disabled sports organizations.

Diabetes Monitor

Contains information about diabetes, including exercise and nutrition suggestions for diabetics.

World Health Network: Exercise and Aging

This site of the American Academy of Anti-Aging Medicine presents numerous articles about exercise and aging.

Fit Pregnancy

Your guide to having a healthy pregnancy with expert information for moms-to-be on prenatal nutrition and exercise.

HealthNet

Contains information on weight training, low-back disorders, exercise programming, heart health, nutrition, mind and body issues, sports medicine, managing stress, wellness, men's health, women's health, diabetes, and arthritis.

Healthfinder

This search engine of the most respected health organization in the world, the National Institutes of Health, enables you to find the latest information on any health-related topic.

References

1. Fransen, M. Dietary weight loss and exercise for obese adults with knee osteoarthritis: Modest weight loss targets, mild exercise, modest effects. *Arthritis and Rheumatology* 50(5):1366–1369, 2004.

2. Jakicic, J. M. Exercise in the treatment of obesity. *Endocrinology and Metabolic Clinics of North America* 32(4):967–980, 2003.

3. American College of Sports Medicine. Position stand: The recommended quantity and quality of exercise for developing and maintaining cardiorespiratory and muscular fitness, and flexibility in healthy adults. *Medicine and Science in Sports and Exercise* 30:975–991, 1998.

4. Centers for Disease Control and Prevention. *National Diabetes Fact Sheet: National Estimates and General Information on Diabetes in the United States,* revised edition. Atlanta: U.S. Department of Health and Human Services, 2004.

5. Steyn, N. P., Mann, J., Bennett, P. H., Temple, N., Zimmet, P., Tuomilehto, J., Lindstrom, J., and Louheranta, A. Diet, nutrition and the prevention of type 2 diabetes. *Public Health and Nutrition* 7(1A):147–165, 2004.

6. Ryan, A. S. Insulin resistance with aging: Effects of diet and exercise. *Sports Medicine* 30(5):327–346, 2000.

7. Tudor-Locke, C. E., R. C. Bell, and A. M. Meyers. Revisiting the role of physical activity and exercise in the treatment of type II diabetes. *Canadian Journal of Applied Physiology* 25(6):466–492, 2000.

8. Ruderman, N. D., J. Devlin, and S. Schneider. *Handbook of Exercise in Diabetes.* Alexandria, VA: American Diabetes Association, 2001.

9. Kelley, D. E., and B. H. Goodpaster. Effects of exercise on glucose homeostasis in type II diabetes mellitus. *Medicine and Science in Sports and Exercise* 33(6 Suppl):S495–S501, 2001.

10. McGavock, J. M., Eves, N. D., Mandic, S., Glenn, N. M., Quinney, H. A., and Haykowsky, M. J. The role of exercise in the treatment of cardiovascular disease associated with type 2 diabetes mellitus. *Sports Medicine* 34(1):27–48, 2004.

11. Wing, R. R., M. G. Goldstein, K. J. Acton, L. L. Birch, J. M. Jakicic, J. F. Sallis, D. Smith-West, R. W. Jeffery, and R. S. Surwit. Behavior science research in diabetes: Lifestyle changes related to obesity, eating behavior, and physical activity. *Diabetes Care* 24(1):117–123, 2001.

12. Storms, W. W. Review of exercise-induced asthma. *Medicine and Science in Sports Exercise* 35(9):1464–1470, 2003.

13. Paisley, T. S., Joy, E. A., and Price, R. J. Exercise during pregnancy: a practical approach. *Current Sports Medicine Reports* 2(6):325–330, 2003.

14. Spirduso, W. W., and D. L. Cronin. Exercise dose-response effects on quality of life and independent living in older adults. *Medicine and Science in Sports and Exercise* 33(6 Suppl):S598–S608, 2001.

15. Marcell, T. J. Sarcopenia: Causes, consequences, and preventions. *Journal of Gerontology* 58(10):M911–M916, 2003.

Exercise Training and Special Populations: Pregnant Women and Individuals with Asthma

NAME _____ DATE _____

Use the following laboratory to design an exercise prescription for a pregnant woman and to test your knowledge of the exercise considerations for those with asthma.

PREGNANCY AND EXERCISE

Pregnancy places special demands on a woman due to the developing fetus's need for calories, protein, vitamins, minerals, and a stable physiological environment. To protect mother and fetus, a consultation with a physician is recommended prior to initiating an exercise program. Exercise of mild to moderate intensity affords numerous health benefits to pregnant women.

Design a regular exercise program (at least three days per week) for a woman in her second trimester. Keep in mind that she should avoid exercise in the supine position, and she should emphasize non–weight-bearing activities. Provide detail about the type of activity and duration of the exercise session. (Example: Monday could be lap swimming at a moderate pace for 20 minutes). Don't forget to include specific rest days.

Sun.	Mon.	Tue.	Wed.	Thu.	Fri.	Sat.

ASTHMA AND EXERCISE

1. What are some of the benefits of regular exercise for asthmatics?

_____

_____

2. Can you think of an exercise that individuals with asthma should not participate in? Why?

_____

_____

_____

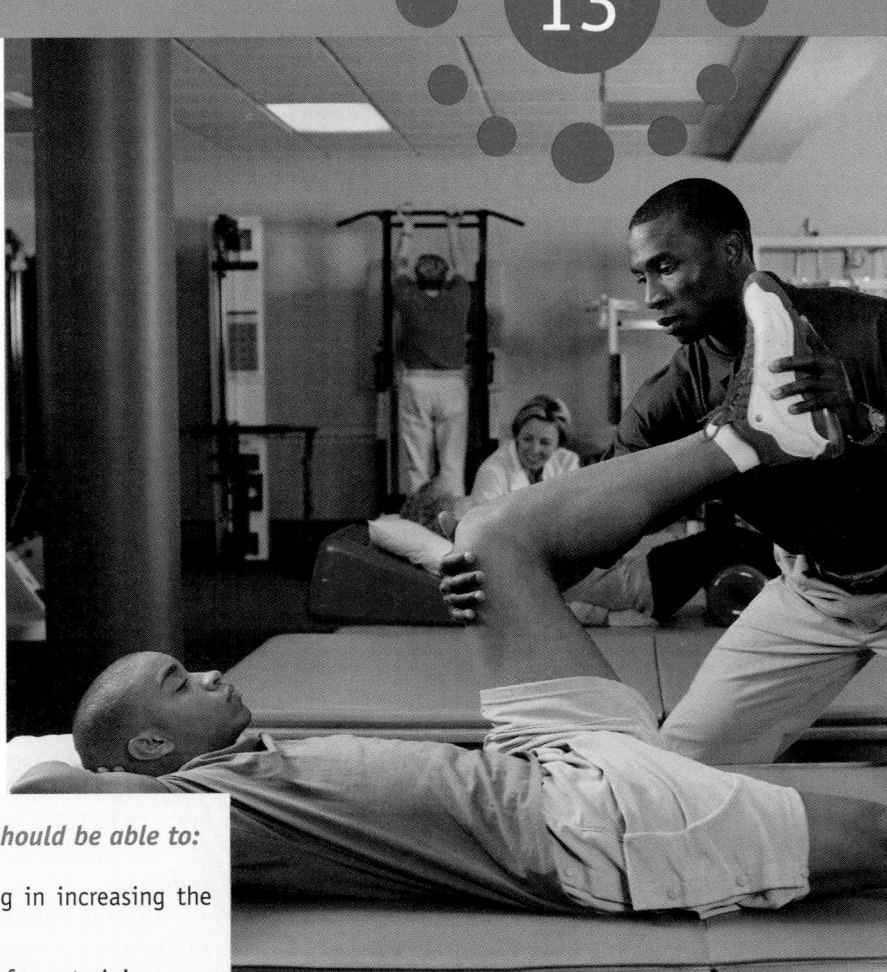

13

After studying this chapter, you should be able to:

1. Discuss the role of overtraining in increasing the risk of exercise-related injury.

2. List the signs and symptoms of overtraining.

3. Define acute and delayed-onset muscle soreness.

4. Discuss possible causes of muscle strains and ways in which they can be avoided.

5. Define tendonitis, and discuss how it should be treated.

6. Discuss ligament sprains and how to avoid them.

7. Describe the most common injuries to the lower extremities.

8. Outline a general plan for reducing the incidence of exercise-related injuries.

9. Discuss the general guidelines for the treatment of injuries.

10. Define cryokinetics, and discuss its use in the rehabilitation process.

Prevention and Rehabilitation of Exercise-Related Injuries

People in the United States are now participating in fitness programs in record numbers. In addition, new types of physical activities have evolved in recent years, ranging from bungee jumping, roller blading, snowboarding, paragliding, and windsurfing. Unfortunately, many of these activities carry inherent risks for injury. For example, in the United States, about 20 million weekend athletes and another 10 million school children experience sports injuries each year (1). For runners, the incidence of injuries has been reported to range from 25% to 75% depending upon various intrinsic and extrinsic factors (Table 13.1).

Although many exercise-related injuries can be prevented, almost everyone who engages in regular physical activity is going to experience one or more injuries during his or her lifetime. In this chapter we discuss the cause, prevention, and treatment of exercise-related injuries.

☀ The Risk and Causes of Injury from Increased Physical Activity

Because running is involved in most physical activities, let's first examine the risk of injury involved with this mode of exercise. More than one-third of runners develop orthopedic injuries serious enough to reduce weekly running mileage (2). Approximately 60% of those injuries involve the foot and knee. One of the major factors responsible for this type and number of injuries is the severity of stress on the legs and feet. In fact, the impact of the foot on the running surface is approximately 2.5 times the body weight of the runner (2). In addition, the incidence of injury increases with running mileage (2). The following rule of thumb may help you gauge your risk of injury due to running: If you run 15 miles a week, you can expect one injury every 2 years. Although many factors have been blamed for the injuries encountered by runners, there is convincing evidence that only a few play a significant role in causing injuries.

The factors most closely correlated with running injuries are improper training techniques, inadequate shoes, and alignment abnormalities in the legs and feet (2). Although all of these factors should be considered, the most important factor seems to be improper training techniques; they account for two-thirds of all injuries (3).

Improper training techniques not only are responsible for increased injuries (3), but also are responsible for the **overtraining syndrome,** a major cause of exercise-related injuries. Overtraining results from too much exercise and not enough recovery time between workouts. The signs and symptoms may include increased resting heart rate, reduced appetite, weight loss, irritability, disturbed sleep, elevated blood pressure, frequent injuries, increased incidence of colds and flu, and chronic fatigue.

To prevent overtraining, a good rule of thumb is to increase your exercise intensity or duration no more than 10% over a 2-week period. In addition, listen to your body. If you notice any of the overtraining signs or symptoms, reduce your training intensity and/or duration and increase your rest intervals. Avoidance of overtraining can greatly reduce your chance of injury and help maintain a positive attitude about fitness.

Although little can be done about some alignment abnormalities in the legs and feet, a change in shoes can help prevent injury in many cases. Approximately one-third of runners experience a decrease in injuries after changing to proper shoes (2) because they provide increased cushioning and support for the arch of the foot. Reductions in injuries also occur with the use of shoes specially designed for such activities as tennis or aerobic dance.

Since it initially became popular in the early 1970s, aerobic dance has also become associated with high rates of injury. From its original form consisting of routines combining dance and calisthenic-type exercises, it has evolved into specialized aerobic programs such as water aerobics, low-impact aerobics, step aerobics, and specific dance aerobics. Approximately one-half of all participants in traditional aerobic dance classes report injuries (4), which occur at a rate of approximately one injury per 100 hours of dancing. One study found that more than three sessions per week, improper shoes, and nonresilient surfaces were the primary causes of injury (4).

Thus, improper exercise techniques (e.g., excessive distance or duration, drastic changes in the exercise routine) are the major causes of injuries. Excessive distance or duration may cause wear to tissues, such as connective tissue in joints, while drastic changes in training routines may put greater stress on tissues and result in injury by tearing tissues. For a brief discussion of the role of nutrition in repair of exercise-induced injuries, see Nutritional Links to Health and Fitness.

---

overtraining syndrome A phenomenon in which too much exercise and not enough recovery time between workouts results in exercise-related injuries. The signs and symptoms may include increased resting heart rate, reduced appetite, weight loss, irritability, disturbed sleep, elevated blood pressure, frequent injuries, increased incidence of infections, and chronic fatigue.

TABLE 13.1
Risk Factors for Sports Injuries

Intrinsic Risk Factors	Extrinsic Risk Factors
Age—risk increases with age	Environmental factors (terrain, surface, weather)
Body size and composition (weight, body fat)	Equipment (footwear, clothing)
Physical fitness—risk greater in unfit individuals	Type of activity—greater risk in competitive activities
Bone density and structure—your specific anatomy may predispose you to injuries	Intensity and amount of activity—intense activity and fatigue cause more injuries
Gender (sex hormones, menarche age)—women at greater risk of injury than men	Warm-up—some evidence to suggest warm-up before exercise decreases risk
Muscle flexibility and strength—less flexibility and strength predispose you to risk	

Source: Murphy, D. F., Connolly, D. A., and Beynnon, B. D. Risk factors for lower extremity injury: A review of the literature. British Journal of Sports Medicine 37(1):13-29, 2003.

IN SUMMARY

- Running injuries occur primarily in the foot and knee, due to the severe stress placed on the legs and feet. The factors most closely associated with running injuries are improper training techniques, inadequate shoes, and alignment problems in the legs and feet.

- Factors associated with injuries in aerobic dance are: participation in more than three sessions per week, improper shoes, and nonresilient surfaces.

- The one factor that increases the likelihood of exercise-related injury the most is overtraining.

Common Injuries: Cause and Prevention

Although many injuries can occur as a result of exercise, some are more common than others. This section discusses the cause and prevention of many general types of injuries associated with exercise training.

BACK PAIN

CAUSE   One of the most important health concerns in the United States is back pain. Over 50% of the population complains of recurring back pain, and over 2 million

Nutritional Links   The Role of Nutrition in Repair of Exercise-Induced Injuries
TO HEALTH AND FITNESS

Nutrition may be important to the repair of exercise-induced injuries in at least two ways. First, repair of damaged muscle involves synthesizing new muscle fibers (to replace damaged fibers removed by the body's repair systems), and this growth process requires that an individual's dietary intake of protein provides enough of the amino acids needed as the building blocks for the new fibers. This does not mean that supplemental dietary protein is required to achieve adequate repair of damaged muscle. You can assure that you have enough protein for repairing damaged muscle by simply following the dietary guidelines discussed in Chapter 7.

The second way that nutrition may affect the repair of injury involves the role of antioxidants in minimizing the extent of injury-induced damage. Immediately after an injury, a variety of chemicals are released in the injured area. Among them are free radicals and various substances that cause inflammation, which in preparing the area for eventual rebuilding causes additional tissue destruction. Antioxidants may play a role in limiting the extent of injury by acting as a scavenger of the free radicals released during both the injury and the early stages of the repair process.

Although much more research is needed in this area to understand the role of nutrition in the repair of injury, one thing is clear: It is obviously wise to ensure that you consume the RDA of all vitamins and minerals each and every day.

people are unable to work because of it (5). Among the many causes of back pain are improper lifting techniques, weak muscles, poor posture, and bone disorders (Table 13.2). Treatments include painkillers, muscle relaxants, antiinflammatory drugs, bracing, traction, bed rest, surgery, and therapeutic exercises. Even without any form of treatment, approximately 80% of back patients recover spontaneously (5). Thus, it is not clear whether the treatments for back pain only serve to lessen the pain or are in fact beneficial in speeding recovery.

Back problems are of critical concern when beginning an exercise program. Depending on the exact nature of the problem, exercise may be extremely helpful or extremely harmful. You should attempt to find the cause of any back problems before starting an exercise program. It is possible that certain types of exercise may compound the problem and thus should be avoided.

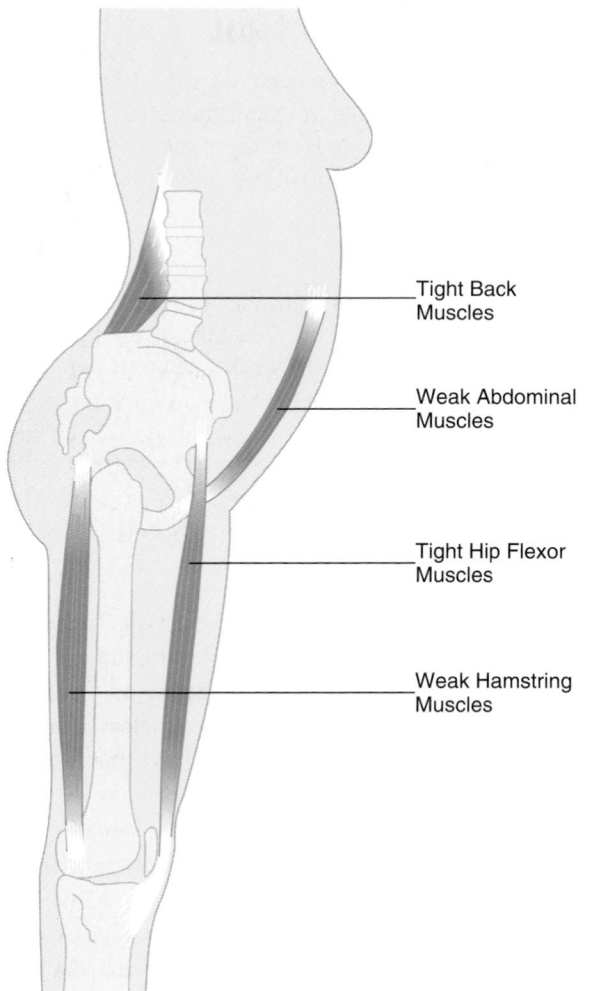

FIGURE 13.1
Major muscles involved in posture and their typical conditions during poor posture. The muscle imbalances shown here lead to poor posture, which can result in back pain.

Tight Back Muscles

Weak Abdominal Muscles

Tight Hip Flexor Muscles

Weak Hamstring Muscles

TABLE 13.2
Risk Factors for Back Pain

In most cases, back pain is preventable. A knowledge of the following factors, which lead to a higher-than-normal risk of recurring back pain, may help in alleviating back pain or preventing future back problems.

Poor posture
Improper lifting of heavy loads
Frequent bending from the waist
Weak lower back muscles
Weak abdominal muscles
Being overweight
Lack of flexibility in lower back
Lack of flexibility in hamstring muscles
Quick, jerking movements of the spine
Osteoporosis
Increasing age

Exercise has been effectively used in pain clinics for treating back pain (6). In addition, exercise can be used to prevent or correct some back problems by strengthening weak muscles and stretching the stronger ones. If you have a problem with your back, consult your physician before beginning an exercise program in order to determine what complications or benefits may result from your exercise program.

PREVENTION Exercise can play a key role in preventing back pain. Exercises to increase flexibility and strength, reduce body fat, improve muscle balance between the abdominal and back muscles, and prevent osteoporosis can decrease your risk of developing back problems (6). In addition, in consultation with your physician you may decide that these exercises can help alleviate back pain that you may already be experiencing.

If muscles on one side of a joint are stronger than those on the other side, the resulting imbalance of forces can pull the associated body parts out of alignment. You should do exercises that strengthen the longer, weakened muscles and stretch the short, stronger ones. For example, individuals with an exaggerated curvature in the lower back will need to strengthen the abdominal muscles and stretch the muscles of the lower back and hips (Figure 13.1).

Use the following guidelines to help prevent the irritation of back problems or to prevent the onset of back pains:

- Maintain a healthy body weight and body composition. Obesity puts great strain on the lower back.
- Warm up before engaging in any physical activity.
- Do exercises to strengthen the abdominal muscles.

- Do exercises to stretch the lower back and hamstring muscles.
- When lying down, lie on your side with your knees and hips bent. Try to avoid lying on your back, but if you do, place a pillow under your knees.
- During prolonged standing, try to take the strain off of the lower back by propping one foot on an object such as a rail or box, which bends the leg at the hip and knee.
- Avoid quick, jerking movements of the spine.
- Do not overextend the neck or lower back or overflex the neck.
- Avoid stretching the long/weak muscles, especially the abdominal muscles.
- Be especially careful when being passively stretched by another person. Avoid passive back or neck stretches or any ballistic passive stretches (Chapter 6).
- Avoid movements that place forces on spinal disks, such as extending and rotating the spine simultaneously, trunk and neck circling, and double leg lifts.
- Avoid forceful hyperextension and flexion of the spine.
- Avoid improper lifting. Squat to lift any object, and never bend at the waist.

ACUTE MUSCLE SORENESS

CAUSE **Acute muscle soreness** may develop during or immediately following an exercise session that has been too long or too intense. Even though popular belief has linked the buildup of lactic acid to acute muscle soreness, lactic acid is not the cause of this type of soreness (7). Instead, it is more likely caused by other alterations in the chemical balance within muscle, increased fluid accumulation in muscle, or injury to muscle tissue.

PREVENTION Exercise that is more strenuous or prolonged than normal is likely to cause the aforementioned changes that result in acute muscle soreness. Novice exercisers should be particularly cautious in this regard when beginning an exercise training program. These changes can be further prevented by gradually beginning and ending each exercise session. All exercise sessions should begin slowly with a warm-up period of 5 to 15 minutes (Chapter 3) to allow muscles to increase their internal temperature slowly to avoid damage during the more stressful exercise training session. Finally, a postexercise cool-down regimen is

important in allowing the muscles to return to their normal, pre-exercise physiological condition.

DELAYED-ONSET MUSCLE SORENESS

CAUSE **Delayed-onset muscle soreness (DOMS)** develops within 24 to 48 hours of a bout of exercise that is excessive in duration or intensity (8). It is also common following new or unique physical activities that use muscle groups unaccustomed to exercise. For example, it is not unusual for a runner to experience soreness in the upper body following the initiation of a weight-training program.

The cause of soreness in DOMS is likely microscopic tears in the muscle (8), which cause swelling and pain. Many investigators believe that this type of injury occurs primarily during the lengthening phase of muscular contraction (eccentric portion of the contraction; Chapter 5). The damage apparently is due to the greater force placed on the muscle during this phase of the contraction. For example, downhill running (which emphasizes such contractions) by an individual unaccustomed to this type of exercise will generally produce soreness in the leg muscles within 24 to 48 hours after the exercise session. Similarly, in people unaccustomed to walking up and down steps, DOMS also occurs 24 to 48 hours after such exercise.

PREVENTION As with acute muscle soreness, DOMS can be prevented by refraining from exercise that is more strenuous or more prolonged than normal. Start with a warm-up and limit both the intensity and duration of the first several workouts. Remember that eccentric contractions are more likely to result in muscle damage than are concentric (shortening) contractions. Therefore, in the beginning stages of an exercise program, try to avoid heavy weights for exercises that involve large amounts of eccentric contractions (e.g., walking down steps, running downhill, and performing certain movements during weight lifting).

acute muscle soreness A condition that may develop during or immediately following an exercise session that has been too long or too intense; is likely caused by alterations in the chemical balance within muscle, increased fluid accumulation in muscle, or injury to muscle tissue.
delayed-onset muscle soreness (DOMS) A condition that develops within 24 to 48 hours after an exercise session that is excessive in duration or intensity; is common following new or unique physical activities that use muscle groups unaccustomed to exercise.

(a)   **(b)**   **(c)**

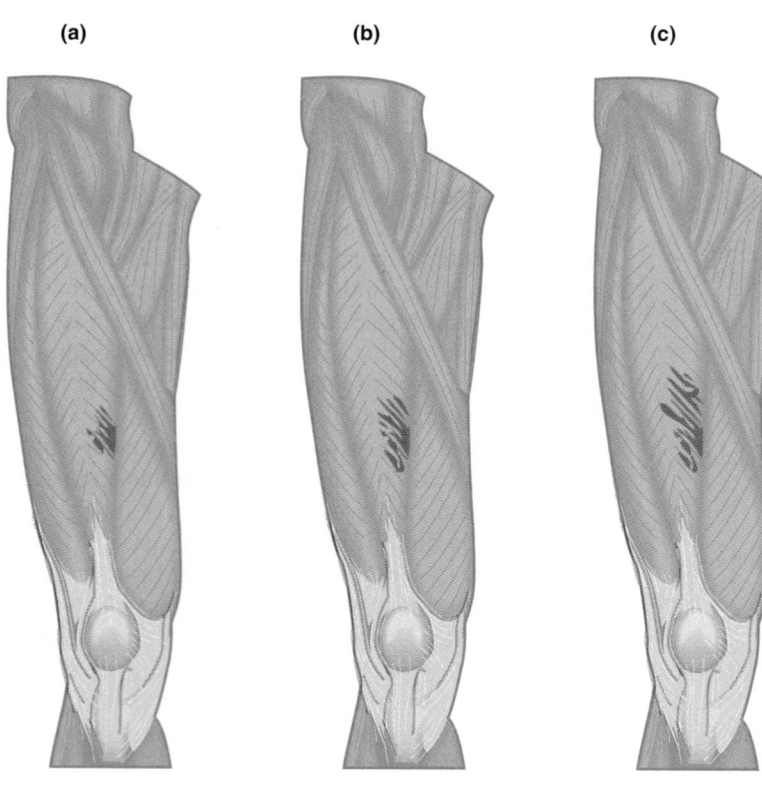

1st Degree   2nd Degree   3rd Degree

FIGURE 13.2
The extent of muscle damage in the three categories of muscle strains. (a) First-degree strain with minimal disruption of muscle fibers. (b) Second-degree strain with significant tearing and hemorrhage. (c) Third-degree strain with complete tear and loss of function.

MUSCLE STRAINS

CAUSE   If a muscle is overstretched or forced to shorten against an extremely heavy weight (as when lifting a heavy box), muscle fibers may be damaged. This damage, which is referred to as a **strain**, can range from a minor separation of fibers to a complete tearing of fibers (9). The following classification system has been developed for categorizing the degree of muscle damage due to strain:

1st Degree Strain: Only a few muscle fibers are stretched or torn (Figure 13.2a). Movement is painful, but a full range of motion is still possible.

2nd Degree Strain: Many muscle fibers are torn (Figure 13.2b), and movement is extremely painful and limited. The torn area may be apparent as a soft, sunken area in the muscle. Swelling may occur around the tear due to hemorrhage (bleeding).

---

strain   Damage to a muscle that can range from a minor separation of fibers to a complete tearing of the muscle.
tendonitis   Inflammation or swelling of a tendon; one of the most common exercise-related injuries.

3rd Degree Strain: The muscle is torn completely (Figure 13.2c). The tear can be in the belly of the muscle, in the tendon, or at the point where the tendon attaches to the bone. Movement is generally impossible. Initial pain is intense but quickly subsides because nerve fibers are also damaged. Surgery is usually necessary for repair.

PREVENTION   Because strains occur when muscles must generate excessive force, it is logical that strains can be prevented by limiting the amount of stress placed on muscles. But note that it is not possible to predict just how much force is needed to cause muscle damage, and that warm muscles are more pliable (that is, more easily stretched and less likely to tear) than cold muscles. Therefore, before lifting a heavy object or engaging in any activity that requires quick, jerking movements, go through a thorough warm-up for 5 to 15 minutes. Even though a good warm-up should prevent muscle strains, remember that muscle contractions that are more strenuous than normal may result in DOMS.

TENDONITIS

CAUSE   Tendons are the tissue that connect muscles to bone. **Tendonitis**, which is the inflammation or swelling of a tendon, is one of the most common exercise-related injuries (9). As muscles shorten and pull on tendons, the tendons move across other tendons, muscles, and soft tissue. This movement, if unaccustomed, can cause irritation and swelling in the tendon. Once tendonitis develops, pain associated with movement is the first symptom. Swelling, redness, and warmth generally follow. Tendonitis can occur in a number of areas, such as the elbow and shoulder, and is a common injury of runners, tennis players, and weight lifters.

PREVENTION   Tendonitis is generally caused by strenuous, prolonged muscle contractions to which an individual is unaccustomed. Therefore, the best prevention of tendonitis is to avoid overuse. If you feel tendon pain or discomfort during a workout, stop exercising. This will prevent further irritation and reduce the severity of tendon damage. If you cannot stop using the muscle and tendon causing the pain, follow the measures for the management of injuries discussed at the end of this chapter.

LIGAMENT SPRAINS

CAUSE   A **sprain** is caused by damage to a ligament (9). Ligaments are tough, inelastic bands of connective tissue that connect the bones, provide joint support, and determine the direction and range of motion of joints. Ligament damage can occur if excessive force is applied to a joint. One of the most common sites of ligament damage is the ankle. When walking or running on an uneven surface it is easy to "turn" the ankle, which means that the ankle joint is rotated such that much of the body weight is placed on the side of the foot. Because the ankle joint is not designed to rotate to that degree, the stress on the joint causes the ligaments to be damaged. Like muscle strains, the degrees of ligament damage are classified as follows:

1st Degree: Stretching and separation of a limited number of ligament fibers, resulting in minor instability of the joint (Figure 13.3a). Minor pain and swelling likely result.

2nd Degree: Tearing and separation of a significant number of ligament fibers (Figure 13.3b). Moderate instability of the joint with definite pain, swelling, and stiffness occur.

3rd Degree: Total tearing or separation of the ligament, causing major instability of the joint (Figure 13.3c). Nerves may be damaged and pain may subside quickly. Considerable swelling generally occurs.

PREVENTION   The development of lightweight metal alloys have made it possible to construct braces that provide added support to joints and therefore offer

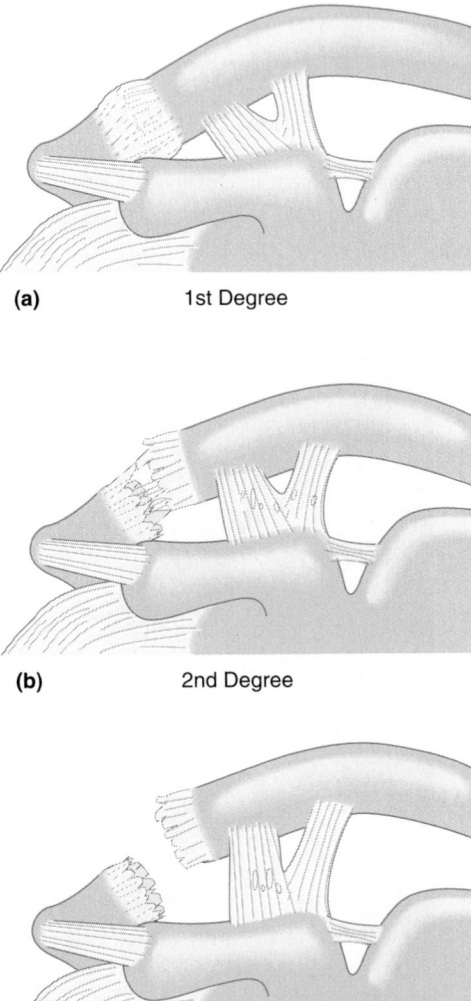

(a)   1st Degree

(b)   2nd Degree

(c)   3rd Degree

FIGURE 13.3
The extent of damage in the three categories of sprains, which involve damage to the ligaments that support the joint. (a) First-degree sprain with minimal disruption of tendons in the shoulder. (b) Second-degree sprain with severe tearing and loss of joint stability. (c) Complete separation.

some protection from ligament damage. These braces are commonly used in football, a sport recognized for inducing knee damage. Without these expensive, high-tech devices, the best protection against torn ligaments is to refrain from activities that may subject a joint to high stress, including tennis, soccer, racquetball, and basketball. In addition, if you have a particular joint that has been injured previously or is weak, work to

sprain Damage to a ligament that occurs if excessive force is applied to a joint.

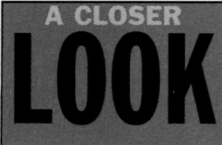

Arthroscopic Surgery: A High-Tech Approach to Joint Repair

Whenever severe ligament or cartilage damage occurs around a joint, as commonly happens to the knee in football, soccer, and basketball players, the usual remedy is surgery. Traditional surgical techniques require the surgeon to cut the joint open in order to repair it, causing additional trauma to the joint and resulting in prolonged recuperation and rehabilitation. Now, however, a commonly used surgical technique called **arthroscopic surgery** allows surgeons to repair joint injuries without causing undue trauma to the joint.

In arthroscopic surgery, surgeons use only two or three small incisions to gain entry into the damaged joint. Through these incisions they insert small micro-optic devices to allow them to see inside the joint, as well as a microsurgery tube that enables them to cut and remove small pieces of damaged tissue and to sew the remaining tissue together. Because the surgeons need make only a few minor incisions, less surgical damage translates into less pain and shorter recovery and rehabilitation times than occur with conventional surgical techniques.

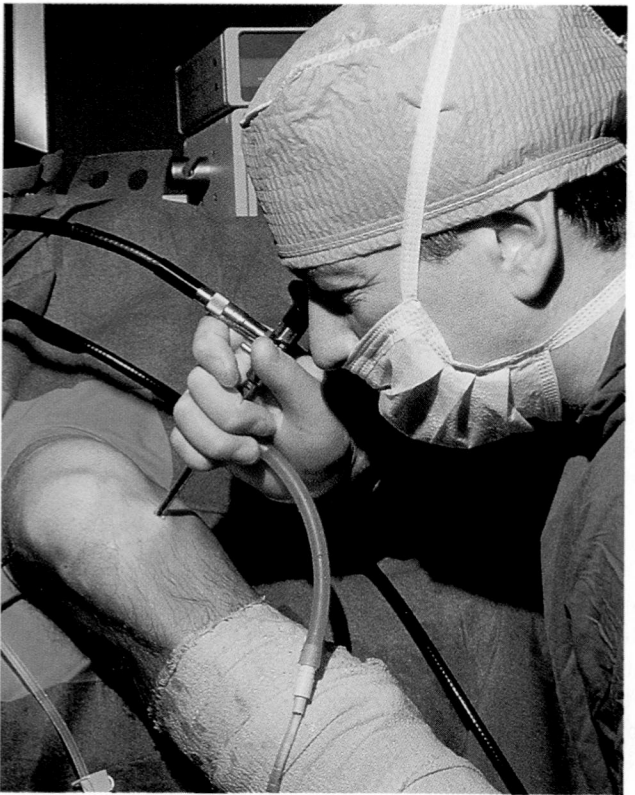

Arthroscopic surgery is relatively painless and requires much less recovery time than conventional surgery, which requires opening the joint capsule.

maintain maximum strength in the muscles surrounding the joint, because strong muscles provide additional support.

TORN CARTILAGE

CAUSE Cartilage is a tough connective tissue that forms a pad on the end of bones in certain joints, such as the elbow, knee, and ankle. Cartilage acts as a shock absorber to cushion the weight of one bone on another and to provide protection from the friction due to joint movement. Although this pad is made of the toughest of connective tissue, it can be damaged and torn (9). Unusually high forces or unusual movements can cause tearing of cartilage, which results in joint pain. This type of injury, and severe ligament damage as well, normally requires surgical correction. To learn about a high-tech procedure for repairing damaged joints, see A Closer Look above.

PREVENTION The only preventive measure for torn cartilage is eliminating those activities that are likely to cause the problem. Again, activities that may result in torn cartilage include any that produce excess stress on the joint or forceful movements that take the joint outside its normal range of motion.

arthroscopic surgery A common surgical procedure that can repair joint injuries without causing undue trauma to the joint.

☀ IN SUMMARY

- Back pain can be the result of many factors and usually subsides without any medical intervention. In some cases exercise can play an important role in preventing back pain and rehabilitating back problems. Exercises to increase flexibility and strength, reduce body fat, improve muscle balance between the abdominal and back muscles, and prevent osteoporosis can decrease your risk of developing back problems.

- Acute muscle soreness, which occurs during or immediately after exercise, may be due to muscle damage, accumulation of fluid within the muscle, and/or chemical imbalances within the muscle itself.

- Delayed-onset muscle soreness (DOMS) usually occurs 24 to 48 hours after an exercise session. Eccentric exercise increases the chances that DOMS will occur.

- When muscle is forced to contract against excessive resistance, the resulting damage to muscle fibers is called a strain. Such damage can range from a minor separation of fibers to a complete tear in the muscle.

- Tendonitis, which is inflammation of a tendon, is one of the most common of all overuse problems associated with physical activity.

- A sprain is cause by damage to a ligament, a type of connective tissue that provide support for joints. In contrast, torn cartilage is damage to the tough connective tissue that provide cushioning between the ends of bones.

☀ Common Injuries to the Lower Extremities

We have discussed the cause and prevention of several general exercise-related injuries. Because many fitness programs involve weight-bearing activities such as running, walking, and aerobic dance, let's take a closer look at some specific injuries involving the legs.

In general, walking does not result in a large number of injuries. However, more than one-third of all runners develop one or more leg injuries as a result of overtraining. Further, recent studies have reported that approximately 50% of all participants in aerobic dance classes develop leg injuries. Most of these running and dance injuries occur in the foot and the knee as a result of the stress placed on the legs and feet. The force of the foot landing on the running surface (or dance floor) is approximately 2.5 times greater than the body weight of the person. In the case of a 150-pound

runner, the amount of force generated when the foot strikes the pavement is 375 pounds! It is easy to see how injuries might occur with this level of stress. In the following paragraphs we discuss the cause and prevention of the most common lower extremity injuries.

PATELLA-FEMORAL PAIN SYNDROME

CAUSE   **Patella-femoral pain syndrome (PFPS)** is a common exercise-induced injury that is manifest as pain behind the patella, or knee cap (9). Also known as "runner's knee" or *chondromalacia*, PFPS may account for almost 10% of all visits to sports injury clinics, or 20–40% of all knee problems (10). Although the precise causes of PFPS remain unclear, the condition results when the patella gets "off track" (Figure 13.4), which causes excessive wear of the patella and pain. Among the several factors that predispose an individual to PFPS are misalignments of the thigh muscles that extend the knee, overuse or prolonged immobilization of the muscles, acute trauma, obesity, and genetics.

When these factors are present, the increased forces and repetitive movements of exercise result in pain and may result in cracking and popping sounds during movement. Over time and with increased use, the articular (joint) cartilage may begin to degenerate, which eventually may lead to osteoarthritis.

PREVENTION   PFPS can be prevented by avoiding stress on the knee due to excessive amounts of running, jumping, aerobic dancing, and stair climbing. Further, the chances of developing PFPS can be reduced by strengthening the front thigh muscles (quadriceps); this improves the tracking of the patella and reduces wear on the patellar surface.

The two best exercises seem to be knee extension exercises over the last 20° of extension and/or isometric contractions of the quadriceps muscles with the leg fully extended (try to press the back of the knee to the floor while lying on your back) (9). Remember, avoid unnecessary stresses on the knee, such as squatting, and excessive amounts of activities such as running, jumping, step aerobics, and stair climbing.

Finally, proper athletic footwear may reduce the chances of developing PFPS. If you develop any of the symptoms of PFPS, see your physician or a podiatrist to

---

patella-femoral pain syndrome (PFPS)   A common exercise-induced injury, sometimes called "runner's knee," that is manifest as pain behind the knee cap (patella); may account for almost 10% of all visits to sports injury clinics, or 20–40% of all knee problems; also known as chondromalacia.

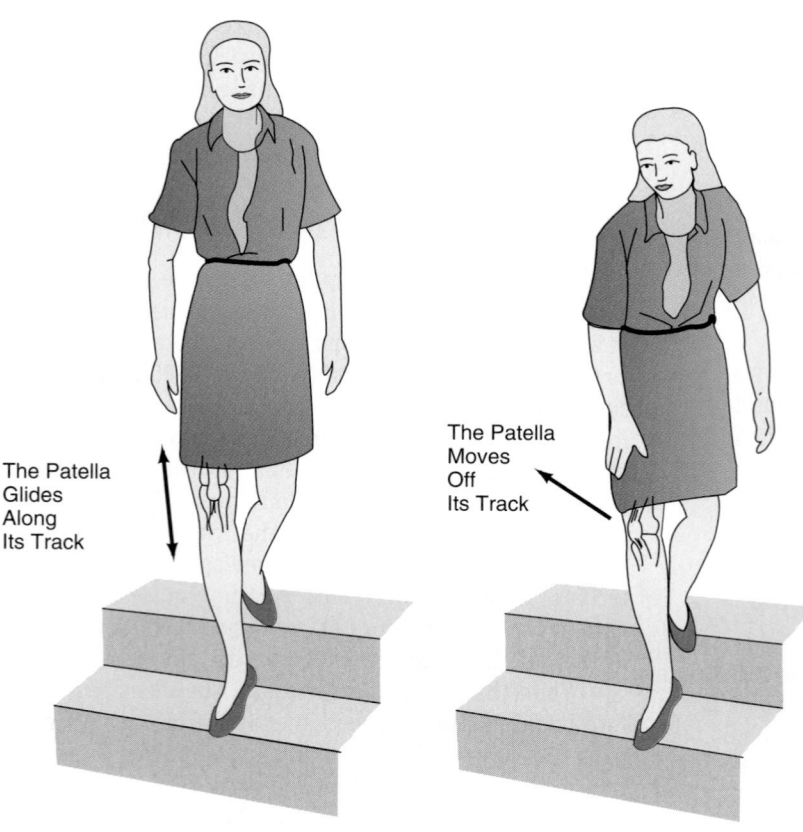

The Patella Glides Along Its Track

The Patella Moves Off Its Track

FIGURE 13.4
When the thigh muscles pull correctly (left), the knee cap stays in place and glides easily in its track. With PFPS (right), the thigh muscles pull unevenly and the knee cap gets "off track." This results in uneven pressure on the back of the knee cap, which causes excessive wear and pain.

discuss the possibility that footwear may be contributing to the problem.

TREATMENT An aggressive rehabilitation program that includes quadriceps exercises, rest, and antiinflammatory drugs has proved beneficial for over 70% of PFPS patients. Although ice neither prevents PFPS nor rehabilitates the joint, it (like antiinflammatory agents) may provide some relief from the pain and inflammation.

SHIN SPLINTS

CAUSE *Shin splints* is a generic term referring to pain associated with injuries to the front of the lower leg (9). Three of the most common injuries that cause shin splints are strain and irritation of one or several muscles and tendons located in the lower leg (Figure 13.5); inflammation of tissue connecting the two bones of the lower leg, the tibia and the fibula; and microscopic breaks (called *stress fractures;* discussed next) in either the tibia or the fibula.

stress fractures Tiny cracks or breaks in the bone.

PREVENTION Shin splints can be avoided by running on soft surfaces; by wearing well-padded, shock-absorbing shoes; and by slowly advancing exercise intensity from walking to running. If shin pain develops, it could be due to a fracture or break of bones and therefore should not be regarded lightly. High-impact activities such as running should be stopped; substitute low-impact activities such as cycling or swimming. Stretching muscles located in the front and back of the lower leg may help prevent the problem.

STRESS FRACTURES

CAUSE **Stress fractures** are tiny cracks or breaks in bone. Although stress fractures can occur in any leg bone, the long bones of the foot extending from the bones in the heel to the toes (the metatarsal bones) are especially susceptible (Figure 13.6). Indeed, these are the most common sites of stress fractures in the body. Stress fractures result from excessive force applied to the leg and foot during running or other types of weight-bearing activities (11). The most likely candidates for this injury are individuals with high arches or poor flexibility of the lower body, and people who increase training intensity or duration too rapidly.

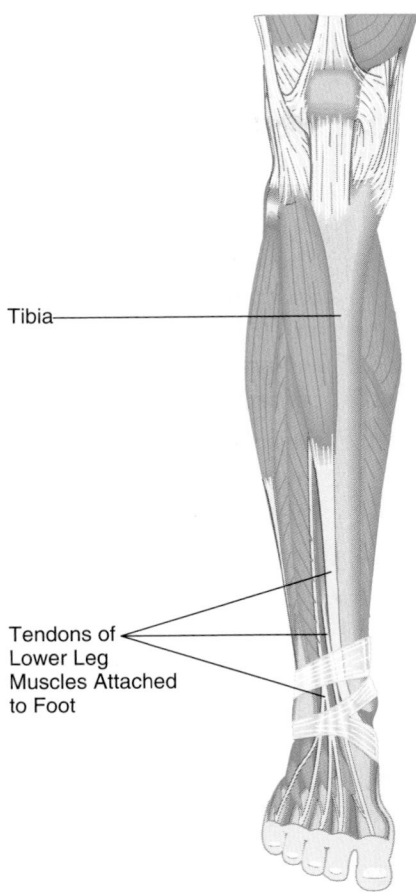

FIGURE 13.5
Locations of the muscles and tendons that are often irritated in shin splints.

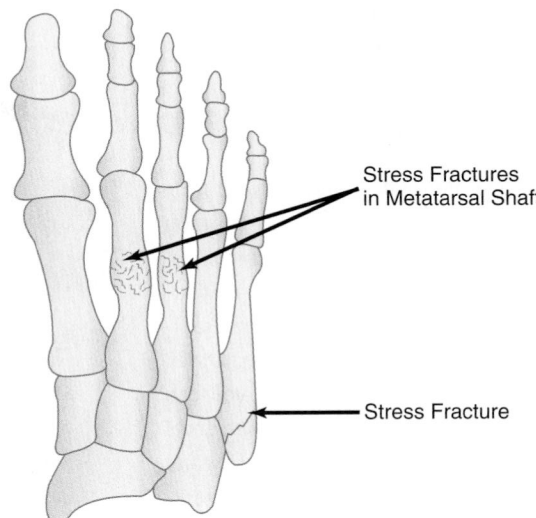

FIGURE 13.6
Some sites of metatarsal stress fractures, which can result in pain during any weight-bearing movement.

PREVENTION   People with high arches should seek exercise advice from their physicians or a podiatrist (foot specialist), who might prescribe arch supports, which aid in preventing a stress-related problem. Again, a key factor in preventing stress fractures is to avoid overtraining by increasing your training load gradually. Remember, increase your exercise intensity or duration no more than 5–10% per week. Often, a lack of flexibility in the hips and the back of the legs will cause the body's weight to be shifted such that some bones become chronically overloaded and fracture. Thus, maintaining flexibility in the back of the legs and hips will reduce your chances of developing a stress fracture. If pain in the foot or leg makes you suspect a stress fracture, stop activities that involve the injured area. See your physician to get an X-ray of the area. If a stress fracture is present, only rest can assist the healing process.

IN SUMMARY

- Common injuries to the lower extremities include (1) PFPS, in which the articular cartilage on the back of the knee cap (patella) may be damaged by chronic use during exercise; (2) shin splints, a condition that encompasses several different injuries to the front of the lower leg; and (3) stress fractures, which are microscopic breaks in the bone.

Reducing Your Risk of Injury

To this point we have discussed the causes and prevention of some general and specific exercise-related injuries. Here we summarize five key ways to reduce your risk of injury due to exercise training.

1. Engage in a program of muscle-strengthening exercises using all major muscle groups. Maintaining a balance of muscular strength around joints will prevent muscular imbalance and reduce the incidence of injury.

2. Warm up before and cool down after all workouts. Remember: Stretching during the warm-up may help prevent injuries, and stretching during the cool-down will help maintain flexibility.

3. Use the proper footwear. Good shoes are obviously important for activities such as running and aerobic dance and can reduce your chance of injury.

4. Do not overtrain! The most important factor in promoting exercise-related injuries is improper training techniques. Gradual progression of exercise intensity and duration is essential in preventing injuries.

5. Incorporate the proper amount of recovery time into your training routine. Rest is an important part of any successful training program.

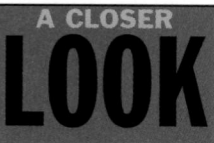

Can Deep Water Running Help Your Recovery?

With an injury that prevents you from exercising, the benefits of training are quickly reversed. Your cardiovascular fitness decreases measurably after two to three weeks without training. However, it is now well accepted that, with reduced training, you can maintain your fitness at a high level for several months. The intensity and specificity of "cross-training" workouts are most important in determining how much fitness you lose when you take time off from exercise training. Of course, you need to find a method of cross training that will allow your injury to heal. Depending on the injury, you may be able to perform various types of cross training such as cycling, rowing, or using a cross-country skiing simulator to maintain your exercise program while your injury heals. Since these methods provide some load on your muscles, you should use them for optimal effect. Unfortunately, some leg injuries are aggravated by these exercises. But, with most leg injuries, you can safely run in the water. Deep water running with a flotation vest provides an excellent training stimulus, and more closely simulates land running than many of the other cross-training options. Running in the wa-

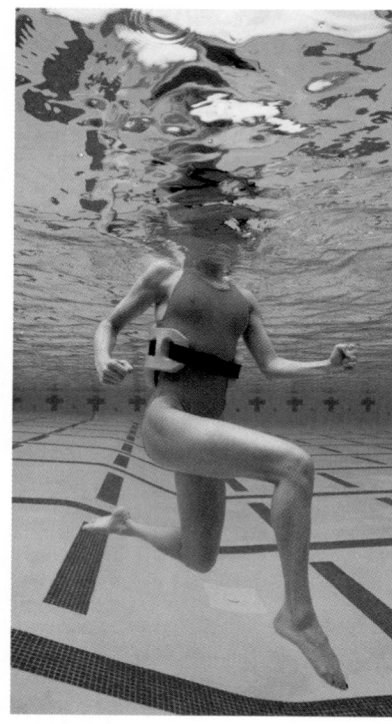

ter is a total body exercise that works your legs, trunk, and arms, and stresses your cardiovascular system.

Aerobic performance is maintained with deep-water running for up to six weeks in trained endurance athletes, and sedentary individuals can actually improve their fitness level. In addition, there is some evidence of improvement in anaerobic measures

and in upper body strength in individuals engaging in deep-water running. A reduction in spinal loading also constitutes a role for deep-water running in the prevention of injury. Here are some of the specific benefits you can derive from deep water running:

- Maintenance of or improvement in running performance.

- You can simulate any type of running workout with the support of the water.

- Easy to simulate interval training since the water adds resistance to your limbs.

- Reduces muscle soreness with strenuous workouts because you eliminate eccentric contractions.

- Effective in maintaining body composition since you can maintain high levels of energy expenditure and burn calories.

- Provides a workout to upper body musculature.

- Strengthening of hip adductors/abductors, lower leg musculature, feet, and abdominal muscles.

- Improvement in flexibility when a stretching routine is included.

To assess your exercise program with respect to the risks of injury it may pose, see Laboratory 13.1 on p. 367.

☼ Management of Injuries

As mentioned earlier, almost everyone who engages in regular physical activity will experience some type of injury. In the following sections we discuss injury treatment and provide an overview of the rehabilitation process.

Any injury that results in extreme pain or the possibility of a broken bone should be examined by a physician, who will likely take X-rays to determine if there are any broken bones. The following treatment regimen should be followed for less severe injuries (strains, sprains, tendonitis, and so on).

INITIAL TREATMENT OF INJURIES

The objectives of the initial treatment of exercise-related injuries are to decrease pain, limit swelling, and

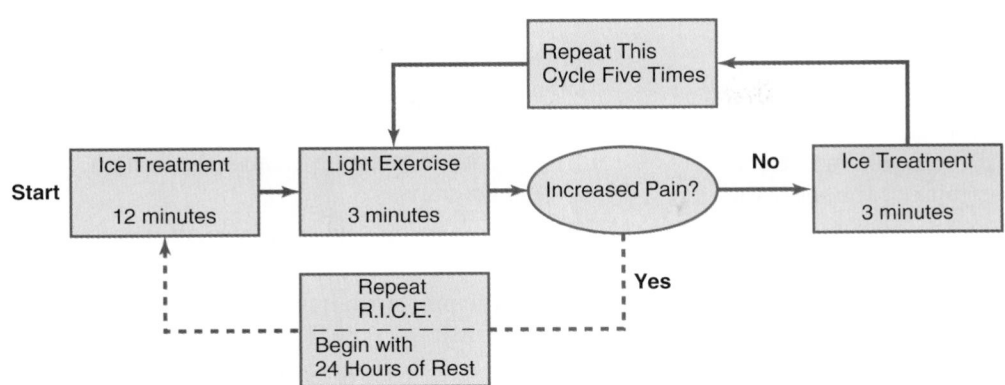

FIGURE 13.7
The steps of the cryokinetics procedure for rehabilitating injuries.

prevent further injury (9). These objectives can be met by a combination of rest, ice, compression, and elevation. The acronym **R.I.C.E.** (R-rest, I-ice, C-compression, E-elevation) is an easy way to remember this treatment protocol. The elements of R.I.C.E. should be applied as soon as possible after the injury. The logic behind using it is as follows.

Rest is required to prevent further injury. Movement of injured tissues will aggravate the injury and result in further damage. Any movement that causes pain should be avoided.

Application of ice to an injury reduces swelling by reducing blood flow to the cooled area. Minimizing swelling around an injury will reduce the pain and lead to more rapid healing. Ice should be placed in a cloth wrap to guard against skin damage due to frostbite and be applied for 30-minute periods, three to four times a day for 2 days after the injury.

Compression of the injured area also reduces swelling. The amount of compression applied is important. It should be enough to reduce fluid collection around the damaged area but should not be severe enough to inhibit blood flow. Snugly wrapping the injured area with an elastic bandage is sufficient to control swelling. Placing a bag of ice in the last two or three wraps of the elastic bandage incorporates pressure and cools at the same time.

Finally, while resting, it is beneficial to elevate the injured area, above the level of the heart if possible. Elevation reduces blood pressure and may therefore reduce swelling. Approximately 3 days following the injury, start an exercise rehabilitation program, as outlined in the next section. If you have any doubts about whether the injury is ready for rehabilitation, delay another 24 to 48 hours.

REHABILITATION

The rehabilitation of minor injuries occurs naturally. That is, after an injury has healed and swelling has subsided, most people will begin to move the injured

area at a rate that depends on the pain involved. As the pain subsides, more movement can occur, until a normal range of motion is restored. However, this rehabilitation regimen has several drawbacks. First, it is very slow. Depending on the injury, the natural rehabilitation process may take five to ten times as long as an aggressive rehabilitation program. Second, the damaged area may be reinjured because many people attempt to return to full use of the injured area too quickly. This secondary injury results in much greater damage than the first injury and can even weaken the tissue and lead to recurring injuries throughout life. Third, for many types of injury, the lack of an aggressive rehabilitation program can prevent the return of full function because the scar tissue that develops limits the normal range of motion. Fortunately, these problems may be overcome by an active rehabilitation process.

A relatively new rehabilitation technique that is implemented after the R.I.C.E. procedures have been followed is called **cryokinetics** (12). It uses approximately 12 minutes of ice application followed by 3 minutes of light exercise followed by another 3 minutes of cold. The 3 minutes of exercise and 3 minutes of ice should be repeated for five cycles. Exercising of the injured limb during this treatment must be guided by the pain associated with its use. Start with an exercise intensity that provides little or no pain. Intensity can be increased gradually as long as no increase in pain occurs. If pain increases during the cryokinetic therapy, stop the treatment and resume the R.I.C.E. procedures until the pain subsides (Figure 13.7).

R.I.C.E. An acronym representing a treatment protocol for exercise-related injuries. It stands for a combination of **R**est, **I**ce, **C**ompression, and **E**levation.
cryokinetics A relatively new rehabilitation technique that is implemented after healing has been completed. It incorporates alternating periods of treatment using ice, exercise, and rest.

The initial management of an injury is critical and determines the time required for completion of the rehabilitation process. For example, a regimen of cryokinetics initiated after a third degree ankle sprain (2–3 days postinjury) results in complete recovery within 2 weeks. In contrast, if the cryokinetic treatment starts late (5–7 days postinjury), the recovery may take 4 to 5 weeks.

As pain subsides and the range of motion returns, full recovery may be accelerated if a program of weight training and flexibility exercises is added to the treatment process. This is especially true for muscle injuries because the healing process may cause the muscle to shorten and thereby limit flexibility. A key point to remember is that an injury that does not heal properly may cause recurring pain during activity and may persist for years. Therefore, for stubborn injuries, seeking the treatment advice of a trained professional (athletic trainer, physical therapist, or physician) is often recommended.

☀ IN SUMMARY

- To reduce your risk of developing an exercise-related injury, follow these guidelines:
  (1) Engage in a program of muscle strengthening exercises to maintain balance in strength around joints.
  (2) Warm up before and cool down after each workout.
  (3) Use the proper equipment (especially proper footwear).
  (4) Increase exercise intensity and duration slowly throughout your exercise training program.
  (5) Maintain the proper rest-to-exercise ratio. Do not overtrain!
- For treating injuries, remember the R.I.C.E. protocol: rest, ice, compression, and elevation.
- A recent and effective technique for injury rehabilitation, called cryokinetics, uses alternating periods of icing, exercise, and rest.

Summary

1. Injuries associated with running occur primarily in the foot and knee because of the excessive stress placed on the legs and feet. The factors most closely associated with running injuries are improper training techniques, inadequate shoes, and alignment problems in the legs and feet.

2. Factors associated with injuries in aerobic dance are more than three sessions per week, improper shoes, and nonresilient surfaces.

3. Overtraining is the greatest risk to developing an exercise-related injury.

4. Back pain is a multifactoral problem that usually subsides without any medical intervention. Exercise, however, can play an important role in preventing back pain and rehabilitating some back problems. Exercises to increase flexibility and strength, reduce body fat, improve muscle balance between the abdominal and back muscles, and prevent osteoporosis can decrease your risk of developing back problems.

5. Acute muscle soreness may occur during or immediately after an exercise session. This type of injury may be due to muscle damage, accumulation of fluid within the muscle, and/or chemical imbalances within the muscle itself.

6. Delayed-onset muscle soreness (DOMS) sometimes occurs 24 to 48 hours after an exercise session. Eccentric exercise increases the chances that DOMS will occur.

7. When a muscle is forced to contract against excessive resistance, fibers are damaged. This damage is referred to as a strain and can range from a minor separation of fibers to a complete tear.

8. Tendonitis is one of the most common of all overuse problems associated with physical activity. The term literally means inflammation of a tendon.

9. A sprain is caused by damage to a ligament, a type of connective tissue that provides support for joints. In contrast, torn cartilage refers to damage to the tough, connective tissue that serves as a cushioning pad between the ends of bones.

10. Common injuries to the lower extremities include PFPS, in which the articular cartilage on the back of the knee cap (patella) may be damaged by chronic use during exercise; shin splints, a condition that encompasses several different injuries to the front of the lower leg; and stress fractures, which are microscopic breaks in the bone.

11. The following guidelines can help you reduce your risk of developing an exercise-related injury:
    - Engage in a program of muscle-strengthening exercises to keep a balance in strength around joints.
    - Warm up before and cool down after each workout.
    - Use the proper equipment (especially proper footwear).

- Increase exercise intensity and duration slowly throughout your exercise training program.
- Maintain the proper rest-to-exercise ratio. Do not overtrain!

12. For treating injuries, remember the R.I.C.E. protocol: rest, ice, compression, and elevation.

13. Recently, an effective new technique for injury rehabilitation called cryokinetics has come into use. This treatment calls for alternating periods of cold applications, exercise, and rest.

Study Questions

1. Discuss the risks of injury involved in running.

2. What are considered the primary causes of running injuries?

3. Discuss the risks of injury associated with aerobic dance, and the factors thought to cause the injuries.

4. Differentiate between acute and delayed-onset muscle soreness.

5. Compare and contrast a strain and a sprain.

6. Define tendonitis and describe the best method of prevention/treatment.

7. What is the cause of PFPS, and how should it be treated?

8. What causes shin splints, and how can they be prevented?

9. List the guidelines that should be followed to minimize the risk of injury from increased physical activity.

10. Define the R.I.C.E. protocol, and discuss its use.

11. Discuss the use of cryokinetics as a rehabilitation technique.

12. Define the following terms:
    arthroscopic surgery
    cartilage
    ligament
    stress fracture
    overtraining syndrome

Suggested Reading

Chou, L. H., V. Akuthota, D. F. Drake, S. D. Toledo, and S. F. Nadler, Sports and performing arts medicine. Lower-limb injuries in endurance sports. *Archives of Physical Medicine and Rehabilitation.* 2004 March 85(3 Suppl 1):S59–66, 2004.

Clarkson, P. M., and D. J. Newham. Association between muscle soreness, damage, and fatigue. *Advances in Experimental Medicine and Biology* 384:457–469, 1995.

Frontera, W., D. Dawson, and D. Slovik. *Exercise in Rehabilitation Medicine.* Champaign, IL: Human Kinetics, 1999.

Herbert, R. D., and M. Gabriel. Effects of stretching before and after exercising on muscle soreness and risk of injury: Systematic review. *British Medical Journal* 325(7362): 468, 2002.

Houglum, P. *Therapeutic Exercise for Athletic Injuries.* Champaign, IL: Human Kinetics, 2001.

Hreljac, A. Impact and overuse injuries in runners. *Medicine and Science in Sports and Exercise* 36(5):845–849, 2004.

Reilly, T., C. N. Dowzer, and N. T. Cable. The physiology of deep-water running. *Journal of Sports Sciences* 21(12): 959–972, 2003.

Thacker, S. B., J. Gilchrist, D. F. Stroup, and C. D. Kimsey. The prevention of shin splints in sports: A systematic review of literature. *Medicine and Science in Sports and Exercise* 34(1):32–40, 2002.

For links to the web sites below visit The Total Fitness and Wellness Website at www.aw-bc.com/powers.

About.com

Provides information about many aspects of fitness, health benefits of exercise, and wellness.

WebMD

Provides information about prevention and treatment of exercise-related injuries.

FamilyDoctor.com

Provides information on basic exercise injuries and sports safety.

Fitness Files

Contains information concerning fitness fundamentals, flexibility and contraindicated exercises, exercise nutrition, and the treatment of exercise injuries.

The Running Page

Contains information about racing, running clubs, places to run, running-related products, running magazines, and treating running-related injuries.

Meriter Fitness

Presents information concerning injury prevention and treatment, weight training, flexibility, exercise prescriptions, and more.

References

1. Radomski, M. Sports injuries. *Wellness Options.* Vol. 6, p. 52, 2003.

2. Murphy, D. F., D. A., Connolly, and B. D. Beynnon. Risk factors for lower extremity injury: A review of the literature. *British Journal of Sports Medicine* 37(1):13–29, 2003.

3. Duffey, M. J., D. F. Martin, D. W. Cannon, T. Craven, and S. P. Messier. Etiologic factors associated with anterior knee pain in distance runners. *Medicine and Science in Sports and Exercise* 32(11):1825–1832, 2000.

4. Macintyre, J., and E. Joy. Foot and ankle injuries in dance. *Clinics in Sports Medicine* 19(2):351–368, 2000.

5. Devereaux, M. W. Low back pain. *Primary Care* 31(1):33–51, 2004.

6. Maher, C. G. Effective physical treatment for chronic low back pain. *Orthopedic Clinics of North America* 35(1): 57–64, 2004.

7. Powers, S., and E. Howley. *Exercise Physiology: Theory and Application to Fitness and Performance*, 2nd ed. Dubuque, IA: McGraw-Hill, 2004.

8. Connolly, D.A., S. P. Sayers, and M. P. McHugh. Treatment and prevention of delayed onset muscle soreness. *Journal of Strength and Conditioning Research* 17(1):197–208, 2003.

9. Prentice, W. E. *Rehabilitation Techniques for Sports Medicine and Athletic Training*, 4th Ed., Dubuque, IA, McGraw-Hill, 2004.

10. Adirim, T. A., and T. L. Cheng. Overview of injuries in the young athlete. *Sports Medicine* 33(1):75–81, 2003.

11. Boden, B. P., D. C. Osbahr, and C. Jimenez. Low-risk stress fractures. *American Journal of Sports Medicine* 29(1):100–111, 2001.

12. Bleakley, C., S. McDonough, and D. MacAuley. The use of ice in the treatment of acute soft-tissue injury: A systematic review of randomized controlled trials. *American Journal of Sports Medicine* 32(1):251–61, 2004.

Prevention of Injuries During Exercise

NAME _____ DATE _____

The following lab is designed to help you identify and eliminate ways in which your exercise program may cause injuries.

DIRECTIONS

For the following measures associated with the prevention of injury, place a check by those you have incorporated into your exercise program (and in some cases, into your life in general). For any measure not checked, write in the space provided exactly what changes you plan to implement to reduce or eliminate the risks associated with that measure.

Preventive Measure   **Changes to Implement**

_____ Proper shoes for the activity worn   _____

_____ Proper warm-up included   _____

_____ All muscle groups involved in the activity stretched _____

_____ Over-stretching of the neck and back avoided   _____

_____ Extension and rotation of the spine avoided   _____

_____ Lifting of extremely heavy objects avoided   _____

_____ Quick, jerking movements avoided   _____

_____ All muscle groups involved in the activity
       strengthened and balanced   _____

_____ Training program properly designed   _____

_____ Appropriate frequency of exercise used   _____

_____ Appropriate intensity of exercise used   _____

_____ Appropriate duration of exercise used   _____

_____ Proper exercise techniques used   _____

_____ (For running) firm, level surface used   _____

_____ Proper cool-down included   _____

_____ Device for supporting muscle or joint used
       (if training cannot be suspended)   _____

Flexibility and Back Pain Risk

NAME _____ DATE _____

Back pain is a multifactoral problem that is preventable in most cases. There are many sources of back pain, including improper lifting techniques, weak muscles, poor posture, inflexibility, and bone disorders. The following tests will assess the flexibility in your lower back, hamstrings, and hip flexors. Choose a partner and use extreme caution in applying force.

TEST 1: BACK TO WALL

Stand with your back against a wall so that your head, shoulders, calves, and heels are all touching the wall. Try to flatten your neck and the hollow of your back by pressing your buttocks down. Your partner should be able to place just a hand between the wall and the small of your back.

Pass _____   Fail _____

INTERPRETATION

If this space is greater than the thickness of a flattened hand, you may have lumbar lordosis (increased curvature in the lower back with a forward pelvic tilt) with shortened lumbar and hip flexor muscles.

To correct or prevent lumbar lordosis, flexibility exercises to lengthen the hip flexor muscles, as well as strength and endurance exercises for the abdominal muscles, are generally recommended.

TEST 2: STRAIGHT LEG LIFT

Lie on your back with your hands behind your neck. Your partner will kneel on your left side and stabilize your right leg by placing his/her right hand on your knee. With his/her left hand, your partner should grasp your left ankle and raise your left leg as near to a right angle (90°) as possible. In this position, your lower back should be in contact with the floor and your right leg should remain straight and on the floor. Repeat this test on the opposite side.

Left side: Pass _____   Fail _____

Right side: Pass _____   Fail _____

INTERPRETATION

If your left leg bends at the knee, your hamstring muscles are short. If your back arches and/or your right leg does not remain on the floor, short lumbar muscles, hip flexors, or both are implicated.

To correct this condition, stretch the hamstrings using exercises such as the one-leg stretch shown in Chapter 6 Sample Flexibility Exercises (6.3a and 6.3b). The lower back stretch shown in 6.4a and 6.4b can be used to lengthen the lumbar muscles.

(continued on next page)

TEST 3: KNEE TO CHEST

(No partner needed) Lie on your back on a table or bench with your right leg extended beyond the edge of the table (about one-third of your thigh is off the table). Bring your left knee to your chest and grasp the back of your thigh, pulling down tightly toward your chest. Your right thigh should remain in contact with the table. Repeat this test on the opposite leg.

Left side: Pass _____   Fail _____

Right side: Pass _____   Fail _____

INTERPRETATION

If your right thigh lifts off the table while you hug your knee to your chest, a tight right hip flexor muscle is indicated.

To stretch the right hip flexor, place the left knee directly above the left ankle and stretch the right leg backward so the right knee touches the floor. Press your pelvis forward and downward. Do not bend your front knee more than 90°. Repeat on the opposite side to stretch the left hip flexor.

SUMMARY

Awareness of flexibility problems may help you alleviate back pain or prevent future back discomfort. Remember that exercises designed to increase flexibility and strength, reduce body fat, improve muscle balance between the trunk flexors and extensors, and prevent osteoporosis can decrease your risk of developing back problems.

14

Prevention of Cancer

After studying this chapter, you should be able to:

1. Define cancer.

2. Discuss the incidence of cancer in the United States.

3. List the most common types of cancer.

4. Identify factors that influence your risk of developing cancer.

5. Discuss several types of occupational carcinogens.

6. Outline ways to reduce your risk of skin cancer due to exposure to ultraviolet light.

7. Discuss the roles of diet and exercise in reducing your cancer risk.

8. Explain how free radicals increase your risk of cancer.

ancer is the second leading cause of death in the United States, and the number of deaths from cancer is increasing steadily. Current predictions are that cancer will strike approximately three of every four families, and it was estimated that during 2004 over 1.3 million new cases of cancer would be diagnosed in the United States (1). Cancer can strike at any age, although it occurs more frequently in older people. Current statistics forecast that about 25% of all U.S. citizens will eventually develop cancer (1).

Although the number of cases is on the rise, the development of new detection and treatment regimens means that cancer need not necessarily be a death sentence today. According to the American Cancer Society, more than 8 million Americans alive today have successfully survived cancer. The key to survival is early detection. If more cancers were diagnosed earlier, over one-half of cancer patients could be saved! The best aids to early detection of cancer are the seven warning signs listed in A Closer Look.

Many experts believe that the rise in cancer may be linked to cancer-causing chemicals in water and food supplies as well as to dangerous lifestyle habits such as smoking, eating high-fat diets, drinking excessively, and sunbathing (1–3). This chapter provides information about the various types of cancers and how to reduce your risk of developing cancer. Let's begin with an overview of what cancer is.

☀ What Is Cancer?

Cancer, which is the uncontrolled growth and spread of abnormal cells, is not a single disease but a collection of over 100 different but related diseases that can occur in almost every tissue and organ in the body (4, 5). Groups of these abnormal cells, called **tumors,** can be either benign or malignant. Generally, benign tumors are not serious health threats because the cells in them grow and divide relatively slowly and remain localized. In contrast, cells of malignant tumors are cancer cells; they grow rapidly and out of control, and they often spread to other locations throughout the body. As cancer cells divide unchecked, the malignant tumor grows in size and invades neighboring tissue. The growing cancer cells interfere with normal organ function, which may eventually result in organ failure, which can be fatal.

The crucial difference between benign tumor cells and cancer cells is that cancer cells can spread through-

---

cancer A collection of over 100 different diseases that can influence almost every body tissue. Cancer is the uncontrolled growth and spread of abnormal cells.
tumor A group of abnormal cells. A tumor can be either benign or malignant (cancerous).

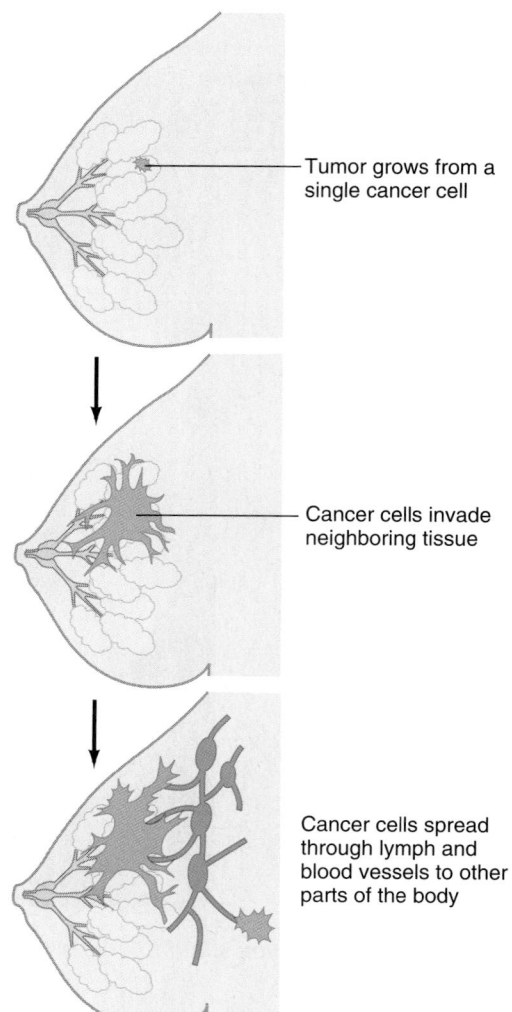

Tumor grows from a single cancer cell

Cancer cells invade neighboring tissue

Cancer cells spread through lymph and blood vessels to other parts of the body

FIGURE 14.1
Growth and metastasis of a malignant breast tumor.

out the body—a process called metastasis. Thus, for example, cancer cells that arise in the breast may invade breast tissue and eventually spread (metastasize) to other organs (Figure 14.1). Metastasis significantly reduces a cancer patient's chances of survival both because more organs are affected and because it is more difficult to treat cancer when it is in more than one location.

When an abnormal growth is discovered in the body, the only way to determine if the growth is a benign or malignant tumor is through biopsy. A biopsy is the surgical removal of a small sample of the tumor for subsequent laboratory analysis.

TYPES OF CANCER

Cancer can develop in almost any organ (4). Skin cancers are more common than cancers of any other organ (1). Other common sites for cancer include the mouth, lung, stomach, colon, kidney, liver, prostate gland, and breast (Figure 14.2). After skin cancer, the most

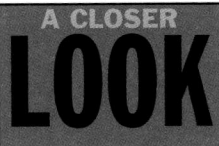

The Seven Warning Signs of Cancer

The best way to survive cancer is to detect it at the earliest possible moment, and early detection can be easier if you know the seven warning signs of cancer. One way to remember them is that each warning sign begins with the first letter of the words in the following sentence:

I Loathe **C**ancer, **T**he **B**ig **B**ad **S**courge.

Indigestion or loss of appetite that persists

Lumps or thickening in the breast or on the lips or tongue

Change in size or color of a wart or mole

Throat problems: nagging or persistent cough or hoarseness and difficulty in swallowing

Bleeding that is unexplained from the bowel, nipples, or vagina, or unexplained blood in the urine

Bowel or bladder habits that change in an obvious way

Sores that do not heal or heal only slowly

If you develop any of these signs, see a physician immediately for a cancer screening test.

Estimated New Cases*		Estimated Deaths*	
Male	**Female**	**Male**	**Female**
Prostate 230,110	Breast 215,990	Lung & Bronchus 91,930	Lung & Bronchus 68,510
Lung & Bronchus 93,110	Lung & Bronchus 80,660	Prostate 29,900	Breast 40,110
Colon & Rectum 73,620	Colon & Rectum 73,320	Colon & Rectum 28,320	Colon & Rectum 28,410
Urinary Bladder 44,640	Uterine Corpus 40,320	Pancreas 15,440	Ovary 16,090
Melanoma of the Skin 29,900	Ovary 25,580	Leukemia 12,990	Pancreas 15,830
Non-Hodgkin's Lymphoma 28,850	Non-Hodgkin's Lymphoma 25,520	Non-Hodgkin's Lymphoma 10,390	Leukemia 10,310
Kidney 22,080	Melanoma of the Skin 25,200	Esophagus 10,250	Non-Hodgkin's Lymphoma 9,020
Leukemia 19,020	Urinary Bladder 15,600	Liver 9,450	Uterine Corpus 7,090
Oral Cavity 18,550	Pancreas 16,120	Urinary Bladder 8,780	Multiple Myeloma 5,640
Pancreas 15,740	Cervix 10,520	Kidney 7,870	Brain 5,490
All Sites 699,560	All Sites 668,470	All Sites 290,890	All Sites 272,810

*Excluding basal and squamous cell skin cancer and carcinoma in situ, except urinary bladder.

FIGURE 14.2
Leading sites of new cancer cases and deaths—2004 estimates.
Source: Cancer Facts and Figures, 2004, p. 10 Reprinted by permission of the American Cancer Society, Inc. Modification is prohibited.

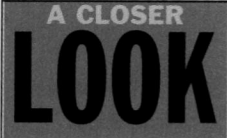

Breast Self-Examination

HOW TO EXAMINE YOUR BREASTS

The best time for a woman to examine her breasts is when the breasts are not tender or swollen. Women who are pregnant, breast-feeding, or have breast implants can also choose to examine their breasts regularly.

1. Lie down and place your right arm behind your head. The exam is done while lying down, not standing up, because when lying down the breast tissue spreads evenly over the chest wall and it is as thin as possible, making it much easier to feel all the breast tissue.

2. Use the finger pads of the three middle fingers on your left hand to feel for lumps in the right breast. Use overlapping dime-sized circular motions of the finger pads to feel the breast tissue.

3. Use three different levels of pressure to feel all the breast tissue. Light pressure is needed to feel the tissue closest to the skin; medium pressure to feel a little deeper; and firm pressure to feel the tissue closest to the chest and ribs. A firm ridge in the lower curve of each breast is normal. If you're not sure how hard to press, talk with your doctor or nurse. Use each pressure level to feel the breast tissue before moving on to the next spot.

4. Move around the breast in an up and down pattern starting at an imaginary line drawn straight down your side from the underarm and moving across the breast to the middle of the chest bone. Be sure to check the entire breast

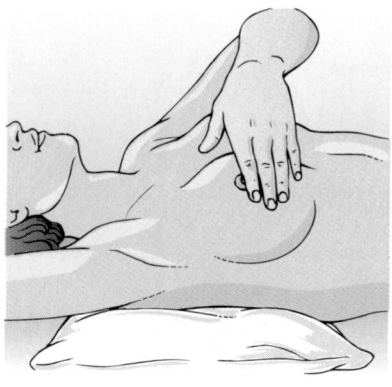

area going down until you feel only ribs and up to the neck or collar bone (clavicle).

There is some evidence to suggest that the up and down pattern (sometimes called the vertical pattern) is the most effective pattern for covering the entire breast without missing any breast tissue.

5. Repeat the exam on your left breast, using the finger pads of the right hand.

6. While standing in front of a mirror with your hands pressing firmly down on your hips, look at your breasts for any changes of size, shape, contour, or dimpling. (The pressing down on the hips position contracts the chest wall muscles and enhances any breast changes.)

7. Examine each underarm while sitting up or standing and with your arm only slightly raised so you can easily feel in this area. (Raising your arm straight up tightens the tissue in this area and makes it difficult to examine.)

Source: American Cancer Society, "Breast Awareness and Self-Examination," 2004, www.cancer.org/docroot/CRI/content/CRI_2_4_3X_Can_breast_cancer_be_found_early_5.asp?sitearea=

---

common types of cancer are prostate cancer in men and breast cancer in women (1). Over 95% of all breast cancers are discovered by women themselves; a routine breast self-examination should be a monthly practice for all women (A Closer Look, above).

Although most cancers occur in people over the age of 40, testicular cancer is one of the most common cancers in young men (1). In general, testicular tumors are first noticed as a painless enlargement of the testis. Accordingly, all young men should routinely examine their testicles (A Closer Look on the following page).

Recently, the largest increase in cancer has been in a deadly form of skin cancer known as malignant melanoma (1). The increase in this type of cancer is likely due to the diminishing layer of ozone in the earth's atmosphere, which protects us from the sun's ultraviolet rays. These rays are the primary cause of skin cancers.

In addition, there has been a tremendous increase in lung cancer in both men (90%) and women (500%) since 1960 (1). The reason for the increased incidence of lung cancer in men is unknown but may be linked to poor air quality (i.e., airborne carcinogens) in many cities. The rise in lung cancer in women is likely due to the rise in the number of female smokers over this time period. The increase is significant because lung cancer is very dangerous, resulting in more deaths among both men and women than any other form of cancer.

HOW DO NORMAL CELLS BECOME CANCEROUS?

Cell growth and division is controlled by DNA located within the cell. Normal DNA carefully regulates cell growth and division so that is occurs in a slow and

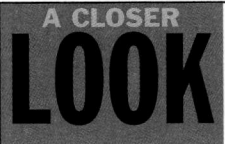

Testicular Self-Examination

Cancer of the testes is one of the most common forms of cancer in men 15 to 34 years of age (1), and it accounts for 12% of all deaths in this group. In 1990 the American Cancer Society listed the following warning signals for testicular cancer:

- A slight enlargement of one of the testicles
- A change in the consistency of a testicle
- A dull ache in the lower abdomen or groin (may not occur in all cases of testicular cancer)
- The sensation of dragging and heaviness in a testicle

Because the key to surviving testicular cancer is early detection, all young men should perform a monthly self-examination, which is best performed shortly after a warm shower or bath, when the skin of the scrotum

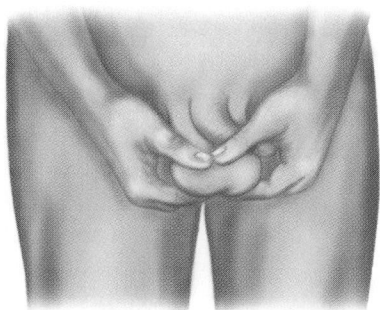

(the sac surrounding the testicle) is most relaxed. The examination is performed by rolling each testicle between the thumb and fingers (see the figure in this box). Lumps are generally found on the side or front of the testicle. Even though the presence of a lump does not necessarily indicate cancer, if you feel any lumps you should call your physician immediately to schedule a medical exam.

Source: Testicular Self Examination, by the National Cancer Institute of Health, Publication No. 93-2636, 1992.

Testicular self-examination.

---

steady fashion. Cancer occurs when DNA is damaged and cell division increases out of control.

DNA damage that results in cancer can occur in response to a number of environmental agents. These cancer-causing agents, called **carcinogens,** include radiation, chemicals, drugs, and other toxic substances (4). When a carcinogen enters the cell, it damages the DNA, which results in a normal cell becoming an abnormal cancer cell (Figure 14.3).

☀ IN SUMMARY

- Cancer is not a single disease but is a collection of diseases that can influence almost every body tissue. Cancer is the uncontrolled growth and spread of abnormal cells; a group of these abnormal cells is called a tumor.
- Common sites for cancers include the skin, colon, lungs, prostate, breasts, and bladder.
- Cancer-causing agents are called carcinogens; common carcinogens include radiation, chemicals, drugs, and other toxic substances.

CANCER RISK FACTORS

The cause of specific cancers is often unknown, but studies have revealed that a variety of carcinogens can damage normal cells and start the cancer process. A number of factors play a role in determining your cancer

risk (1, 6–8); heredity, race, radiation exposure, viruses, tobacco use, alcohol use, occupational carcinogens, ultraviolet light, and diet are all considered cancer risk factors (Figure 14.4). Let's discuss each separately.

HEREDITY If a close relative (such as a father or mother) has had cancer, your chances of developing cancer are three times greater than average (6, 7). Although the exact link between heredity and cancer remains unclear, cancers of the breast, stomach, colon, prostate, uterus, ovaries, and lungs appear to run in families. Whether these family patterns of increased cancer risk are due to genetics or the fact that people in the same family experience similar environmental risks remains unclear.

RACE Both the incidence of cancer and the cancer death rates are higher among blacks than among whites (6, 7). Over the past 40 years, cancer death among blacks rose at approximately 50%, versus a 10% increase for whites (1). The reason for the higher

---

carcinogens Cancer-causing agents, which include radiation, chemicals, drugs, and other toxic substances.

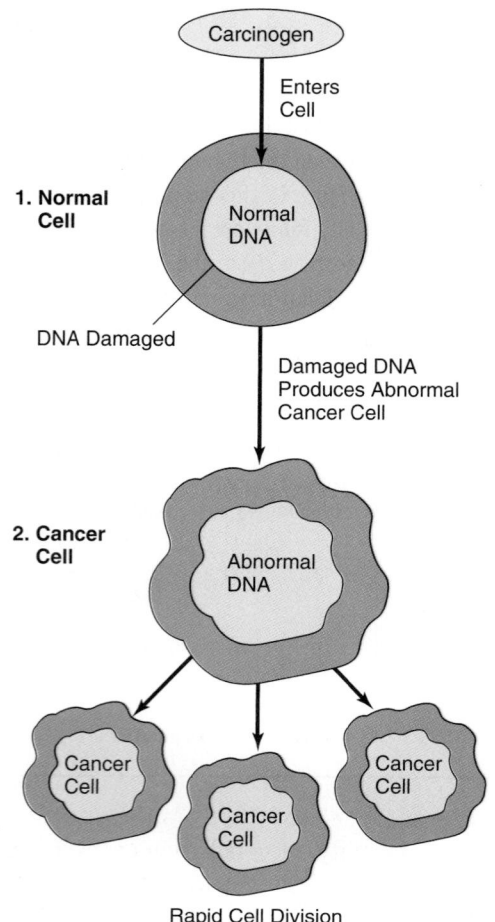

FIGURE 14.3
The transformation of a normal cell into a cancer cell. Entry of a carcinogen into the cell is followed by damage of the DNA.

death rate in blacks is unclear, but it may be linked to the fact that cancers in whites are often detected at an earlier, more treatable stage. Fitness and Wellness for All provides a few statistics on the role of race in various cancer risks.

RADIATION   Up to 5% of all cancers may be caused by radiation exposure due to medical X-rays, occupational exposure through computer monitors, and environmental radiation (8). Further, many modern conveniences that emit electromagnetic fields, such as electric blankets, and low-frequency radio waves, such as those associated with cellular telephones, have been implicated in causing cancer.

VIRUSES   It is clear that viruses are linked to many cancers (1, 8). Viruses can cause cancer by invading the cell and damaging DNA. Research has demonstrated that viruses play a role in several blood cancers (leukemias) as well as cancers of the lymphatic system (lymphomas). In addition, evidence suggests that viruses can cause liver, cervical, nose, and pharynx cancer.

TOBACCO   Tobacco use is the single largest cause of cancer deaths (approximately 25%) (6, 7, 9). Heavy smokers are 15 to 25 times more likely to die of cancer than are nonsmokers (1, 8, 9). Although the major cancer risk of smoking is the increased chance of developing lung cancer, smoking also causes an increased risk for oral cancers (of the mouth, pharynx, larynx, and esophagus), as well as of pancreas and bladder cancer (8, 9). The average life expectancy for a chronic smoker is 7 years shorter than for a nonsmoker.

The risk of developing lung cancer and other smoking-related cancers is related to the total lifetime exposure to cigarette smoke (31–33). This is measured by several factors such as the number of cigarettes smoked each day and the number of years a person has smoked. In short, the risk of developing smoking-related cancer is greatest in heavy smokers with a long history of smoking.

Even if you don't smoke, new evidence shows that secondhand tobacco smoke is also carcinogenic. Thus, you should avoid both active smoking and inhaling

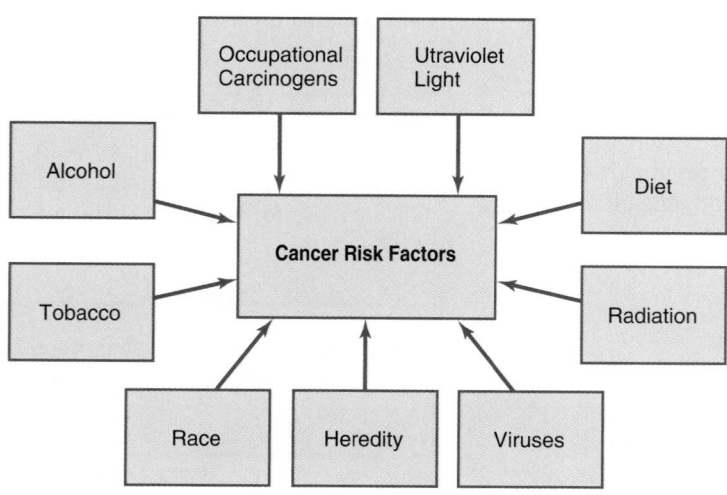

FIGURE 14.4
Cancer risk factors.

Race and the Risk of Cancer in the United States

Over 1.2 million Americans will be diagnosed with cancer this year, and during that time over 550,000 Americans are expected to die from cancer. Overall, African Americans are more likely to develop cancer than are individuals of any other racial or ethnic group in this country. During the 1990s, the cancer rates were approximately 443 per 100,000 individuals among African Americans, 403 per 100,000 among whites, 279 per 100,000 among Asians/Pacific Islanders, 275 per 100,000 among Hispanics, and 153 per 100,000 among American Indians.

The increased likelihood that African Americans will develop cancer is also apparent in the rates for specific types of cancer. African Americans have the highest incidence of colon, rectum, and lung cancers in the United States, and African-American men are 50% more likely to develop prostate cancer than men of any other racial or ethnic group in America. Moreover, the cancer death rates are also greatest among African Americans, who are 33% more likely to die of cancer than are Asians/Pacific Islanders, American Indians, and Hispanics.

---

smoke from others. Cigarettes are not the only risk from tobacco; pipes, cigars, and smokeless tobacco also increase the risk for oral cancers.

ALCOHOL   Heavy use of alcohol increases the risk for oral, esophagus, liver, and breast cancer (10). Combining drinking and smoking creates an even greater risk for developing cancer. Even moderate drinking has been linked to an increased risk of breast cancer in women.

OCCUPATIONAL CARCINOGENS   Factory workers and people living near factories may have an increased risk of cancer due to specific types of chemicals used or produced by the factory. Industrial chemicals known to be carcinogenic include benzene, nickel, chromate, asbestos, and vinyl chloride (8).

One of the most common occupational carcinogens is asbestos, a substance formerly used in the building and automobile industries. People who work with radioactive substances may also have increased risk for cancer. Working with coal tars, as in the mining professions, or working near airborne carcinogens, such as in the auto painting business, is also dangerous. Many chemicals used to kill weeds (herbicides) and insects (pesticides) contain potential carcinogens and are found in excessive amounts in some water supplies.

ULTRAVIOLET LIGHT   Exposure to the sun or to artificial tanning lights is a major contributor to an increased risk for skin cancer (1, 8). Ultraviolet radiation from these two sources is responsible for over 700,000 new cases of skin cancer each year. Tanning machines and sunlamps produce ultraviolet rays and present as much risk as do the sun's rays. Some tanning salons claim that their equipment emits ultraviolet light at different wavelengths than sunshine and is therefore

less dangerous. This is not true! If a sunlamp causes you to tan or burn, it is just as dangerous as the sun.

DIET   According to the National Academy of Sciences, diet is implicated in 60% of the cancers in women and 40% of the cancers in men (11). A high-fat diet has been linked to breast, colon, and prostate cancer, and it contributes to obesity, which in turn increases the risk for colon, breast, and uterine cancer. In addition, salt-cured, smoked, and nitrite-cured foods have been linked to cancers of the esophagus and stomach.

☀ **IN SUMMARY**

- Even though the cause of many specific cancers is often unknown, many cancer risk factors have been identified.
- Important factors that play a role in determining your risk for developing cancer include heredity, race, radiation, viruses, tobacco use, alcohol consumption, occupational carcinogens, exposure to ultraviolet light, and dietary factors.

CANCER PREVENTION

Recall from our earlier discussion of heart disease that we can control selected risk factors for CHD. Many cancers can be prevented in the same way—with lifestyle changes. Indeed, approximately 80% of all cancers are related to lifestyle and environmental factors (1, 8, 30). According to the National Cancer Institute, people who lead a healthy lifestyle have only about one-third to one-half the rate of cancer deaths compared with the general population. Thus, with a change in lifestyle and avoidance of environmental factors that increase your risk, you can prevent many cancers. The first step in reducing your risk of cancer is to identify which cancer

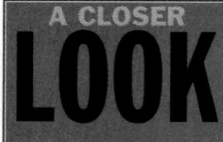

Early Detection of Skin Cancer

Skin cancer remains the most common type of cancer. Fortunately, many types of skin cancer are curable if detected and treated early. The key to early detection is self-examination. This exam should be performed monthly and should include the entire body, particularly those areas of the body exposed to the sun. When examining your skin, begin by examining your moles. Almost everyone has moles and while the vast majority of moles are harmless, a change in a mole's appearance is a sign that you should see your doctor. When examining moles, use the simple ABCD rule to help you remember the important signs of melanoma and other skin cancers.

- **A** is **Asymmetry:** Note if one-half of a mole does not match the other half.
- **B** is for **Border:** Notice if the border of the mole is irregular, ragged, or notched.
- **C** is for **Color:** Take note if the color of the mole is not the same all over. That is, does the mole have differing shades of black, brown, and sometimes patches of red or white.
- **D** is for **Diameter:** Notice if the diameter of the mole is larger than 6 millimeters (about the size of a pencil eraser). Importantly, note if the mole appears to be growing in size.

It is important to appreciate that some skin cancers may not fit the ABCD rule described above, so it is particularly important for you to notice any changes in skin lesions or the appearance of a new skin lesion. Other warning signs of skin cancer are as follows:

- A sore that does not heal.
- A new growth of any kind.
- Spread of pigment from the border of a spot to surrounding skin.
- Redness or a new swelling beyond the border of a mole.
- Change in sensation on the skin, such as itchiness, tenderness, or pain.
- Change in the surface of a mole, such as scaliness, oozing, bleeding, or the appearance of a bump or nodule.

If you observe any of these changes in your skin, schedule an appointment with your physician as soon as possible to have this potential problem evaluated. Remember that many skin cancers can be successfully treated; however, early detection is the key in treatment of any cancer.

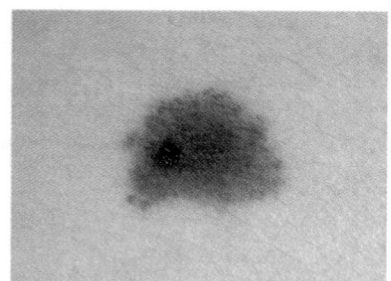

(a)

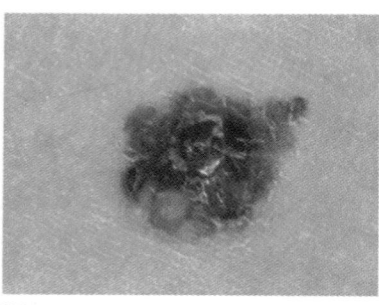

(b)

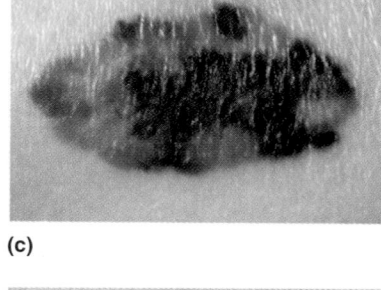

(c)

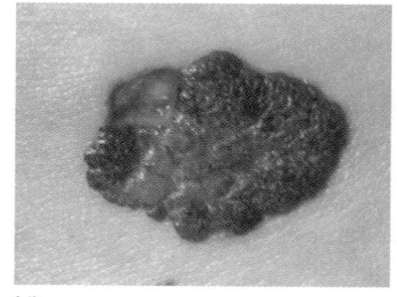

(d)

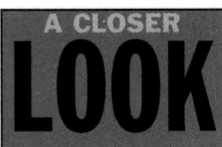

Protect Your Skin from Ultraviolet (UV) Rays

Lotions containing a sunscreen—a substance that protects the skin from UV radiation—should be applied approximately 30 minutes prior to exposure, because the protective ingredients require several minutes to be absorbed. The sunscreen should have a sun protection factor (**SPF**) of at least 15, which provides you with 15 times greater protection than unprotected skin. To better understand the meaning of SPF, consider the following example. If a fair-skinned person exposed to bright sunlight experiences a sunburn following 10 min-utes of sun exposure, then the use of a sunscreen rated at 15 SPF would increase the amount of time required to burn by a factor of 15. That is, use of a 15 SPF sunscreen would increase the amount of time required for sunburn from 10 minutes to 150 minutes (i.e., 10 minutes $\times$ 15 SPF = 150 minutes). The following guidelines can reduce your risk of developing skin cancer due to overexposure to ultraviolet rays.

1. Stay out of the sun between 10:00 A.M. and 2:00 P.M., when UV rays are the strongest.

2. If you use any skin preparation containing vitamin A (Retin A), stay out of the sun. Retin A skin lotions increase your susceptibility to UV damage.

3. Avoid sunlamps and tanning booths. If sunlamps tan you, they damage your skin.

4. When exercising outdoors or during swimming, use a waterproof sunscreen, and apply it often and in adequate quantities.

5. Avoid sunburn by limiting your sun exposure.

6. Reapply sunscreen often. This particularly applies when swimming or sweating during sun exposure.

---

risk factors apply to you (Laboratory 14.1, p. 385). The next step is to modify those aspects of your environment and lifestyle that increase your chances of developing cancer. Although each individual's heredity (including race) is a given, the following cancer risk factors can be modified.

ALCOHOL   Oral cancer and cancers of the larynx, throat, esophagus, and liver occur more frequently among heavy drinkers of alcohol (8). Because even moderate alcohol consumption has been implicated as a cause of some cancers, it is wise to abstain from alcohol consumption or to at least decrease your consumption to a low level. Remember, combining alcohol and tobacco puts you at even greater risk.

RADIATION   Avoid overexposure to any source of radiation. Medical X-rays, low-frequency radio waves, and other sources of low-level radiation may not be avoidable and are not harmful unless encountered in excess.

TOBACCO   Both cigarette smoking and use of smokeless tobacco increase your risk of cancer. Cigarette smoking is responsible for 87% of all lung cancer cases, and use of chewing tobacco or snuff increases your risk of cancer of the mouth, larynx, throat, and esophagus (8, 9). Cancer risks can be greatly reduced by abstaining from all tobacco products. If you have never used any tobacco products, don't start. If you are using tobacco products, stop. Many of the detrimental effects of tobacco can be reversed if you quit using them. Indeed, quitting smoking can reduce the risk of having lung cancer and other cancers. Importantly, the risk of cancer decreases as the number of years since quitting increases. Even long-term smokers who quit after age 50 substantially reduce their risk of dying early from cancer (32, 33). Therefore, the argument that it is too late to quit smoking because the damage is already done is not true.

OCCUPATIONAL CARCINOGENS   Avoid all industrial pollutants and follow safety procedures in the workplace. In particular, avoid exposure to industrial agents such as radon, dioxins, nickel, chromate, asbestos, and vinyl chloride. If you have questions concerning the carcinogenic risks of chemical exposure in your workplace, contact the Environmental Protection Agency (EPA). The EPA can provide you with a complete list of cancer-causing chemicals and identify those used in your workplace.

ULTRAVIOLET LIGHT   Prolonged exposure to ultraviolet light from any source can damage your skin and increase your risk of cancer (8, 28). Limiting your sun exposure is an obvious way to avoid the carcinogenic effect of ultraviolet light. If you must be exposed to the sun for work or recreation, wear protective clothing and use a sunscreen on exposed skin to block the effects of ultraviolet light (A Closer Look).

Remember, there is no such thing as a safe tan (12). All ultraviolet exposure to your skin can be damaging

---

SPF   Abbreviation for "sun protection factor." A sunscreen with an SPF of 15 provides you with 15 times more protection than unprotected skin.

whether you tan quickly or accumulate it slowly over time. Although the need for protection from the sun is now widely advocated, most people associate such protection with the occasional extreme exposure (e.g., day at the beach) and tend to ignore the long-term day-to-day exposure to the sun. However, studies have shown that over the course of a lifetime, a person will receive tens of thousands of doses of damaging ultraviolet radiation (28). Unfortunately, this cumulative exposure to the sun greatly increases your risk of developing skin cancer (28). Therefore, this cumulative effect of casual sun exposure over the years underscores the need for everyday basic sunscreen protection. How much daily sunscreen protection do you need to reduce your risk of cancer? A definitive answer to this question is not available but research shows that daily use of even low-level sunscreen (i.e., SPF 4–10) can reduce your lifetime ultraviolet exposure by 50% or more (28). See A Closer Look on p. 378 for early warning signs of skin cancer.

DIET Diet is probably the most important factor in controlling your risk of cancer (11). Among the primary nutrients in foods that seem to have a protective effect against cancer are vitamins A, E, and C (13), which appear to protect cells against damage by free radicals (also called *oxygen radicals*). Free radicals are normally produced in cells, but when they are produced in large quantities they promote the development of cancer by binding to DNA, altering its structure and function such that the cell divides rapidly and out of control (Figure 14.5). Recent research has shown that vitamins A, E, and C may reduce the risk of cancer because they are antioxidants, substances that remove free radicals from cells and thus prevent DNA damage. These findings have prompted many cancer experts to recommend a diet that is high in antioxidants (Nutritional Links to Health and Fitness).

Nutritional Links
TO HEALTH AND FITNESS

Foods High in Antioxidants May Reduce Your Risk of Cancer

The antioxidants beta carotene (which the body converts to vitamin A), vitamin C, and vitamin E appear to reduce an individual's risks of cancer (and perhaps of other diseases as well) by neutralizing free radicals (11, 12, 23). Therefore, increasing your dietary intake of antioxidants is an important dietary goal.

Among the best sources of beta carotene are apricots, asparagus, broccoli, carrots, peas, spinach, and tomatoes. Foods that contain substantial amounts of vitamin C include asparagus, broccoli, cauliflower, grapefruit, oranges, peppers, red cabbage, tangerines, and tomatoes. Foods high in vitamin E include vegetable oils, nuts, and seeds; vitamin E is also present in low levels in a variety of other foods.

Nutritionists remain divided on whether you should use vitamin supplements to increase your intake of antioxidants. Even though some researchers have suggested that it is safe to supplement your diet with up to 400 units of vitamin E and up to 500 mg of vitamin C (24), it remains a good idea to consult your physician or dietician before deciding to use vitamin supplements to raise your dietary intake of antioxidants.

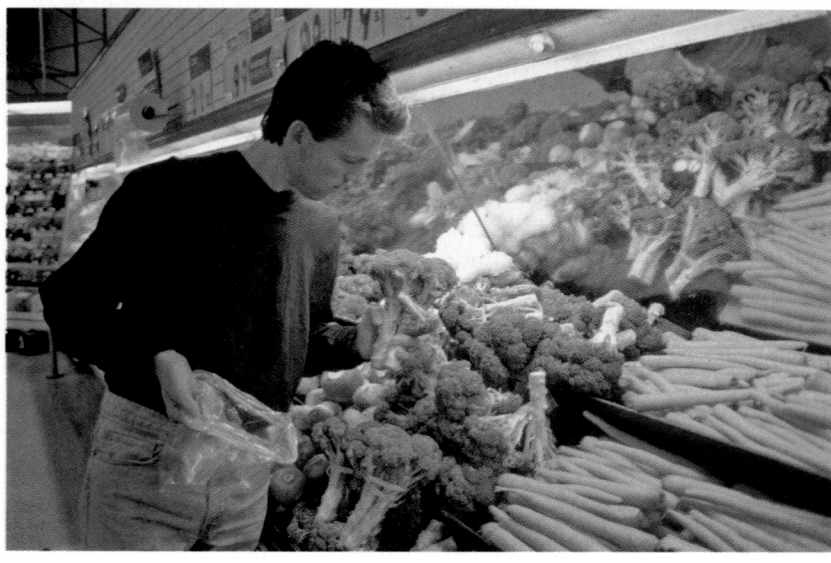

Foods such as broccoli and carrots contain primary nutrients that can protect against cancer.

Cancer Deaths in Men and Women

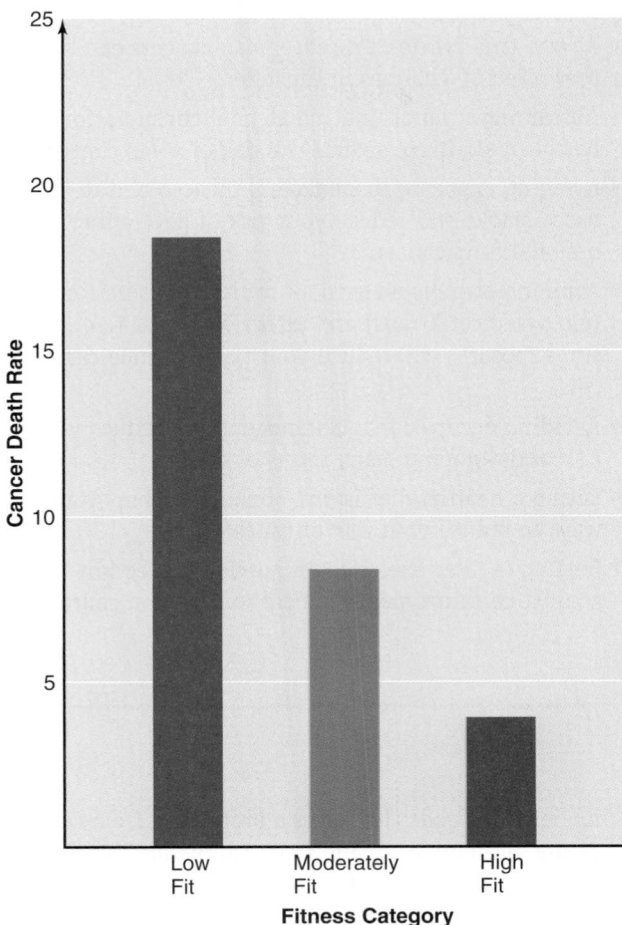

FIGURE 14.5
The declining risks of dying from cancer associated with increased exercise-related fitness. Cancer death rate is expressed as number of deaths per 10,000 men and women per year.

Consumption of a high-fiber diet lowers your risk of colon and rectal cancers. The apparent advantage of a high-fiber diet is that fiber in food increases the frequency of bowel movements, which by decreasing the time the colon and rectum are exposed to dietary carcinogens, reduces the risk of cancer.

Even though dietary fat has been hypothesized to be a risk factor for colon and rectal cancer, recent studies (14–17) suggest that fat per se is not a major risk factor in most cancers. These studies indicate instead that consumption of more than 4 oz of red meat or more than 1 oz of processed meat per day increases your risk of colon and rectal cancers by 12–49%. The biological link between cancer and the ingestion of red meat remains unclear and is the focus of intensive research. For a list of dietary guidelines for lowering your risk of cancer, see Nutritional Links to Health and Fitness on this page.

Nutritional Links
TO HEALTH AND FITNESS

Dietary Guidelines for Lowering Cancer Risk

The American Cancer Society has issued the following nutritional guidelines for lowering your risk of cancer (1):

1. **Avoid obesity.** Sensible eating habits and regular exercise will help you avoid excessive weight gain. Obesity increases your risk of colon, breast, gallbladder, prostate, ovarian, and uterine cancers.

2. **Reduce your fat intake.** Reduce the intake of total dietary fat to less than 30% of total calories consumed, and reduce the intake of saturated fat to less than 10% of total calories. A high-fat diet increases your risk of breast, colon, and prostate cancers.

3. **Eat more high-fiber foods.** Regular consumption of cereals, fresh fruits, and vegetables is recommended. Increasing your fiber intake may reduce your risk of colon cancer.

4. **Include foods rich in vitamins A, C, and E in your daily diet.** These vitamins may reduce your risk of cancer by removing free radicals. See Nutritional Links to Health and Fitness on p. 380 for a list of foods containing these vitamins.

5. **Include cruciferous vegetables in your diet.** Research has shown that cabbage, broccoli, brussels sprouts, kohlrabi, and cauliflower may help reduce the incidence of certain types of cancers. Why these particular vegetables reduce cancer risk is unclear and continues to be the subject of active research.

6. **Eat salt-cured, smoked, and nitrate-cured foods in moderation.** Numerous studies have reported a high incidence of cancer in people who consume large quantities of these foods.

7. **Keep alcohol consumption moderate.** High consumption of alcohol increases the risk of cancers of the mouth, larynx, throat, esophagus, and liver.

EXERCISE REDUCES THE RISK OF CANCER

Some studies (2, 18–22, 28) have provided evidence that regular exercise may provide some protection against dying from cancer (Figure 14.5). The best evidence comes from studies demonstrating that people who engage in regular exercise have a lower incidence of colon cancer (21). In addition, some reports suggest that exercise training reduces the occurrence of breast and uterine cancer in women (20).

The primary debate about how exercise protects against cancer centers around the question, "Does exercise alter the immune system to reduce the formation of cancer cells?" Tumors are normally formed in everyone from time to time, but the immune system typically destroys the abnormal cells before they increase in number. Therefore, a strong immune system acts to reduce the risk of cancer, whereas a weak immune system may increase your risk of cancer. Although numerous studies suggest that physically active individuals have an increased resistance to infection (25) and a decreased incidence of certain forms of cancer (2, 18–20), scientific evidence that indicates that exercise positively alters the immune system is limited (26, 27). Therefore, it may be that factors other than adaptation of the immune system are responsible for the observation that exercise is associated with a reduced risk of cancer.

☀ IN SUMMARY

- As was true for heart disease, may cancers can be prevented by changes in lifestyle.
- Abstaining from or limiting alcohol consumption has been shown to reduce the risk of some cancers.
- Avoiding exposure to smokeless tobacco and to tobacco smoke will reduce your risk of developing oral and lung cancer.
- Avoiding overexposure to all sources of radiation (e.g., medical X-rays) and ultraviolet light (e.g., sun exposure) will reduce your risk for some cancers.
- Avoiding occupational carcinogens will reduce your risk of developing many forms of cancer.
- Eating a healthy diet is one of the most important ways to reduce your risk of cancer.
- Getting regular exercise can provide protection against certain types of cancer (e.g., colon cancer).

Summary

1. The diseases known as cancers are major killers, and the incidence of these diseases is increasing. Currently, cancer is the number two cause of death in the United States.

2. Cancer is the uncontrolled growth and spread of abnormal cells. Groups of abnormal cells can form a tumor, which can be classified as either benign (abnormal growth but not life threatening) or malignant (consist of cancerous cells, which are life threatening because they will eventually spread to other tissues and disrupt organ function).

3. Carcinogens are cancer-causing agents.

4. Skin cancer is the most common type of cancer. Other common sites of cancer include the mouth, lung, colon, stomach, liver, bone, prostate gland, and breast.

5. Normal cells become cancerous when DNA becomes damaged, which results in uncontrolled cell division.

6. Heredity, race, radiation, viruses, tobacco, alcohol, occupational carcinogens, ultraviolet light, and a low-fiber diet are factors that increase your risk of developing cancer. Cancer risk can be lowered by reducing your exposure to radiation, tobacco, alcohol, ultraviolet light, and occupational carcinogens.

7. Approximately 80% of all cancers are related to lifestyle and environmental factors.

8. Diet is probably the most important factor in controlling your risk of cancer. Among the primary nutrients in foods that offer a protection from cancer are vitamins A, E, and C, which reduce the risk of cancer by removing free radicals.

9. Exercise has been shown to reduce the risk of colon, uterine, and breast cancer.

Study Questions

1. Define the following terms:
   cancer
   carcinogen
   tumor

2. What is the most common type of cancer?

3. How do normal cells become cancerous?

4. List nine cancer risk factors.

5. What does SPF stand for, and how is it defined?

6. Exercise has been shown to reduce the risk of which types of cancer?

7. What is an antioxidant? How do antioxidants reduce the risk of cancer?

8. What types of cancer are linked to tobacco use?

9. Name five occupational carcinogens.

10. Discuss the signs of skin cancer.

11. Outline the dietary guidelines for reducing your risk of cancer.

Suggested Reading

American Cancer Society. *2004 Cancer facts and figures.* Atlanta: American Cancer Society, 2004.

Bauman, A. Updating the evidence that physical activity is good for health: An epidemiological review 2000–2003. *Journal of Science and Medicine in Sports* 7:6–19, 2004.

Bostwick, D. G. The American Cancer Society: Prostate Cancer Atlanta: American Cancer Society, 1999.

Eyre, H. et al. Preventing cancer, cardiovascular disease, and diabetes. *Stroke* 35:1–12, 2004.

Nole, G., and A. Johnson. An analysis of cumulative lifetime solar ultraviolet radiation exposure and the benefits of daily sun protection. *Dermatology Therapy* 17: 57–62, 2004.

Tannock, I., and R. P. Hill. *The Basic Science of Oncology.* St. Louis: McGraw-Hill, 1998.

Thune, I., and A. Furberg. Physical activity and cancer risk: Dose-response and cancer, all sites and site specific. *Medicine and Science in Sports and Exercise* 33: S530–S550, 2001.

Stix, G. Overcoming self: A company tries to turn the immune system against cancer. *Scientific American* 291:40–41, 2004.

Willett, W. Diet and cancer: One view at the start of the millennium. *Cancer, Epidemiology, Biomarkers and Prevention* 10:3–8, 2001.

For links to the web sites below visit The Total Fitness and Wellness Website at www.aw-bc.com/powers.

Mayo Clinic Health

Provides wide-ranging information about cancer and many other health-related issues.

American Medical Association

Presents many sources of information about a wealth of medical problems, including cancer.

WebMD

Contains information on a wide variety of diseases and medical problems, including cancer.

American Cancer Society

Includes up-to-date information, including cancer statistics, risk factors, and current treatments.

References

1. American Cancer Society. *2004 Cancer Facts and Figures.* Atlanta: American Cancer Society, 2004.

2. Gerhardsson, M., S. E. Norell, H. Kiviranta, N. L. Pedersen, and A. Ahlbom. Sedentary jobs and colon cancer. *American Journal of Epidemiology* 123:775–780, 1986.

3. *The Cancer Process.* Philadelphia, PA: The American Institute for Cancer Research, November 1991.

4. Robbins, S., and V. Kumar. *Basic Pathology.* Philadelphia: W. B. Saunders, 1997.

5. Tannock, I., and R. P. Hill, eds. *The Basic Science of Oncology.* St. Louis: McGraw-Hill, 1998.

6. American Cancer Society, Texas Division. *Cancer: Assessing Your Risk.* Dallas: American Cancer Society, 1982.

7. Greenwald, P. Assessment of risk factors for cancer. *Preventive Medicine* 9:260–263, 1980.

8. National Cancer Institute. *Cancer rates and risks.* U.S. Dept. of Health and Human Services. NIH Publication No. 85-691, Bethesda, MD, 1985.

9. Fielding, J. Smoking: Health effects and controls. *New England Journal of Medicine* 313:491–497, 1985.

10. Rothman, K. The proportion of cancer attributable to alcohol consumption. *Preventive Medicine* 9:174–179, 1980.

11. *Surgeon General's Report on Nutrition and Health.* Washington, DC: Diane Publishing Co., 1994.

12. Donatelle, R., and L. Davis. *Access to Health: Brief Second Edition.* Englewood Cliffs, NJ: Prentice Hall, 1996.

13. Kanter, M. Free radicals and exercise: Effects of nutritional antioxidant supplementation. *Exercise and Sport Science Reviews* 23:375–397, 1995.

14. Willett, W. C. Diet and cancer. *Oncologist* 5:393–404, 2000.

15. Sandu, M., I. White, and K. McPherson. Systematic review of prospective cohort studies on meat consumption and colorectal cancer risk: A meta-analytical approach. *Cancer, Epidemiology, Biomarkers and Prevention* 10:439–496, 2001.

16. Norat, T., and E. Roboli. Meat consumption and colorectal cancer: A review of epidemiological evidence. *Nutritional Reviews* 59:37–47, 2001.

17. Willett, W. Diet and cancer: One view at the start of the millennium. *Cancer, Epidemiology, Biomarkers and Prevention* 10:3–8, 2001.

18. Vena, J. E., S. Graham, M. Zielezny, J. Brasure, and M. K. Swanson. Occupational exercise and risk of cancer. *American Journal of Clinical Nutrition* 45:318–327, 1987.

19. Paffenbarger, R. S., R. T. Hyde, A. L. Wing, and C. C. Hsieh. Physical activity, all-cause mortality of college alumni. *New England Journal of Medicine* 314:605–613, 1986.

20. Frisch, R. E., G. Wyshak, N. L. Albright, et al. Lower prevalence of breast cancer and cancers of the reproductive system among former college athletes compared to non-athletes. *British Journal of Cancer* 52:885–891, 1985.

21. Blair, S., H. Kohl, R. Paffenbarger, D. Clark, K. Cooper, and L. Gibbons. Physical fitness and all-cause mortality: A prospective study of healthy men and women. *Journal of American Medical Association* 262:2395–2401, 1989.

22. Thune, I., and A. Furberg. Physical activity and cancer risk: Dose-response and cancer, all sites and site specific. *Medicine and Science in Sports and Exercise* 33:S530-S550, 2001.

23. Leeds, M. *Nutrition for Healthy Living.* Boston: WCB-McGraw-Hill, 1998.

24. Clarkson, P. Vitamins and trace minerals. In *Ergogenics,* D. Lamb and M. Williams, eds. Madison, WI: Brown and Benchmark, 1991.

25. Nash, M. Exercise and immunology. *Medicine and Science in Sports and Exercise* 26:125–127, 1994.

26. Woods, J., and M. Davis. Exercise, monocyte/macrophage function, and cancer. *Medicine and Science in Sports and Exercise* 26:147–157, 1994.

27. Shepard, R., S. Rhind, and P. Shek. The impact of exercise on the immune system: NK cells, interleukins 1 and 2, and related responses. *Exercise and Sport Sciences Reviews* 23:215–241, 1995.

28. Bauman, A. Updating the evidence that physical activity is good for health: An epidemiological review 2000–2003. *Journal of Science and Medicine in Sports* 7:6–19, 2004.

29. Nole, G., and A. Johnson. An analysis of cumulative lifetime solar ultraviolet radiation exposure and the benefits of daily sun protection. *Dermatology Therapy* 17:57–62, 2004.

30. Eyre, H. et al. Preventing cancer, cardiovascular disease, and diabetes. *Stroke* 35:1–12, 2004.

31. Edwards, R. The problem of tobacco smoking. *British Medical Journal* 328:217–219, 2004.

32. Westmaas, J., and T. Brandon. Reducing risk in smokers. *Current Opinion Pulmonary Medicine* 10:284–288, 2004.

33. Stein, C., and G. Colditz. Modifiable risk factors for cancer. *British Journal of Cancer* 90:299–303, 2004.

Determining Your Cancer Risk

NAME _____ DATE _____

The purpose of this laboratory is to increase your awareness of your risk of developing all forms of cancer. Complete the following questions by putting a check under either "Yes" or "No."

The more times you put a check under "Yes," the more risk factors you have for developing cancer. If you checked "Yes" even once, you should take steps to modify your lifestyle and reduce your risk for cancer. For some specific information about lowering your cancer risks, see the text.

	Yes	No
1. Do you have a family history of cancer?	_____	_____
2. Do you have a fair complexion?	_____	_____
3. Are you regularly exposed to occupational carcinogens or various types of radiation?	_____	_____
4. Is your skin regularly exposed to excessive sunlight?	_____	_____
5. Do you consume more than 4 oz of red meat or 1 oz of processed meat per day?	_____	_____
6. Do you regularly eat smoked foods?	_____	_____
7. Is your diet low in fiber?	_____	_____
8. Are you obese?	_____	_____
9. Do you consume an excessive amount of alcohol?	_____	_____
10. Do you use tobacco products or breathe secondhand tobacco smoke?	_____	_____

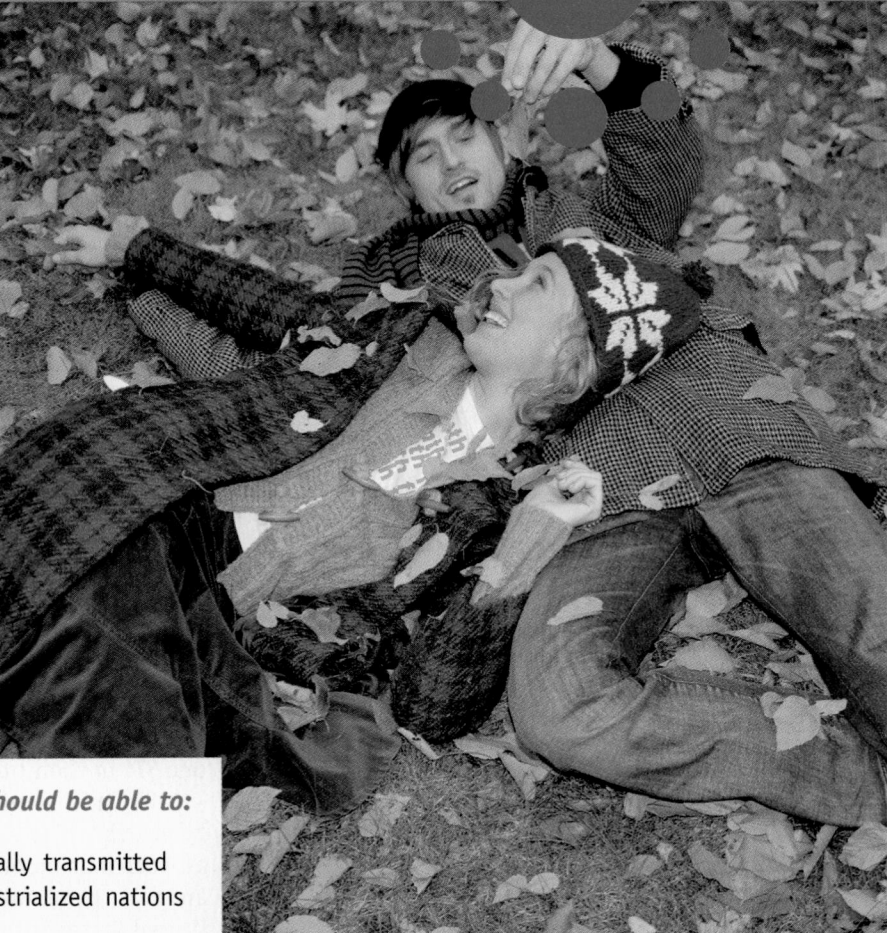

15

After studying this chapter, you should be able to:

1. Compare the incidence of sexually transmitted infections (STIs) between industrialized nations and developing countries.

2. Discuss the progressive stages of acquired immunodeficiency syndrome (AIDS) and explain why prevention of AIDS is essential.

3. Describe how the human immunodeficiency virus (HIV) is transmitted from individual to individual.

4. Outline how the following STIs are transmitted from individual to individual: trichomoniasis, chlamydia, hepatitis B, gonorrhea, venereal warts, genital herpes, and syphilis.

5. List and outline the symptoms and treatments of the most common sexually transmitted infections in the United States.

6. Identify the guidelines to reduce your risk of acquiring sexually transmitted infections.

Sexually Transmitted Infections

Throughout this book we have discussed factors that influence your health and well-being. An important risk factor that can negatively affect health and wellness is **sexually transmitted infections (STIs).** Because of the large number of young people impacted by STIs, one of the national health objectives for Healthy People 2010 is to promote responsible sexual behavior among adolescents. This chapter discusses STIs as a health threat and discusses ways to reduce your risk of contracting a sexually transmitted infection.

☼ Sexually Transmitted Infections

STIs have been called a "hidden epidemic" that is posing serious economic and health consequences to the United States (28). The Federal Institute of Medicine has issued the warning that STIs represent a growing threat to the nation's health and national action is urgently needed to decrease the growing rate of STIs (30). STIs are a challenge to public health because of their "hidden" nature. That is, STIs are often "silent" diseases because early symptoms are often ignored and untreated. Further, although STIs can be diagnosed through medical testing, routine screening programs are not widespread and social stigmas about STIs often prevent infected individuals from visiting healthcare professionals for testing (30). Therefore, many cases of STIs go unreported, resulting in an underestimation of the total number of people infected with STIs.

Current estimates indicate over 15 million people in the United States are infected each year by one or more STIs (1, 28). In fact, compared with other countries, the rate of STIs in the United States far exceeds those of every other industrialized nation (28). A complete explanation for this fact is not available; however, it seems likely that a lack of education and public awareness of the dangers of STIs play a role in the high incidence of STIs in the United States.

The United States is not the only country that STIs pose a significant health threat. Indeed, STIs also pose a major health problem in many other countries (see Fitness and Wellness for All). STIs are generally spread through sexual contact. More than 25 different STIs have been identified, and statistics reveal that one in

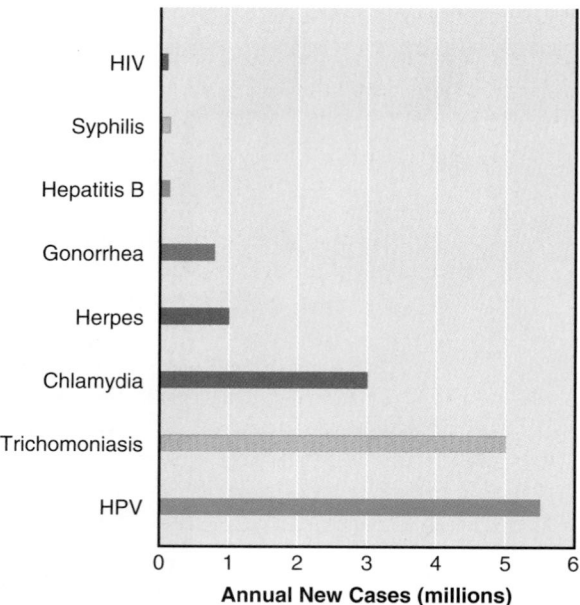

Most Common STIs in the United States

Annual New Cases (millions)

FIGURE 15.1
The most common STIs in the United States as estimated by annual new cases of the infection.
Key for abbreviations: HIV—human immunodeficiency virus; HPV—human papillomavirus
Source: Data are from the Centers for Disease Control and Prevention (12).

four people in the United States will contract at least one STI in their lifetime.

While it is well known that STIs pose a significant health threat to Americans, it is also clear that STIs are an economic burden as well. Indeed, current estimates are that the annual comprehensive cost of STIs in the United States is in excess of $12 billion. Some of the most common STIs in the United States include acquired immunodeficiency syndrome (AIDS), trichomoniasis, chlamydia, hepatitis B, gonorrhea, venereal warts, genital herpes, and syphilis (2) (Figure 15.1). Because of its important worldwide health ramifications, we begin our discussion of STIs with a detailed look at AIDS.

AIDS

In the early 1980s, physicians in San Francisco, Los Angeles, and New York began noticing repeated occurrences of rare diseases among young and previously healthy men. It was quickly determined that these problems were the result of a severely impaired immune system. Even before the virus responsible for the breakdown in the immune system was discovered, this disease was given the name **Acquired Immunodeficiency Syndrome** or **AIDS** (28). The explanation for the choice of AIDS as a name for this disorder is as follows (28):

A —The disease is not inherited but must be *acquired*

---

sexually transmitted infections (STIs) A group of more than 25 infections that are generally spread through sexual contact.
AIDS A fatal disease that develops from infection by the human immunodeficiency virus, or HIV.

I —*Immuno*, because the virus affects the immune system (your immune system is responsible for protection against infectious diseases and cancer)

D —*Deficiency*, because the body's immune system is deficient

S —*Syndrome*, because the symptoms of AIDS occur together

The virus that causes AIDS was discovered in the mid-1980s and named human immunodeficiency virus (HIV). A virus is a tiny infectious agent that cannot live independently and must invade a host cell to survive. When HIV enters the bloodstream, immune cells rush to the virus in an attempt to destroy this invading agent. However, upon entry into the bloodstream, HIV enters circulating immune cells and uses these cells as a host to replicate itself. Importantly, the entry of HIV into immune cells eventually disarms these cells and impairs the body's ability to fight infections. Over time, the level of HIV in the blood increases and the immune system gradually becomes weaker and weaker resulting in immunodeficiency and the development of AIDS. Later in this chapter, we will discuss the difference between HIV and full-blown AIDS.

INCIDENCE OF AIDS Current estimates are that over a million people in the United States are infected with HIV, and this number is growing every day (3–8). Moreover, the number of deaths from AIDS is also increasing each year. In fact, AIDS is one of the leading causes of death in American men ages 25 to 44, and the fourth leading cause of death among women in the same age group (9). In the beginning of the AIDS epidemic in the United States, the disease was predominant among homosexuals; however, the incidence of AIDS among heterosexual Americans is on the rise. For more details on who's becoming infected with AIDS, see Figure 15.2 for a look at the race and gender distributions of new HIV infections in the United States.

AIDS/HIV is not only a major health problem in the United States; the number of people infected with HIV is increasing all over the world. It is currently estimated that over 40 million people worldwide are infected with HIV, over 28 million of them in Africa alone (Figure 15.3). Clearly, AIDS/HIV is a global health threat that will create great socioeconomic problems for future generations.

STAGES OF HIV INFECTION

Many people infected with HIV are often unaware that they carry the virus because symptoms may not appear for months or even years after infection. Evidence now suggests that in many cases the virus may remain dormant in the body for five to ten years before creating health problems (2, 5, 10). After this incubation

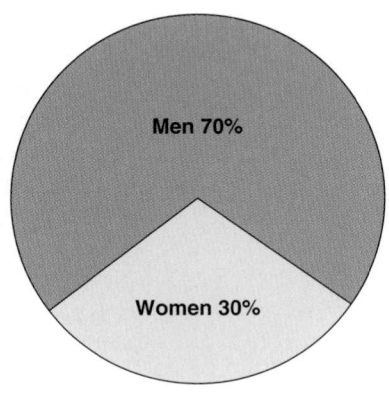

(a) Estimates of Annual New Infections by Gender

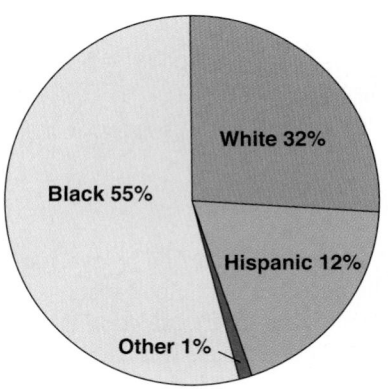

(b) Estimates of Annual New Infections by Race

FIGURE 15.2
Each year over 40,000 Americans become infected with HIV. The pie charts above indicate that certain groups of Americans are becoming infected with HIV disproportionately compared to their proportion of the U.S. population. For example, even though men make up about half of the population, 70% of new HIV infections each year occur in men (a). Moreover, although African Americans account for only 13% of the U.S. population, more than half of all new HIV infections occur in that group (b).
Source: Data are from the Centers for Disease Control and Prevention (12).

period, the virus begins to multiply and eventually damages specific cells within the immune system. Because an impaired immune system is incapable of preventing infections, from the common cold to cancer, the body becomes vulnerable to a variety of diseases. When serious disease symptoms appear due to HIV infection, the individual has developed AIDS.

Once an individual is infected with HIV, the natural course of the infection progresses into AIDS in three stages (Figure 15.4) (25). The first stage after HIV enters the body is the silent stage. During this stage, there are no physical symptoms and the only evidence of HIV is the development of HIV antibodies in the blood. Typically, HIV antibodies are formed within two weeks after infection with HIV, but it can take up to

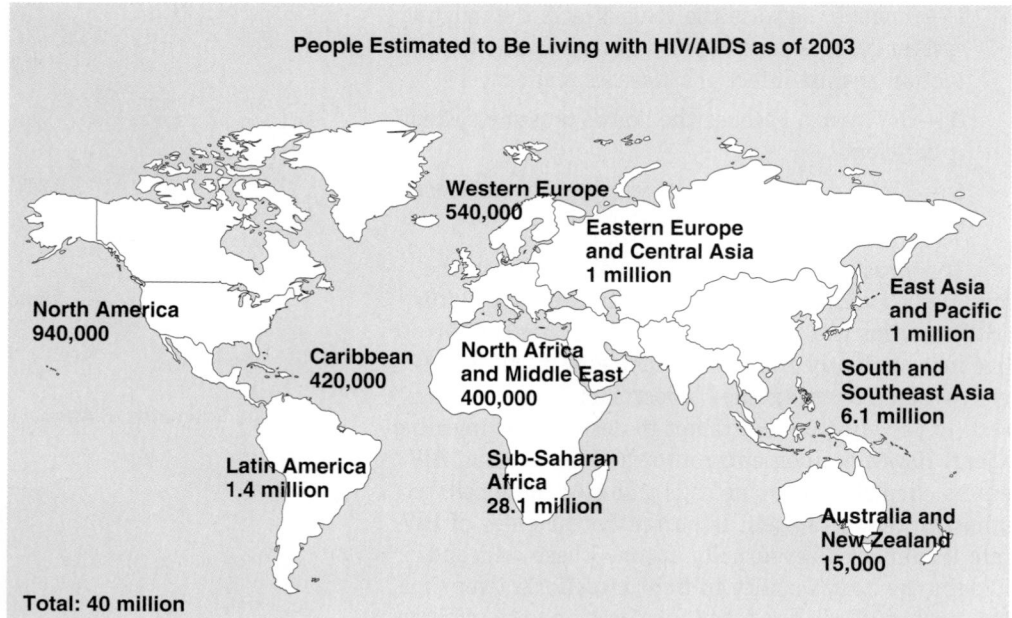

FIGURE 15.3
Estimated number of people living with AIDS/HIV around the world as of 2004.
Source: Data are from the United Nations, 2004

six to eight weeks before antibody levels are high enough to be detected by a blood test.

The second phase of HIV infection is called the symptomatic infection stage. This stage consists of several symptoms that may include constant fatigue, fever, weight loss, swollen lymph nodes, and sore throat. Symptoms that develop later include night sweats, chronic infections, skin disorders, and ulcers of the membranes lining the nose, mouth, and other body cavities.

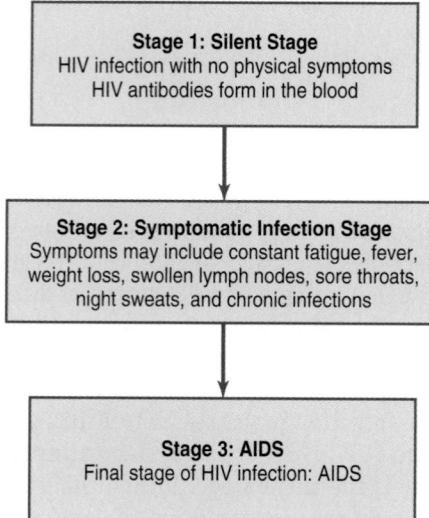

FIGURE 15.4
Stages in the development of AIDS. See text for a detailed description of this process.

Unless medical research can develop a cure for HIV, all HIV-infected individuals will eventually progress to the third and final stage of HIV infection, AIDS. AIDS is characterized by all of the general symptoms associated with the second phase of HIV infection plus one or more opportunistic diseases such as pneumonia or selected types of cancer such as Kaposi's sarcoma (see Table 15.1). Moreover, in this final stage of HIV infection, it is common for HIV to cross the blood-brain barrier and cause personality changes, deterioration of memory and judgment, and brain tumors (25, 28).

While AIDS is a fatal disease, people now live with AIDS for many years (25). This is possible because of improved medications coupled with superior clinical management of the disease. In recent years, the National Institutes of Health has devoted millions of research dollars toward the development of a cure for AIDS. Because of this investment in AIDS research, scientific progress has led some researchers to conclude that eventually AIDS will be considered a chronic disease (i.e., like hypertension or diabetes) that can be controlled by appropriate medical treatment (25). See A Closer Look "The Search for a Cure for AIDS" for more information about AIDS research.

MYTHS ABOUT THE TRANSMISSION OF HIV The many myths about how HIV is transmitted creates unnecessary fears in many people. This fear has caused some individuals to avoid any type of contact with infected individuals. Therefore, while it is critically important to understand how HIV can be transmitted, it is also important to know how HIV cannot be transmitted. In the following paragraphs we dispel some of the

FITNESS AND WELLNESS FOR ALL

STIs Are a Worldwide Problem

Sexually transmitted diseases (STIs) are a major health problem in countries around the world. Nonetheless, the incidence of STIs varies widely with some countries reporting a relatively low incidence whereas other countries report a high prevalence of STIs (20–23, 25). For example, the incidence of STIs tends to be relatively low in many highly industrialized countries whereas STIs constitute a large health risk for most developing countries (20). In this regard, it is currently estimated that each year there are over 340 million new cases of curable STIs around the world and that over 75% (i.e., 255 million) of these cases occur in developing countries (20).

The reasons for the differences in the incidence of STIs between industrialized and developing countries are numerous and complex. For example, it has been commonly assumed that a lack of education is a major factor contributing to the high incidence of STIs in developing countries. However, this is not always the case. For instance, a 1998 study by the World Health Organization reports that the sub-Saharan Africa region has the highest incidence of HIV infection in the world. However, the majority of HIV infections occur in the most literate men and women of this region (25).

What is the explanation for this surprising finding? A complete answer is not currently available but it is possible that, in some regions of the world, more education is associated with economic and cultural changes that result in behaviors that increase the risk of developing STIs (25). For example, increased education may result in a better job with higher income to support high-risk behaviors such as paying for prostitutes or maintaining a number of different sexual partners.

In summary, STIs remain a worldwide health problem with over 340 million new cases of curable STIs reported each year. However, the incidence of STIs varies widely around the world with the highest relative incidence of STIs occurring in developing countries. The explanation for these country-by-country differences is complex and requires additional study for a more complete understanding.

myths about the transmission of HIV. You *cannot* get HIV from any of the following:

- **Causal contact with HIV-infected individuals.** Normal household or social contact does not transmit HIV. Shaking hands, hugging, or providing personal care such as bathing, feeding, or dressing are unlikely to transmit HIV.

- **Contact with inanimate objects.** HIV cannot live outside of the body. Therefore, HIV cannot survive on toilet seats, drinking fountains, countertops,

---

TABLE 15.1
Common Opportunistic Diseases Associated with the Development of AIDS

Disease	Symptoms of Disease
Kaposi's sarcoma (type of cancer)	Brown or purple lesions on the skin that resemble bruises but do not heal
Primary lymphoma of the brain (type of cancer)	Headaches, loss of memory, personality changes, impaired vision
Tuberculosis (bacterial infection)	Fever, night sweats, fatigue, cough, weight loss
Pneumocytsis carinii pneumonia (rare form of pneumonia)	Chest pain, dry cough, difficulty breathing
Ctytomegalovirus (viral infection)	Viral infection that can occur in the lung, gastrointestinal tract, or central nervous system; symptoms vary depending upon the location of the infection
Atypical mycobacterium (bacterial infection)	High fever, night sweats, fatigue, weakness

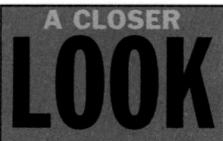

A CLOSER LOOK

The Search for a Cure for AIDS

Current estimates are that more than 40 million people worldwide are infected with AIDS. Without a cure for this disease, these people will typically die within 7–12 years after acquiring the virus. Therefore, there is an urgent need for both an effective anti-AIDS vaccine and treatment strategies to cure this disorder. The challenge to cure AIDS is being met by the medical research community as scientists around the world are currently working to develop drug treatment strategies to prevent AIDS and to cure patients currently infected with the virus (17, 18). A major problem confronting scientists in the treatment for AIDS is the fact that the virus is capable of mutating into many different viral strains. That is, the virus is capable of changing its characteristics. This shifting face of the virus makes the development of a drug to kill all strains of the virus extremely difficult. How much time will be required to find a complete cure for AIDS is currently unknown. Nonetheless, recent advances in the treatment for AIDS have diminished the mortality and morbidity of the disease. Many scientists remain optimistic that a cure for the AIDS virus will be found within a decade (17, 18).

---

doorknobs, or other areas. If a surface becomes infected with blood or semen containing HIV, alcohol, bleach, Lysol, or hydrogen peroxide can disinfect the surface.

- **Sports participation.** To date, there are no documented cases of HIV transmission via sports. Further, HIV is not found in sweat of HIV-positive individuals and HIV exists in limited quantities in tears. Finally, according to the Centers for Disease Control and Prevention, there is limited risk of contracting HIV during contact sports even when bleeding occurs.

- **Saliva.** Although there is a slight risk of contracting the HIV virus by contact with saliva, the risk is extremely small. Indeed, there is no evidence that HIV has ever been transmitted from one person to another by kissing or by drinking from water fountains or beverage containers used by HIV-infected individuals.

- **Swimming pools, hot tubs, or whirlpool baths.** HIV cannot live or replicate in water. Therefore, HIV cannot be transmitted by contact with water contained in hot tubs, whirlpools, or swimming pools.

- **Contact with animals.** Household pets and farm animals cannot contract the HIV virus. Therefore, these animals cannot spread HIV to humans.

- **Insect bites.** Studies reveal that biting insects such as mosquitoes, biting flies, and bedbugs cannot transmit the HIV virus.

HOW HIV IS TRANSMITTED Now that we have dispelled the common myths about HIV transmission, let's discuss how HIV *can be* transmitted from individual to individual. A key point to remember is that for HIV to replicate in the body, the virus must have entry into the bloodstream. Therefore, any exchange of body fluids such as blood, semen, or vaginal secretions is a possible mode for transmission of HIV. The three most common modes of HIV transmission are the following:

- Vaginal or anal intercourse without using a condom.
- Sharing of needles contaminated with HIV-infected blood during injected drug use, tattoos, or body piercing.
- Passage of the virus from mother to fetus in the uterus (20–50% chance) or in blood during delivery.

In addition to these common modes of HIV transmission, the virus can also be transmitted from an HIV-infected mother to a baby by breast-feeding. Moreover, it is also possible to transmit the virus by the sharing of sex toys if they are not properly disinfected and cleaned. Finally, HIV can be transmitted through accidental contamination when infected blood enters the body through the mucus membranes of the eyes or mouth or through breaks in the skin (i.e., cuts, abrasions, or punctures).

☀ IN SUMMARY

- Every year millions of people in the United States are infected by one or more sexually transmitted infections (STIs).
- The most common STIs in the United States include AIDS, chlamydia, gonorrhea, pelvic inflammatory disease, venereal warts, herpes, and syphilis.
- AIDS is a fatal disease that develops from infection by the human immunodeficiency virus (HIV).
- Americans are becoming disproportionately infected with the disease with 70% of the new HIV infections occurring in men. Further, although

African Americans make up only 13% of the U.S. population, approximately 55% of all new cases of AIDS in the United States impact this group.

- At present, there is no cure for AIDS. Nonetheless, many scientists remain optimistic that a cure for the AIDS virus will be found within a decade.

TRICHOMONIASIS

OVERVIEW AND INCIDENCE   *Trichomonas vaginalis* is a one-celled organism (protozoan) that infects the vaginal or urinary mucosa to cause a vaginal infection called **trichomoniasis (trick)**. Trichomoniasis is a very common infection that infects approximately 5 million people each year (28). Although sexual intercourse is a common mode of transmission for this infection, trichomoniasis can be contracted by prolonged exposure to moisture (e.g., exposure to wet bathing suits or other clothing infected with trichomonas vaginalis) (28). Indeed, trichomonas vaginalis is a very hardy organism that can live for several hours on wet towels or toilet seats (25, 28). Since trichomoniasis can be contracted by means other than sexual intercourse, this infection is often referred to as a sexually related infection.

Again, a common mode of transmission of trichomoniasis is by vaginal intercourse or sexual contact with an infected person. Women can acquire the disease from infected men or women whereas men usually acquire the disease from infected women (28).

SYMPTOMS AND TREATMENT

Most men and women experience symptoms of infection within days after contact with trichomonas vaginalis. For women, common symptoms include the following:

- Yellow-green (often foamy) vaginal discharge with a strong odor
- Irritation and itching of the genital area
- Pain or irritation during intercourse

Men may experience the following symptoms:

- Irritation inside the penis
- Discharge from the penis
- Burning sensation during urination or after ejaculation

Trichomoniasis can be diagnosed by a simple medical test. When trichomoniasis is detected in a woman, her sexual partner(s) should also be treated for this infection because the infection can be passed back and forth between partners (called the ping-pong effect). Infection with trichomoniasis can be treated systemically with drugs and some topical agents may also be

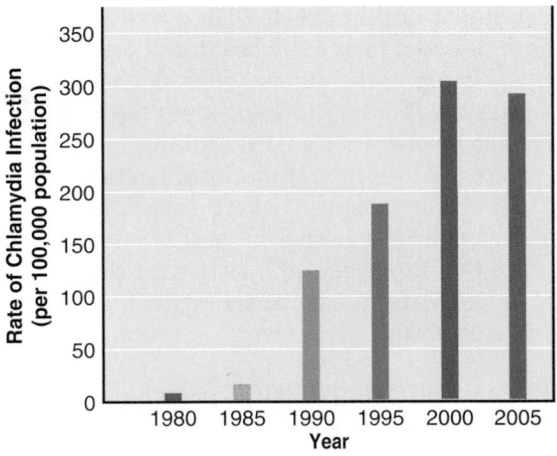

FIGURE 15.5
Reported rates of chlamydia in the United States from 1980–2005. Notice the rapid rise in chlamydia infections during the 20-year period from 1980–2000.
Source: Data are from the Centers for Disease Control and Prevention.

effective (25). Although trichomoniasis is not generally considered a life-threatening infection, prolonged and untreated trichomoniasis is associated with an increased risk of cancer (25). Therefore, if you possess symptoms of this infection, seek medical attention immediately.

CHLAMYDIA

OVERVIEW AND INCIDENCE   **Chlamydia** is one of the most common STIs among heterosexual people worldwide (2). The disease is caused by a bacterial infection within the reproductive organs and is spread through vaginal, anal, and oral sex. The incidence of chlamydia infection in the United States experienced a rapid growth during 1980–2000 (Figure 15.5). A report from the Centers for Disease Control and Prevention reveals that chlamydia is the most common bacterial infection in the United States with over 3 million new cases of chlamydia occurring each year (11, 12). Equally alarming is the estimate that about 20% of all college students may have chlamydia (1). The good news is that the infection rates of chlamydia in the United States may be on the decline (Figure 15.5) (12).

---

trichomoniasis (trick)   A vaginal infection caused by a one-celled protozoan called *Trichomonas vaginalis.*

chlamydia   The most common sexually transmitted disease among heterosexuals in the United States; is caused by a bacterial infection within the reproductive organs and is spread through vaginal, anal, and oral sex.

Recall that Healthy People 2010 is a national health initiative designed to improve health and prevent the spread of disease in the United States. One important goal of Healthy People 2010 is to reduce the incidence of STIs. The Healthy People 2010 objective for chlamydia is to reduce the incidence of this infection to less than four cases of chlamydia per 100,000 people. As you can see in Figure 15.5, achieving this goal is a formidable task since the current rate of infection for chlamydia in the United States is approximately 275 cases per 100,000 individuals.

SYMPTOMS AND TREATMENT Symptoms of chlamydia often go unnoticed and may vary among individuals. In fact, over 75% of the women and 50% of the men infected do not develop symptoms and are unaware that they carry the bacteria. For both men and women, early symptoms occur within 7–21 days after infection. Early symptoms of infection in women may include the following:

- Unusual vaginal discharge
- A burning sensation when urinating
- Unexplained vaginal bleeding between menstrual periods

Later symptoms, typically occurring several months after infection include the following:

- Lower back pain
- Lower abdominal pain
- Pain during intercourse
- Low-grade fever

Up to 50% of all males infected with chlamydia do not develop symptoms when first infected. However, several months after infection, the following symptoms may occur:

- Unusual discharge from the penis
- Burning sensation when urinating
- Low-grade fever
- Pain and swelling of the testicles

---

pelvic inflammatory disease (PID) An inflammatory infection of the lining of the abdominal and pelvic cavities; common symptoms include pain in the lower abdominal cavity, fever, and menstrual irregularities.

hepatitis B A viral infection that attacks the liver. Hepatitis B can be transmitted by sexual intercourse with an infected person and at present, no cure exists for this disease.

Chlamydia can be diagnosed by a blood test or a Pap smear, where the bacteria responsible for the infection are grown in a tissue culture. Fortunately, chlamydia can be cured by administration of antibiotics. If untreated, chlamydia can result in infertility in both men and women. Further, untreated chlamydia in women can lead to **pelvic inflammatory disease (PID),** an inflammatory infection of the lining of the abdominal and pelvic cavity. Common symptoms of pelvic inflammatory disease include pain in the lower abdominal cavity, fever, and menstrual irregularities. If you suspect that you are infected by chlamydia or any other STI, see your physician immediately as early treatment is important to prevent potentially serious long-term health consequences.

⁂ IN SUMMARY

- Trichomoniasis (trick) is a common STI caused by infection with a protozoan called trichomonas vaginalis.

- Symptoms of trick include a yellow-green vaginal discharge for women and a discharge from the penis for men.

- Chlamydia is the most common STI among heterosexuals and is caused by a bacterial infection within the reproductive organ; this infection is spread through vaginal, anal, and oral sex. Chlamydia is curable by treatment with antibiotics.

- Symptoms of chlamydia vary among individuals. Unfortunately, over 75% of the women and 50% of the men infected do not develop symptoms and are unaware that they carry the bacteria.

HEPATITIS B

OVERVIEW AND INCIDENCE Current estimates are that over 80,000 people in the United States are infected with a virus that attacks the liver and results in **hepatitis B** (28). The virus that causes hepatitis B can be transmitted by contact with infected blood, blood products, semen, vaginal secretions, and saliva (25). Consequently, high-risk groups for contracting hepatitis B include individuals who have a job that involves handling human blood, and people who have sexual intercourse with infected persons (28). Further, your risk of contracting hepatitis B is higher if you engage in sexual relations with more than one partner (25). Individuals who are at risk for contracting hepatitis B are often advised to be vaccinated against the disease.

Hepatitis is a disorder that promotes an inflammatory response in the liver resulting in a decrease in normal liver function. The liver is a required organ that performs numerous bodily functions such as the regulation of blood glucose between meals, production of bile, and detoxification of the blood. Because the liver performs many functions essential for life, severe liver dysfunction can be life threatening (32). Therefore, hepatitis B is a very serious disease.

SYMPTOMS AND TREATMENT Approximately 30% of the individuals infected with hepatitis B do not develop symptoms (28). In the remaining 70% of hepatitis B–infected individuals, a variety of symptoms may be present. Common symptoms include the following (32):

- Jaundice (eyes or skin turns yellow)
- Reduced appetite
- Nausea
- Vomiting
- Stomach and/or joint pain
- Chronic fatigue

Although the mortality rate for hepatitis B is typically lower than some other forms of hepatitis, it is estimated that over 5,000 people die each year in the United States from this disease (28). Therefore, based upon both the symptoms of the disease and the mortality risk, hepatitis B is a serious and debilitating disorder.

Hepatitis B is diagnosed by a blood test for antibodies that are indicative of infection with the hepatitis B virus. Unfortunately, there is currently no cure for hepatitis B (28). Therefore, prevention of this disease is critical. Once hepatitis B is diagnosed, the treatment consists of rest and consumption of amounts of fluid to insure adequate hydration. For some with the hepatitis B virus, the liver can become severely compromised; for those who do develop severe liver disease from hepatitis B infection, two drugs (alpha interferon and lamivudine) have been shown to be effective in reducing symptoms (28). Medical research aimed at developing a cure for hepatitis B continues and hopefully, a cure for this disease will be forthcoming.

GONORRHEA

OVERVIEW AND INCIDENCE Gonorrhea (also known as "drip" or " the clap") is another common STI, and it is estimated that over 400,000 cases of gonorrhea will be reported in the United States each year (12). In comparison to other STIs, the incidence of gonorrhea ranks this STI as the second highest communicable bacterial infection. Only chlamydia is more prevalent. Fortunately, however, the rate of gonorrhea infection in the United States has declined over the past 25 years (Figure 15.6). The Healthy People 2010 goal for gonorrhea is to reduce the incidence of this infection from the current annual rate of approximately 140 infections per 100,000 people to less than 20 infections per 100,000 individuals.

The bacterium that causes gonorrhea is called *Neisseria gonorrhoeae* and grows well within mucous membranes in the body. This bacterium cannot grow outside the body because it requires a warm and moist environ-

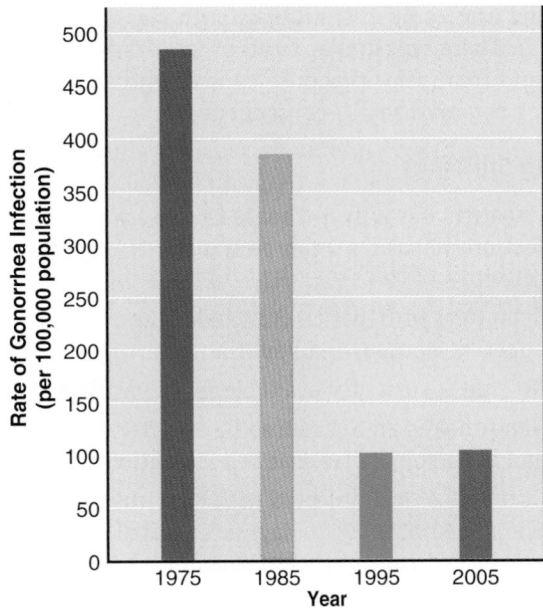

FIGURE 15.6
Reported rates of gonorrhea in the United States from 1980–2005. Notice the decline in gonorrhea infections during the period from 1975–1995.
Source: Data are from the Centers for Disease Control and Prevention.

ment. Therefore, gonorrhea cannot be spread by contact with toilet seats, doorknobs, or other inanimate objects. However, gonorrhea can be transmitted through vaginal, anal, and oral sex.

SYMPTOMS AND TREATMENT Over 80% of men develop symptoms within 2–10 days after sexual contact with an infected person. Typical symptoms include a milky discharge from the penis and painful urination (13). Moreover, in some men, lymph glands in the groin become inflamed and swollen (25, 28). In contrast, only 20% of women infected with gonorrhea develop symptoms. When symptoms are present, they include painful urination and an occasional fever (13). The lack of symptoms in women poses a serious problem because the woman is unaware that she has been infected and may continue to spread the disease to sex partners.

Gonorrhea can be diagnosed by a tissue culture of the discharge from the penis or vagina and is curable by treatment with antibiotics. When diagnosed early and treated with appropriate medication, gonorrhea can be easily cured (25). However, untreated gonorrhea may spread to the prostate, testicles, kidney, and blad-

---

gonorrhea A common sexually transmitted disease; can be transmitted through vaginal, anal, and oral sex; is caused by a bacterial infection and is curable by antibiotics.

der and can result in sterility in both men and women (2, 13). Therefore, similar to all other STIs, early detection and treatment of gonorrhea is essential to prevent serious negative health consequences.

☀ IN SUMMARY

- Hepatitis B is a liver disease caused by a viral infection. Hepatitis B can be transmitted by sexual activity.
- Symptoms of Hepatitis B include jaundice, reduced appetite, nausea, and vomiting.
- No cure is currently available for hepatitis B.
- Gonorrhea is an STI caused by a bacterial infection and is curable by treatment with antibiotics.
- Over 80% of men infected with gonorrhea develop symptoms within 2–10 days after sexual contact with an infected person; typical symptoms include a milky discharge from the penis and painful urination.
- In contrast to men, only 20% of women infected with gonorrhea develop symptoms. When symptoms are present, they include painful urination and occasional fever.

VENEREAL WARTS

OVERVIEW AND INCIDENCE　**Venereal warts** (also known as genital warts) are caused by a small group of viruses called human papilloma viruses (1, 2, 13). Human papilloma virus refers to a group of over 100 different strains of viruses; over 30 of these strains can infect the genitals (28). Infection generally occurs through sexual contact with an infected individual; after exposure, the virus penetrates the skin or mucous membranes of the genitals or anus, and warts appear within 3–9 weeks (1, 2, 13, 25).

The incidence of venereal warts in the United States is relatively high. Indeed, current estimates are that over 20 million women in the United States are infected

with the human papilloma virus (25). Moreover, it is predicted that over 75% of their sexual partners are also infected (25). The incidence of venereal warts varies across the population with the highest rate of occurrence in people between 19–30 years of age (28). In particular, studies suggest that the incidence of venereal warts in college students is extremely high. For example, a study at the University of California at Berkeley found that almost 50% of the female college students examined for a routine gynecological exam were positive for infection with human papilloma virus (29).

SYMPTOMS AND TREATMENT　On portions of the external genitals that are dry (such as the penis), warts may develop as a series of small itchy bumps on the skin and may range in size from that of a pinhead to that of a pencil eraser. Men can detect these warts by routinely examining their genitals for suspicious growths. If, however, the warts are inside the reproductive tract, symptoms may be absent. In women, a physician can often detect these warts during a routine Pap smear.

Treatment for venereal warts may take several forms. Warts can be treated with several different types of medication, which results in the warts drying up within a few days, or they can be removed by cryosurgery (freezing them), laser surgery, or excision surgery. It is important to note that removal of the wart does not always remove the virus from the individuals system (28). In fact, because the virus can remain dormant in cells, in some cases, warts can reappear within months or even years after treatment (28). Unfortunately, the extent to which an individual can spread the virus after the visible warts have been removed is currently unknown.

Do venereal warts present a serious health threat? Not always. Many genital warts will disappear without medical treatment. The greatest risk from venereal warts is that, in women, untreated warts increase their risk of uterine and cervical cancer. Exactly how venereal warts result in cancer is unclear. Nonetheless, what is known is that within five years after infection, about 30% of all untreated warts result in a precancerous growth. If this precancerous growth remains untreated, 70% will lead to cancer (2, 13).

GENITAL HERPES

OVERVIEW AND INCIDENCE　**Herpes** is a general term for a family of diseases that are caused by viral infections. The herpes simplex virus causes genital herpes infections. The herpes simplex virus is not a single virus but is a family of more than 70 herpes viruses (2, 28). In the 1960s it was discovered that two specific forms of herpes simplex virus generally cause genital herpes;

---

venereal warts　Warts caused by a small group of viruses called human papilloma viruses; infection generally occurs through sexual contact with an infected individual; after exposure, the virus penetrates the skin or mucous membranes of the genitals or anus, and warts appear within 6–8 weeks; also known as genital warts.

herpes　A general term for a family of diseases caused by viral infections; is highly contagious and can be transmitted through any form of sexual contact (e.g., hand-to-genital contact, oral sex, or intercourse).

these viruses are labeled as type I herpes simplex virus (HSV-1) and type II herpes simplex virus (HSV-2) (28). In general, type 1 infections are more common above the waist (e.g., sores on the lips or mouth) whereas type 2 infections are more common below the waist (e.g., genital lesions) (28).

Genital herpes is highly contagious and can be transmitted through any form of sexual contact (such as hand-to-genital contact, oral sex, or intercourse). The incidence of genital herpes in the United States is greatest among white teens and young adults (28). Over 1 million new cases of herpes were reported in the United States during 2004 and it is estimated that genital herpes affects approximately 45 million Americans, which represents about 17% of the population of the United States (12, 28). The current national health initiative (i.e., Healthy People 2010) has set a goal of reducing the incidence of herpes infection from 17% to less than 14% of the population (31).

SYMPTOMS AND TREATMENT   For most people infected with the herpes simplex virus, the initial infection is the most severe (28). The first symptoms of herpes infection generally appear within 3–20 days after exposure to the virus (25, 28). Symptoms of herpes vary from sores (blisters) on the mouth, rectum, and genitals, to fever and swollen glands. Interestingly, symptoms may disappear and then reappear without warning. Indeed, while symptoms may come and go, the virus remains in the body for life.

At present, there is no cure for herpes, but newly developed drugs show promise. Although treatment with cold-sore medication reduces the pain and irritation of the sore, remember that rubbing anything on the herpes blister increases the chance of spreading herpes-laden fluids to other body parts or to other people.

SYPHILIS

OVERVIEW AND INCIDENCE   **Syphilis** is a well-known STI that can be transmitted through direct sexual contact. Each year thousands of new cases of syphilis are reported in the United States (12). Like chlamydia and gonorrhea, syphilis is caused by a bacterial infection. The bacterium responsible for syphilis is a spiral-shaped bacteria called *Treponema pallidum*. This bacterium requires a warm and moist environment such as the genitals or the mucous membranes of the mouth to survive.

SYMPTOMS AND TREATMENT   The symptoms of untreated syphilis vary because the disease generally progresses through four stages: 1) primary syphilis; 2) secondary syphilis; 3) latent syphilis; and 4) tertiary syphilis. The early symptoms of stage one (primary syphilis) generally include a painless sore,

called a **chancre,** located at the initial site of infection (such as the penis, vaginal walls, or mouth). The size of the chancre may vary, but it is often about the size of a dime. In both men and women, this chancre will completely disappear in 3–6 weeks.

Within 6 weeks after the disappearance of the chancre, secondary symptoms associated with stage two syphilis appear. These include a skin rash or white patches on the mucous membranes of the mouth, throat, or genitals. Hair loss may also occur, lymph glands may become swollen, and infectious sores may develop around the mouth or genitals.

If syphilis is not treated, stage-two symptoms typically disappear and stage three—latent syphilis—begins. During this phase of the syphilis infection, the infected person may not experience symptoms or they may experience symptoms that are vague and difficult to diagnose without a blood test to screen for the bacteria (25).

Stage four—tertiary syphilis—is rarely seen in the United States because medical treatment usually prevents the disease from progressing to this stage. Nonetheless, if untreated, the infected individual may spend several years in stage-three syphilis (i.e., without symptoms) while the syphilis infection is slowly spreading to organs throughout the body leading to stage four—tertiary syphilis. This last stage of untreated syphilis may result in heart damage, blindness, deafness, paralysis, and mental disorders (28).

Syphilis can be diagnosed with a blood test and can be cured by antibiotics (2, 13, 28). However, because of the progressive nature of this infection, early treatment of syphilis is important to prevent serious and long-term health problems.

✸ IN SUMMARY

- Venereal warts are caused by human papilloma viruses that are typically spread by sexual contact with an infected individual.

- Venereal warts are treatable in several ways including medication and surgery to remove the warts.

- The greatest risk from venereal warts is that untreated warts in women will increase their risk of uterine and cervical cancer.

- Herpes is a viral STI that can be transmitted through

---

chancre   A sore that appears at the site of infection in stage one syphilis.

syphilis   A sexually transmitted disease that can be transmitted through direct sexual contact; is caused by a bacterial infection and can be cured with antibiotics.

any form of sexual contact; symptoms generally include sores on the mouth, rectum, and genitals.

- At present, there is no cure for the herpes virus.
- Syphilis is an STI caused by a bacterial infection and can be treated with antibiotics.
- Syphilis infections progress through four stages: Stage one—primary syphilis; Stage two—secondary syphilis; Stage 3—Latent syphilis; and Stage four—Tertiary syphilis
- Symptoms of untreated syphilis vary depending upon the stage of the infection; early symptoms in stages one and two may include a painless sore followed by hair loss, swollen lymph glands, and infectious sores around the mouth or genitals.

OTHER STIs

In addition to the previously discussed STIs, numerous other sexually transmitted infections also exist. In this section, we present a brief discussion of three common but less serious STIs.

PUBIC LICE   Pubic lice, commonly known as crabs, are parasites that infect the pubic area. Pubic lice are usually transmitted from person to person by sexual contact but can also be transmitted by infected bed linen, clothes, or even toilet seats. These organisms grip pubic hair and feed on blood from tiny blood vessels in the surrounding skin. Once an infection occurs, pubic lice reproduce and the numbers of lice in the infected area grows. When large numbers of lice are present, they can be visualized as brown spots on pubic hairs and the surrounding skin.

As the pubic lice feed on skin in the pubic area, they irritate the skin and blood, causing itching and sometimes swelling. Fortunately, both over-the-counter and prescription skin creams are available to eliminate pubic lice. While one treatment with a topical cream may be sufficient to be curative, it is also important to wash all infected clothing and bed linen.

SCABIES   **Scabies** is caused by a parasite (i.e., tiny mite) that infects the skin between the fingers, on the wrist, under the breasts, and the pubic area. Once an infection occurs, the female mite burrows under the skin causing irritation and itching. Close contact (including sexual contact) with an infected individual can spread these parasites. Note, unlike pubic lice, scabies is rarely

---

scabies   Scabies is caused by a parasite (i.e., tiny mite) that can infect skin between the fingers, on the wrist, under the breasts, and the pubic area.

---

contracted by clothing, bedding, or toilet seats (25).

A physician can diagnose scabies by scraping the infected area and performing a microscopic test to determine if mites are present. Once diagnosed, scabies is often treated with a prescription medication called Kwell (28). Typically, one or more treatments result in the complete removal of the invading mites.

CANDIDASIS   Candidasis, also called yeast infection, is a common form of vaginitis (inflammation of the vagina) caused by a fungus called *Candida albicans* (28). While this fungus is normally found in small quantities in the vagina, a rapid growth of the fungus results in a "yeast infection" that is characterized by itching, discomfort, and a thick vaginal discharge (28). This fungus can be spread from person to person by sexual contact and this infection can also manifest itself in the mouth and throat. Candidasis requires different treatments depending on the location of the infection, but is curable regardless of location with the appropriate medication.

See A Closer Look on p. 399 for answers to additional questions about STIs.

☀ IN SUMMARY

- Pubic lice, or "crabs," are parasites that infect the pubic area. Pubic lice can be transmitted from person to person by sexual contact.
- Scabies is an STI caused by a tiny mite that can infect skin between fingers, under the breast, and in the pubic area.
- Candidasis (yeast infection) is a common form of vaginitis that can be sexually transmitted.

☀ Reducing Your Risk for Sexually Transmitted Infections

There is no cure for AIDS or herpes, and although treatment methods exist for many other STIs, prevention is clearly the best approach. The keys to preventing STIs are education and responsible action. Laboratory 15.1 will help you evaluate your risks of contracting an STI by making you aware of attitudes and behaviors that increase the risk of infection via sexual activity. In the following sections, we discuss several steps that you can take to avoid infection with an STI.

ABSTINENCE

Complete abstinence from sexual activity is the only certain way to prevent STIs. As discussed previously, STIs can be transmitted by oral and anal sex. Therefore, avoidance of all forms of sexual activity is required to

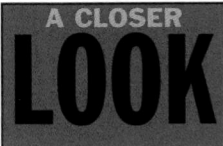

Answers to Frequently Asked Questions About STIs

Are STIs becoming more common or less common in the United States?

It depends on the STI. While the estimated incidence of HIV/AIDS is holding constant at about 40,000 new cases per year, the number of new cases of gonorrhea and genital herpes is increasing. Fortunately, the rates of new cases of chlamydia and syphilis have declined in the past several years.

Which STIs are the most serious for women?

Although HIV/AIDS is a serious problem in women, they bear a larger burden than do men with respect to gonorrhea, chlamydia, and venereal warts because they suffer more frequent and more serious complications from those infections (12). For example, 10–20% of women with gonorrhea or chlamydia will develop a very serious complication—pelvic inflammatory disease,

which can lead to serious pelvic pain and infertility. Furthermore, women infected with venereal warts have an increased risk of cervical cancer. Finally, women infected with an STI during pregnancy can experience early onset of labor and premature birth, which is the leading cause of infant death and disability in the United States.

Who should get tested for HIV?

Anyone who is at risk for HIV infection should get tested. You are at risk if (1) you have had unprotected sex with anyone who has not been involved in a long-term, mutually monogamous relationship with you, or (2) either you or your partner has had unprotected sex with other people during the past several years, or (3) you have shared needles or syringes with anyone for injecting drugs, or (4) you received a blood transfusion before 1985.

Getting tested for HIV if you are at risk is important because many people carrying HIV don't know they are infected, and because early treatment for HIV can improve the outcome of the infection. Testing is available from several sources, including any physician, your student health clinic, Planned Parenthood, and your local public health department. Taking the test itself is simple: It involves only taking a small blood sample that is sent to a laboratory for analysis. Costs of these tests are generally between $50 and $100. Another option—home testing kits—is available from several manufacturers. All these home testing kits provide a sterile lancet (needle) for pricking your finger to obtain a few drops of blood, and a sterile storage container for sending the blood sample to a lab for analysis. Whenever choosing a home testing kit, select only those clearly marked as approved by the federal Food and Drug Administration (FDA).

---

eliminate all risk of contracting an STI. While abstinence is an option for some people, for many people abstinence is not an acceptable means of avoiding STIs. Therefore for individuals not willing to refrain from sexual activity, other strategies to prevent STIs are available.

MONOGAMY

Maintaining a monogamous relationship with a sexual partner that is not infected with an STI is another way to avoid STIs. The key to success with this strategy is that both partners must be free of STIs and that the relationship must remain monogamous. Failure of one member of the relationship to maintain monogamy will increase the risk of contracting an STI. While monogamy can reduce your risk of STIs, this strategy can be problematic.

USE OF LATEX CONDOMS (MALES)

The pores of latex condoms are too small to allow the transmission of many STIs. Therefore, consistent and proper use of a latex condom by males during all sexual activity (e.g., oral or anal sex, vaginal intercourse) will

reduce your risk of contracting an STI.

How effective are latex condoms in preventing the transmission of STIs? A study by the American Public Health Association revealed that use of latex condoms during sexual activities is effective against the transmission of HIV and gonorrhea in both men and women (33). Further, although definitive evidence is not available, it appears likely that the use of male condoms will also reduce the risk of other STIs including syphilis and chlamydia (34). Nonetheless, latex condoms will not prevent the transmission of certain types of STIs such as scabies and pubic lice. Moreover, genital ulcer diseases and genital herpes infections can occur in areas not covered by condoms (25). Therefore, while condom use will reduce your risk for many types of STIs, use of male condoms will not provide absolute protection against all STIs (33, 34).

FEMALE CONDOMS

A laboratory study conducted by the Centers for Disease Control and Prevention (CDC) indicates that female condoms are effective mechanical barriers against viruses including HIV (34). From these studies, the CDC has

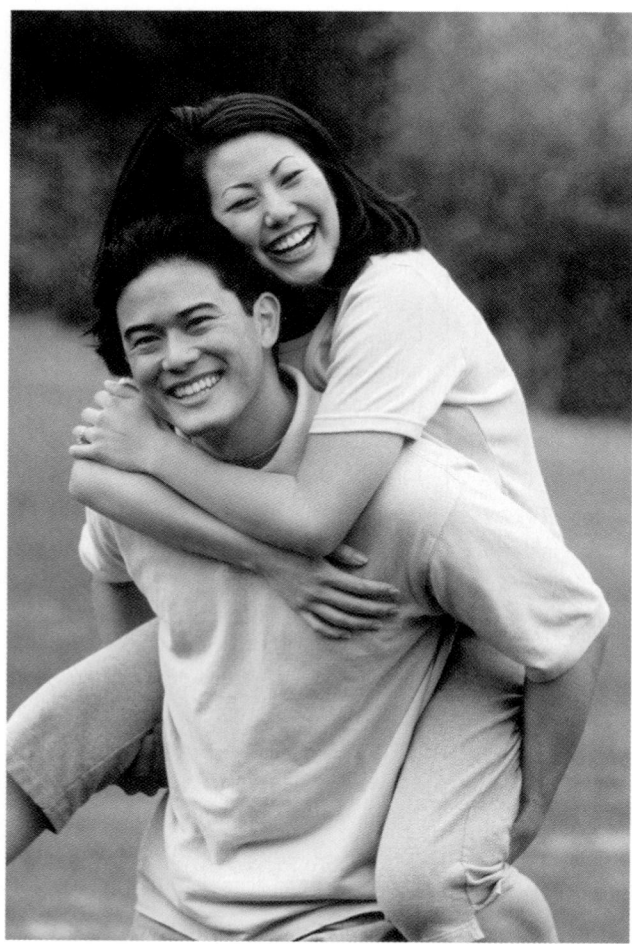

Maintaining a monogamous relationship with an STI-free partner is a strategy to prevent the contraction of an STI.

LIMITING THE NUMBER OF SEXUAL PARTNERS

Limiting your number of sexual partners will decrease your risk of contracting an STI (25). The rationale behind this statement is simple: increased numbers of sexual partners increases your odds of being exposed to an STI. Therefore, limiting your number of sexual partners is a wise behavior to reduce your risk of STIs.

DISCUSS STIs WITH SEXUAL PARTNERS

Prior to engaging in sexual activity with a new partner, you should discuss the concern of becoming infected with an STI with this individual. This discussion should include talks about whether they have been recently medically screened for an STI or whether they have engaged in high-risk behaviors (e.g., multiple sexual partners) that would increase their risk of being infected with an STI. This kind of conversation can lead to a mutual concern for prevention of STIs and in some cases, result in the decision to refrain from sexual activity until medical screening for STIs has been completed (25).

AVOID USE OF DRUGS AND ALCOHOL

The use of psychoactive drugs and alcohol prior to engaging in sexual activity can impair your reasoning and increase your risk of engaging in risky sexual activity and/or the failure to use condoms during sex. Therefore, because drugs and alcohol weaken your ability to reason, you should refrain from the use of drugs or alcohol to reduce your risk of contracting STIs.

OTHER PROTECTIVE MEASURES

In addition to the previously discussed actions to prevent STIs, there are several other steps that you can take to reduce your risk of contracting an STI. These include:

- Inspect yourself and your partner for signs of STIs
- Do not share needles, scissors, or razors
- Wash your genitals before and after sex
- Do not handle towels, wet bedding, or underclothing that have been in contact with an individual suspected to be infected with an STI

If you suspect that you have been exposed to an STI, you should contact your physician immediately for medical screening. Never try to diagnose an STI yourself and do not delay seeking medical attention if you develop symptoms of any STI. Clearly, early diagnosis and treatment of an STI is essential to ensure that an STI does not lead to long-term health problems. Importantly, if you learn that you are infected with an STI, you should immediately inform all of your sexual partners.

concluded that when used consistently and correctly, female condoms may reduce the risk of STIs including HIV (34). However, clinical studies proving that female condoms prevent the spread of STIs are not currently available. Nonetheless, the CDC recommends that when male condoms cannot be used, sexual partners should consider the use of female condoms to reduce the risk of STIs (34).

NONOXYNAL-9

Vaginal spermicides containing nonoxynal-9 are not effective against preventing most STIs including gonorrhea, HIV, or chlamydia (28). In fact, evidence indicates that nonoxynal-9 can increase the risk of contracting STIs by irritating the vaginal or anal lining and increasing the ease of infectious agents of gaining entry into the body (28). Therefore, the CDC has issued a warning that condoms containing nonoxynal-9 should be avoided (28).

Indeed, failing to tell a partner about your infection with an STI increases the risk of the spread of STIs to others.

☀ **IN SUMMARY**

- Avoidance of sexual activity (abstinence) is the only absolute means of preventing sexually transmitted infections

- Limit your number of sexual partners
- Use latex condoms to reduce your risk of contracting an STI
- Avoid the use of drugs or alcohol prior to engaging in sexual activities
- Discuss STIs with sexual partners

Summary

1. Every year, millions of people in the United States are infected by one or more sexually transmitted infections (STIs).

2. Some of the most common sexually transmitted infections include AIDS, chlamydia, gonorrhea, hepatitis B, venereal warts, herpes, and syphilis.

3. AIDS is a fatal disease that develops from infection by the human immunodeficiency virus (HIV).

4. All STIs require medical treatment. Successful treatments for chlamydia, gonorrhea, venereal warts, and syphilis are available.

5. Chlamydia is a common STI among heterosexuals and is caused by a bacterial infection within the reproductive organs; it is spread through vaginal, anal, and oral sex.

6. Gonorrhea is an STI caused by a bacterial infection and is curable by treatment with antibiotics.

7. Venereal warts result from the spread of human papilloma viruses by sexual contact.

8. Herpes is caused by a virus that can be transmitted through any form of sexual contact. At present, there is no cure for the herpes virus.

9. Syphilis is caused by a bacterial infection and can be treated with antibiotics.

10. Hepatitis B is a liver disease caused by a viral infection and can be transmitted by sexual activity.

11. Most STIs can be avoided by following "safe sex" guidelines including limiting your number of sexual partners, using condoms, and avoiding high-risk behaviors.

Study Questions

1. Name the seven most common STIs in the United States.

2. Which of the most common STIs are currently incurable?

3. Discuss the relationship between venereal warts and uterine or cervical cancer.

4. Describe the symptoms of AIDS and state the status of research aimed at curing this deadly disease.

5. Discuss the three stages of AIDS beginning with infection with HIV leading to the final stage.

6. Outline the symptoms of chlamydia, trichomoniasis, hepatitis B, and gonorrhea. Do gender differences exist in symptoms of these STIs?

7. List the common symptoms of venereal warts, herpes, and syphilis. Are symptoms for these STIs similar between men and women?

8. Identify the treatments available for all of the common STIs in the United States.

9. Outline ways to reduce your risk of contracting STIs.

10. Which STIs are the most serious for women?

11. Which STIs are becoming more common in the United States?

12. Discuss who should get tested for STIs.

Suggested Reading

Anderson, B. *Reproductive Health*. Sudbury, MA: Jones and Bartlett, 2005.

Donatelle, R. *Access to Health*, 9th ed. San Francisco: Benjamin Cummings, 2006.

Fields, R. *Drugs in Perspective*. St. Louis: McGraw Hill, 2004.

Greenberg, J., C. Bruess, and D. Haffner. *Exploring the Dimensions of Human Sexually*. Sudbury, MA: Jones and Bartlett, 2004.

Pruitt, B., and J. Stein. *Decisions for Healthy Living*. San Francisco: Benjamin Cummings, 2004.

HIV/AIDS Update. Atlanta: Centers for Disease Control and Prevention, 2004.

Tracking the Hidden Epidemics: Trends in STIs in the United States. Atlanta: Centers for Disease Control and Prevention, 2004.

For links to the web sites below visit The Total Fitness and Wellness Website at www.aw-bc.com/powers.

Centers for Disease Control and Prevention

Provides information on a variety of disease-related topics, including the latest statistics on the incidence of and mortality from various diseases in the United States.

American Medical Association

Contains many sources of information about a wide variety of medical problems including alcohol, tobacco, and drug use.

WebMD

Contains information about a wide variety of diseases and medical problems including alcohol, tobacco, and drug use.

References

1. Donatelle, R., and L. Davis. *Access to Health,* 9th ed. San Francisco: Benjamin Cummings, 2006.

2. Daniels, D., R. Hillman, S. Barton, and D. Goldmeir. *Sexually Transmitted Disease and AIDS.* London: Springer-Verlag, 1993.

3. HIV/AIDS Surveillance Report. Atlanta: Centers for Disease Control and Prevention, 9:(1), 1997.

4. AIDS. Statistics from the Centers for Disease Control and Prevention 7:1691–1693, 1993.

5. Nevid, J. *201 Things You Should Know About AIDS.* Boston: Allyn and Bacon, 1993.

6. Rosenberg, P., and M. Gail. Uncertainty in estimates of HIV prevalence derived by back calculation. *Annals of Epidemiology* 1:105–115, 1990.

7. Biggar, R., and P. Rosenberg. HIV infection/AIDS in the U.S. during the 1990's. *Clinical Infectious Diseases* 17(Suppl.): S219–S223, 1993.

8. HIV/AIDS Update. Atlanta: Centers for Disease Control and Prevention, 2001.

9. Hamm, R., H. Donnell, and W. Watkins. An update on the epidemiology of AIDS in Missouri. *Missouri Medicine* 91:132–136, 1994.

10. Watanabe, M. AIDS: 20 years later. *The Scientist* 15:1, 2001.

11. Incidence of Sexually Transmitted Diseases in the U.S. Atlanta: Centers for Disease Control and Prevention, 1996.

12. Tracking the Hidden Epidemics: Trends in STIs in the United States 2000. Atlanta: Centers for Disease Control and Prevention, 2001.

13. Robbins, S., and M. Angell. *Basic Pathology.* Philadelphia: W. B. Saunders, 1997.

14. Hales, D. *An Invitation to Health,* 8th ed. San Francisco, CA: Benjamin Cummings, 1998.

15. NIDA. Keeping your body healthy. www.drugabuse.gov/DrugPages/Risky.html.2004.

16. US Department of Health and Human Services. *Healthy People 2010.* 2nd ed. With understanding and improving health and objectives for improving health. Washington DC: US Department of Health and Human Services, 2000.

17. Mullins, J., D. Nickle, L. Heath, A. Rodrigo, and G. Lerch. Immunogen sequence: The fourth tier of AIDS vaccine design. *Expert Reviews in Vaccines* 3:S151–S159, 2004.

18. Srivastava, I., J. Ulmer, and S. Barnett. Neutralizing antibody responses to HIV: Role of protective immunity and challenges for vaccine design. *Expert Reviews of Vaccines* 3:S33–S52, 2004.

19. Jackson, D., G. Dallabetta, and R. Steen. Sexually transmitted infections: Prevention and management. *Clinical Occupational and Environmental Medicine* 4:167–188, 2004.

20. Maynaud, P., and D. Mabey. Approaches to the control of sexually transmitted infections in developing countries. *Sexually Transmitted Infections* 80: 174–182, 2004.

21. Fenton, K., and C. Lowndes. Recent trends in the epidemiology of sexually transmitted infections in European Union. *Sexually Transmitted Infections* 80:255–263, 2004.

22. Lowndes, C., and K. Fenton. Surveillance systems for STIs in the European Union: Facing a changing epidemiology. *Sexually Transmitted Infections* 80:264–271, 2004.

23. Brown, A. E. et al. Recent trends in HIV and other STIs in the United Kingdom. *Sexually Transmitted Infections* 80:159–166, 2004.

24. Holmes, K., R. Levine, and M. Weaver. Effectiveness of condoms in preventing sexually transmitted diseases. *Bulletin of the World Health Organization* 82:454–461, 2004.

25. Greenberg, J., C. Bruess, and D. Haffner. *Exploring the Dimensions of Human Sexuality.* Sudbury, MA: Jones and Bartlett, 2004.

26. Anderson, B. *Reproductive Health.* Sudbury, MA: Jones and Bartlett, 2005.

27. Mulvihill, M., M. Zelman, P. Holdaway, E. Tompary, and J. Turchany. *Human Diseases: A Systemic Approach.* Upper Saddle River, NJ: Prentice Hall, 2001.

28. Strong, B., C. DeVault, B. Sayad, and W. Yarber. *Human Sexuality.* St. Louis: McGraw-Hill, 2005.

29. Bauer, H. et al. Genital human papillomavirus infection in female university students as determined by a PCR-method. *Journal of the American Medical Association* 265:472–477, 1991.

30. Eng, T., and W. Butler (eds.) *The Hidden Epidemic: Confronting Sexually Transmitted Diseases.* Washington, D.C.: National Academy Press, 1997.

31. Healthy People 2010. National Health Promotion and disease prevention objectives. PHS, 2001.

32. Nowak, T., and A. Handford. *Essentials of Pathophysiology.* St. Louis: McGraw-Hill, 1999.

33. American Public Health Association. Condoms proved effective against HIV transmission. *The Nation's Health* (4) September, 2001.

34. Centers for Disease Control and Prevention. Sexually transmitted diseases treatment guidelines. *Mortality and Morbidity Report* 51:1–80, 2002.

Inventory of Attitudes and Behaviors Toward Sexually Transmitted Infections (STIs)

NAME _____ DATE _____

This laboratory is designed to assist you in identifying attitudes and behaviors that increase your risk of contracting an STI. Remember, all STIs are preventable and your attitude and behavior determines your risk of being infected. Please read the following statements about sexual attitudes and behaviors and identify whether each statement is "true or false" for you. After completion of this exercise, go to the key at the bottom of the page and compute your level of risk for contracting an STI.

TRUE OR FALSE

_____ 1. I maintain a monogamous sexual relationship with a trusted partner.

_____ 2. I never engage in sexual activities without the use of a condom.

_____ 3. I never use alcohol or other drugs prior to sexual activities.

_____ 4. I am knowledgeable about the health risks associated with STIs.

_____ 5. I have a thorough knowledge about how all STIs are transmitted.

_____ 6. I *do not* share needles or syringes to inject drugs.

_____ 7. I am concerned about the risk of contracting an STI.

_____ 8. I always discuss STIs and "safe sex" with new partners prior to having sexual relations.

_____ 9. I always avoid sexual contact if I believe there is any risk of contracting an STI.

_____ 10. I believe that responsible "safe sex" is one of the best ways to reduce the chances of getting an STI.

SCORING AND INTERPRETATION

Count the number of "false" answers to all 10 statements and calculate your risk level for contracting an STI as follows:

0 false answers = low risk for infection with STI
1–3 false answers = high risk for infection with STI
4 or more false answers = very high risk for infection with STI

After calculating your risk for contracting STIs, please review all of the statements that you answered with a "false" answer and take action to correct this attitude or behavior so that you can respond to these statements with a "true" answer in the future. Answer the following questions to help you evaluate your sexual practices and think about STI prevention.

(continued on next page)   **403**

List three ways to bring up the subject of STIs with a new partner. How would you ask whether he or she has been exposed to any STIs or engaged in any risky behaviors?

_____

_____

_____

_____

_____

List three ways to bring up the subject of condom use with your partner. How might you convince someone who does not want to use a condom?

_____

_____

_____

_____

_____

_____

If you had an STI in the past that you might still possibly pass on (e.g., herpes), how would you tell your partner(s), and what precautions would you take during each act of sexual activity?

_____

_____

_____

_____

_____

16

Addictive Substances

After studying this chapter, you should be able to:

1. Define substance abuse and addiction.

2. Outline the acute effects of alcohol, marijuana, and cocaine on the body.

3. List several guidelines that can be used to maintain control over alcohol use.

4. Outline the behavioral and physiological effects of alcohol as a function of the level of alcohol in the blood.

5. Discuss the long-term health consequences of alcohol, marijuana, and cocaine use.

6. Describe the addictive properties of tobacco and the impact of prolonged tobacco use on health.

7. Describe the acute effects of caffeine on the body.

8. Outline products that contain caffeine and list the pros and cons of caffeine use.

9. Identify ways to reduce your risk of drug use.

Drugs play a significant role in modern society. On the positive side, the medical application of drugs in the prevention and treatment of diseases is critical to maintain wellness. For example, the appropriate use of antibiotics, hypertension medications, cancer treatment drugs, and cholesterol medications can maintain health and extend the life span of people. On the negative side, abuse of drugs is a major risk to wellness and can impose a major burden on families and society as a whole. Indeed, one of the most serious problems facing society in the twenty-first century is the abuse of psychoactive drugs (i.e., drugs designed to alter the mind or behavior). Psychoactive drugs in common use today include alcohol, cocaine, marijuana, and tobacco. Unfortunately, misuse of these drugs has and continues to damage many millions of lives worldwide. This chapter will discuss commonly used psychoactive drugs and describe ways to avoid drug abuse. We begin with a discussion of addiction.

☀ Addiction

Historically, the term **addiction** has been defined as a compulsive psychological need for a drug. More recently, the definition of addiction has been expanded to include a psychological need for other behaviors as well (6). For example, while drug use is a classic illustration of addiction, many other addictive behaviors exist, such as addictions to gambling, spending money, or eating.

The cause of addiction is complex and, in general, there appears to be no single cause for addiction. That is, addictions are often the result of numerous causes. For example, personal characteristics such as poor coping skills, environment (e.g., interaction with people using drugs), and heredity can all play a role in the development of addiction. In some cases of addiction, addictive behaviors such as drug abuse or gambling trigger the release of chemicals (e.g., neurotransmitters such as dopamine) in the brain leading to a psychological "rush" or the sensation of pleasure (22). Nonetheless, the fact that brain chemistry plays a role in the development of some addictions does not release individuals from the responsibility of avoiding an addictive behavior. Indeed, in addition to brain chemistry, lifestyle and personality traits also play an important role in the development of an addiction. Therefore, making personal decisions not to experiment with potentially addictive behaviors (e.g., drug use) is the key to

prevention. Further, recognizing the difference between a healthy habit and an addictive unhealthy behavior is important in the prevention of addiction. Addictive behaviors with potentially negative consequences are often associated with the following traits (6):

- **Reinforcement leading to craving.** Repeated behaviors that produce pleasurable emotional states reinforce the behavior. This repeated reinforcement can lead to a craving to engage in a particular behavior.

- **Loss of control.** Addictive behaviors lead to a loss of self-control and the individual loses the ability to resist engaging in the activity.

- **Escalation.** Many addictive behaviors are associated with an increased need for the addictive behavior. That is, as the addictive behavior is repeated, higher levels of the substance or activity is required to provide the same level of satisfaction.

- **Negative outcomes.** In all cases, addictive unhealthy behavior is associated with negative consequences such as impairment in physical or mental health.

Recognizing that you are engaging in a behavior that contains one or more of the above traits is essential to prevent the development of an addictive behavior. Therefore, if you are engaging in a behavior associated with any of the above traits, stop and consider carefully if this behavior should be stopped to avoid addiction. Remember, prevention of addiction is much easier to achieve than treatment for addiction.

☀ IN SUMMARY

- Addiction is a compulsive psychological need for a drug or other behaviors.
- Addictions are often the result of numerous causes including personal characteristics such as poor coping skills, your environment, and heredity.
- Recognizing the difference between a healthy habit and an addictive unhealthy behavior is important in the prevention of addiction.

☀ Substance Abuse

Alcohol abuse and the use of illegal drugs are two of the biggest substance problems in the United States today. Millions of Americans abuse alcohol and use illegal (recreational) drugs such as cocaine or marijuana (1, 4, 9–12). (See Fitness and Wellness for All, p. 414.) Unfortunately, alcohol or recreational drug abuse can lead to drug addiction (also called **chemical dependency**). Further, abuse of alcohol or recreational drugs increases your risk of accidents and may damage your

---

addiction A compulsive psychological need for a drug or behavior.
chemical dependency A term for drug addiction.
substance abuse Abuse of any drug such as alcohol, tobacco, and cocaine.

health. Over the past 10 years, several new substances have arrived on the drug scene, and some drugs that have been popular for years are still in vogue (A Closer Look, p. 408). Nonetheless, the most commonly abused drugs in the United States continue to be alcohol, marijuana, cocaine, and tobacco, which are discussed in forthcoming sections.

Recognition of substance abuse is an essential first step toward finding a solution to the problem. The American Psychiatric Association defines **substance abuse** as one or more of the following traits (6):

- Recurrent drug use resulting in a failure to perform major responsibilities at work, home, or school
- Continued drug use despite social or personal problems caused by the effects of the drug
- Recurrent drug use in a situation where the drug imposes physical danger to the individual (drug use before driving a car)
- Recurrent legal problems associated with drug use

Note that many people who engage in intermittent use of drugs may not exhibit any of the above traits on a regular basis. Nonetheless, intermittent drug use has been shown to lead to chronic substance abuse and is a warning sign to stop this type of undesired behavior before the problem escalates.

RISK OF DRUG ADDICTION

What factors influence your risk of developing an addiction to drugs? The answer is complex because numerous factors influence your risk of developing drug dependence. In brief, the key factors that determine your risk for drug addiction are the type of drug used, genetics, your psychological makeup, and social factors.

Drugs vary in their potential for dependency. Figure 16.1 illustrates the relative addiction risk of commonly used psychoactive drugs. For example, using tobacco products poses a great risk for the development of dependency because nicotine is a highly addictive drug. Similarly, drugs like crack, alcohol, heroin, and cocaine are also highly addictive. By contrast, drugs such as marijuana and LSD are relatively less addictive.

Genetic factors may also influence your risk of developing a dependency on drugs. Research indicates that differences in brain chemistry and metabolism make some individuals more vulnerable to drug dependence (22). At present, the precise differences in brain chemistry and metabolism that contribute to increased risk of drug dependence remain unclear and this topic remains an active area of research (22).

Psychological risk factors for drug dependence include an inability to cope with stress or rejection, a strong need for excitement, and a tendency toward impulsive behavior. In this regard, people may turn to drugs to avoid coping with stress, rejection, or depres-

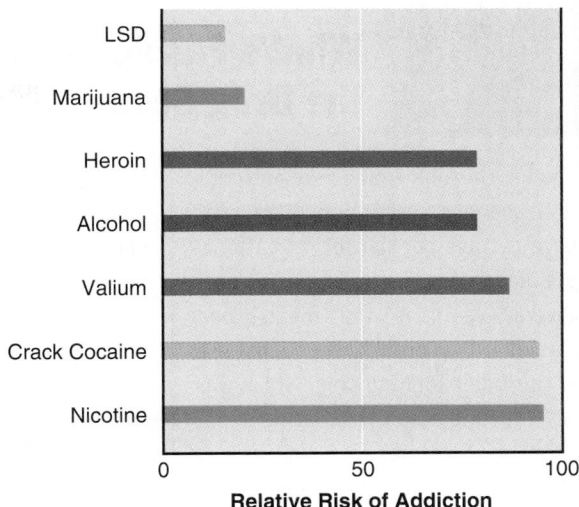

FIGURE 16.1
This figure illustrates the relative addiction risk of several commonly used psychoactive drugs. The numbers on the bottom are dimensionless and reflect the relative risk of addiction across drugs. Note that nicotine ranks as one of the most addictive drugs whereas the risk of developing an addiction to LSD ranks considerable lower.

sion. Several social risk factors for drug dependency also exist. For instance, easy access to drugs, strong peer pressure to use drugs, drug use in your family, and poverty are important social factors that increase your risk of developing a dependency on drugs.

☼ IN SUMMARY

- Drug abuse (substance abuse) is a global problem.
- Alcohol abuse and the use of illegal drugs are two of the biggest substance abuse problems in the United States.
- Key factors that determine your risk for drug addiction are the type of drug used, genetics, your psychological makeup, and social factors.
- Drugs vary in their potential for dependency. Highly addictive drugs include nicotine, crack, alcohol, and heroin.

ALCOHOL

Alcohol (ethyl alcohol) is the most widely used recreational drug in U.S. society, and the most popular drug on college campuses—used twice as much as marijuana and five times as much as cocaine (3). It is estimated that over 85% of college students in the United States use alcohol and, unfortunately, some 20–28% abuse it (3). Although many people consume alcohol to "get high," in reality alcohol is a central nervous system depressant that slows down the function of the brain. This depressive effect of alcohol results in impaired vision, slowed reaction time, and impaired motor

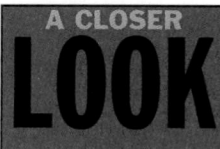

What's Fashionable on the Drug Scene Today?

Among the numerous new prescription and nonprescription drugs that have become popular for recreational use among Americans during the past several years is the prescription painkiller OxyContin®. The illegal use of this habit-forming drug, which was developed to ease the suffering of patients with painful diseases such as cancer, has grown markedly across the United States in recent years. Its addictive qualities have led to abuse among some recreational users; many have overdosed on this powerful painkiller, and others have turned to crime to feed their habits.

Another group of drugs that have widespread popularity—the so-called "club drugs"—includes some new drugs and some drugs that have been in recreational use for decades. Among the most common club drugs, which are used by young adults at all-night dance parties such as "raves" or "trances," are Ecstasy, GHB, ketamine, Rohypnol, methamphetamine, and LSD. The use of these drugs can cause serious health problems (see the table below), and in some cases their use can be fatal (15, 16). Moreover, when taken in combination with alcohol, the dangers associated with using club drugs are multiplied.

Drug (chemical name)	Slang or street names	Route of administration	Acute effects on body	Long- or short-term health effects
Methylene-dioxymethampheta-mine (MDMA)	Ecstasy, XTC, X, Adam, Clarity, Lover's Speed	Orally (tablet or capsule)	Acts as a stimulant; increases heart rate and blood pressure	Because it is neuro-toxic, use results in permanent damage to neurons (nerve cells)
Gammahydroxybu-tyrate (GBH)	Grievous Bodily Harm, G, Liquid ecstasy, Georgia Home Body	Orally; can be in liquid, white powder, tablet, or capsule forms	Acts as an intoxicating sedative (central nervous system depressant); increases release of growth hormone, so is sometimes used by body builders to build muscle	Overdose can occur quickly; symptoms include nausea, vomiting, and loss of consciousness; large overdoses can be fatal
Ketamine	Special K, K, Vitamin K, Cat valiums	Orally or smoked with marijuana or tobacco; produced in liquid form or as white powder	Acts as an anesthetic that produces dream-like states and hallucinations	High doses can cause amnesia, impaired motor function, depression, and fatal respiratory problems
Rohypnol	Roofies, Rophies, Roche, Forget-me Pill	Orally; produced in tablet form that easily dissolves in water	Acts as a sedative; produces drowsiness	Acute adverse effects include decreased blood pressure, confusion, and loss of memory
Methamphetamine	Speed, Ice, Chalk, Meth, Crystal, Crank, Fire, Glass	Orally; produced as a white powder	Can produce excited speech, increased physical activity levels, and agitation	Chronic use can lead to memory loss, aggression, psychotic behavior, and cardiac and nervous system damage
Lysergic Acid Diethylamide (LSD)	Acid, Boomers, Yellow Sunshine	Orally; produced in tablet, capsule, or liquid form	Acute effects include dilated pupils, increased heart rate and body temperature, sweating, dry mouth, and loss of appetite	Long-term use can result in psychotic behavior and hallucinations

---

TABLE 16.1
Behavioral and Physiological Effects of Alcohol
These physiological effects of alcohol were derived from reference 19.

Blood alcohol concentration (%)	Behavioral and physiological effects of alcohol	Hours required to metabolize alcohol
0.0–0.05	Increase in relaxation, feeling of euphoria, and decreased alertness.	2–3
0.05–0.10	Reduced social inhibition and impairment in reaction time and motor skills. This level of alcohol may significantly impact driving skills. Many states define legally drunk as a BAC of 0.08% or higher.	4–6
0.10–0.15	Increased impairment in reaction time and motor skills. Loss of peripheral vision.	6–10
0.15–0.30	Difficulty in walking, slurred speech, impaired pain perception, and impairment in other sensory perceptions.	10–24
More than 0.30	Can result in unconsciousness. Death possible at BAC levels of 0.35% or more. These levels of BAC are generally achieved by binge drinking.	More than 24

Source: Data from E. Ogden and H. Moskowitz, "Effects of Alcohol and Other Drugs on Driver Performance." Traffic Injury Prevention, September 5(3):185–198, 2004.

---

coordination (20). Overconsumption of alcohol also impairs your judgment. By decreasing the fear of danger, it can encourage risk-taking behaviors (such as driving too fast), which increases the likelihood of accidents (20). Drinking too much can also increase your risk of using poor judgment in social situations and in making decisions concerning sexual behavior.

The blood level of alcohol determines the magnitude of central nervous system depression by the drug. The blood alcohol concentration (BAC) is determined by the amount of alcohol consumed, your body weight, and the rate of alcohol metabolism by your body. For example, if two men that differ in body weight (e.g., 200 pounds vs. 150 pounds) consume the same amount of alcohol, the smaller individual will have the higher BAC. Alcohol is metabolized in the liver and, in general, the body can remove 0.3 ounce of alcohol per hour. In practical terms, this rate of removal is approximately half of one drink (i.e., one beer, one glass of wine, or one cocktail). Therefore, if an individual drinks slow, consuming less than one drink per hour, he or she can maintain a relatively low BAC. In contrast, an individual who drinks rapidly, consuming more than two drinks per hour, will increase his or her blood alcohol level, leading toward intoxication.

Even low doses of alcohol can have significant behavioral and physiological effects (Table 16.1). For instance, relatively small amounts of alcohol in your blood can decrease your level of alertness and increase your risk of injury (20). Higher doses lead to more unpleasant effects such as impaired motor skills and

slowed reaction times (19). These negative physiological effects of alcohol form the basis for state laws regarding the legal level of blood alcohol for driving. Indeed, since 0.05–0.10% BAC results in significant impairment in reaction times and motor skills, many states have established 0.08–0.10% BAC or above as the legal definition for alcohol intoxication (19).

Chronic abuse of alcohol over a period of years can result in liver disease (e.g., cirrhosis), damage to the nervous system, and an increased risk of certain cancers (2). Development of liver disease due to years of drinking may eventually result in total liver failure and

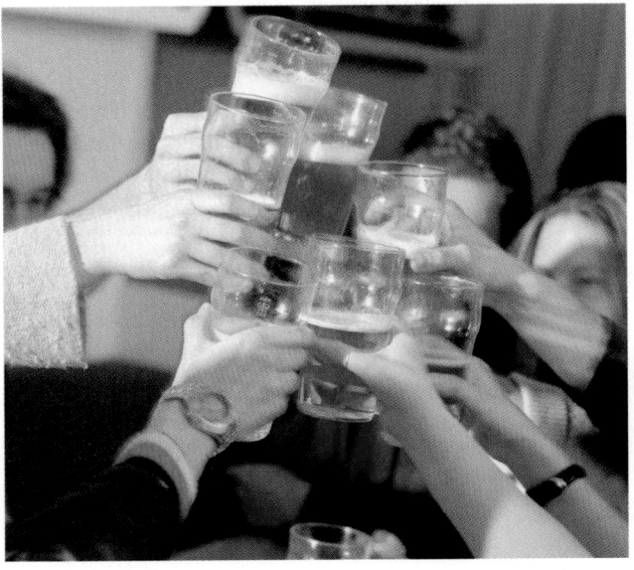

Social drinking and alcohol use is common on college campuses.

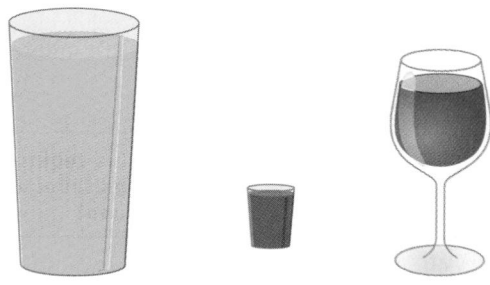

FIGURE 16.2
Ethyl alcohol is the psychoactive ingredient of all alcoholic beverages. In general, a 12-ounce beer, a 1.5 ounce cocktail drink, and a 5-ounce glass of wine contain approximately the same amount of ethyl alcohol (0.6 ounce).

death. The damage to the nervous system that results from alcohol abuse is often localized to the left side of the brain, which is responsible for written and spoken language, logic, and mathematical skills. The degree of brain damage that occurs appears to be directly related to the amount of alcohol consumed (2). Further, repeated irritation of the gastrointestinal system by alcohol has been linked to cancers of the esophagus, stomach, mouth, tongue, and liver. Another and often overlooked problem linked to chronic consumption of alcohol is undernutrition (Nutritional Links to Health and Fitness, above).

Addiction to alcohol is usually a slowly developing condition that can happen to anyone. Research into the cause of alcoholism has revealed that addiction to alcohol may have hereditary, psychological, and environmental components. Unfortunately, the details of how and why alcoholism begins are still somewhat a mystery.

You can assess your drinking habits by answering the questions in Laboratory 16.1 on p. 417. If you feel that you might be drinking too much, seek professional help from your physician or organizations such as Alcoholics Anonymous. Using the following guidelines will assist you in maintaining control over your drinking habits (1, 3):

- Know your limits and stay within them. If you are at a party and feel that you are drinking too much, learn to say "no," and switch to a nonalcoholic beverage.

marijuana A plant mixture (stems, leaves, or seeds) from either the Cannabis sativa or Cannabis indica (hemp) plants. The active chemical in marijuana that produces physical effects is tetrahydrocannabinol (THC); the higher the THC concentration in marijuana, the greater the effect.

Nutritional Links
TO HEALTH AND FITNESS
Alcohol Abuse and Undernutrition

Undernutrition is commonly associated with chronic alcohol abuse because the presence of alcohol repeatedly irritates the gastrointestinal system. Over time, the continued irritation of the gastric lining resulting from the consumption of alcohol often impairs appetite, and the ensuing lowered food intake forces the body to function on a diet that is deficient in both calories and essential nutrients. The resulting undernutrition can, in extreme cases, promote a loss of muscle mass and abnormal functioning of many body organs.

The best approach to dealing with this alcohol-related problem is to seek professional help for alcoholism. In many cases the cessation of alcohol abuse eliminates the alcohol-induced reduction in appetite, and the individual's return to normal eating habits provides the calories and nutrients needed for improved health. In severe cases of alcohol-related undernutrition, the advice of a physician and/or a nutritionist is required.

- When drinking, stick to the rule of less than 0.3 ounce (i.e., one drink) of alcohol per hour. This will reduce the likelihood that you will become physically or mentally impaired by alcohol.
- Wine, beer, and mixed drinks are less intoxicating than straight liquor. Stick to these more dilute drinks instead of the higher-alcohol beverages.
- Eating and drinking at the same time will slow down the rate of alcohol absorption and reduce your chance of becoming impaired. Never drink on an empty stomach.
- When leaving a party or bar after drinking, don't drive; call a cab or have someone else drive you home. The best course of action is to never drink and drive.

MARIJUANA

Use of marijuana became popular in the United States in the 1960s, and it remains one of the most popular illegal drugs among college students (1, 4). **Marijuana** is a plant mixture (stems, leaves, or seeds) from either the *Cannabis sativa* or *Cannabis indica* (hemp) plants that is either ingested or smoked. The active chemical

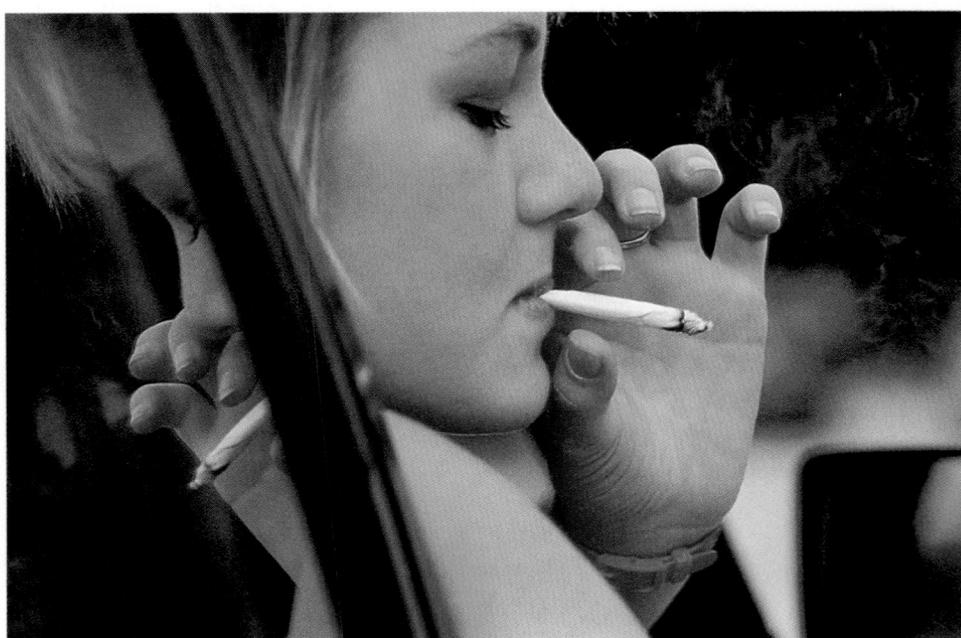

Smoking marijuana may increase your risk of accidents and health damage.

in marijuana that produces physical effects is tetrahydrocannabinol (THC). The higher the THC concentration in the marijuana, the greater the effect. The THC content in marijuana varies between 0.5% and 3.0%, and the average percentage of THC in marijuana sold in the United States is about 1.0% (4).

Marijuana can be used in many forms. It can be brewed and drunk as a tea, or it can be baked into cookies or brownies. However, marijuana is most often smoked in pipes or by rolling the marijuana into cigarettes. Effects are generally felt within 15 to 30 minutes and usually disappear within 2 to 3 hours.

Marijuana is classified as a stimulant, and its immediate effects are increased heart rate and blood pressure, bloodshot eyes, and dry mouth and throat. Recent evidence suggests that acute use of marijuana increases the risk of stroke in male adolescent users (23). Use of marijuana also impairs motor coordination and may increase your risk of accidents. Further, acute use of marijuana alters the normal function of memory centers in the brain. This memory loss resembles that observed in normal aging. However, whether these changes in function put long-term marijuana users at risk for early mental disorders is not clear.

Long-term use of marijuana presents several dangers. First, consistent users of marijuana may become psychologically dependent on its use. Further, regular smoking of marijuana causes lung damage similar to that caused by smoking tobacco (4). The effect of long-term marijuana use on the heart is not well known; however, many investigators believe that marijuana

increases the workload on the heart, which may eventually result in damage.

COCAINE

The use of **cocaine** (coke) in the United States increased dramatically during the 1980s, and current estimates are that over 5 million Americans use the drug (1). Recent estimates are that Americans spend over $38 dollars a year on the purchase of cocaine (13). Further, a recent survey suggests that as many as 6% of college students have also experimented with cocaine (1). This makes cocaine the third most widely used drug by college students.

Cocaine is a powerful stimulant derived from the leaves of the South American coca shrub, which grows primarily in the Andes Mountains. Cocaine, which is extracted from the coca leaves using a multistep process, produces a white powder (similar to sugar in appearance). Varying the extraction process can produce several different forms of cocaine, such as crack cocaine, rock cocaine, or freebase cocaine.

---

cocaine A powerful stimulant derived from the leaves of the South American coca shrub, which grows primarily in the Andes Mountains. Cocaine, which is extracted from the coca leaves using a multistep process, produces a white powder.

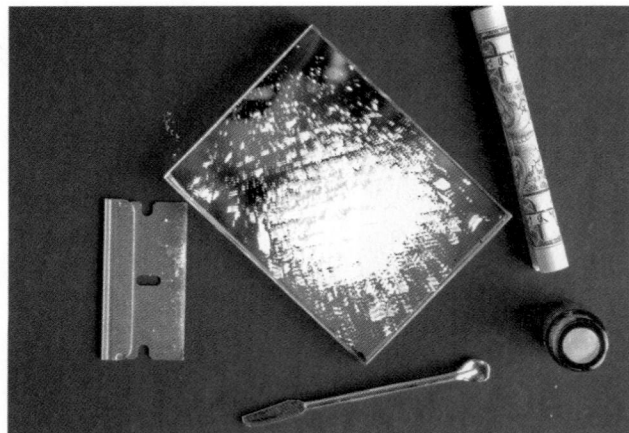

One of the most common methods of cocaine administration is snorting.

Cocaine can be used in several ways. Common uses include snorting (sniffing cocaine into the nose), smoking, and intravenous injection. All routes of administration result in a rapid and short-lived high that generally lasts from 5 to 20 minutes. Cocaine is a highly addictive drug; when the cocaine high disappears, the user wants more. Spending over $1500 per day for cocaine is not uncommon for an addict. As a result of their addiction, cocaine addicts often suffer psychological damage, which eventually contributes to loss of jobs and financial ruin.

The immediate physiological effects of cocaine are varied. The drug is both an anesthetic and a central nervous system stimulant (21). Cocaine use increases heart rate and blood pressure (14, 21). Other effects include a feeling of euphoria, heightened self-confidence,

---

nicotine The additive and psychoactive drug in tobacco plants.

---

and increased alertness (21). In large doses, cocaine is extremely dangerous, and numerous deaths have resulted from overdoses. Further, long-term cocaine use may damage the heart, brain, and respiratory system.

Treatment for cocaine addiction requires professional help. To assist cocaine addicts, the National Institute for Drug Abuse (NIDA) has established toll-free hotlines (1-800-COCAINE). If you or anyone you know uses cocaine, seek professional help at once. Cocaine addiction is a serious problem that requires immediate attention. For more information on drug treatment programs consult the National Institute of Drug Abuse website listed at the end of this chapter.

☀ IN SUMMARY

- The most common recreational drug in American society is alcohol and it is estimated that over 85% of college students drink alcohol.
- Relatively low levels of blood alcohol (i.e., 0.05–0.10%) can impair both reaction time and motor skills resulting in a diminished ability to drive.
- Marijuana remains the most popular illegal drug with college students.
- Cocaine, a powerful stimulant derived from the leaves of coca plants, is the third most popular drug used by college students.
- Club drugs are a group of drugs used by young adults at all-night dance parties. Common club drugs include Ecstasy, GHB, Rohypnol, ketamine, methamphetamine, and LSD.

TOBACCO

Nicotine, contained in tobacco products, is the most heavily used addictive drug in the United States. In 2003, 30% of the U.S. population 12 and older (>72 million people) used tobacco at least once a

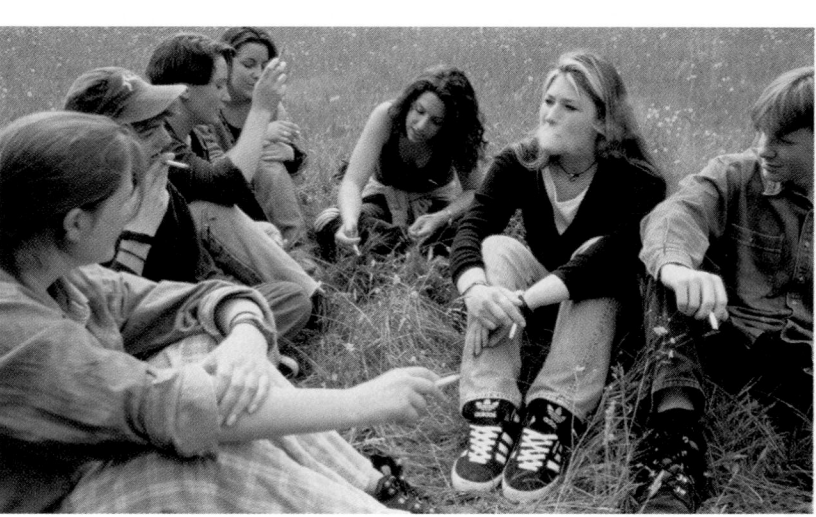

Cigarette smoking remains popular, especially among college students facing new stresses and peer influence.

month (13). This number includes 14 million people of college age (i.e., 18–25 years old). The good news is that smoking rates for young Americans are no longer climbing and have declined slightly from the peaks reached in the late 1990s. Nonetheless, use of tobacco products in the United States continues to involve a large number of Americans.

Cigarette smoking has been the most popular method of nicotine use since the beginning of the twentieth century (13). Unfortunately, cigarettes and other forms of tobacco use are associated with major health risks. This fact prompted the U.S. Surgeon General to issue a national warning that cigarettes and other forms of tobacco use (e.g., cigars, pipes, and chewing tobacco) are addictive and that nicotine is the drug in tobacco that causes the addiction (13). This report also stated that smoking was a major cause of stroke and heart attacks and was the third leading cause of death in the United States. Further, regular tobacco use increases the risk of several forms of cancer including lung cancer (13). In fact, statistics from the Centers for Disease Control and Prevention indicate that tobacco use remains the leading preventable cause of death in the United States, causing more than 440,000 deaths each year and resulting in an annual cost of more than $75 billion in direct medical costs (13).

Nicotine is absorbed readily from tobacco smoke in the lungs and it does not matter whether the smoke is from cigarettes, cigars, or pipes (13). Moreover, inhalation of secondhand smoke also results in the absorption of nicotine. Nicotine is also absorbed in the mouth when tobacco is chewed. With regular use of tobacco, nicotine can accumulate in the body and remain for several hours (13).

Why is nicotine so addictive? The reason for the addiction is that nicotine provides an almost immediate "psychological kick" to the body because it causes the release of epinephrine from the adrenal cortex (an endocrine gland in the body) (14). This stimulates the central nervous system and increases both heart rate and blood pressure (14). This psychological stimulation is rapidly lost, which leads to both depression and fatigue, leading the abuser to seek more nicotine.

Addiction to nicotine results in withdrawal symptoms when a person tries to stop smoking. For example, studies indicate that when chronic smokers were deprived of cigarettes for 24 hours, they had increased anger, hostility, aggression, and a loss of social cooperation (13). Further, people suffering from nicotine withdrawal take longer to regain emotional equilibrium following exposure to stress (13). Moreover, during periods of abstinence from smoking, smokers show a wide range of physical and mental impairments such as impaired psychomotor skills (i.e., movement coordination) and impaired cognitive functions (13).

While behavior modification approaches to smoking cessation were discussed in Chapter 10, it is important

TABLE 16.2
Caffeine Content of Popular Foods and Drug Prescriptions

Food or drug preparation	Serving size	Caffeine (mg)
Coffee (drip method)	5 oz cup	110–150
Coffee (instant)	5 oz cup	40–108
Coffee (decaffeinated)	5 oz cup	2–5
Tea (bag or loose; 5 min brew)	5 oz cup	20–50
Cocoa (mix)	5 oz cup	6
Milk chocolate	1 oz serving	6
Baking chocolate	1 oz serving	35
Mountain Dew (soft drink)	12 oz serving	54
Coca Cola (soft drink)	12 oz serving	46
Dr. Pepper (soft drink)	12 oz serving	40
Pepsi Cola (soft drink)	12 oz serving	38
No Doz tablets	1 tablet or capsule	100
Vivarin tablets	1 tablet or capsule	200

Source: Data collected from Consumers Union, FDA, National Coffee Association, Physicians Desk Reference for non-Prescription Drugs, 1983.

to mention that studies have revealed that some of the most successful long-term smoking cessation programs involve not only behavioral treatment but also use pharmacological treatment as well (13). Most of these pharmacological treatments involve using nicotine gum or the use of transdermal patches (i.e., patches placed on the skin) to deliver nicotine during the initial stages of smoking cessation. The success of smoking cessation treatment varies widely across studies. Generally, the rates of relapse for smoking cessation are highest in the first few weeks after smoking cessation and diminish greatly after about three months (13). So, if you smoke, it is possible to stop. Begin this process by reviewing approaches to behavioral modification in Chapter 10 and start your smoking cessation program today!

USE OF CAFFEINE

Caffeine is a stimulant found in a wide variety of common foods including coffee, tea, and coca (Table 16.2). It seems likely that caffeine is the most frequently

caffeine A stimulant found in a wide variety of common foods such as coffee, tea, and chocolate.

FITNESS AND WELLNESS FOR ALL

The Pervasiveness of Drug Abuse in America

Drug use and abuse occurs in people of all ages, educational and income levels, and ethnic groups. Still, research shows that some people are more likely to try illegal drugs and are consequently at greater risk for drug abuse. For example, young males with risk-taking personalities and a strong apathy toward school are at high risk for experimenting with drugs (12). Social factors that increase an individual's risk for drug abuse include frequent exposure to drug users, easy access to drugs, and poverty. In contrast, drug use is less common in individuals who are independent thinkers and are not easily influenced by their peers. Further, compared to individuals who are uninterested in schoolwork, individuals who attend school regularly and earn good grades are less likely to try illegal drugs.

---

ingested psychoactive drug in the world (24). Caffeine stimulates the central nervous system by stimulating a variety of brain centers resulting in increased alertness and decreased drowsiness (15, 16). In fact, caffeine has been shown to reduce fatigue and improve performance during prolonged endurance exercise (e.g., running a marathon) (18). Evidence that caffeine may improve endurance exercise performance has prompted the International Olympic Committee to consider banning high blood levels of caffeine during performance in the Olympic games (14).

Similar to other habit-forming drugs, chronic use of caffeine can lead to mild addiction (15, 16). In this regard, abrupt discontinuation of caffeine intake can result in severe headache, fatigue, irritability, and gastrointestinal distress. Nonetheless, cessation of caffeine use has been shown to be considerably easier to achieve than cessation of other stimulants, such as nicotine (17).

The question of whether caffeine use is associated with negative health consequences remains controversial. At present, there is no clear consensus as to whether long-term use of caffeine poses a significant health risk. However, a recent review concluded that moderate daily intake of caffeine (less than 400 mg/day) is not associated with adverse health effects (24). Nonetheless, it is clear that high doses of caffeine (i.e., 200 mg or more) can increase both heart rate and blood pressure and, in some people, caffeine increases the risk of abnormal heart rhythms (15, 16). Further, for people unaccustomed to caffeine use or when caffeine is consumed in large doses, caffeine can produce tremors, nervousness, restlessness, and insomnia. Therefore, if you consume caffeine as a part of your regular diet, it is wise to use caffeine in moderation. See Table 16.2 for a listing of the caffeine content of common foods, beverages, and drug preparations.

☀ IN SUMMARY

- Nicotine, the psychoactive drug in tobacco products, is one of the most addictive drugs available.
- Use of tobacco can lead to an addiction to nicotine and prolonged use of tobacco products can lead to numerous health problems including an increased risk of heart disease and cancer.
- Caffeine is a central nervous system stimulant that can reduce fatigue and improve alertness.
- Caffeine is addictive and withdrawal from caffeine use can result in headaches and other side effects.
- It is currently unclear if prolonged use of caffeine poses significant health risks.

☀ Say "No" to Drugs

Drug abuse cuts across all segments of the U.S. population (Fitness and Wellness for All). Avoiding drug use requires self-discipline and control. Several steps can help protect you from the temptation to use drugs (1, 3, 17):

1. Increase your self-esteem. Take pride in yourself and your achievements; this will boost your confidence and improve your ability to say "no" to drugs.
2. Learn how to cope with stress. When stressed, use one or more of the stress management techniques discussed in Chapter 10 (such as exercise or progressive relaxation).
3. Develop numerous interests. Develop interest in hobbies or sports that provide you with pleasure.
4. Practice assertiveness. Becoming assertive is an important key to learning to say "no" to drugs.

Summary

1. Alcohol, nicotine (tobacco products), marijuana, and cocaine are the most widely used and abused drugs in the United States.

2. Use of alcohol, marijuana, and cocaine increases your risk of accidents, and prolonged use of these substances may result in psychological dependence, addiction, and damaged health.

3. Alcohol is the single most common recreational drug used in the United States.

4. Chronic abuse of alcohol can result in liver disease, damage to the nervous system, and increased risk of certain cancers.

5. Blood alcohol concentrations of 0.05–0.10% can result in a significant reduction in reaction time and impaired motor skills.

6. Long-term use of marijuana may result in psychological dependence and may increase your risk of cardiopulmonary diseases (similar to tobacco smoking).

7. Cocaine is a highly addictive drug that, when taken in large doses, can be lethal.

8. Use of tobacco can lead to an addiction to nicotine and prolonged use of tobacco products can lead to numerous health problems including increased risk of heart attack, stroke, and cancer.

9. Caffeine is a central nervous system stimulant found in numerous common foods and beverages. Whether chronic consumption of caffeine is a significant health risk is currently unclear.

10. You can decrease your risk of using drugs by increasing your self-esteem, learning how to cope with stress, developing numerous interests, and practicing assertiveness.

Study Questions

1. Define and discuss the terms *substance abuse* and *addiction*.

2. Outline those factors that determine the risk of developing an addiction to drugs.

3. Discuss the short-term and long-term effects of alcohol use.

4. Describe the changes in behavior and physiological function that occur as blood alcohol levels increase.

5. What is the most widely used recreational drug in America?

6. List four steps that can help you feel less tempted to use drugs.

7. Discuss the short-term and long-term effects of marijuana use.

8. Describe the physiological response to the use of cocaine.

9. List the physiological responses to caffeine.

10. Outline steps that you can take to decrease your risk of drug use.

Suggested Reading

Donatelle, R. *Access to Health,* 9th edition. San Francisco: Benjamin Cummings, 2006.

Fields, R. *Drugs in Perspective.* St. Louis: McGraw-Hill, 2004.

Powers, S., and E. Howley. *Exercise Physiology: Theory and Application to Fitness and Performance.* St. Louis: McGraw-Hill, 2004.

Pruitt, B., and J. Stein. *Decisions for Healthy Living.* San Francisco: Benjamin Cummings, 2004.

Wilson, H. *Drugs, Society, and Behavior.* St. Louis: McGraw-Hill, 2004.

Wilson, H. *Drugs and Substance Abuse.* St. Louis: McGraw-Hill, 2001.

For links to the web sites below visit The Total Fitness and Wellness Website at www.aw-bc.com/powers.

American Medical Association

Contains many sources of information about a wide variety of medical problems including alcohol, tobacco, and drug use.

WebMD

Contains information about a wide variety of diseases and medical problems including alcohol, tobacco, and drug use.

Higher Education Center for Alcohol and Other Drug Prevention

Presents information about alcohol and drug abuse on college campuses; also contains web links to other related organizations.

National Institute on Drug Abuse

This comprehensive site contains information about commonly abused drugs, the incidence of drug abuse in the United States, and where to find help with rehabilitation from drug dependency.

References

1. Donatelle, R. *Access to Health,* 9th edition. San Francisco: Benjamin Cummings, 2006.

2. Robbins, S., and M. Angell. *Basic Pathology.* Philadelphia: W. B. Saunders, 1997.

3. Hales, D. *An Invitation to Health,* 8th ed. Redwood City: Benjamin Cummings, 1998.

4. Liska, K. *Drugs and the Human Body,* Englewood Cliffs, NJ: Prentice Hall, 2000.

5. National Institute on Drug Abuse. Community drug alert bulletin on club drugs. July 7, 2001.

6. American Psychiatric Association. *Diagnostic and Statistical Manual of Mental Disorders.* Washington, DC: American Psychiatric Association, 1994.

7. Fields, R. *Drugs in Perspective.* St. Louis: McGraw-Hill, 2004.

8. Pruitt, B., and J. Stein. *Decisions for Healthy Living.* San Francisco: Benjamin Cummings, 2004.

9. Wilson, H. *Drugs, Society, and Behavior.* St. Louis: McGraw-Hill, 2004.

10. Wilson, H. *Drugs and Substance Abuse.* St. Louis: McGraw-Hill, 2001.

11. Werch, C. et al. A sport-based intervention for preventing alcohol use and promoting physical activity among adolescents. *Journal School Health* 73:380–388, 2003.

12. Ginn, S. Relationships among alcohol consumption, drug use, and goal orientation among college students in the southeastern USA. *Psychological Reports* 94:411–421, 2004.

13. National Institute on Drug Abuse. Info facts. www .drugabuse.gov. US Department of Health and Human Services, 2004.

14. Powers, S., and E. Howley. *Exercise Physiology: Theory and Application to Fitness and Performance.* St. Louis: McGraw-Hill, 2004.

15. Powers, S., and S. Dodd. Caffeine and endurance performance: A review. *Sports Medicine* 2:165–174, 1985.

16. Dodd, S., R. Herb, and S. Powers. Caffeine and exercise performance: An update. *Sports Medicine* 15:14–23, 1993.

17. Glantz, M., and C. Hartel (eds.) *Drug Abuse: Origins and Interventions.* Washington, DC: APA Publications, 1999.

18. Maughan, R. Dietary supplements. *Journal of Sports Sciences* 22:95–113, 2004.

19. Ogden, E., and H. Moskowitz. Effects of alcohol and other drugs on driver performance. *Traffic Injury Prevention* 5:185–198, 2004.

20. Sindelar, H., N. Barnett, and A. Spirito. Adolescent alcohol use and injury: A summary and critical review of the literature. *Minerva Pediatrics* 56:291–309, 2004.

21. White, S., and C. Lambe. The pathophysiology of cocaine abuse. *Journal of Clinical Forensic Medicine* 10:27–39, 2003.

22. Cannon, C., and M. Bseikri. Is dopamine required for natural reward? *Physiology of Behavior* 81:741–748, 2004.

23. Geller T., L. Loftis, and D. Brink. Cerebellar infarction in adolescent males associated with acute marijuana use. *Pediatrics* 113:e365–370, 2004.

24. Nawrot, P., S. Jordan, J. Eastwood, J. Rotstein, A. Hugenholtz, and M. Feeley. Effects of caffeine on human health. *Food Additives and Contamination* 20:1–30, 2003.

Alcohol Abuse Inventory

NAME _____ DATE _____

This laboratory is designed to increase your awareness of your drinking habits. For this inventory to provide a valid assessment of your drinking behaviors, you must answer each question honestly.

DIRECTIONS

Please check under "Yes" or "No" for each of the following questions regarding your use of alcohol.

		Yes	No
1.	Do you often drink alone?	_____	_____
2.	When drinking, do you often worry about running out of alcoholic beverages?	_____	_____
3.	Do you drink alcohol on a daily basis?	_____	_____
4.	When stressed, do you immediately drink alcohol to reduce your stress levels?	_____	_____
5.	Do you crave alcohol during all parts of the day?	_____	_____
6.	Do you have trouble saying "no" to drinking at a party?	_____	_____
7.	Do you sometimes have trouble remembering what you did the night before?	_____	_____
8.	Does your drinking impair your school or job performance?	_____	_____
9.	Does your drinking impair your ability to use good judgment or cause you to have accidents?	_____	_____
10.	Do you ever lie about how much you drink to friends or family?	_____	_____

Answering "Yes" to only one of the questions above suggests that you may be drinking too much. Answering "Yes" to two questions is a clear warning sign that you may have or are in the process of developing an alcohol abuse problem. Answering "Yes" to three or more questions indicates that you have a serious alcohol abuse problem, and that you should seek professional help.

(continued on next page)

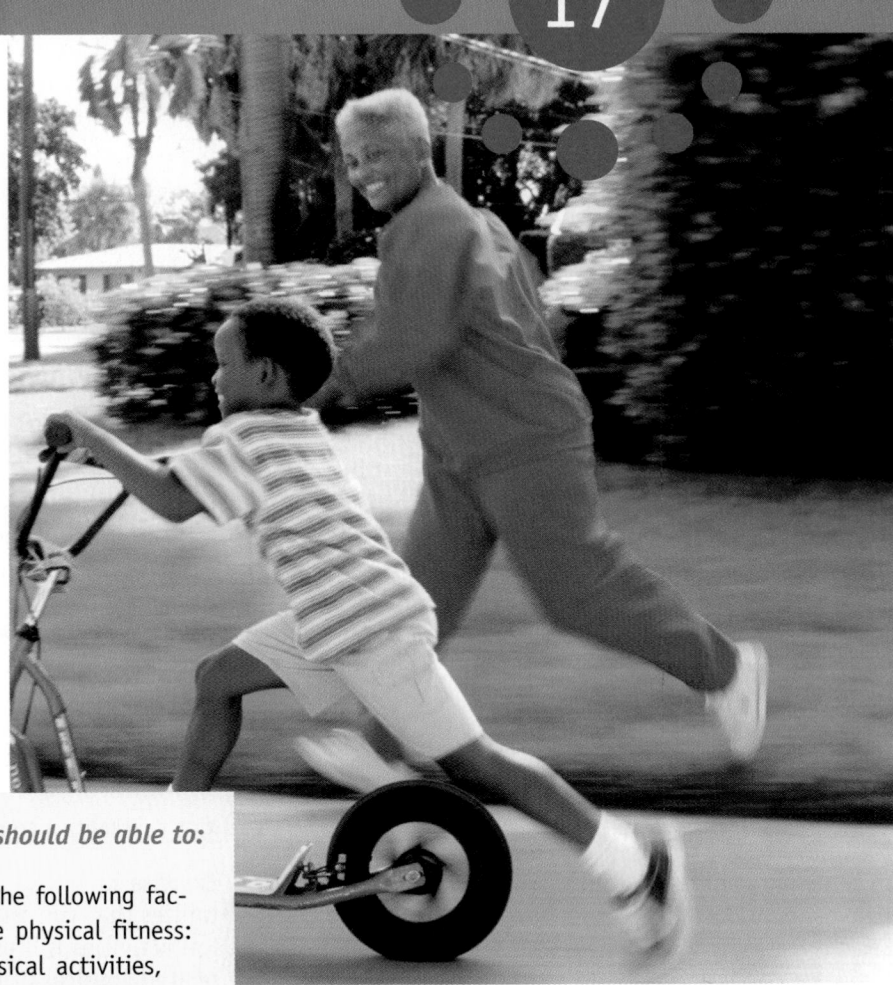

17

Lifetime Fitness
and Wellness

After studying this chapter, you should be able to:

1. Discuss the importance that the following factors play in achieving lifetime physical fitness: goal setting, selection of physical activities, planning exercise sessions, monitoring fitness progress, and social support.

2. Outline several common misconceptions about physical fitness.

3. Discuss the key factors to consider when choosing a health club.

4. List age-related changes in fitness and wellness and describe actions that you can take to maintain fitness and wellness throughout the life span.

5. Describe strategies for choosing a personal physician and list the regularity of routine medical check-ups for your age group and gender.

6. List the keys to success for achieving lifetime wellness.

Exercise must be performed regularly throughout your life to achieve the exercise-induced benefits of physical fitness and wellness. Fitness cannot be stored! If you stop exercise, you will lose fitness and begin to lose the health and wellness benefits derived from regular exercise.

Identical to exercise, good health behaviors and a healthy diet must be practiced on a daily basis to achieve a lifetime of wellness. For example, healthy dietary habits to reduce the risk of heart disease and cancer must be followed every day rather than one or two days a week. This chapter suggests strategies for maintaining a lifetime fitness and wellness program. We also consider key factors in choosing an exercise facility (i.e., health club) and discuss important issues related to health care decisions.

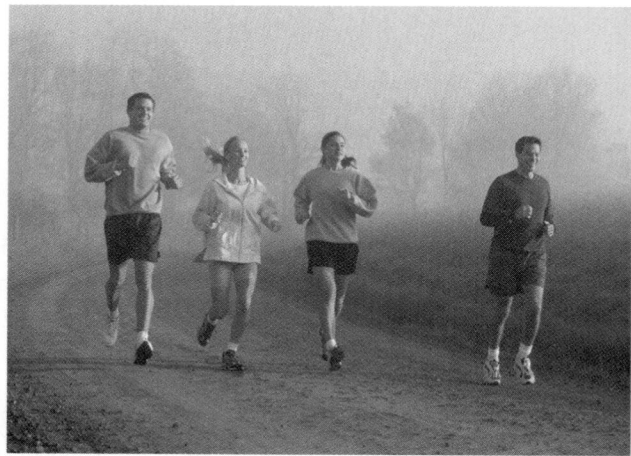

Exercising with friends makes workouts more fun.

☀ Exercise Adherence: Lifetime Fitness and Wellness

Studies have shown that over 60% of adults who start an exercise program quit within the first month (1). In contrast, people who start an exercise program and continue to exercise regularly for at least 6 months have an excellent chance of maintaining a regular exercise routine for years to come (1). Thus, the first 6 months of your exercise program are critical in determining your lifetime adherence to exercise. The significance of exercising regularly for several months is probably linked to the fact that 2 to 6 months of training are generally required to bring about significant improvements in both fitness and body composition (i.e., fat loss). This positive feedback, once achieved, provides a strong incentive to continue exercising.

Beginning a lifetime exercise program requires a strong personal commitment to physical fitness and application of the principles of behavior modification to change from a sedentary lifestyle to an active lifestyle. In the next sections we discuss several factors that will assist you in maintaining a lifetime commitment to physical activity.

GOAL SETTING FOR ACTIVE LIFESTYLES

Although the first step in beginning a successful exercise program is desiring to be physically fit, the second step is establishing both short-term and long-term fitness goals (goal setting was introduced in Chapter 1 and discussed in detail in Chapter 3). Your goals should be based on your personal needs and desire for fitness, and they should be realistic. Goal setting provides a target to shoot for and adds an incentive to maintain regular exercise habits. Goals can be either maintenance goals or improvement goals. For example, a realistic short-term improvement goal for cardiorespiratory

fitness might be to decrease your 1.5-mile run time from 15 minutes to 14 minutes during your first 6 months of training. In contrast, a short-term maintenance goal might be to average 20 miles of running per week during the first year of training. A key point to remember about fitness goals is that they should be modified from time to time to accommodate any changes in your fitness needs and to allow you to correct any unrealistic goals you may have set.

SELECTING ACTIVITIES

Exercise should be fun! You should choose exercise activities that you enjoy. However, not all enjoyable physical activities will promote improvement in health-related physical fitness. Which sports or activities provide the best training effect to improve physical fitness? Table 17.1 evaluates the fitness potential of a variety of popular sports and activities. Note that no one activity is rated as being excellent in promoting all aspects of fitness. To achieve total physical fitness, you should participate in several activities.

Another key consideration is the availability and convenience of the activity. Regardless of how much you enjoy a particular activity, if it is not convenient, your chances of regular participation are greatly reduced. For example, suppose you enjoy swimming but the pool closest to your home or school is 10 miles away, and to make matters worse, the pool hours of operation conflict with your daily schedule. In combination, these two factors decrease your chances of successfully using swimming as your primary mode of regular exercise. The solution to this problem is simple. Continue to swim when you have the opportunity, but choose another convenient activity that you enjoy as your regular exercise mode. Remember, selecting a convenient and enjoyable activity will

TABLE 17.1
Fitness Evaluation of Various Activities and Sports

| Sport/Activity | Fitness Ranking | | | | |
	Cardiorespiratory Endurance	Upper Body Muscular Strength and Endurance	Lower Body Muscular Strength and Endurance	Flexibility	Caloric Expenditure (calories/min)
Aerobic dance	Good	Good	Good	Fair	5–10
Badminton	Fair	Fair	Good	Fair	5–10
Baseball	Poor	Fair	Fair	Fair	4–6
Basketball	Good	Fair	Good	Fair	10–12
Bowling	Poor	Fair	Poor	Fair	3–4
Canoeing	Fair	Good	Poor	Fair	4–10
Football (flag/touch)	Fair	Fair	Good	Fair	5–10
Golf (walking)	Poor	Fair	Good/fair	Fair	2–4
Gymnastics	Poor	Excellent	Excellent	Excellent	3–4
Handball	Good	Good/fair	Good	Fair	7–12
Karate	Fair	Good	Good	Excellent	7–10
Racquetball	Good/fair	Good/fair	Good	Fair	6–12
Running	Excellent	Fair	Good	Fair	8–15
Skating (ice)	Good/fair	Poor	Good/fair	Good/fair	5–10
Skating (roller)	Good/fair	Poor	Good/fair	Fair	5–10
Skiing (alpine)	Fair	Fair	Good	Fair	5–10
Skiing (nordic)	Excellent/good	Good	Good	Fair	7–15
Soccer	Good	Fair	Good	Good/fair	7–17
Tai Chi	Good/fair	Good/fair	Good/fair	Fair	5–9
Tennis	Good/fair	Good/fair	Good	Fair	5–12
Volleyball	Fair	Fair	Good/fair	Fair	4–8
Waterskiing	Poor	Good	Good	Fair	4–7
Weight training	Poor	Excellent	Excellent	Fair	4–6
Yoga	Poor	Poor	Poor	Excellent	2–4

Source: From Getchell, B. Physical Fitness: A Way of Life. Copyright © 1992. Reprinted by permission of Allyn and Bacon.
Lan, C. S. Chen, and J. Lai. Tai Chi. American Journal of Chinese Medicine 32:151–160, 2004.
Taylor-Pillae, R. and E. Foelicher. Effectiveness of Tai Chi in improving aerobic capacity: A meta analysis. Journal of Cardiovascular Nursing 19:48–57, 2004.

greatly increase your chances of maintaining a regular exercise program.

PLANNING EXERCISE SESSIONS

Exercise sessions should be systematic and connected to your exercise goals (2, 3). This is particularly true during the first several weeks of an exercise program. To achieve your objectives, you must train on a regular basis.

Choosing a regular time to exercise helps to make it a habit. Some fitness instructors suggest that morning exercise is superior to exercise at other times of the day; however, there is no scientific evidence to support the notion that there is an optimal time of day to

exercise. This is fortunate, because individual preferences for a daily exercise time vary. Some people prefer to exercise in the morning hours, whereas others may prefer a noon workout. Choose a time that works for you; the key to exercising regularly is to choose a convenient time to work out and stick with it.

MONITORING PROGRESS

Monitoring your progress in achieving or maintaining physical fitness is an important factor in providing feedback and motivation to continue. You can monitor your progress in at least two ways. First, maintain a training log to provide feedback concerning the amount

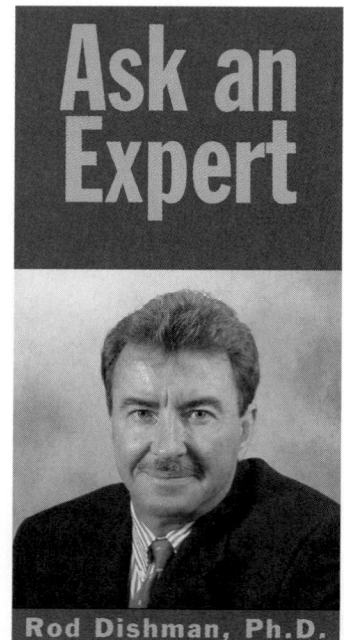

Ask an Expert

Rod Dishman, Ph.D.

Exercise Adherence

Dr. Dishman is professor of exercise science and Director of the Exercise Psychology Laboratory at the University of Georgia, Athens, GA. He is one of the world's leading experts in exercise psychology and issues related to exercise adherence. Dr. Dishman has published numerous scientific papers, books, and book chapters related to exercise adherence. In the following interview, Dr. Dishman addresses several questions related to adherence to regular exercise.

Q: **What factors can help me stay motivated to maintain a regular exercise program?**

A: Make exercise your top priority by actions, not just intentions. Schedule a time and pick a place to exercise. Many people find exercise at lunchtime or at the end of the day invigorating; however, most inactive people prefer relaxation. Also, strong intentions often weaken by day's end, and people may feel fatigued and want to rest, not exert. If the later scenario describes you, exercise early in the day.

If you lack the self-motivation to carry out exercise goals, pick other activities or rewards that are important to you and make a commitment not to indulge yourself until daily exercise goals are met. Also, keep a record to ensure that you don't conveniently forget or lie to yourself when you don't meet exercise goals.

Engineer your environment to make it hard to talk yourself out of exercising. Put exercise equipment near your bed at night, so you see it first thing in the morning. Keep exercise gear in your car or at work for availability whenever exercise opportunities arise.

Contrary to popular belief, there is little evidence that high level fitness is needed for health benefits. Moderate exertion seems effective too. Pick a type of exercise you most enjoy, a time that best fits your schedule, and an intensity that is pleasurable.

Don't judge the benefits of your exercise by fitness gains alone. Research confirms that moderate exercise can have calming and mood elevating effects and may even improve sleep.

Q: **How important is fitness goal setting as a motivating factor for beginning an exercise program?**

A: Specific, long-term exercise goals are important to get an exercise program started. Goals don't have to be fully realistic. An idealized goal that you might not be able to reach can nevertheless be a good exercise incentive; however, you must plan a series of shorter term step-by-step goals that are attainable and can bring you closer to your ultimate objective. Distant goals should not change, but immediate daily goals can and often should be flexible. Avoid the abstainer's fallacy that there is only one rigid, unyielding plan that will work for you.

Q: **Is it possible to develop a psychological dependence on exercise and, therefore, develop an addiction to exercise?**

A: In the 1970s, William P. Morgan of the University of Wisconsin described eight cases of running addiction, when a commitment to running exceeded prior commitments to work, family, social relations, and medical advice. Similar cases have been labeled as positive addiction, runner's gluttony, fitness fanaticism, athlete's neurosis, obligatory running, and exercise abuse. Little is understood, however, about the origins, valid diagnosis, or the mental health impact of abusive exercise.

of exercise performed. For example, a daily training log can help you monitor the number of miles run, the amount of weight lifted, total calories expended during exercise, any changes in body weight, and so on. A number of commercially available training diaries and computer programs are available.

A second means of monitoring your fitness progress is through periodic fitness testing (Chapter 2). Fitness testing provides positive feedback when fitness levels are improving. This type of information is a useful motivational tool and should be a part of every fitness program.

SOCIAL SUPPORT

Social support is another key factor in many successful exercise programs. Enjoying interaction with friends or colleagues during exercise or in the locker room before or after a workout is an important part of making exercise fun. See Fitness-Wellness Consumer for some tips on choosing a health club. Beginning an exercise program with a friend is an excellent way to start exercising on a regular basis, provided that both individuals share the same commitment to improving personal fitness.

PEERS AS ROLE MODELS

Your personal commitment to exercise can be positively influenced by peers who serve as good role models for

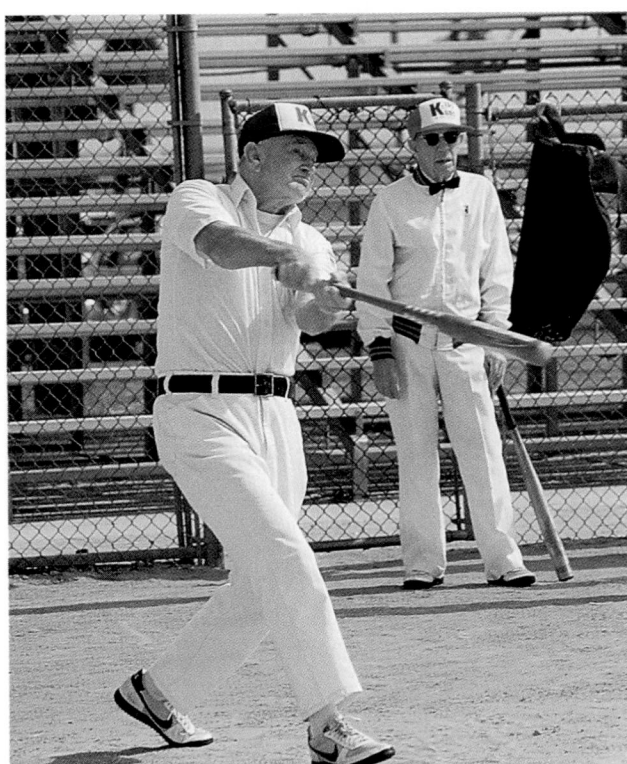

Aging may change your physical activity needs over the course of a lifetime.

FITNESS-WELLNESS CONSUMER

Health Clubs: Choosing a Fitness Facility

While it isn't necessary to join a fitness club to become physically fit, many people prefer exercising in the social environment provided by a club. However, before choosing a fitness facility, consider the following recommendations (4, 5):

- Investigate the variety of fitness programs available in your community before deciding to join any fitness club. Explore not only commercial fitness facilities, but also programs offered by your local YMCA or university.

- Consider the club's location. Is the facility convenient to your home or to work?

- Check the club's reputation with the Better Business Bureau. Inquire how long the club has been in business and if clients have registered complaints.

- Make several trial visits to investigate the cleanliness of the locker rooms, the quality of exercise equipment, and how many people use the facility at your desired workout time.

- Inquire about the qualification of the fitness instructors. It is important to ensure that the club's fitness instructors are well trained. See A Closer Look on p. 424 for what a "fitness expert" truly is.

- Consider the club's approach to fitness and training. Does it provide routine physical fitness tests and health screening services (e.g., blood pressure measurement)? Do instructors routinely spend time with members, or are members required to seek out instructors to obtain assistance?

- Avoid signing a long-term contract with any fitness club. Be wary of contract clauses that waive either the club's liability for injury to you or your right to defend yourself in court.

- Avoid clubs that advertise overnight fitness or quick weight loss. After reading the first eight chapters of this book, you already know that these types of claims are false.

the benefits of exercise. Most of us know individuals who exercise regularly and look terrific as a result of proper training and diet. These role models can be motivational to people who are beginning an exercise program.

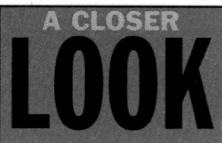

What Is a Fitness Expert?

Even though there is presently no standard definition of "fitness expert," anyone who has earned an advanced degree (such as an M.S. or a Ph.D.) in exercise science, kinesiology, or exercise physiology from a reputable university can generally be considered a fitness expert. Moreover, many trained professionals in health education, physical education, and nutrition may also qualify as fitness experts. Although individuals with bachelor's degrees in exercise science may have a sufficient background to answer many fitness-related questions, the more advanced the degree, the more knowledgeable the individual should be about exercise and fitness.

Exercise scientists who are actively conducting research in exercise physiology and are active in such professional organizations as the American Physiological Society or the American College of Sports Medicine are generally the best sources of valid information, especially concerning more technical matters. Additionally, physicians with postgraduate training in exercise physiology or a strong personal interest in preventive medicine are also good sources of scientifically based fitness information.

If you having difficulty finding a local fitness expert who can answer your questions, contact the American College of Sports Medicine (P.O. Box 1440, Indianapolis, IN 46206-1440) for the name of a fitness expert near you.

CHANGING PHYSICAL ACTIVITY NEEDS

As we age, our needs for and interest in physical activity often change. It is thus important to modify your fitness program throughout your life. For instance, while some people engage in a single activity such as basketball over the course of several years, many people lose interest in repeating the same daily activity. When this occurs, it becomes important to find other activities that interest you. Many physical activity options exist, so individuals should remain flexible in their exercise habits and be willing to modify their programs as the need arises. Maintaining enthusiasm for exercise is the foundation of lifetime fitness. See A Closer Look below for some strategies that can help you adhere to a lifetime exercise program.

☀ IN SUMMARY

- Over 60% of adults who start an exercise program quit within the first month.
- People who start an exercise program and exercise regularly for at least 6 months have an excellent chance of maintaining a regular exercise routine for years to come.
- Setting exercise goals, selecting enjoyable exercise activities, planning exercise sessions, monitoring fitness progress, exercising with friends, and adjusting your activity as you age are all important aspects of your lifetime adherence to exercise.

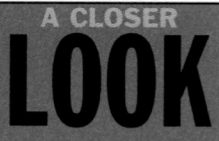

The Keys to Success in Exercise Adherence

Maintaining a regular program of exercise requires motivation and a lifetime commitment to exercise. The following positive steps (6, 7) are the keys to successfully adhering to a lifetime exercise program.

- Strive to maintain your desire and motivation to be physically fit.
- Establish both short-term and long-term fitness goals.
- Choose exercise activities that are fun.

- Select activities and/or places to work out that are convenient.
- Schedule time every day for a workout.
- Exercise with a friend.
- Associate with peers who are positive physical fitness role models.
- Adjust your exercise training routine as you age or as your exercise interests change.

☀ Diet and Fitness Products: Consumer Issues

The fitness boom in the United States has brought an explosion of fitness and diet books and magazines, as well as a huge number of companies that produce exercise equipment. Although some fitness books and magazines are written by experts, many are written by individuals with little formal training in exercise physiology. Unfortunately, books and articles written by nonexperts often convey misinformation, and some of these writings have created many exercise myths. Further, many exercise products are not useful in promoting physical fitness or weight loss. In the next several sections we discuss some key consumer issues related to exercise and weight loss.

COMMON MISCONCEPTIONS ABOUT PHYSICAL FITNESS

There are numerous misconceptions about exercise, weight loss, and physical fitness, and to thoroughly discuss them would require hundreds of pages of text. So, even though debunking all exercise myths is beyond the scope of this book, we can dispel some of the most common ones.

HAND WEIGHTS The popularity of handheld weights has increased rapidly in the past several years. Some manufacturers claim that using hand weights will greatly increase arm and shoulder strength. Although carrying hand weights will increase the energy expenditure during exercise, 1- to 3-pound hand weights do not promote significant strength gains (particularly in college-age individuals).

Further, there are some concerns about the use of hand weights. First, gripping them may increase blood pressure (10). Individuals with high blood pressure should seek a physician's advice about the use of hand weights during exercise (6, 8). Hand weights may also aggravate existing elbow or shoulder arthritis. Finally, some aerobics instructors have banned hand weights in large classes because of the potential danger of hitting someone with an outstretched hand.

RUBBER WAIST BELTS AND SPOT REDUCTION

Recall that spot reduction of body fat is the concept of being able to lose body fat from a specific body location. Numerous myths exist concerning the spot reduction effects of such practices as wearing nylon suits or rubber waist bands, as well as exercise focused on a specific body area (e.g., sit-ups). The bottom line is that no method of spot reduction is effective in removing fat from a specific body area (Chapter 8). Although exercise can assist in creating a negative caloric balance

Nutritional Links
TO HEALTH AND FITNESS

Do Nutritional Ergogenic Aids Promote Physical Fitness?

The popular fitness literature is replete with claims that nutritional supplements improve physical fitness and build muscle mass. The following nutritional products are popular supplements that are often used by athletes or fitness enthusiasts:

Amino acids	Organ extracts
Bee pollen	Vitamin supplements
Gelatin	Wheat germ oil
Mineral supplements	Yeast

Do any of these supplements improve physical fitness or performance? The answer is "no" if you are eating a nutritionally balanced diet. Volumes of research clearly show that nutritional supplements do not improve physical fitness in well-fed, healthy individuals. (See reference 8 at the end of the chapter for a review.)

and therefore promote fat loss, the loss of fat occurs throughout the body and is not localized to one particular area.

ERGOGENIC AIDS A drug or nutritional product that improves physical fitness and exercise performance is called an **ergogenic aid.** Numerous manufacturers market products that they claim promote strength and cardiovascular fitness. The popularity of these products usually stems from their reported use by champion athletes, but the key concern for the consumer is whether ergogenic aids promote fitness.

Only limited scientific evidence supports the notion that nutritional ergogenic aids promote fitness or increase athletic performance in humans (Nutritional Links to Health and Fitness). However, both anabolic steroids and the drug Clenbuterol have proved to increase muscle mass in animals (11, 12). Although this may seem to be good news for people who want to increase their muscle mass, the bad news is that both drugs have been shown to be harmful to health. Recent evidence has shown that prolonged use of both drugs

ergogenic aid A drug or nutritional product that improves physical fitness and exercise performance.

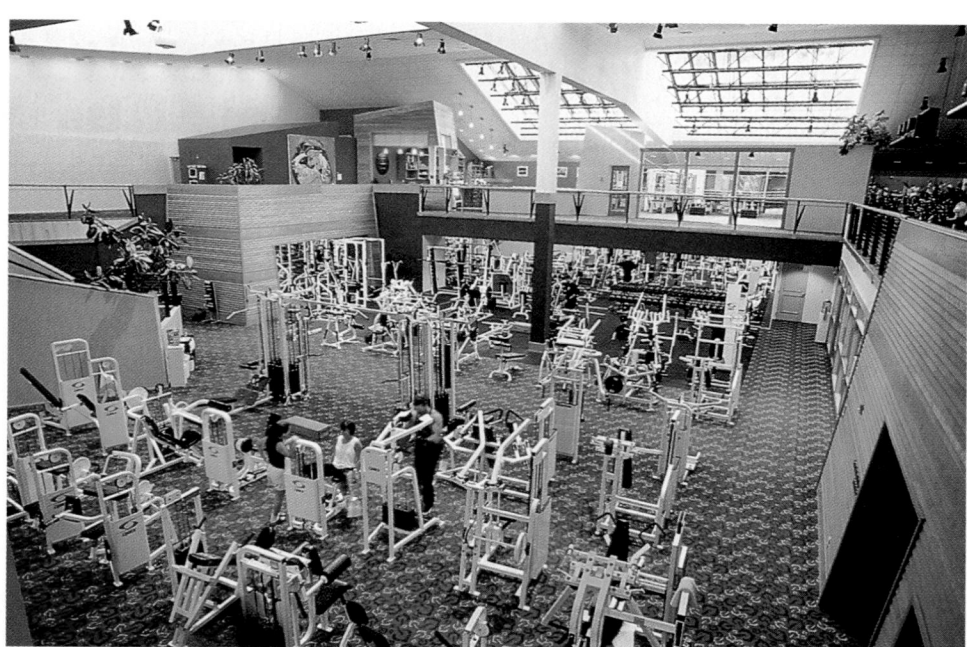

Examine the features of a health club carefully before joining.

may result in serious organ damage and, in some cases, death (13, 14). See references 15 and 16 at the end of the chapter for reviews on these topics.

EXERCISE EQUIPMENT   Many types of exercise equipment are available. Every week, magazine and television ads promote a "new" exercise device designed to trim waistlines and build huge muscles overnight. In truth, there are no "miracle" exercise devices capable of promoting such changes. In fact, there is really no need to buy *any* exercise devices to promote fitness. A well-rounded fitness program can be designed without exercise equipment. However, if you want to purchase exercise equipment for home use, buy from a reputable and well-established company (9). Beware of mail-order products, and examine the product before you buy (9). When in doubt about the usefulness of an exercise product, consult a fitness expert.

PASSIVE EXERCISE DEVICES   A **passive exercise** machine is a motor-driven device designed to move or vibrate the body without any muscular activity. Passive

---

passive exercise Movement performed on a motor-driven device designed to move or vibrate the body without any muscular activity. Passive exercise devices come in many forms, including rolling machines, vibrating belts, pillows, and passive motion tables, but they do not improve physical fitness or promote weight loss.

---

exercise devices come in many forms, including rolling machines, vibrating belts, pillows, and passive motion tables. Manufacturers claim that passive exercise devices improve physical fitness and assist in weight loss. Unfortunately, there is no such thing as effortless exercise. Passive exercise devices do not improve physical fitness or promote weight loss (17).

HOT TUBS, SAUNAS, AND STEAMBATHS   Hot tubs, saunas, and steambaths are popular attractions at many health clubs. Although they may improve mental attitudes by promoting relaxation, none promotes fat loss or improves physical fitness. While water loss due to perspiration will reduce your body weight temporarily, it does not result in fat loss. Further, the weight will return as soon as you replace the lost fluids by eating and drinking.

There are also potential dangers in the use of saunas, steambaths, and hot tubs. One of the major problems concerns the regulation of blood pressure. All of these forms of heat stress increase blood flow to the skin to promote cooling; this reduces blood return to the heart and may reduce blood flow to the brain, resulting in fainting. Therefore, when using a sauna, hot tub, or steambath, note the following precautions (9):

- Seek a physician's advice before using hot baths if you suffer from heart disease, hypertension, diabetes, kidney disease, or chronic skin problems, or if you are pregnant.

- Don't use hot bath facilities when you are alone; someone should be present to get emergency help if you develop a health problem, such as fainting.

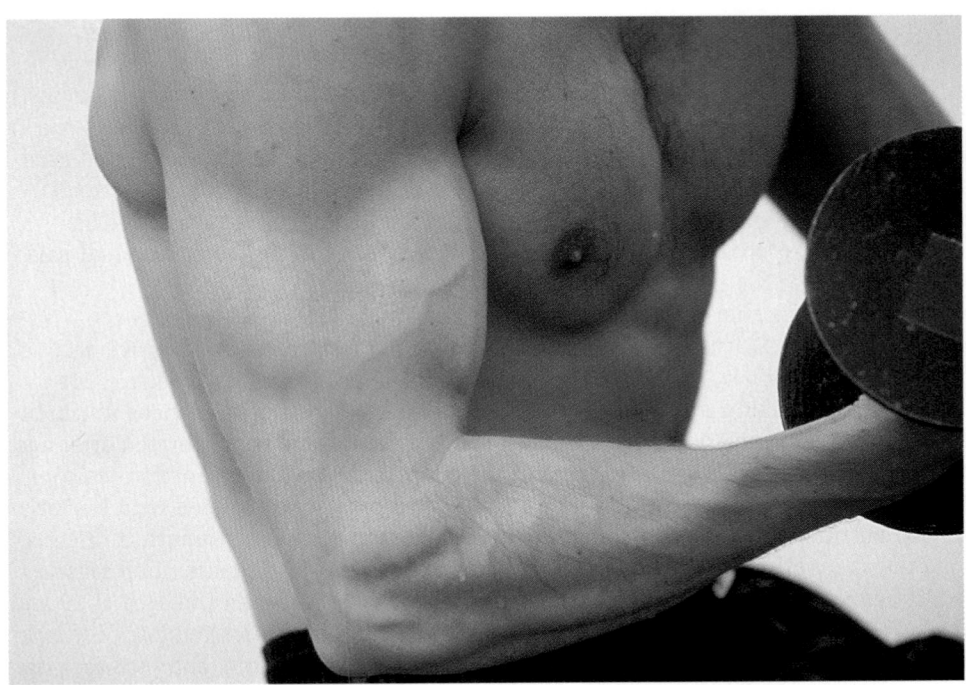

Having a championship physique does not make an individual a fitness expert.

- Don't wear jewelry in hot baths (the metal will absorb heat and may burn your skin).
- Don't drink alcohol prior to or while bathing because alcohol may increase your risk of fainting during heat exposure.
- Don't exercise in a sauna, hot tub, or steam bath. The combination of exercise and a hot environment may result in overheating.
- Do not enter a sauna, hot tub, or steambath immediately following vigorous exercise. Entering a steambath without cooling down after exercise increases your risk of fainting.
- The duration of stay and recommended temperatures of saunas, steambaths, and hot tubs are as follows:

  Sauna: Air temperature should not exceed 190°F (~88°C) and the stay in sauna should not exceed 15 minutes.

  Steambath: Air temperature should not exceed 120°F (~38°C) and the stay in steambath should not exceed 10 minutes.

  Hot tub (or whirlpool): Water temperature should not exceed 100°F (~38°C) and the stay in hot tub should not exceed 15 minutes.

FITNESS BOOKS AND MAGAZINES   Book stores generally have numerous fitness-related publications on their shelves. Although many fitness books have been written by experts in the field of exercise science, others have been written by individuals with little or no formal training in exercise physiology. Dozens of fitness books and magazine articles have been written by models, movie stars, body builders, and even professional or Olympic athletes who have no academic training in exercise science. Clearly, having athletic talent or a good physique does not make an individual a fitness expert.

How do you evaluate the credibility of a fitness or weight control book? After reading and studying this book, you should be able to distinguish between fitness facts and fiction. For example, beware of texts that promise overnight results or quick, effortless weight loss. If you have doubts about the validity of a new fitness text, contact a local fitness expert for advice.

☀ IN SUMMARY

- Numerous misconceptions exist concerning physical fitness.
- Wearing rubber waist belts will not result in spot reduction of fat.
- Passive exercise devices do not improve physical fitness and will not promote weight loss.
- Although hot tubs, saunas, and steambaths are relaxing, they will not promote loss of body fat.

☀ Aging: A Challenge for Physical Fitness and Wellness

Age-related changes in physiological function were introduced in Chapter 12. In this chapter, we expand our discussion of aging and identify ways to slow age-related changes in our bodies and minds. Aging is a normal process that begins when we reach adult maturity and continues through old age (called senescence). It is well documented that human aging results in numerous physiological changes (23–26). The cause of human aging has been a topic of investigation for many years. While numerous theories exist to explain the cause of aging, none of these theories completely explains all of the physical and mental changes that occur (26). Therefore, experts in aging now believe that the aging process results from a combination of factors including genetics, environment, diet, and lifestyle (15, 26).

While it is impossible to stop the aging process, by practicing good health habits, it is possible to sustain physical fitness and wellness over the course of the entire life span. Maintaining physical fitness and wellness from maturity through old age has been termed "successful aging" and is the result of good nutrition, engaging in regular exercise, and applying the many other healthful living practices described throughout this book. In the next two sections, we describe both physical and mental changes that occur during normal human aging and discuss actions that can be taken to achieve successful aging. We begin with a discussion of the physiological changes your body undergoes as you age.

AGE-RELATED CHANGES IN YOUR BODY

As mentioned above, aging is a normal process that results in gradual and numerous changes in both body and mind; in youth, all of the body's organ systems function at a higher level than is required for optimal function. Therefore, a gradual and small age-related decrease in organ system function does not impair our ability to function until these changes reach a very drastic level. In the following sections, we outline some of the most important age-related changes that occur during the life span.

CARDIOVASCULAR SYSTEM Aging is associated with a decrease in the heart's maximal pumping capacity (maximal cardiac output) primarily due to a decline in maximal heart rate (Chapter 4). Further, aging results in a progressive buildup of fatty plaque in blood vessels resulting in a "hardening of the arteries" (called arteriosclerosis, Chapter 9). This hardening of the arteries may also contribute to a gradual increase in blood pressure resulting in age-related high blood pressure (hypertension).

PULMONARY SYSTEM In the absence of lung disease, age-related changes in pulmonary function are generally small and do not compromise our ability to supply oxygen to the body.

BONE AND JOINT HEALTH Aging results in a gradual loss of bone strength due to a decrease in bone mineral mass (osteoporosis). Therefore, aging results in soft bones that are at risk for fractures. This age-related change in bone is gradual and typically begins in both men and women around age 20. However, the loss of bone mass in women is greatly accelerated after menopause due to the decline in circulating estrogen. Aging also results in a loss of connective tissue between joints that may result in inflammation and pain during movement (arthritis).

MUSCLE MASS Aging results in a progressive decline in muscular strength in both men and women. Note, however, that the rate of age-related changes in muscular strength is not constant and is accelerated after age 50. Loss of skeletal muscle mass and function (sarcopenia) is a major health problem associated with human aging. Age-related loss of muscular strength is directly related to losses in skeletal muscle mass; total muscle mass declines by about 40% between the ages of 20 and 80. This is important because age-related loss of muscle mass reduces mobility, independence, and increases the risk of falls in the elderly. Importantly, falls in the elderly are associated with a high risk of bone fractures due to age-related osteoporosis. Because skeletal muscles generate the force required to maintain bone mass, an age-related loss of muscle results in a vicious cycle, contributing to the increased loss of bone mass in the elderly.

SKIN Numerous age-related changes in skin occur. In general, aging results in reduced oil production, changes in the connective tissue, and altered pigmentation in the skin. Collectively, these changes appear as dry, spotted, and wrinkled skin.

VISION Around age 40 or so, many people experience changes in their vision. These changes may include the inability to focus on close objects (presbyopia), impaired night vision, and a loss of depth perception.

TASTE AND SMELL Aging results in a decline in both the sensation of taste and smell due to changes in the cells (on the tongue and in the nose) responsible for these senses. These changes are important and may contribute to the loss of appetite associated with old age.

BRAIN AND CENTRAL NERVOUS SYSTEM Like all other organ systems in the body, the brain and central nervous system experience age-related changes. These changes occur due to a loss of brain cells (neurons) and a decrease in neurotransmitters. One of the more obvious changes in brain function with aging is a gradual loss of memory.

HAIR Hair is typically thickest at age 20 and begins to decrease in thickness during the aging process.

Further, as cells at the base of hair follicles age, they produce less pigment and hair color begins to fade, giving way to "gray" hair.

DELAYING THE AGING PROCESS: SUCCESSFUL AGING

While the aging process cannot be stopped, it is clear that many characteristics of aging are not due to aging per se, but occur due to lifestyle choices. For example, due to neglect and abuse of our body and mind, the aging process can be accelerated resulting in a faster decline in function that would occur if these abuses were absent. A few simple lifestyle choices that you can make every day will make large differences in your ability to achieve successful aging and maintain wellness. While these healthy living suggestions have been discussed throughout this book, the following list summarizes the key lifestyle factors that contribute to maintaining wellness throughout the life span.

MAINTAIN A LIFELONG PROGRAM OF REGULAR PHYSICAL EXERCISE   The importance of regular exercise has been emphasized throughout this book. Regular aerobic exercise will maintain a healthy cardiovascular system whereas a program of weight training will uphold muscular strength and assist in maintaining healthy bones. Importantly, regular exercise will also assist in maintaining a healthy body weight and will make a vast difference in your vitality and energy level as you age.

EAT A HEALTHY DIET   A major focus of this book has been the importance of a healthy diet in maintaining wellness. A varied diet, low in calories and fat, is essential to maintain a healthy body weight and reduce the risk of both heart disease and cancer. As discussed in Chapter 7, a healthy diet should focus on fresh fruits and vegetables, whole grains, and lean portions of poultry and fish.

MAINTAIN A HEALTHY WEIGHT   Obesity increases your risk of many diseases (Chapter 8). Therefore, maintaining a healthy body composition is an essential goal to achieve a lifetime of wellness.

EXERCISE YOUR MIND   The brain is a "plastic organ" that is capable of being "enhanced" by increased mental activity. Likewise, a lack of mental activity can cause brain function to decline. Therefore, to prevent your brain from "wasting away" as a part of the aging process, you should continue to challenge your mind by a lifelong program of learning consisting of reading, thinking/problem solving, intelligent conversation, and listening.

AVOID SUBSTANCE ABUSE   As discussed in Chapter 16, abuse of alcohol and other drugs can have very negative consequences on health and wellness. Moreover, smoking and the use of other tobacco products greatly increase your risk of cardiovascular disease and certain types of cancer. Therefore, avoidance of substance abuse is an important lifestyle choice that will greatly improve your ability to achieve successful aging and wellness.

REDUCE STRESS   Recognizing and reducing stress in your daily life is essential to maintain wellness. So, reduce your stress levels, get adequate amounts of sleep, and practice the relaxation techniques discussed in Chapter 10.

PROTECT YOUR SKIN AND EYES FROM SUN DAMAGE   Chronic exposure to UV rays from the sun can damage your skin and your eyes. Long-term exposure to UV rays can cause premature aging and increase the risk of skin cancer. Further, UV exposure can impair your vision by increasing the risk of cataracts (cloudy appearance within the lens of the eye). Therefore, protect your skin from sun damage by using sunscreen and wearing protective clothing (long sleeves, hats, etc.). Protect your eyes from UV damage by wearing sunglasses with UV protection within the lens.

GET REGULAR MEDICAL CHECKUPS   Regular visits with your doctor are important for early detection and treatment of disease and will be discussed in more detail in the next section.

☀ Informed Health Care Choices

Maintaining wellness over the course of a lifetime requires good personal decisions about managing your personal health care. This requires personal knowledge about health and exercise, seeking advice from medical and nutritional professionals when necessary, and taking personal responsibility for making informed health care decisions. Indeed, being an informed patient is the key to intelligent use of the health care system. In the following sections, we discuss several important health care issues including how to choose a personal physician, deciding when to see a doctor versus self-treatment, and the timing of regular checkups and tests. We begin with a discussion of how to choose a personal physician.

CHOOSING A PERSONAL PHYSICIAN

Choosing a personal physician is an important decision. Everyone, regardless of age, needs a good reliable physician for common medical problems that arise from time

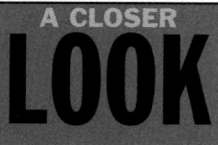

Glossary of Medical Specialists

Medical specialists are doctors that have received focused training in a specific area of medicine. These doctors have had several additional years of training (above a normal residency) and have passed rigorous board exams in their chosen area of expertise. The following list describes the most common types of medical specialists.

Anesthesiologist Specializes in the delivery of anesthesia during surgery and monitors the patient's immediate recovery following surgery.

Cardiologist Diagnoses and treats diseases of the heart and blood vessels.

Dermatologist Specializes in care and treatment of skin diseases.

Emergency room specialist Specializes in the care and treatment of trauma patients and acute illnesses.

Gastroenterologist Diagnoses and treats diseases of the digestive system and liver.

Hematologist A hematologist specializes in disorders of the blood.

Internist Specializes in the non-surgical treatment of adults. Major areas of medical interest may include heart disease, cancer, diabetes, and arthritis.

Neurologist Diagnoses and treats disorders of the brain and nervous system.

Neurosurgeon Specializes in surgical treatment of disorders of the brain and nervous system.

Obstetrician/gynecologist A gynecologist specializes in the treatment of the reproductive systems of women whereas an obstetrician specializes in the treatment of pregnant women and delivering babies.

Oncologist Specializes in the treatment of cancer.

Otorhinolaryngologist Specializes in diagnosis and treatment of problems in the ear, nose, and throat.

Pediatrician A pediatrician specializes in the treatment of children.

Physiatrist Specializes in physical medicine and rehabilitation.

Psychiatrist Treats behavior disorders using both psychotherapy and medications.

Radiologist Specializes in the use of imaging technology (e.g., x-rays, ultrasound, etc.) to diagnose diseases (e.g., cancer) and injuries (e.g., broken bones).

Surgeon Specializes in the use of surgery to diagnose and treat diseases. A general surgeon may perform a wide variety of surgical procedures whereas some surgeons specialize in a specific area of surgery (e.g., cardiovascular surgery, plastic surgeon, etc.).

Urologist Diagnoses and treats problems associated with the urinary tract in men and women, and in reproductive disorders in men.

---

to time. Using the emergency room or walk-in medical clinics for basic medical care is often a mistake and can be expensive (27). While emergency room physicians are trained to take care of emergencies, they may not be the best choice for routine health care (27). Further, while walk-in medical clinics are well prepared to take care of day-to-day health care problems, these clinics will not know your medical history. Therefore, choosing a primary care physician who will maintain your medical history on file, and is competent to recognize and treat a full range of medical problems, is essential for optimal use of the health care system.

How do you choose a personal physician? In general, there are two basic types of doctors to choose from: (1) family practitioners; and (2) internists. Family practitioners are physicians that have completed a three-year residency (training after medical school) and are trained in a wide variety of medical topics. Family practitioners are capable of treating most acute and chronic illnesses for people of all ages. However, for complicated illnesses, family practitioners will often refer patients to the appropriate medical specialist (see A Closer Look for details on medical specialists).

Internists are doctors who specialize in adult medical problems. Like family practitioners, internists complete a three-year residency after medical school and are required to pass a rigorous examination to receive specialty certification (27). Internists receive advanced medical training in areas such as heart disease, cancer, diabetes, and arthritis. However, similar to family practitioners, complicated diseases may require that an internist refer patients to a specialist for further evaluation.

Once you make the decision to choose either a family practitioner or an internist, you should do some investigating before selecting a specific doctor. In making your choice, consider the following factors (27):

- **Medical training and background.** You should investigate the physician's education and professional background, including hospital privileges (which hospital the physician uses), and board certification. Ask friends and other physicians for recommendations about the doctor's technical skills.
- **Physician availability.** Is the doctor available? If you have an urgent medical need, will he or she make arrangements to see you the day you call their office? Further, will the doctor be available to talk to you on the phone and return phone calls promptly?
- **Medical philosophy.** What is the physician's medical philosophy? Will he or she treat each illness seriously, or dismiss all of your medical problems? Will he or she prescribe medication every time you have a medical complaint?
- **Is the doctor with a group or solo?** f the doctor is in a solo private practice, does he or she have other doctors that can treat your medical problems when your personal physician is away?
- **Bedside manner.** Finding a personal physician that you are comfortable with is very important. Moreover, most people seek a doctor that is caring and concerned about the patient's health. Finally, it is important that you have complete confidence that you will receive an informed and carefully considered opinion from your doctor.
- **Medical payment requirements.** What kind of payment is required? Do you have to pay the fee directly, or will the doctor's office bill your insurance company or accept Medicare?

DECIDING WHEN TO SEE A DOCTOR

When personal medical problems arise, how do you make the decision to see a doctor or rely on self-treatment? This is often a difficult question to answer. Nonetheless, in general, the decision to seek professional medical help should be guided by your medical history and the nature and duration of the symptoms. For example, if you have a history of serious medical problems and develop symptoms of a previous disorder, being proactive and seeking medical help immediately is the correct action.

On the other hand, if you are healthy and develop symptoms of an illness but are unsure of the significance of your symptoms, call your physician and ask medical advice over the phone. If your physician is not available, ask to speak to a nurse or physician assistant associated with your doctor. Often these medical professionals can provide you with guidance about whether you need to seek treatment immediately or monitor your symptoms at home.

Clearly, for any symptom that is severe, persistent, or recurring, you should see your physician immediately. Further, you should seek rapid medical attention if you have any of the following injuries or symptoms: suspicion of a broken bone, severe bleeding, deep wound, severe burns, chest pain, shortness of breath, poisoning/drug overdose, and/or sudden loss of consciousness (27).

TIMING OF REGULAR MEDICAL CHECKUPS AND MEDICAL TESTS

How often should you schedule physical exams and other routine medical screening tests? The answer to this question varies as a function of your age, occupation, lifestyle, and medical history. Nonetheless, general guidelines exist for both men and women and are presented in Table 17.2. In general, most medical experts believe that routine physical exams for adults should begin at age 18 and continue throughout the life span (27, 28). While Table 17.2 offers general guidelines on how often men and women should have a physical exam or particular screening test, this information may differ based on your medical history or your risk for certain diseases. Indeed, the recommendations provided in Table 17.2 are for individuals of average risk and do not replace the advice of your doctor (28).

EFFECTIVE COMMUNICATION WITH YOUR DOCTOR IS IMPORTANT

The rapport between a patient and doctor plays an important role in the quality and effectiveness of treatment. Effective communication is a critical part of establishing a positive relationship between the patient and physician. Here are some guidelines for getting the most from your visit to the doctor.

PREPARE FOR YOUR APPOINTMENT IN ADVANCE
Studies reveal that 70% of correct medical diagnoses depend on what you tell your doctor about your symptoms (27). Therefore, prior to your visit, you should write down a concise list of your symptoms. Try not to leave anything out of your list; what you think is a minor detail may be very important.

DURING THE APPOINTMENT   Bring any medications that you are taking to your appointment and mention any current medical treatments. Feel free to ask questions. No question is a dumb question. You are entitled to a diagnosis provided in terms that you understand.

TABLE 17.2
Medical Check-Ups: Your Examination Timetable

This chart provides general guidelines for physical exams and routine medical tests for both men and women. Note that these guidelines are for men and women of average health risks only and do not replace the advice of your doctor. Information obtained from references (27–29).

Age	Sex	Test	Frequency
18 and over	M/F	Complete physical	Every 1–3 years
	M/F	Blood pressure	Every 1–3 years
	M/F	Blood lipid (cholesterol) profile	Every 1–3 years
	F	Pelvic exam	Annually
	F	Pap smear	Every 1–3 years
	F	Breast exam	Annually
40 and over	M/F	Visual acuity, glaucoma	Every 3 years
	M	Fecal occult blood test	Annually
	M	Digital rectal exam	Annually
	F	Mammogram	Annually
50 and over	M/F	Sigmoidoscopy	Every 5 years
	M/F	Colonoscopy	Every 10 years
	F	Fecal occult blood test	Annually
65 and over	M/F	Visual acuity, glaucoma	Annually
	M/F	Hearing	Annually

If you are unclear about any part of your diagnosis and proposed treatment, ask your physician to provide another explanation of your problem and the proposed treatment. If you want more details about your condition, ask your doctor to recommend reading material and become an educated patient. Finally, prior to leaving the doctor's office, make certain that you are sure about what the next steps are for your treatment (i.e., return for another visit, more tests, and/or obtain a prescription).

☀ Lifetime Commitment to Wellness

The primary objective of this book is to provide the knowledge and skills required to maintain a lifetime program of proper nutrition, good health behaviors, and exercise to achieve total wellness. This educational process began in Chapter 1 by introducing the concept of wellness as well as a discussion of the health benefits of exercise. Chapter 1 also permitted the opportunity to assess your lifestyle and identify areas that require modification. Subsequent chapters have discussed important contributors to wellness such as regular physical activity, good nutrition, weight control, stress management, and modifying unhealthy behaviors.

It is important to appreciate that achieving wellness is a lifetime proposition that requires daily attention to maintain healthy behaviors. The choice to maintain a healthy lifestyle and achieve wellness is yours to make. The time to make lifestyle changes and a commitment to wellness is now so review your current health behaviors that require modification (see lifestyle assessment in Chapter 1) and take action today to achieve a lifetime of wellness. See A Closer Look "Keys to Success in Lifetime Wellness" for reminders of the important steps in maintaining total wellness throughout your lifetime.

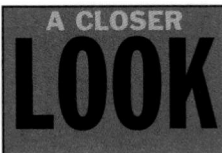

Keys to Success in Lifetime Wellness

Maintaining a regular program of good health behavior, exercise, and healthy dietary practices to achieve "total wellness" requires motivation and a lifetime commitment to a healthy lifestyle. Keys to success in adhering to a lifetime wellness program include the following:

- A desire to achieve wellness
- Establish both short- and long-term wellness goals

- Maintain a regular schedule of wellness activities (e.g. exercise, healthy diet, and relaxation)
- Schedule routine medical check-ups and screening tests as recommended by your physician
- Remain informed about changing medical opinion about good health behaviors, nutrition, and exercise programs to sustain wellness

- Schedule time in every day for exercise and relaxation
- Associate with peers who are positive "wellness" role models
- Forgive yourself when you commit wellness lifestyle errors; when these events occur, simply make the necessary behavioral adjustments to get back on the correct path to sustain wellness
- Expect to be successful in achieving a lifetime of wellness; a positive attitude is essential for lifetime wellness

Summary

1. Exercise must be performed regularly throughout your life to achieve the benefits of physical fitness, wellness, and disease prevention.

2. Over 60% of the adults who start an exercise program quit within the first month. However, evidence exists that people who start an exercise program and continue to exercise for 6 months have an excellent chance of maintaining a regular fitness routine for years.

3. The following are important aspects of maintaining a lifetime commitment to physical activity: goal setting, activity selection, regularity of exercise sessions, monitoring your progress, social support, peers as role models, and modifying your physical activity program as a result of aging.

4. Before choosing a health club, you should consider the following factors: Check the club's reputation with the local Better Business Bureau before joining; investigate programs offered throughout your community before deciding to join a particular club; before joining any facility, examine the membership contract carefully; in general, avoid clubs that advertise "overnight" fitness or weight loss success; and arrange to make several trial visits to the facility before joining. Several visits to the facility will provide you with answers regarding whether the locker room facilities are well maintained and clean, the exercise machines are in good working order, the club employees are well trained and eager to answer your fitness-related questions, and the facil-

ity is not overcrowded during the hours that you plan to use the club.

5. There is no standard definition of a *fitness expert*. However, a fitness expert is, generally, someone who has earned an advanced degree in exercise science, kinesiology, or exercise physiology.

6. Numerous exercise misconceptions exist. After studying this book you should be able to distinguish between fact and fiction. If you have doubts about the validity of a new fitness product or textbook, contact a local fitness expert for advice.

7. Maintaining a regular program of good health behavior, exercise, and healthy dietary practices to achieve wellness requires motivation and a lifetime commitment to a healthy lifestyle.

Study Questions

1. Outline the key factors that play a role in maintaining a regular program of exercise.

2. List five points to consider when choosing a health club.

3. Give your definition of a *fitness expert*.

4. Numerous exercise misconceptions exist. Discuss the misconceptions associated with yoga, the use of hand weights, the use of rubber weight belts to lose body fat, and nutritional ergogenic aids.

5. What factors should be considered when purchasing exercise equipment?

6. List several precautions that should be considered when using hot tubs, saunas, or steambaths.

7. Do passive exercise devices promote physical fitness and weight loss? Explain your answer.

8. What percentage of people who start an exercise program quit within the first month?

9. Discuss the importance of activity selection in maintaining physical fitness.

10. List five activities that are considered to be good or excellent modes of promoting cardiorespiratory fitness.

11. Identify eight key elements that lead to success in adhering to a lifetime wellness program.

12. Discuss the major age-related changes in fitness and wellness and describe actions that you can take to maintain fitness and wellness throughout the life span.

13. Describe strategies for choosing a personal physician.

14. Outline a recommendation for the regularity of routine medical check-ups for your age group and gender.

15. List nine keys to success for achieving lifetime wellness.

Suggested Reading

Booth, F. W., and M. V. Chakravarthy. Cost and consequences of sedentary living: New battleground for an old enemy. *President's Council on Physical Fitness and Sports Research Digest*, 3:16, 2002.

Edlin, G., and E. Golanty. *Health and Wellness.* Sudbury, MA: Jones and Bartlett, 2004.

Franks, B., E. Howley, and Y. Iyriboz. *The Health Fitness Handbook.* Champaign, IL: Human Kinetics, 1999.

Health clubs: What to look for. *Consumer Reports.* February, 34, 1999.

Mayo Clinic Family Health Book. New York: HarperResource, 2003.

Nieman, D. *Exercise Testing and Prescription.* St. Louis: McGraw-Hill, 2002.

Powers, S. and E. Howley. *Exercise Physiology: Theory and Application to Fitness and Performance.* 5th ed. St. Louis: McGraw-Hill, 2004.

For links to the web sites below visit The Total Fitness and Wellness Website at www.aw-bc.com/powers.

American College of Sports Medicine

Contains information about aging, exercise, health, and fitness.

WebMD

Includes the latest information on a variety of health-related topics, including diet, exercise, and stress; also contains links to other sites on nutrition, fitness, and wellness topics.

American Council on Exercise

A nonprofit organization that provides information on a variety of topics related to exercise and fitness.

President's Council on Physical Fitness and Sports

Provides information concerning a wide range of subjects related to exercise and fitness.

American Medical Association

Contains many sources of information about a wide variety of medical and health issues.

Mayo Clinic

Contains information about a wide variety of diseases and medical issues. Further, this site is a good source for information about aging, nutrition, and choosing health care providers.

References

1. Dishman, R., ed. *Exercise Adherence: Its Impact on Public Health.* Champaign, IL: Human Kinetics, 1988.

2. Getchell, B. *Physical Fitness: A Way of Life,* 5th ed. Needham Heights, MA: Allyn and Bacon, 1998.

3. Howley, E., and B. D. Franks. *Health Fitness: Instructors Handbook.* Champaign, IL: Human Kinetics, 1997.

4. Balady, G. Health clubs: Are they right for you? *Harvard Men's Health Watch,* November 6, 1998.

5. Health clubs: What to look for. *Consumer Reports,* February, 1999.

6. Dishman, R. *Advances in Exercise Adherence.* Champaign, IL: Human Kinetics, 1994.

7. Resnick, B. Testing a model of exercise behavior in older adults. *Research in Nursing and Health* 24:83–89, 2001.

8. Clarkson, P. Vitamins and trace minerals. In *Ergogenics,* D. Lamb and M. Williams, eds. Madison, WI: Brown and Benchmark, 1991.

9. Corbin, C. *Concepts of Fitness and Wellness: A Comprehensive Lifestyle Approach.* St. Louis: McGraw-Hill, 2003.

10. Graves, J., M. Pollock, S. Montain, A. Jackson, and J. O'Keefe. The effect of hand-held weights on the physiological response to walking exercise. *Medicine and Science in Sports and Exercise* 19:260–265, 1987.

11. Criswell, D., S. Powers, and R. Herb. Clenbuterol-induced fiber type transition in the soleus of adult rats. *European Journal of Applied Physiology* 74:391–396, 1996.

12. Heitzman, R. The effectiveness of anabolic agents in increasing rate of growth in farm animals: Report on experiments in cattle. In *Anabolic Agents in Animal Production,* F. Lu and J. Rendell, eds. Stuttgart, Germany: Georg Thieme, 1976.

13. Palmer, R., M. Delday, D. McMillan, B. Noble, P. Bain, and C. Maltin. Effects of the cyclo-oxygenase inhibitor, fenbufen, on clenbuterol-induced hypertrophy of cardiac and skeletal muscle of rats. *British Journal of Pharmacology* 101:835–838, 1990.

14. Taylor, W., S. Snowball, C. Dickson, and M. Lesna. Alterations in liver architecture in mice treated with anabolic androgens and dimethylnitrosamine. *NATO Advanced Study Institute Series, Series A* 52:279–288, 1982.

15. Powers, S., and E. Howley. *Exercise Physiology: Theory and Application to Fitness and Performance,* 5th ed. St. Louis: McGraw-Hill, 2004.

16. Lamb, D., and M. Williams. *Ergogenics: Enhancement of Performance in Exercise and Sport.* Vol. 4. Madison, WI: Brown and Benchmark, 1991.

17. Martin, A. D., and G. Kauwell. Continuous assistive-passive exercise and cycle ergometer training in sedentary women. *Medicine and Science in Sports and Exercise* 22: 523–527, 1990.

18. McArdle, W., V. Katch, and F. Katch. *Essentials of Exercise Physiology.* Philadelphia: Lippincott Williams and Wilkins, 2004.

19. McGlynn, G. *Dynamics of Fitness: A Practical Approach.* Dubuque, IA: Wm. C. Brown, 1998.

20. Pollock, M., and J. Wilmore. *Exercise in Health and Disease,* 3rd ed. Philadelphia: W. B. Saunders, 1999.

21. Lan, C., S. Chen, and J. Lai. Tai Chi. *American Journal of Chinese Medicine* 32:151–160, 2004.

22. Taylor-Pillae, R., and E. Foelicher. Effectiveness of Tai Chi in improving aerobic capacity: A meta analysis. *Journal of Cardiovascular Nursing* 19:48–57, 2004.

23. Doherty, T. Aging and sarcopenia. *Journal of Applied Physiology* 95:1717–1727, 2003.

24. Powers, S., J. Quindry, and K. Hamilton. Aging, exercise, and cardioprotection. *Annuals of New York Academy of Sciences* 1019:462–470, 2004.

25. Demirel, H., K. Hamilton, R. Shanely, N. Tumer, M. Koroly, and S. Powers. Age and attenuation of exercise-induced cardioprotection. *American Journal of Physiology* 285:H1609–1615, 2004.

26. Harman, D. The free radical theory of aging. *Antioxidants and Redox Signaling* 5:557–561, 2003.

27. Margen, S. (Editor). *The Wellness Encyclopedia.* Boston: Houghton Mifflin Company, 1995.

28. *Mayo Clinic Family Health Book.* New York: HarperResource, 2003.

29. Thomas, M., S. Habermann, S. Rajkumar, S. Randall, M. Edson, C. Scott, M. Litin, K. Amit, M. Ghost, and D. McCallum. Mayo Clinic Internal Medicine Board Review. Philadelphia: Lippincott Williams and Williams, 2004.

Wellness Profile

NAME _____ DATE _____

After reading *Total Fitness and Wellness*, you should be equipped with the knowledge and skills you need to lead a healthy, fit lifestyle. Take the opportunity now to examine your strengths in six areas of wellness. Write your top three strengths for each factor of wellness below.

PHYSICAL WELLNESS

Maintaining overall physical health and participating in physical activities. Examples of strengths include endurance, balance, and flexibility.

_____

_____

_____

EMOTIONAL WELLNESS

Possessing a positive self-concept and dealing appropriately with your feelings. Strengths may include self-confidence, trust, and optimism.

_____

_____

_____

INTELLECTUAL WELLNESS

Retaining knowledge, thinking critically about issues, making sound decisions, and finding solutions to problems. Examples include inquisitiveness, curiosity, and dedication.

_____

_____

_____

SOCIAL WELLNESS

Developing lasting relationships with family and friends, and contributing to the community. Strengths in this area would be compassion and friendliness.

_____

_____

_____

(continued on next page)

ENVIRONMENTAL WELLNESS

Protecting yourself from environmental hazards and minimizing your negative impact on the environment. Behaviors such as recycling and carpooling are strengths in this aspect of wellness.

_____

_____

_____

Is there an aspect of wellness that you need to develop more fully? If so, which one? What can you do now to improve this wellness factor in your life?

_____

_____

_____

_____

_____

_____

Evaluating Fitness Products

NAME _____ DATE _____

The benefits of exercise are numerous. However, many media sources claim to sell "quick" and "miraculous" products for health and fitness. Some advertisements claim that "just a few minutes a day" are needed to lose weight, tone muscles, and trim inches. However, we know that true fitness requires effort. Complete this activity to practice thinking critically about fitness advertisements.

Find three examples of misleading or false claims on fitness or health products. You can find examples in popular magazines, television or radio ads, or other media sources. Answer the following questions for each of your products.

1. What is misleading or false about the fitness claims?

_____

_____

_____

2. Why is this statement false?

_____

_____

_____

3. Is it written by an expert in the field of exercise and physical fitness?

_____

_____

_____

4. Are the benefits of the product reasonable?

_____

_____

_____

5. Does the claim use gimmick words like "quick," "spot reduce," or "just minutes a day?"

_____

_____

_____

6. Are the advertisers trying to help you or just sell their product?

_____

_____

_____

Keep these ideas in mind to avoid being the victim of fitness rip-offs. If a product sounds too good to be true, it probably is.

APPENDIX A

Healthy People 2010

Healthy People is a national health promotion and disease prevention initiative developed and coordinated by the U.S. Department of Health and Human Services, Office of Disease Prevention and Health Promotion. The goal of *Healthy People 2010* is to improve the health of all Americans, eliminate disparities in health across populations, and increase the length and quality of life in the U.S. These goals can be achieved by meeting numerous health-related objectives. Selected *Healthy People 2010* objectives include:

- Increase the proportion of people who engage in daily physical activity
- Reduce activity limitation due to chronic back conditions
- Reduce cigarette smoking among people
- Increase the consumption of fruits and vegetables
- Reduce the lung cancer death rate
- Reduce the melanoma death rate
- Reduce the number of college students that engage in heavy drinking of alcoholic beverages
- Reduce the number of people who experience adverse health effects from stress each year
- Reduce the number of overweight people of ages 20 and older

Nutritional Content of Common Foods and Beverages

The following table of nutrient values is taken from the evaluEat diet analysis software that is a supplement to this text. The foods in the table shown here are just a fraction of the foods provided in the software. When using the software, you can quickly find these by entering the EvaluEat code in the search field. Values are obtained from the USDA Nutrient Database for Standard References, Release 16. A "0" indicates that nutrient value is determined to be zero; a blank space indicates that nutrient information is not available.

Amt = serving amount; **Wt** = weight; **Ener** = energy; **Prot** = protein; **Carb** = carbohydrate; **Fiber** = dietary fiber; **Fat** = total fat; **Sat** = saturated fat; **Chol** = cholesterol; **Calc** = calcium; **Iron** = iron; **Sodi** = sodium

EvaluEat Code	Food Name	Amount	Wt (g)	Ener (kcal)	Prot (g)	Carb (g)	Fiber (g)	Fat (g)	Sat (g)	Chol (g)	Calc (mg)	Iron (mg)	Sodi (mg)
Grains													
18001	Bagel, Plain/Onion/Poppy/Sesame, enriched	1 bagel (4" dia)	89	244.75	9.345	47.526	2.047	1.424	0.196	0	65.86	3.168	475.26
18013	Biscuit, Plain or Buttermilk, refrig dough, baked, reduced fat	1 biscuit (2-1/4" dia)	21	62.79	1.638	11.634	0.399	1.092	0.272	0	3.99	0.649	304.71
18035	Bread, Mixed Grain/7-Grain/Whole Grain	1 slice, large	32	80	3.2	14.848	2.048	1.216	0.258	0	29.12	1.11	155.84
18041	Bread, Pita, White, enriched	1 pita, large (6-1/2" dia)	60	165	5.46	33.42	1.32	0.72	0.1	0	51.6	1.572	321.6
18042	Bread, Pita, Whole Wheat	1 pita, large (6-1/2" dia)	64	170.24	6.272	35.2	4.736	1.664	0.262	0	9.6	1.958	340.48
18044	Bread, Rye - Pumpernickel	1 slice, regular	26	65	2.262	12.35	1.69	0.806	0.114	0	17.68	0.746	174.46
18047	Bread, Raisin, enriched	1 slice	26	71.24	2.054	13.598	1.118	1.144	0.281	0	17.16	0.754	101.4
18064	Bread, Wheat (includes wheat berry)	1 slice	25	65	2.275	11.8	1.075	1.025	0.223	0	26.25	0.827	132.5
18055	Bread, Wheat, reduced kcal	1 slice	23	45.54	2.093	10.028	2.76	0.529	0.079	0	18.4	0.681	117.53
18069	Bread, White, commercially prep, crumbs/cubes/slices	1 slice	25	66.5	1.91	12.653	0.6	0.822	0.179	0	37.75	0.935	170.25
18057	Bread, White, reduced kcal	1 slice	23	47.61	2.001	10.189	2.231	0.575	0.126	0	21.62	0.734	104.19
43100	Breakfast bars, oats, sugar, raisins, coconut (include granola bar)	1 cup	186	863.04	18.228	124.062	5.766	32.736	23.603	0	111.6	5.915	517.08
8053	Cereal, 100% Bran (wheat bran & barley)	.333 cup (1 NLEA serving)	29	83.23	3.683	22.678	8.294	0.609	0.087	0	22.04	8.1	120.93
8037	Cereal, Granola (oats & wheat germ) homemade	1 cup	122	597.8	18.141	64.599	10.492	29.719	5.535	0	95.16	5.185	26.84
8284	Cereal, Low Fat Granola with Raisins/Kellogg	.667 cup (1 NLEA serving)	55	201.3	4.4	44	2.75	2.75	0.825	0	23.1	1.65	135.3
8180	Cereal, Oats, Regular/Quick/Instant, ckd w/salt	1 cup	234	145.08	6.084	25.272	3.978	2.34	0.421	0	18.72	1.591	374.4
8157	Cereal, Wheat, Puffed, fortified	1 cup	12	43.68	1.764	9.552	0.528	0.144	0.024	0	3.36	3.804	0.48
8147	Cereal, Wheat, Shredded, large biscuit	2 biscuits (1 NLEA serving)	46	156.4	5.235	36.138	5.336	1.104	0.207	0	20.24	1.509	5.52
18620	Cracker, Original Premium Saltine Crackers/Nabisco	1 serving	14	58.8	1.526	9.954	0.364	1.428	0.259	0	27.02	0.727	177.8
18621	Cracker, Ritz/Nabisco	1 serving	16	78.72	1.152	10.272	0.304	3.664	0.627	0	23.52	0.648	124.16
18235	Cracker, Whole Wheat	10 Triscuit Bits	10	44.3	0.88	6.86	1.05	1.72	0.339	0	5	0.308	65.9
18258	English Muffin, Plain/Sourdough, enriched	1 muffin	57	133.95	4.389	26.22	1.539	1.026	0.148	0	99.18	1.425	264.48
20029	Grain, Couscous, ckd	1 cup, cooked	157	175.84	5.95	36.455	2.198	0.251	0.046	0	12.56	0.597	7.85
20038	Grain, Oats	1 cup	156	606.84	26.348	103.381	16.536	10.764	1.899	0	84.24	7.363	3.12
20037	Grain, Rice, Brown, Long grain, ckd	1 cup	195	216.45	5.031	44.772	3.51	1.755	0.351	0	19.5	0.819	9.75

EvaluEat Code	Food Name	Amount	Wt (g)	Ener (kcal)	Prot (g)	Carb (g)	Fiber (g)	Fat (g)	Sat (g)	Chol (g)	Calc (mg)	Iron (mg)	Sodi (mg)
20345	Grain, Rice, White, Long grain, enriched,ckd w/salt	1 cup	158	205.4	4.25	44.509	0.632	0.442	0.122	0	15.8	1.896	603.56
22005	Macaroni and Cheese Dinner, Kraft Original Flavor, unprepared	1 NLEA Serving (makes about 1 cup prepared)	70	259	11.34	47.53	1.47	2.59	1.26	9.8	92.4	2.562	561.4
20100	Macaroni, enriched, cooked	1 cup elbow shaped	140	197.4	6.678	39.676	1.82	0.938	0.133	0	9.8	1.96	1.4
18274	Muffin, Blueberry, commercially prep	1 medium	113	313.01	6.215	54.24	2.938	7.345	1.579	33.9	64.41	1.819	505.11
18279	Muffin, Corn, commercially prep	1 medium	113	344.65	6.667	57.517	3.842	9.492	1.53	29.38	83.62	3.175	588.73
18283	Muffin, Oatbran	1 medium	113	305.1	7.91	54.579	5.198	8.362	1.228	0	71.19	4.746	444.09
20113	Noodles, Chinese, Chow Mein	1 cup	45	237.15	3.771	25.893	1.755	13.842	1.973	0	9	2.128	197.55
20110	Noodles, Egg, enriched, ckd w/salt	1 cup	160	212.8	7.6	39.744	1.76	2.352	0.496	52.8	19.2	2.544	11.2
18293	Pancakes, Plain, homemade	1 pancake (4" dia)	38	86.26	2.432	10.754	3.686	0.806	22.42	83.22	0.684	166.82	
20121	Pasta, Spaghetti, enriched, ckd w/o salt	1 cup	140	197.4	6.678	39.676	2.38	0.938	0.133	0	9.8	1.96	1.4
20125	Pasta, Spaghetti, Whole Wheat, ckd	1 cup	140	173.6	7.462	37.156	6.3	0.756	0.139	0	21	1.484	4.2
43572	Popcorn, microwave, low fat and sodium	1 cup	148	634.92	18.648	108.617	21.016	14.06	2.094	0	16.28	3.374	725.2
18349	Roll, French	1 roll	38	105.26	3.268	19.076	1.216	1.634	0.366	0	34.58	1.03	231.42
18350	Roll, Hamburger/Hot Dog, Plain	1 roll	43	119.97	4.085	21.264	0.903	1.862	0.47	0	59.34	1.428	205.97
18348	Roll, Hamburger/Hot Dog, Whole Wheat	1 medium (2-1/2" dia)	36	95.76	3.132	18.396	2.7	1.692	0.301	0	38.16	0.871	172.08
18353	Roll, Hard/Kaiser	1 roll (3-1/2" dia)	57	167.01	5.643	30.039	1.311	2.451	0.345	0	54.15	1.87	310.08
19015	Snack, Granola Bar, Hard, Plain	1 bar (1 oz)	28	131.88	2.828	18.032	1.484	5.544	0.664	0	17.08	0.826	82.32
19020	Snack, Granola Bar, Soft, Plain	1 bar (1 oz)	28	124.04	2.072	18.844	1.288	4.816	2.027	0.28	29.4	0.717	77.84
19034	Snack, Popcorn, air-popped	1 cup	8	30.56	0.96	6.232	1.208	0.336	0.046	0	0.8	0.213	0.32
19051	Snack, Rice Cake, brown rice, Plain	2 cakes	18	69.66	1.476	14.67	0.756	0.504	0.103	0	1.98	0.268	
22901	Tortellini, pasta with cheese filling	1 cup	236	724.52	31.86	110.92	4.484	17.063	8.496	99.12	358.72	3.54	811.84
18449	Tortilla, Corn, w/o salt, ready to cook	1 tortilla, medium (approx 6" dia)	26	57.72	1.482	12.116	1.352	0.65	0.087	0	45.5	0.364	2.86
18364	Tortilla, Flour, ready-to-cook	1 tortilla medium (approx 6" dia)	46	149.5	4.002	25.576	1.518	3.266	0.803	0	57.5	1.518	219.88
18360	Tortilla, Taco Shell, baked	1 large (6-1/2" dia)	21	98.28	1.512	13.104	1.575	4.746	0.681	0	33.6	0.525	77.07
18365	Waffle, Plain/Buttermilk, frozen, ready-to-heat	1 waffle square	39	97.89	2.301	15.054	0.858	3.042	0.505	12.48	86.19	1.657	291.72

Protein Sources

43212	Bacon bits, meatless	1 cup	186	885.36	59.52	53.196	18.972	25.199	7.542	0	187.86	269.7	
16104	Bacon, vegetarian, meatless	1 strip	5	15.5	0.534	0.316	0.13	1.476	0.231	0	1.15	0.121	73.25
16006	Beans, Baked, Plain or Vegetarian, canned	1 cup	254	236.22	12.167	52.121	12.7	1.143	0.295	0	127	0.737	1008.38

EvaluEat Code	Food Name	Amount	Wt (g)	Ener (kcal)	Prot (g)	Carb (g)	Fiber (g)	Fat (g)	Sat (g)	Chol (g)	Calc (mg)	Iron (mg)	Sodi (mg)
16015	Beans, Black, mature seeds, boiled w/o salt	1 cup	172	227.04	15.239	40.781	14.964	0.929	0.239	0	46.44	3.612	1.72
16029	Beans, Kidney, mature seeds, canned	1 cup	256	207.36	13.312	38.093	8.96	0.794	0.115	0	69.12	3.149	888.32
16033	Beans, Kidney, Red, mature seeds, boiled w/o salt	1 cup	177	224.79	15.346	40.356	13.098	0.885	0.127	0	49.56	5.204	3.54
16070	Beans, Lentils, mature seeds, boiled w/o salt	1 cup	198	229.68	17.86	39.857	15.642	0.752	0.105	0	37.62	6.593	3.96
16110	Beans, Soy, mature seeds, roasted w/salt	1 cup	172	810.12	60.578	57.706	30.444	43.688	6.319	0	237.36	6.708	280.36
16162	Beans, Soy, Tofu, Mori-Nu, silken, firm	1 slice	84	52.08	5.796	2.016	0.084	2.268	0.341	0	26.88	0.865	30.24
16051	Beans, White, mature seeds, canned	1 cup	262	306.54	19.021	57.483	12.576	0.76	0.194	0	191.26	7.834	13.1
16137	Beans, Hummus, Garbanzo or Chick Pea Spread, homemade	1 tbsp	15	26.55	0.729	3.018	0.6	0.312	0.168	0	7.35	25.95	
13012	Beef, All Cuts, All Grades, lean (1/4" trim) cooked	3 oz	85	183.6	25.143	0	0	8.424	3.222	73.1	7.65	2.542	56.95
13004	Beef, All Cuts, All Grades, lean & fat (1/4" trim) cooked	3 oz	85	259.25	22.049	0	0	18.309	7.259	74.8	8.5	2.227	52.7
13306	Beef, Ground, lean, broiled, welldone	3 oz	85	238	23.97	0	0	14.994	5.891	85.85	10.2	2.082	75.65
13313	Beef, Ground, regular, broiled, welldone	3 oz	85	248.2	23.12	0	0	16.541	6.503	85.85	10.2	2.329	79.05
7933	Chicken breast, oven-roasted, fat-free, sliced	1 serving 2 slices	42	33.18	7.052	0.911	0	0.164	0.055	15.12	2.52	0.134	456.54
5009	Chicken, Broiler or Fryer, meat & skin, roasted	1 cup, chopped or diced	140	334.6	38.22	0	0	19.04	5.306	123.2	21	1.764	114.8
5012	Chicken, Broiler or Fryer, meat only, no skin, fried	1 cup, chopped or diced	140	306.6	42.798	2.366	0.14	12.768	3.444	131.6	23.8	1.89	127.4
5013	Chicken, Broiler or Fryer, meat only, no skin, roasted	1 cup, chopped or diced	140	266	40.502	0	0	10.374	2.856	124.6	21	1.694	120.4
43128	Chicken, meatless	1 cup	186	416.64	43.97	6.77	6.696	13.528	3.385	0	65.1	100.44	
22904	Chili con carne w/beans, canned entree	1 serving	222	255.3	20.18	24.487	8.214	8.147	2.109	24.42	66.6	3.308	1032.3
22720	Chili, Vegetarian Chili w/beans, canned entree/Hormel	1 cup	247	205.01	11.93	38.013	9.88	0.692	0.124	0	96.33	3.458	778.05
1143	Egg Substitute, liquid	1 cup	251	210.84	30.12	1.606	0	8.308	1.654	2.51	133.03	5.271	444.27
1128	Egg, Whole, fried	1 large	46	92.5	6.27	0.405	0	1.975	210.2	27.1	0.911	93.8	
1129	Egg, Whole, hard-cooked	1 large	50	77.5	6.29	0.56	0	5.305	1.633	212	25	0.595	62
1131	Egg, Whole, poached	1 large	50	73.5	6.265	0.38	0	0.679	1.543	211	26.5	66.5	
1132	Egg, Whole, scrambled	1 large	61	101.26	6.765	1.342	0	7.448	2.244	214.72	43.31	0.732	170.8
15187	Fish, Bass, Freshwater, cooked w/dry heat	3 oz	85	124.1	20.553	0	0	1.156	0.851	73.95	87.55	1.623	76.5
15011	Fish, Catfish, Channel, breaded & fried	3 oz	85	194.65	15.377	6.834	0.595	2.826	2.795	68.85	37.4	1.215	238
15016	Fish, Cod, Atlantic, baked/broiled (dry heat)	3 oz	85	89.25	19.406	0	0	0.248	0.143	46.75	11.9	0.417	66.3
15034	Fish, Haddock, baked or broiled (dry heat)	3 oz	85	95.2	20.604	0	0	0.263	0.142	62.9	35.7	1.148	73.95

EvaluEat Code	Food Name	Amount	Wt (g)	Ener (kcal)	Prot (g)	Carb (g)	Fiber (g)	Fat (g)	Sat (g)	Chol (g)	Calc (mg)	Iron (mg)	Sodi (mg)
15037	Fish, Halibut, Atlantic & Pacific, baked or broiled (dry heat)	3 oz	85	119	22.687	0	0	0.799	0.354	34.85	51	0.91	58.65
15087	Fish, Salmon, Sockeye w/bone, canned,drained	3 oz	85	130.05	17.399	0	0	6.214	1.397	37.4	203.15	0.901	457.3
15086	Fish, Salmon, Sockeye, baked or broiled (dry heat)	3 oz	85	183.6	23.214	0	0	9.325	1.629	73.95	5.95	0.468	56.1
15102	Fish, Snapper, baked or broiled (dry heat)	3 oz	85	108.8	22.355	0	0	1.462	0.31	39.95	34	0.204	48.45
15128	Fish, Tuna Salad	1 cup	205	383.35	32.882	19.29	0	18.983	3.165	26.65	34.85	2.05	824.1
15126	Fish, White Tuna, canned in H₂O, drained	3 oz	85	108.8	20.077	0	0	2.525	0.673	35.7	11.9	0.825	320.45
15124	Fish, White Tuna, canned in oil, drained	3 oz	85	158.1	22.551	0	0	6.868	1.088	26.35	3.4	0.553	336.6
7945	Frankfurter, beef, heated	1 serving	52	169.52	6.001	1.96	0	15.319	5.947	29.12	6.24	0.811	600.08
17002	Lamb, Domestic, Choice, Composite, lean & fat (1/4" trim) ckd	3 oz	85	249.9	20.842	0	0	17.799	7.506	82.45	14.45	1.598	61.2
7043	Lunch Meat, Beef, thin slices	1 oz	28.35	50.18	7.969	1.619	0	1.089	0.468	11.624	3.119	0.765	407.957
7007	Lunch Meat, Bologna (Beef)	1 slice	28	87.08	2.876	1.114		7.893	3.118	15.68	8.68	0.308	302.4
7079	Lunch Meat, Turkey Breast Meat	1 slice	28	26.88	2.044	3.822	0.56	0.378	0.118	3.36	3.08	0.33	47.04
16097	Peanut Butter, chunky w/salt	2 tbsp	32	188.48	8.022	6.749	2.112	15.904	3.066	0	16.96	0.653	150.4
16098	Peanut Butter, smooth w/salt	2 tbsp	32	191.68	7.99	5.894	1.888	16.73	3.209	0	15.04	0.602	160
16390	Peanuts, All Types, dry roasted w/o salt	1 oz	28.35	165.848	6.713	6.098	2.268	14.079	1.954	0	15.309	0.641	1.701
16090	Peanuts, All Types, dry roasted w/salt	1 oz	28.35	165.848	6.713	6.098	2.268	14.079	1.954	0	15.309	0.641	230.486
22903	Pizza, Pepperoni, frozen	1 serving	146	400.04	16.191	36.208	2.336	21.112	7.066	33.58	0	2.613	878.92
22902	Pizza, Sausage & pepperoni, frozen	1 serving	146	385.44	15.768	36.179	2.336	19.695	6.336	30.66	191.26	2.774	854.1
10124	Pork Bacon, Cured, broiled, pan-fried, or roasted	1 slice, cooked	8	43.28	2.963	0.114	0	3.342	1.099	8.8	0.88	0.115	184.8
10188	Pork Composite (leg,loin/shoulder/sparerib) Fresh, lean&fat, ckd	3 oz	85	232.05	23.434	0	0	14.603	5.287	77.35	21.25	0.935	52.7
10220	Pork, Ground, Fresh, ckd	3 oz	85	252.45	21.837	0	0	17.655	6.562	79.9	18.7	1.097	62.05
7019	Sausage, Chorizo (Pork & Beef)	1 link (4" long)	60	273	14.46	1.116	0	22.962	8.628	52.8	4.8	0.954	741
7919	Sausage, Turkey, breakfast links, mild	1 serving	56	131.6	8.635	0.874	0	10.13	4.002	33.6	17.92	0.599	327.6
16107	Sausage, Vegetarian, Meatless	1 link	25	64.25	4.633	2.46	0.7	4.54	0.732	0	15.75	0.93	222
15159	Shellfish, Clams, boiled/steamed (moist heat)	20 small	190	281.2	48.545	9.747	0	3.705	0.357	127.3	174.8	53.124	212.8
15158	Shellfish, Clams, breaded & fried	3 oz	85	171.7	12.104	8.781		9.477	2.281	51.85	53.55	11.824	309.4
15137	Shellfish, Crab, Alaskan King, boiled/steamed	1 leg	134	129.98	25.929	0	0	2.064	0.178	71.02	79.06	1.018	1436.48
15148	Shellfish, Lobster, Northern, boiled/steamed (moist heat)	3 oz	85	83.3	17.425	1.088	0	0.502	0.091	61.2	51.85	0.331	323
15168	Shellfish, Oyster, Eastern, breaded & fried	6 medium	88	173.36	7.718	10.226		11.07	2.813	71.28	54.56	6.116	366.96
15245	Shellfish, Oyster, Eastern, Farmed, raw	6 medium	84	49.56	4.385	4.645	0	1.302	0.372	21	36.96	4.855	149.52

EvaluEat Code	Food Name	Amount	Wt (g)	Ener (kcal)	Prot (g)	Carb (g)	Fiber (g)	Fat (g)	Sat (g)	Chol (g)	Calc (mg)	Iron (mg)	Sodi (mg)
15171	Shellfish, Oyster, Pacific, raw	1 medium	50	40.5	4.725	2.475	0	1.15	0.255	25	4	2.555	53
15151	Shellfish, Shrimp, boiled/steamed (moist heat)	4 large	22	21.78	4.6	0	0	0.238	0.064	42.9	8.58	0.68	49.28
15150	Shellfish, Shrimp, breaded & fried	4 large	30	72.6	6.417	3.441	0.12	3.684	0.626	53.1	20.1	0.378	103.2
43133	Soyburger	1 cup	186	332.94	33.313	24.924	8.556	11.104	1.337	0	53.94	3.906	1023
42130	Turkey bacon, cooked	1 ounce	28.34	108.259	8.389	0.879	0	7.907	2.351	27.773	2.551	0.598	647.569
5220	Turkey, Fryer/Roaster, Breast, no skin, roasted	1 unit (yield from 1 lb ready-to-cook turkey)	87	117.45	26.152	0	0	0.644	0.209	72.21	10.44	1.331	45.24
5208	Turkey, Fryer/Roaster, Dark Meat w/skin, roasted	1 unit (yield from 1 lb ready-to-cook turkey)	106	192.92	29.351	0	0	7.484	2.247	124.02	28.62	2.47	80.56
5206	Turkey, Fryer/Roaster, Light Meat w/skin, roasted	1 unit (yield from 1 lb ready-to-cook turkey)	123	201.72	35.387	0	0	5.633	1.538	116.85	22.14	1.98	70.11
5306	Turkey, Ground, cooked	1 patty (4 oz, raw)	82	192.7	22.435	0	0	10.783	2.78	83.64	20.5	1.583	87.74
17089	Veal, Composite, lean & fat, cooked	3 oz	85	196.35	25.585	0	0	9.682	3.638	96.9	18.7	0.978	73.95
43134	Vegetarian fillets	1 cup	186	539.4	42.78	16.74	11.346	33.48	5.299	0	176.7	3.72	911.4
43137	Vegetarian meatloaf or patties	1 cup	186	366.42	39.06	14.88	8.556	16.74	2.65	0	53.94	3.906	1023
43136	Vegetarian stew	1 cup	186	228.78	31.62	13.02	2.046	5.58	0.883	0	57.66	2.418	744
Dairy													
43276	Cheese spread, cream cheese base	1 cup	186	548.7	13.206	6.51	0	53.196	33.517	167.4	132.06	2.102	1251.78
1009	Cheese, Cheddar	1 cup, shredded	113	455.39	28.137	1.446	0	37.448	23.834	118.65	814.73	0.768	701.73
1012	Cheese, Cottage, Creamed, large or small curd	4 oz	113	116.39	14.114	3.028	0	5.096	3.224	16.95	67.8	0.158	457.65
1015	Cheese, Cottage, Lowfat, 2% fat	4 oz	113	101.7	15.526	4.102	0	2.181	1.38	9.04	77.97	0.181	458.78
1014	Cheese, Cottage, Nonfat, Uncreamed, Dry, large or small curd	4 oz	113	96.05	19.515	2.091	0	0.475	0.308	7.91	36.16	0.26	14.69
1017	Cheese, Cream	1 tbsp	14.5	50.605	1.095	0.386	0	5.056	3.185	15.95	11.6	0.174	42.92
1186	Cheese, Cream, fat free	1 ounce	28.34	27.206	4.084	1.644	0	0.385	0.255	2.267	52.429	0.051	154.453
1168	Cheese, Cheddar or Colby, low fat	1 cup, shredded	113	195.49	27.516	2.158	0	0.251	4.906	23.73	468.95	74.58	
1019	Cheese, Feta	1 oz	28.35	74.844	4.029	1.16	0	0.168	4.237	25.232	139.766	17.577	
1035	Cheese, Provolone	1 oz	28.35	99.509	7.252	0.607	0	0.218	4.842	19.562	214.326	39.123	
1040	Cheese, Swiss	1 oz	28.35	107.73	7.635	1.525	0	0.276	5.04	26.082	224.249	21.83	
1028	Cheese, Mozzarella, Part Skim Milk	1 oz	28.35	72.009	6.878	0.785	0	4.513	2.867	18.144	221.697	0.062	175.487
1026	Cheese, Mozzarella, Whole Milk	1 oz	28.35	85.05	6.285	0.621	0	6.336	3.729	22.397	143.168	0.125	177.755
1032	Cheese, Parmesan, grated	1 tbsp	5	21.55	1.923	0.203	0	1.431	0.865	4.4	55.45	0.045	76.45
42205	Cheese, pasteurized process, cheddar or american, fat-free	1 cup	186	275.28	41.85	24.924	0	1.488	0.937	20.46	1281.54	0.521	2842.08

EvaluEat Code	Food Name	Amount	Wt (g)	Ener (kcal)	Prot (g)	Carb (g)	Fiber (g)	Fat (g)	Sat (g)	Chol (g)	Calc (mg)	Iron (mg)	Sodi (mg)
1037	Cheese, Ricotta, Part Skim Milk	1 cup	246	339.48	28.019	12.644	0	19.459	12.12	76.26	669.12	1.082	307.5
1049	Cream, Half and Half	1 tbsp	15	19.5	0.444	0.645	0	1.725	1.074	5.55	15.75	0.011	6.15
1053	Cream, Heavy Whipping	1 cup, whipped	120	414	2.46	3.348	0	1.649	27.638	164.4	78	90	
42185	Frozen yogurts, chocolate, nonfat milk, with low calorie sweetener	1 cup	186	199.02	8.184	36.642	3.72	1.488	0.939	7.44	295.74	0.074	150.66
42187	Frozen yogurts, flavors other than chocolate	1 cup	186	236.22	5.58	40.176	0	6.696	4.326	24.18	186	0.856	117.18
1082	Milk, Lowfat, 1% fat w/added vitamin A	1 cup	244	102.48	8.223	12.176	0	2.367	1.545	12.2	263.52	0.854	122
1104	Milk, Lowfat, 1% fat, Chocolate	1 cup	250	157.5	8.1	26.1	1.25	2.5	1.54	7.5	287.5	0.6	152.5
1085	Milk, Nonfat/Fat Free, Skim w/added Vit A	1 cup	245	83.3	8.257	12.152	0	0.196	0.287	4.9	222.95	1.225	107.8
16120	Milk, Soy, fluid	1 cup	245	120.05	9.188	11.368	3.185	5.096	0.524	0	9.8	1.421	29.4
1077	Milk, Whole, 3.25% fat	1 cup	244	146.4	7.857	11.029	0	7.93	4.551	24.4	246.44	0.073	104.92
1102	Milk, Whole, Chocolate	1 cup	250	207.5	7.925	25.85	2	8.475	5.26	30	280	0.6	150
1180	Sour cream, fat free	1 ounce	28.34	20.972	0.879	4.421	0	0	0	2.551	35.425	0	39.959
1179	Sour cream, light	1 ounce	28.34	38.542	0.992	2.012	0	3.004	1.87	9.919	39.959	0.02	20.121
43261	Yogurt, fruit variety, nonfat	1 cup	186	174.84	8.184	35.34	0	0.372	0.221	3.72	282.72	0.13	107.88
1121	Yogurt, Lowfat w/fruit, 10g protein/8 oz	1 cup (8 fl oz)	245	249.9	10.707	46.673	0	2.646	1.708	9.8	372.4	0.171	142.1
1117	Yogurt, Lowfat, Plain, 12g protein/8 oz	1 cup (8 fl oz)	245	154.35	12.863	17.248	0	3.797	2.45	14.7	448.35	0.196	171.5
1116	Yogurt, Whole Milk, Plain, 8g protein/8 oz	1 cup (8 fl oz)	245	149.45	8.502	11.417	0	7.963	5.135	31.85	296.45	0.123	112.7
Fruits													
9103	Fruit Salad (peach, pineapple, pear, apricot & cherry) canned in juice	1 cup	249	124.5	1.27	32.494	2.49	0.075	0.01	0	27.39	0.623	12.45
9003	Fruit, Apple w/skin, raw	1 large (3-1/4" dia) (approx 2 per lb)	212	110.24	0.551	29.277	5.088	0.36	0.059	0	12.72	0.254	2.12
9007	Fruit, Apple, slices, sweetened, canned, drained	1 cup slices	204	136.68	0.367	34.068	3.468	1	0.163	0	8.16	0.469	6.12
9402	Fruit, Applesauce, canned, sweetened w/added Vit C	1 cup	255	193.8	0.459	50.771	3.06	0.459	0.076	0	10.2	0.892	71.4
9401	Fruit, Applesauce, canned, unsweetened w/added Vit C	1 cup	244	104.92	0.415	27.548	2.928	0.122	0.02	0	7.32	0.293	4.88
9021	Fruit, Apricot, raw	1 apricot	35	16.8	0.49	3.892	0.7	0.136	0.009	0	4.55	0.136	0.35
9038	Fruit, Avocado, California, peeled, raw	1 fruit without skin and seeds	173	288.91	3.391	14.947	11.764	26.659	3.678	0	22.49	1.055	13.84
9040	Fruit, Banana, peeled, raw, mashed/sliced	1 medium (7" to 7-7/8" long)	118	105.02	1.286	26.951	3.068	0.389	0.132	0	5.9	0.307	1.18
9050	Fruit, Blueberries, raw	1 cup	145	82.65	1.073	21.01	3.48	0.479	0.041	0	8.7	0.406	1.45
9070	Fruit, Cherries, Sweet, raw	1 cup, with pits, yields	117	73.71	1.24	18.732	2.457	0.234	0.044	0	15.21	0.421	0

EvaluEat Code	Food Name	Amount	Wt (g)	Ener (kcal)	Prot (g)	Carb (g)	Fiber (g)	Fat (g)	Sat (g)	Chol (g)	Calc (mg)	Iron (mg)	Sodi (mg)
9078	Fruit, Cranberries, raw	1 cup, chopped	110	50.6	0.429	13.42	5.06	0.143	0.012	0	8.8	0.275	2.2
9087	Fruit, Dates, Domestic, Natural, dried	1 cup, pitted, chopped	178	501.96	4.361	133.553	14.24	0.694	0.057	0	69.42	1.816	3.56
9089	Fruit, Figs, raw	1 large (2-1/2" dia)	64	47.36	0.48	12.275	1.856	0.192	0.038	0	22.4	0.237	0.64
9111	Fruit, Grapefruit, Red, White or Pink, peeled, raw	.5 medium (approx 4" dia)	128	40.96	0.806	10.342	1.408	0.128	0.018	0	15.36	0.115	0
9131	Fruit, Grapes, American type (slip skin) raw	1 cup	92	61.64	0.58	15.778	0.828	0.322	0.105	0	12.88	0.267	1.84
9148	Fruit, Kiwifruit (Chinese Gooseberry) peeled, raw	1 fruit without skin, medium	76	46.36	0.866	11.142	2.28	0.395	0.022	0	25.84	0.236	2.28
9176	Fruit, Mango, peeled, raw	1 cup, sliced	165	107.25	0.841	28.05	2.97	0.446	0.109	0	16.5	0.214	3.3
9184	Fruit, Melon, Honeydew, peeled, wedges, raw	1 wedge (1/8 of 6" to 7" dia melon)	160	57.6	0.864	14.544	1.28	0.224	0.061	0	9.6	0.272	28.8
9191	Fruit, Nectarine, raw	1 fruit (2-1/2" dia)	136	59.84	1.442	14.348	2.312	0.435	0.034	0	8.16	0.381	0
9193	Fruit, Olives, Ripe, pitted, canned	1 tbsp	8.4	9.66	0.071	0.526	0.269	0.897	0.119	0	7.392	0.277	73.248
9200	Fruit, Orange, All Varieties, peeled, raw	1 fruit (2-5/8" dia)	131	61.57	1.231	15.392	3.144	0.157	0.02	0	52.4	0.131	0
9226	Fruit, Papayas, peeled, cubed/mashed, raw	1 medium (5-1/8" long x 3" dia)	304	118.56	1.854	29.822	5.472	0.426	0.131	0	72.96	0.304	9.12
9236	Fruit, Peach, peeled, raw	1 medium (2-1/2" dia) (approx 4 per lb)	98	38.22	0.892	9.349	1.47	0.245	0.019	0	5.88	0.245	0
9252	Fruit, Pear, raw	1 pear, medium (approx 2-1/2 per lb)	166	96.28	0.631	25.664	5.146	0.199	0.01	0	14.94	0.282	1.66
9279	Fruit, Plum, raw	1 fruit (2-1/8" dia)	66	30.36	0.462	7.537	0.924	0.185	0.011	0	3.96	0.112	0
9291	Fruit, Prunes, dried	1 prune	8.4	20.16	0.183	5.366	0.596	0.032	0.007	0	3.612	0.078	0.168
9298	Fruit, Raisins, seedless	1 cup (not packed)	145	433.55	4.451	114.811	5.365	0.667	0.084	0	72.5	2.726	15.95
9302	Fruit, Raspberries, raw	1 cup	123	63.96	1.476	14.686	7.995	0.799	0.023	0	30.75	0.849	1.23
9316	Fruit, Strawberries, halves/slices, raw	1 cup, halves	152	48.64	1.018	11.674	3.04	0.456	0.023	0	24.32	0.638	1.52
9326	Fruit, Watermelon, balls, raw	1 cup, balls	154	46.2	0.939	11.627	0.616	0.231	0.025	0	10.78	0.37	1.54

Vegetables

EvaluEat Code	Food Name	Amount	Wt (g)	Ener (kcal)	Prot (g)	Carb (g)	Fiber (g)	Fat (g)	Sat (g)	Chol (g)	Calc (mg)	Iron (mg)	Sodi (mg)
11358	Potatoes, red, flesh and skin, baked	1 potato, large (3" to 4-1/4" dia)	299	266.11	6.877	58.574	5.382	0.449	0.078	0	26.91	2.093	23.92
11356	Potatoes, Russet, flesh and skin, baked	1 potato, large	299	290.03	7.864	64.106	6.877	0.389	0	0	53.82	3.199	23.92
11702	Vege, Artichokes (Globe or French) boiled w/salt, drained	1 artichoke, medium	120	60	4.176	13.416	6.48	0.192	0.044	0	54	1.548	397.2

EvaluEat Code	Food Name	Amount	Wt (g)	Ener (kcal)	Prot (g)	Carb (g)	Fiber (g)	Fat (g)	Sat (g)	Chol (g)	Calc (mg)	Iron (mg)	Sodi (mg)
11705	Vege, Asparagus, boiled w/salt, drained	4 spears (1/2" base)	60	13.2	1.44	2.466	1.2	0.132	0.043	0	13.8	0.546	144
11626	Vege, Bean Sprouts, Mung, mature seeds, sprouted, canned, drained	1 cup	125	15	1.75	2.675	1	0.075	0.02	0	17.5	0.538	175
11723	Vege, Beans, Snap, Green, boiled w/salt, drained	1 cup	125	43.75	2.362	9.863	4	0.35	0.08	0	57.5	1.6	298.75
11734	Vege, Beets, boiled w/salt, drained	.5 cup slices	85	37.4	1.428	8.466	1.7	0.153	0.024	0	13.6	0.672	242.25
11741	Vege, Broccoli Stalks, raw	1 stalk	114	31.92	3.397	5.974	0.399	0.062	0	0	54.72	1.003	30.78
11742	Vege, Broccoli, boiled w/salt, chopped, drained	.5 cup, chopped	78	21.84	2.324	3.947	2.574	0.273	0.042	0	31.2	0.523	204.36
11745	Vege, Brussels Sprouts, boiled w/salt, drained	.5 cup	78	31.98	1.989	6.763	2.028	0.398	0.082	0	28.08	0.936	200.46
11109	Vege, Cabbage Heads, raw	1 cup, chopped	89	21.36	1.282	4.966	2.047	0.107	0.014	0	41.83	0.525	16.02
11751	Vege, Cabbage, boiled w/salt, drained	.5 cup, shredded	75	16.5	0.765	3.345	1.425	0.322	0.04	0	23.25	0.127	191.25
11960	Vege, Carrots, Baby, raw	1 medium	10	3.5	0.064	0.824	0.18	0.013	0.002	0	3.2	0.089	7.8
11757	Vege, Carrots, boiled w/salt, drained	.5 cup slices	78	27.3	0.593	6.412	2.34	0.14	0.023	0	23.4	0.265	235.56
11761	Vege, Cauliflower, boiled w/salt, drained	.5 cup (1" pieces)	62	14.26	1.141	2.548	1.674	0.279	0.043	0	9.92	0.205	150.04
11143	Vege, Celery, raw	1 cup, diced	120	16.8	0.828	3.564	1.92	0.204	0.052	0	48	0.24	96
11765	Vege, Chard, Swiss, boiled w/salt, drained	1 cup, chopped	175	35	3.29	7.227	3.675	0.14	0	0	101.5	3.955	726.25
11768	Vege, Collards, boiled w/salt, drained	1 cup, chopped	190	49.4	4.009	9.329	5.32	0.684	0.089	0	266	2.204	478.8
11908	Vege, Corn, White, Sweet, canned, vacuum/regular pack	.5 cup	105	82.95	2.53	20.412	2.1	0.525	0.081	0	5.25	0.441	285.6
11900	Vege, Corn, White, Sweet, ears, raw	1 ear, large	143	122.98	4.605	27.199	3.861	1.687	0.26	0	2.86	0.744	21.45
11176	Vege, Corn, White, Yellow, Sweet, canned, vacuum/regular pack	.5 cup	105	82.95	2.53	20.412	2.1	0.525	0.081	0	5.25	0.441	285.6
11205	Vege, Cucumber, raw	.5 cup slices	52	7.8	0.338	1.888	0.26	0.057	0.018	0	8.32	0.146	1.04
11783	Vege, Eggplant (Brinjal) boiled w/salt,drained	1 cup (1" cubes)	99	34.65	0.822	8.643	2.475	0.228	0.044	0	5.94	0.248	236.61
11264	Vege, Fungi, Mushrooms, canned, caps/slices, drained	1 can	132	33	2.468	6.719	3.168	0.383	0.05	0	14.52	1.043	561
11260	Vege, Fungi, Mushrooms, slices, raw	1 medium	18	3.96	0.56	0.583	0.216	0.061	0.008	0	0.54	0.094	0.72
11790	Vege, Kale, boiled w/salt, drained	1 cup, chopped	130	36.4	2.47	7.319	2.6	0.52	0.068	0	93.6	1.17	336.7
11251	Vege, Lettuce, Cos/Romaine, raw	1 inner leaf	10	1.7	0.123	0.329	0.21	0.03	0.004	0	3.3	0.097	0.8
11252	Vege, Lettuce, Iceberg, head, raw	1 head, medium	539	53.9	4.366	11.265	5.39	0.593	0.075	0	107.8	1.886	48.51
11803	Vege, Okra, boiled w/salt, drained	.5 cup slices	80	17.6	1.496	3.608	2	0.168	0.036	0	61.6	0.224	4.8
11808	Vege, Parsnip, boiled w/salt, drained	.5 cup slices	78	63.18	1.03	15.233	3.12	0.234	0.039	0	28.86	0.452	191.88
11300	Vege, Peas w/edible pod-Snow/Sugar, raw	1 cup, chopped	98	41.16	2.744	7.399	2.548	0.196	0.038	0	42.14	2.038	3.92
11811	Vege, Peas, Green, boiled w/salt, drained	1 cup	160	134.4	8.576	25.024	8.8	0.352	0.062	0	43.2	2.464	382.4
11308	Vege, Peas, Green, canned, regular pack, drained	1 cup	170	117.3	7.514	21.386	6.97	0.595	0.105	0	34	1.615	428.4

EvaluEat Code	Food Name	Amount	Wt (g)	Ener (kcal)	Prot (g)	Carb (g)	Fiber (g)	Fat (g)	Sat (g)	Chol (g)	Calc (mg)	Iron (mg)	Sodi (mg)
11979	Vege, Pepper, Jalapeno, raw	1 cup, sliced	90	27	1.215	5.319	2.52	0.558	0.056	0	9	0.63	0.9
11333	Vege, Pepper, Sweet, Green, chopped/sliced, raw	1 medium	119	23.8	1.023	5.522	2.023	0.202	0.069	0	11.9	0.405	3.57
11821	Vege, Pepper, Sweet, Red, raw	1 medium	119	30.94	1.178	7.176	2.38	0.357	0.07	0	8.33	0.512	2.38
11833	Vege, Potato, boiled w/o skin & w/salt	1 medium	167	143.62	2.856	33.417	3.34	0.167	0.043	0	13.36	0.518	402.47
11838	Vege, Potato, French Fries, frozen, oven heated, w/salt	10 strips	50	100	1.585	15.595	1.6	3.78	0.631	0	4	0.62	133
11429	Vege, Radish, slices, raw	1 large (1" to 1-1/4" dia)	9	1.44	0.061	0.306	0.144	0.009	0.003	0	2.25	0.031	3.51
11854	Vege, Spinach, boiled w/salt, drained	1 cup	180	41.4	5.346	6.75	4.32	0.468	0.076	0	244.8	6.426	550.8
11457	Vege, Spinach, raw	1 cup	30	6.9	0.858	1.089	0.66	0.117	0.019	0	29.7	0.813	23.7
11857	Vege, Squash, Summer, All Varieties, boiled w/salt, drained	1 cup slices	180	36	1.638	7.758	2.52	0.558	0.115	0	48.6	0.648	426.6
11863	Vege, Squash, Winter, All Varieties, baked w/salt	1 cup, cubes	205	79.95	1.824	17.938	5.74	1.291	0.266	0	28.7	0.677	485.85
11875	Vege, Sweet Potato, baked in skin w/salt	1 medium (2" dia, 5" long, raw)	114	102.6	2.291	23.609	3.762	0.171	0.039	0	43.32	0.787	280.44
11531	Vege, Tomato, Red, canned, whole	1 cup	240	40.8	1.92	9.384	2.16	0.312	0.043	0	74.4	2.328	307.2
11529	Vege, Tomato, Red, ripe, whole, raw	1 cup, chopped or sliced	180	32.4	1.584	7.056	2.16	0.36	0.081	0	18	0.486	9
11897	Vege, Yam, boiled or baked w/salt	1 cup, cubes	136	157.76	2.026	37.509	5.304	0.19	0.039	0	19.04	0.707	331.84
11894	Vegetables, Mixed, frozen, boiled w/salt, drained	.5 cup	91	53.69	2.603	11.912	4.004	0.137	0.028	0	22.75	0.746	246.61

Fast Foods
Breakfast Items

EvaluEat Code	Food Name	Amount	Wt (g)	Ener (kcal)	Prot (g)	Carb (g)	Fiber (g)	Fat (g)	Sat (g)	Chol (g)	Calc (mg)	Iron (mg)	Sodi (mg)
21023	Fast Food, French Toast w/butter	2 slices	135	356.4	10.341	36.045		18.765	7.749	116.1	72.9	1.89	513
21025	Fast Food, Pancakes w/butter & syrup	2 cakes	232	519.68	8.259	90.898		13.99	5.851	58	127.6	2.622	1104.32
21026	Fast Food, Potatoes, Hash Brown	.5 cup	72	151.2	1.944	16.15		9.216	4.324	9.36	7.2	0.482	290.16
21002	Fast Food, Sandwich, Biscuit w/egg	1 biscuit	136	372.64	11.601	31.906	0.816	22.073	4.729	244.8	81.6	2.897	890.8
21003	Fast Food, Sandwich, Biscuit w/egg & bacon	1 biscuit	150	457.5	16.995	28.59	0.75	31.095	7.95	352.5	189	3.735	999
21004	Fast Food, Sandwich, Biscuit w/egg & ham	1 biscuit	192	441.6	20.429	30.317	0.768	27.034	5.914	299.52	220.8	4.55	1382.4
21005	Fast Food, Sandwich, Biscuit w/egg & sausage	1 biscuit	180	581.4	19.152	41.148	0.9	38.7	14.976	302.4	154.8	3.96	1141.2
21007	Fast Food, Sandwich, Biscuit w/egg, cheese & bacon	1 biscuit	144	476.64	16.258	33.422		31.392	11.398	260.64	164.16	2.549	1260
21011	Fast Food, Sandwich, Croissant w/egg & cheese	1 croissant	127	368.3	12.789	24.308		24.701	14.065	215.9	243.84	2.197	551.18
21012	Fast Food, Sandwich, Croissant w/egg, cheese & bacon	1 croissant	129	412.8	16.228	23.646		28.354	15.432	215.43	150.93	2.193	888.81
21013	Fast Food, Sandwich, Croissant w/egg, cheese & ham	1 croissant	152	474.24	18.924	24.198		33.577	17.475	212.8	144.4	2.128	1080.72

EvaluEat Code	Food Name	Amount	Wt (g)	Ener (kcal)	Prot (g)	Carb (g)	Fiber (g)	Fat (g)	Sat (g)	Chol (g)	Calc (mg)	Iron (mg)	Sodi (mg)
Chicken													
21035	Fast Food, Chicken, breaded, fried, dark meat (drumstick or thigh)	2 pieces	148	430.68	30.074	15.703		26.699	7.049	165.76	35.52	1.598	754.8
21036	Fast Food, Chicken, breaded, fried, light meat (breast or wing)	2 pieces	163	493.89	35.713	19.576		29.519	7.844	148.33	60.31	1.483	974.74
21102	Fast Food, Sandwich, Chicken Filet, plain	1 sandwich	182	515.06	24.115	38.693		29.448	8.527	60.06	60.06	4.677	957.32
Burgers													
21092	Fast Food, Sandwich, Cheeseburger (2 patty) plain	1 sandwich	155	457.25	27.667	22.056		28.474	12.997	110.05	232.5	3.41	635.5
21098	Fast Food, Sandwich, Cheeseburger, large, one meat patty w/condiments & veges	1 sandwich	219	562.83	28.185	38.391		32.938	15.039	87.6	205.86	4.665	1108.14
21109	Fast Food, Sandwich, Hamburger, one patty w/condiments & veges	1 sandwich	110	279.4	12.914	27.291		13.475	4.131	26.4	62.7	2.629	503.8
21107	Fast Food, Sandwich, Hamburger, plain	1 sandwich	90	274.5	12.321	30.51		11.817	4.141	35.1	63	2.403	387
Mexican													
21061	Fast Food, Burrito w/beans & cheese	2 pieces	186	377.58	15.066	54.963		11.699	6.849	27.9	213.9	2.269	1166.22
21066	Fast Food, Burrito w/beef	2 pieces	220	523.6	26.598	58.52	0	20.812	10.459	63.8	83.6	6.094	1491.6
21078	Fast Food, Nachos w/cheese	1 portion (6-8 nachos)	113	345.78	9.097	36.33		18.95	7.78	18.08	272.33	1.277	815.86
21080	Fast Food, Nachos w/cheese, beans, ground beef & peppers	1 portion (6-8 nachos)	255	568.65	19.788	55.819	6.327	30.702	12.487	20.4	385.05	2.78	1800.3
21082	Fast Food, Taco	1 large	263	568.08	31.77	41.107	0.333	31.613	17.484	86.79	339.27	3.708	1233.47
Sides/Beverages/Other													
21118	Fast Food, Hot Dog, plain	1 sandwich	98	242.06	10.388	18.032		14.543	5.109	44.1	23.52	2.313	670.32
21033	Fast Food, Ice Cream Sundae, hot fudge	1 sundae	158	284.4	5.641	47.669	0	8.627	5.023	20.54	206.98	0.585	181.7
14346	Fast Food, Milk Beverage, Chocolate Shake/McDonald's	1 medium shake (16 fl oz)	333	422.91	11.322	68.265	6.327	12.321	7.702	43.29	376.29	1.032	323.01
14347	Fast Food, Shake, Vanilla/McDonald's	1 medium shake (16 fl oz)	333	369.63	11.655	59.607	0.333	9.99	6.187	36.63	406.26	0.3	273.06
21130	Fast Food, Onion Rings, breaded, fried	1 portion (8-9 onion rings)	83	275.56	3.702	31.324		15.513	6.953	14.11	73.04	0.847	429.94
21049	Fast Food, Pizza w/cheese	1 slice	63	140.49	7.68	20.5		3.213	1.54	9.45	116.55	0.58	335.79
21050	Fast Food, Pizza w/cheese, meat & veges	1 slice	79	184.07	13.011	21.291		5.364	1.535	20.54	101.12	1.533	382.36
21051	Fast Food, Pizza w/pepperoni	1 slice	71	181.05	10.125	19.866		6.958	2.236	14.2	64.61	0.937	266.96
21138	Fast Food, Potato, French fried w/vegetable oil	1 large	169	577.98	7.267	67.279	5.915	31.147	6.507	0	23.66	1.318	334.62
21105	Fast Food, Sandwich, Fish w/tartar sauce	1 sandwich	158	431.34	16.938	41.017		22.768	5.235	55.3	83.74	2.607	614.62

Beverages

EvaluEat Code	Food Name	Amount	Wt (g)	Ener (kcal)	Prot (g)	Carb (g)	Fiber (g)	Fat (g)	Sat (g)	Chol (g)	Calc (mg)	Iron (mg)	Sodi (mg)
14006	Beverage, Alcoholic, Beer, Light	1 can or bottle (12 fl oz)	354	99.12	0.708	4.602	0	0	0	0	17.7	0.142	10.62
14003	Beverage, Alcoholic, Beer, Regular	1 can	356	117.48	1.068	5.732	0.356	0.214	0	0	17.8	0.071	14.24
14010	Beverage, Alcoholic, Daiquiri, prep from recipe	1 cocktail (2 fl oz)	60	111.6	0.036	4.164	0.06	0.036	0.004	0	1.8	0.054	3
14049	Beverage, Alcoholic, Distilled Spirits, Gin, Vodka, Rum, Whiskey	1 jigger 1.5 fl oz	42	110.46	0	0	0	0	0	0	0	0	0.84
14084	Beverage, Alcoholic, Wine (all table)	1 glass 3.5 fl oz	103	79.31	0.206	3.296	0	0	0	0	8.24	0.36	6.18
14209	Beverage, Coffee, Brewed	1 cup (8 fl oz)	237	9.48	0.332	0	0	1.801	0	0	2.37	0.024	2.37
14201	Beverage, Coffee, brewed, prepared with tap water, decaffeinated	1 cup (8 fl oz)	237	9.48	0.332	0	0	1.801	0	0	2.37	0.024	2.37
14400	Beverage, Cola w/caffeine	1 can 12 fl oz	370	155.4	0.185	39.775	0	0	0	0	11.1	0.074	14.8
14177	Beverage Mix, Chocolate Flavor, dry mix, prep w/milk	1 cup (8 fl oz)	266	226.1	8.592	31.681	1.064	0.495	4.948	23.94	252.7	457.52	
14318	Beverage Mix, Chocolate Malted Milk Powder, no added nutrients, prep w/milk	1 cup (8 fl oz)	265	225.25	8.931	29.68	1.325	0.551	4.99	26.5	259.7	455.8	
14351	Beverage Mix, Strawberry Flavor, dry, prep w/milk	1 cup (8 fl oz)	266	234.08	7.98	32.718	0	0.303	5.081	31.92	292.6	369.74	
14182	Beverage, Chocolate Syrup w/o added nutrients, prep w/milk	1 cup (8 fl oz)	282	253.8	8.657	36.04	0.846	0.485	4.74	25.38	250.98	408.9	
14390	Beverage, Cocoa Mix w/aspartame, dry, low kcal, prep w/H$_2$O	1 packet dry mix with 6 fl oz water	192	55.68	2.419	10.445	0.96	0.013	0	0	90.24	405.12	
14194	Beverage, Cocoa Mix, dry, w/o added nutrients, prep w/H$_2$O	1 oz packet with 6 fl oz water	206	113.3	1.669	23.978	1.03	0.035	0.672	2.06	45.32	201.88	
14419	Beverage, Coffee Mix w/sugar (French) dry, prep w/H$_2$O	6 fl oz H$_2$O & 2 rounded tsp mix	189	56.7	0.567	6.615	0	0.062	2.947	0	7.56	136.08	5.668
14136	Beverage, Soft Drink, Ginger Ale	1 can or bottle (16 fl oz)	488	165.92	0	42.798	0	0	0	0	14.64	0.878	34.16
14145	Beverage, Soft Drink, Lemon-Lime	1 can or bottle (16 fl oz)	491	196.4	0	51.064	0	0	0	0	9.82	0.344	54.01
14153	Beverage, Soft Drink, Pepper type	1 can or bottle (16 fl oz)	491	201.31	0	51.064	0	0.491	0.344	0	14.73	0.196	49.1
14355	Beverage, Tea, Brewed	1 cup (8 fl oz)	237	2.37	0	0.711	0	0	0.005	0	0	0.047	7.11
14553	Beverage, Wine, non-alcoholic	1 fl oz	29	1.74	0.145	0.319	0	0	0	0	2.61	0.116	2.03
9206	Fruit Juice, Orange, fresh	1 cup	248	111.6	1.736	25.792	0.496	0.099	0.06	0	27.28	0.496	2.48
9215	Fruit Juice, Orange, frozen concentrate, unsweetened, prep	1 cup	249	112.05	1.693	26.842	0.498	0.03	0.017	0	22.41	0.249	2.49
9016	Fruit Juice, Apple, canned or bottled, unsweetened w/o added Vit C	1 cup	248	116.56	0.149	28.966	0.248	0.082	0.002	0	18.96	225.15	7.44
9018	Fruit Juice, Apple, frozen concentrate, unsweetened w/o added Vit C, prep	1 cup	239	112.33	0.335	27.581	0.239	0.074	0.047	0	17.36	295.12	16.73

EvaluEat Code	Food Name	Amount	Wt (g)	Ener (kcal)	Prot (g)	Carb (g)	Fiber (g)	Fat (g)	Sat (g)	Chol (g)	Calc (mg)	Iron (mg)	Sodi (mg)
11655	Vegetable Juice, Carrot, canned	1 cup	236	94.4	2.242	21.924	1.888	0.168	0.064	0	56.64	689.12	
11886	Vegetable Juice, Tomato, canned w/o salt	1 cup	243	41.31	1.847	10.303	0.972	0.058	0.019	0	24.3	556.47	

Fats/Sweets/Other

EvaluEat Code	Food Name	Amount	Wt (g)	Ener (kcal)	Prot (g)	Carb (g)	Fiber (g)	Fat (g)	Sat (g)	Chol (g)	Calc (mg)	Iron (mg)	Sodi (mg)
16124	Bean Sauce, Soy (Tamari)	1 tsp	6	3.6	0.631	0.334	0.048	0.003	0.001	0	1.2	12.72	
1001	Butter, Regular (with salt)	1 tbsp	14.2	101.814	0.121	0.009	0	11.518	5.799	30.53	3.408	0.003	81.792
1002	Butter, Whipped (with salt)	1 tbsp	9.4	67.398	0.08	0.006	0	7.624	4.746	20.586	2.256	0.015	77.738
18101	Cake, Chocolate, homemade, w/o icing	1 piece (1/12 of 9" dia)	95	340.1	5.035	50.73	1.52	14.345	5.158	55.1	57	1.53	299.25
18146	Cake, Yellow, homemade, w/o icing	1 piece (1/12 of 8" dia)	68	245.48	3.604	36.04	0.476	9.928	2.668	36.72	99.28	1.115	233.24
43031	Candies, chocolate covered, caramel with nuts	1 cup	186	874.2	17.67	112.846	7.998	39.06	8.662	0	145.08	3.162	44.64
19120	Candy, Milk Chocolate	1 bar 1.55 oz	44	235.4	3.366	26.136	1.496	13.05	6.271	10.12	83.16	1.034	34.76
19126	Candy, Peanuts, milk chocolate coated	10 pieces	40	207.6	5.24	19.76	1.88	13.4	5.84	3.6	41.6	0.524	16.4
19127	Candy, Raisins, milk chocolate coated	10 pieces	10	39	0.41	6.83	0.42	1.48	0.88	0.3	8.6	0.171	3.6
19434	Cheese puffs and twists, corn based, low fat	1 oz	28.35	122.472	2.41	20.511	3.033	3.43	0.595	0.284	101.21	0.363	364.298
18154	Cookie, Brownies, homemade	1 brownie (2" square)	24	111.84	1.488	12.048		6.984	1.757	17.52	13.68	0.442	82.32
18378	Cookie, Chocolate Chip, homemade w/butter	1 cookie, medium (2-1/4" dia)	16	78.08	0.912	9.312		4.544	2.251	11.2	6.08	0.397	54.56
18170	Cookie, Fig Bar	1 individual package (2 oz package containing 2 3" bars)	57	198.36	2.109	40.413	2.622	4.161	0.64	0	36.48	1.653	199.5
18184	Cookie, Oatmeal, homemade w/raisins	1 cookie (2-5/8" dia)	15	65.25	0.975	10.26		2.43	0.485	4.95	15	0.398	80.7
1054	Cream, Whipped Cream Topping, Pressurized	1 tbsp	3	7.71	0.096	0.375	0	0.667	0.415	2.28	3.03	0.002	3.9
4002	Fat, Animal, Lard, Pork	1 tbsp	12.8	115.456	0	0	0	12.8	5.018	12.16	0	0	0
18269	French Toast, homemade w/reduced fat (2%) milk	1 slice	65	148.85	5.005	16.25		7.02	1.77	75.4	65	1.085	311.35
19270	Ice Cream, Chocolate	.5 cup (4 fl oz)	66	142.56	2.508	18.612	0.792	7.26	4.488	22.44	71.94	0.614	50.16
19271	Ice Cream, Strawberry	.5 cup (4 fl oz)	66	126.72	2.112	18.216	0.594	5.544	3.425	19.14	79.2	0.139	39.6
19095	Ice Cream, Vanilla	1 tsp	4.7	33.793	0.042	0.042	0	3.783	0.705	0	1.41	0	
4067	Margarine, Hard, Corn, Soybean-Hydrogenated & Cottonseed-Hydrogenated w/salt	1 tsp	4.7	33.793	0.042	0.042	0	3.783	0.705	0	1.41	0	44.321
4611	Margarine, regular, tub, composite, 80% fat, with salt	1 tbsp	12.8	91.648	0.102	0.077	0	10.291	1.66	0	3.328	0	138.112
1110	Milk Shake, Thick, Chocolate	1 container (10.6 oz)	300	357	9.15	63.45	0.9	8.1	5.043	33	396	0.93	333

EvaluEat Code	Food Name	Amount	Wt (g)	Ener (kcal)	Prot (g)	Carb (g)	Fiber (g)	Fat (g)	Sat (g)	Chol (g)	Calc (mg)	Iron (mg)	Sodi (mg)
1111	Milk Shake, Thick, Vanilla	1 container (11 oz)	313	350.56	12.082	55.558	0	9.484	5.903	37.56	456.98	0.313	297.35
4053	Oil, Vegetable/Salad/Cooking, Olive	1 tbsp	13.5	119.34	0	0	0	13.5	1.816	0	0.135	0.089	0.405
4510	Oil, Vegetable/Salad/Cooking, Safflower, linoleic >70%	1 tbsp	13.6	120.224	0	0	0	13.6	0.844	0	0	0	0
18239	Pastry, Croissant, Butter	1 croissant, mini	28	113.68	2.296	12.824	0.728	5.88	3.265	18.76	10.36	0.568	208.32
18245	Pastry, Danish, Cheese	1 pastry	71	265.54	5.68	26.412	0.71	15.549	4.824	11.36	24.85	1.136	319.5
11942	Pickles, cucumber, fresh, (bread and butter pickles)	1 slice	7	5.39	0.063	1.253	0.105	0.014	0.004	0	2.24	0.028	47.11
18301	Pie, Apple, enriched, commercially prep	1 piece (1/8 of 9" dia)	125	296.25	2.375	42.5	2	13.75	4.746	0	13.75	0.563	332.5
18305	Pie, Blueberry, commercially prep	1 piece (1/8 of 9" dia)	125	290	2.25	43.625	1.25	12.5	2.099	0	10	0.375	406.25
18308	Pie, Cherry, commercially prep	1 piece (1/8 of 9" dia)	125	325	2.5	49.75	1	13.75	3.203	0	15	0.6	307.5
4017	Salad Dressing, 1000 Island, regular, w/salt	1 tbsp	16	59.2	0.174	2.342	0.128	5.61	0.815	4.16	2.72	0.189	138.08
4635	Salad dressing, 1000 Island dressing, fat-free	1 tbsp	14.6	19.272	0.08	4.273	0.482	0.212	0.029	0.73	1.606	0.041	106.434
4636	Salad dressing, Italian dressing, fat-free	1 tbsp	14.6	6.862	0.142	1.278	0.088	0.127	0.043	0.292	4.38	0.058	164.834
4114	Salad Dressing, Italian, regular w/salt	1 tbsp	14.7	42.777	0.056	1.533	0	4.17	0.658	0	1.029	0.093	243.138
4641	Salad dressing, mayonnaise, light	1 tbsp	14.6	47.304	0.128	1.197	0	4.831	0.761	5.11	1.168	0.047	98.258
4026	Salad Dressing, Mayonnaise, regular, Safflower/Soybean Oil, w/salt	1 tbsp	13.8	98.946	0.152	0.373	0	10.957	1.187	8.142	2.484	0.069	78.384
4012	Salad dressing, Miracle Whip Light Dressing/Kraft	1 tbsp	16	36.96	0.096	2.304	0.016	2.976	0.464	4.16	0.8	0.027	131.36
4638	Salad dressing, ranch dressing, fat-free	1 tbsp	14.6	17.374	0.036	3.87	0.015	0.28	0.075	1.022	7.3	0.153	110.23
4640	Salad dressing, ranch dressing, reduced fat	1 tbsp	14.6	32.85	0.15	2.365	0.131	2.526	0.194	3.066	18.25	0.127	136.072
4135	Salad Dressing, Vinegar & Oil, homemade	1 tbsp	16	71.84	0	0.4	0	8.016	1.456	0	0	0	0.16
6930	Sauce, cheese, ready-to-eat	.25 cup	63	109.62	4.227	4.303	0.315	8.373	3.786	18.27	115.92	0.132	521.64
6555	Sauce, hollandaise, with butterfat, dehydrated, prepared with water	1 cup (8 fl oz)	244	224.48	4.441	12.956	0.732	18.593	10.931	48.8	117.12	0.854	1473.76
6931	Sauce, Pasta, Spaghetti/Marinara	1 cup	250	142.5	3.55	20.55	4	5.15	0.737	0	55	1.8	1030
6164	Sauce, Salsa	1 cup	259	72.52	3.289	16.162	4.144	0.622	0.078	0	77.7	2.512	1124.06
4031	Shortening, Vegetable Fat, Soy hydrogenated & Cottonseed hydrogenated	1 tbsp	12.8	113.152	0	0	0	12.8	3.2	0	0	0	0
19002	Snack, Beef Jerky	1 piece, large	20	82	6.64	2.2	0.36	5.12	2.17	9.6	4	1.084	442.6
19003	Snack, Corn Chips, Plain	1 oz	28.35	152.807	1.871	16.131	1.389	9.469	1.29	0	36.005	0.374	178.605
19422	Snack, Potato Chips, light	1 oz	28.35	133.529	2.013	18.966	1.673	5.897	1.179	0	5.954	0.383	139.482
19411	Snack, Potato Chips, Plain, salted	1 oz	28.35	151.956	1.985	14.997	1.276	9.809	3.107	0	6.804	0.462	168.399

EvaluEat Code	Food Name	Amount	Wt (g)	Ener (kcal)	Prot (g)	Carb (g)	Fiber (g)	Fat (g)	Sat (g)	Chol (g)	Calc (mg)	Iron (mg)	Sodi (mg)
19047	Snack, Pretzel, Hard, Plain, salted	10 twists	60	228.6	5.46	47.52	1.92	2.1	0.45	0	21.6	2.592	1029
19056	Snack, Tortilla Chips, Plain	1 oz	28.35	142.034	1.985	17.832	1.843	7.428	1.423	0	43.659	0.431	149.688
6008	Soup, Beef Broth or Bouillon, canned	1 cup	240	16.8	2.736	0.096	0	0.528	0.264	0	14.4	0.408	782.4
6070	Soup, Beef, chunky, canned	1 cup	240	170.4	11.736	19.56	1.44	5.136	2.544	14.4	31.2	2.328	866.4
6413	Soup, Chicken Broth, canned, made w/H2O	1 cup	240	38.4	4.848	0.912	0	1.368	0.384	0	9.6	0.504	763.2
6018	Soup, Chicken Noodle, chunky, canned	1 cup	240	175.2	12.72	17.04	3.84	6	1.392	19.2	24	1.44	849.6
6468	Soup, Vegetarian Vegetable, canned, made w/H2O	1 cup	241	72.3	2.097	11.978	0.482	1.928	0.289	0	21.69	1.084	821.81
6583	Soup, ramen noodle, any flavor, dehydrated, dry	1 container, individual	64	289.92	5.952	41.92	1.536	1.667	4.883	0	10.24	76.8	
19296	Sweet, Honey, strained/extracted	1 tbsp	21	63.84	0.063	17.304	0.042	0	0	0	1.26	0.088	0.84
19283	Sweet, Ice Popsicle	1 bar (1.75 fl oz)	52	37.44	0	9.828	0	0	0	0	0	0	6.24
19297	Sweet, Jams & Preserves	1 tbsp	20	55.6	0.074	13.772	0.22	0.014	0.002	0	4	0.098	6.4
19334	Sweet, Sugar, brown	1 tsp packed	4.6	17.342	0	4.477	0	0	0	0	3.91	0.088	1.794
19335	Sweet, Sugar, granulated, white	1 tsp	4.2	16.254	0	4.199	0	0	0	0	0.042	0	0
19129	Sweet, Syrup, pancake	1 tbsp	20	46.8	0	12.294	0.14	0	0	0	0.6	0.006	16.4
1073	Whipped Dessert Topping, Nondairy, semi solid, frozen	1 tbsp	4	12.72	0.05	0.922	0	1.012	0.871	0	0.24	0.005	1
42135	Whipped topping, frozen, low fat	1 ounce	28.34	62.348	0.85	6.688	0	3.713	3.195	0.567	20.121	0.028	20.405

APPENDIX C

Nutritional Content of Fast Foods*

ARBY'S

BURGER KING

JACK IN THE BOX

KFC

MCDONALD'S

PIZZA HUT

TACO BELL

This appendix is only a list of the main menu offerings. For more menu items and evaluEat codes, see "Fast Foods" in Appendix B.

For more information on the nutritional content of these restaurants' menu items, please visit their websites.

* Source: CyberSoft, Inc. the *NutriBase Nutrition Facts Desk Reference,* 2nd ed. Avery, a member of Penguin Putnam, Inc. © 2001 by Cybersoft, Inc.

Name	Serving Size	Gram weight	Calories	Protein (g)	Carb. (g)	Total Fat (g)	Sat Fat. (g)	% Calories from Fat	Chol. (mg)	Sodium (mg)	Fiber (g)	Sugar (g)	Calcium (mg)	Iron (mg)	Vit. A (IU)	Vit. C (mg)
Arby's																
Arby's – Breakfast																
Egg, Scrambled	1.8 Oz	50	70	6	0	5	2	65.22	220	70	0	0	20	0.72	*	0
French Toastix w/o Powdered Sugar or Syrup (5 Oz)	3 Hotcakes	124	370	7	48	17	4	41.02	0	440	4	*	70	1.80	*	0
Sausage Patty	1.4 Oz	39.70	200	7	1	19	7	84.24	60	290	0	0	0	0.72	*	0
Arby's – Sides																
French Fries, Cheddar Curly	6 Oz	170	450	7.50	52	25	6	48.60	5	1420	0	*	80	2.70	*	12
French Fries, Curly, Medium	4.5 Oz	128	380	5	49	19	4.50	44.19	0	1100	0	*	0	1.80	*	12
French Fries, Homestyle, Medium	5 Oz	142	420	5	57	19	3	40.81	0	830	4	*	0	1.44	*	21
Jalapeno Bites	3.9 Oz	110	330	7	29	21	9	56.76	40	670	2	*	40	0.72	*	1.20
Mozzarella Sticks	4.8 Oz	137	470	18	34	29	14	55.65	60	1330	2	*	400		*	1.20
Onion Petals	4 Oz	113.40	410	4	43	24	3	53.47	0	300	2	*	20	0.72	*	0
Potato Cakes	2 Cakes	85.10	220	2	21	14	3	57.80	0	460	3	*	0	1.08	*	6
Potato, Baked Broccoli 'n Cheddar	13.6 Oz	384	550	14	71	25	13	39.82	50	730	7	*	250	3.96	*	63.60
Arby's – Poultry and Seafood																
Chicken Finger Meal	10.7 Oz	303	880	35	81	47	8	47.69	60	2240	0	*	0	1.80	*	9
Chicken Finger Snack	7.4 Oz	208	610	20	62	32	6	46.75	30	1610	0	*	0	1.80	*	9
Fish Fillet Sandwich	7.9 Oz	223	540	23	51	27	7	45.08	40	880	2	*	80	3.60	*	1.20
Roast Turkey Deluxe, Lowfat	6.9 Oz	196	230	19	33	5	1.50	17.79	25	870	4	*	60	2.70	*	9
Arby's – Sandwiches																
Barbecue Sandwich, Arby-Q	6.6 Oz	186	380	19	42	15	5	35.62	30	990	3	*	100	3.60	*	4.80
Chicken Bacon 'N Swiss Sandwich	7.8 Oz	222	610	37	52	30	9	43.13	75	1620	5	*	200	2.70	*	2.40
Chicken Breast Fillet Sandwich	7.6 Oz	216	560	30	49	28	6	44.37	55	1080	6	*	80	2.70	*	1.20
French Dip Sub	7.1 Oz	200	490	30	43	22	8	40.41	56	1440	3	*	120	6.30	*	1.20
Grilled Chicken Deluxe Sandwich	8.7 Oz	247	420	30	42	16	4	33.33	60	930	3	*	80	2.70	*	12
Grilled Chicken Sandwich, Lowfat	6.3 Oz	179	280	30	33	5	1.50	15.15	50	920	4	*	50	2.52	*	4.80
Italian Sub	10.3 Oz	291	800	28	49	54	16	61.21	85	2610	2	*	350	4.50	*	9

* Values Unavailable.

Name	Serving Size	Gram weight	Calories	Protein (g)	Carb. (g)	Total Fat (g)	Sat Fat. (g)	% Calories from Fat	Chol. (mg)	Sodium (mg)	Fiber (g)	Sugar (g)	Calcium (mg)	Iron (mg)	Vit. A (IU)	Vit. C (mg)
Roast Beef Sandwich, Regular	5.6 Oz	158	400	23	36	20	7	43.27	40	1030	3	*	50	4.50	*	0
Roast Chicken Club	8.4 Oz	239	540	37	39	29	8	46.19	70	1590	3	*	200	2.70	*	2.40
Roast Chicken Deluxe, Lowfat	7 Oz	196	260	23	32	5	1.50	16.98	40	950	4	*	60	2.70	*	9
Turkey Sub	10.7 Oz	303	670	29	49	39	10	52.94	60	2130	2	*	350	4.50	*	9
Arby's – Beverages and Shakes																
Milk	8 Oz	227	120	8	12	5	3	36	20	120	0	*	300	0.36	*	2.40
Orange Juice	10 Oz	283	140	1	34	0	0	0	0	0	0	*	0	0	*	78
Shake, Chocolate	10.3 Oz	292	390	8	69	9	6	20.82	10	270	0	*	250	0.90	*	*
Shake, Jamocha	10.3 Oz	292	380	8	66	9	6	21.49	10	300	0	*	250	0.90	*	*
Shake, Strawberry	10.3 Oz	292	380	8	67	9	6	21.26	10	270	0	*	250	0.90	*	*
Shake, Vanilla	10.3 Oz	292	380	8	67	9	6	21.26	12	270	0	*	250	0.90	*	0
Arby's – Salads																
Salad, Garden, w/ 1 Crouton Packet and 2 Saltine Crackers	10.2 Oz	290	110	9	16	3	0	21.26	0	150	1	*	200	0.36	*	72
Salad, Grilled Chicken, Lowfat	14.2 Oz	401	190	25	16	4	0.50	18	40	530	1	*	200	0.36	*	75
Salad, Roast Chicken, Lowfat	14.2 Oz	401	200	25	16	5	0.50	21.53	40	800	1	*	200	0.36	*	75
Arby's – Breads																
Biscuit w/Margarine	2.8 Oz	78.50	270	5	26	16	3	53.73	0	750	0	*	0	0	*	0
Croissant	2.2 Oz	62	260	6	28	16	10	51.43	20	300	0	*	0	2.70	*	0
Arby's -Dessert and Snacks																
Turnover, Iced Apple	3.4 Oz	96.10	360	4	54	14	3	35.20	0	180	6	*	0	1.44	*	1.20
Turnover, Iced Cherry	3.5 Oz	97.80	350	4	53	14	3	35.59	0	190	0	*	0	1.44	*	4.80
Burger King																
Burger King – Breakfast																
Biscuit w/Egg	1 Sandwich	132	380	11	37	21	5	49.61	140	1010	1	3	60	2.70	200	0
Biscuit w/Sausage	1 Sandwich	130	490	13	36	33	10	60.24	35	1240	1	3	40	2.70	0	0
Biscuit w/Sausage, Egg & Cheese	1 Sandwich	188	620	20	37	43	14	62.93	185	1650	1	4	150	2.70	500	0
French Toast Sticks	5 Sticks	113	440	7	51	23	5	47.15	2	490	3	12	60	1.80	0	0
Burger King – Sides																
French Fries, Medium, Salted	1 Serving	116	400	3	50	21	8	47.13	0	820	4	0	0	0.72	0	0
French Fries, Unsalted, Medium	1 Serving	116	400	3	50	21	8	47.13	0	760	4	0	0	0.72	0	0

* Values Unavailable.

Source: CyberSoft, Inc. *The NutriBase Nutrition Facts Desk Reference.* 2nd ed. Avery, a member of Penguin Putnam, Inc. © 2001 by CyberSoft

Name	Serving Size	Gram weight	Calories	Protein (g)	Carb. (g)	Total Fat (g)	Sat Fat. (g)	% Calories from Fat	Chol. (mg)	Sodium (mg)	Fiber (g)	Sugar (g)	Calcium (mg)	Iron (mg)	Vit. A (IU)	Vit. C (mg)
Hash Brown Rounds, Large	1 Serving	128	410	3	42	26	10	56.52	0	750	4	0	0	1.08	0	0
Onion Rings, Medium	1 Serving	94	380	5	46	19	4	45.60	2	550	4	4	100	0.72	0	0
Cini-Minis, w/o Vanilla Icing	4 Rolls	108	440	6	51	23	6	47.59	25	710	1	20	60	2.70	1000	1.20
Burger King – Chicken																
Chicken Tenders, 5 Piece	5 Pieces	77	230	14	11	14	4	55.75	40	590	0	0	0	0.36	0	0
Patty, BK Broiler Chicken Breast	1 Serving	99	140	21	4	4	1	26.47	90	570	*	*	*	*	*	*
Burger King – Burgers																
Cheeseburger	1 Serving	133	360	21	27	19	9	47.11	60	760	1	4	150	2.70	300	0
Cheeseburger, Bacon	1 Serving	140	400	24	27	22	10	49.25	70	940	1	4	150	2.70	300	0
Cheeseburger, Double Patty	1 Serving	198	580	38	27	36	17	55.48	120	1060	1	5	250	4.50	400	0
Cheeseburger, Double Whopper	1 Serving	374	1010	55	47	67	26	59.64	180	1460	3	8	300	7.20	750	9
Cheeseburger, Whopper	1 Serving	295	760	35	47	48	17	56.84	110	1380	3	8	250	4.50	750	9
Hamburger	1 Serving	120	320	19	27	15	6	42.32	50	520	1	4	80	2.70	100	0
Hamburger, Double Whopper	1 Serving	349	920	49	47	59	21	58.03	155	980	3	8	150	7.20	500	9
Hamburger, Whopper	1 Serving	270	660	29	47	40	12	54.22	85	900	3	8	100	4.50	500	9
Burger King – Sandwiches																
Chick 'n Crisp Sandwich	1 Sandwich	139	460	16	37	27	6	53.41	35	890	3	3	40	1.80	0	0
Chicken Sandwich	1 Sandwich	229	710	26	54	43	9	54.74	60	1400	2	4	100	3.60	0	0
Croissan'wich w/ Sausage & Cheese	1 Sandwich	106	450	13	21	35	12	69.84	45	940	1	3	100	1.80	200	0
Fish Sandwich, BK Big	1 Sandwich	252	720	23	59	43	9	54.13	80	1180	3	4	80	3.60	100	0
Burger King – Beverages and Shakes																
Chocolate Shake, Medium	1 Serving	397	440	12	75	10	6	20.55	30	330	4	67	300	2.70	400	0
Coca Cola Classic®, Medium	22 Fl Oz	660	280	0	70	0	0	0	0		0	70	0	0	0	0
Diet Coke®, Medium	22 Fl Oz	660	1	0	0	0	0	0	0		0	0	0	0	0	0
Sprite®, Medium	22 Fl Oz	682	260	0	66	0	0	0	0		0	66	0	0	0	0
Vanilla Shake, Medium	1 Medium	397	430	13	73	9	5	19.06	30	330	2	66	400	0	100	6
Burger King – Dessert																
Pie, Dutch Apple	1 Serving	113	300	3	39	15	3	44.55	0	230	2	22	0	1.44	0	6

* Values Unavailable.

Name	Serving Size	Gram weight	Calories	Protein (g)	Carb. (g)	Total Fat (g)	Sat Fat. (g)	% Calories from Fat	Chol. (mg)	Sodium (mg)	Fiber (g)	Sugar (g)	Calcium (mg)	Iron (mg)	Vit. A (IU)	Vit. C (mg)
Jack In The Box – Breakfast																
Breakfast Jack Sandwich	1 Sandwich	126	280	17	28	12	5	37.50	190	750	1	3	150	3.60	400	3.60
Breakfast Sandwich, Ultimate	1 Sandwich	243	600	34	39	34	10	51.17	400	1470	2	7	300	3.60	750	6
French Toast Sticks w/Bacon	1 Serving	131	470	12	53	23	4	44.33	30	700	2	10	100	0.72	0	0
Pancake w/Bacon	1 Serving	157	370	12	59	9	2	22.19	30	1020	3	14	80	2.70	0	0
Jack In The Box – Sides																
Egg Rolls	3 Egg Rolls	170	440	15	40	24	6	49.54	35	1020	4	5	80	4.50	750	12
French Fries, Curly Chili Cheese	1 Serving	230	650	14	60	41	12	55.49	25	1760	4	3	150	2.70	750	0
French Fries, Curly Seasoned	1 Serving	125	410	6	45	23	5	50.36	0	1010	4	0	40	1.80	300	0
French Fries, Regular	1 Serving	113	350	4	46	16	4	41.86	0	710	3	0	10	0.72	0	6
Hash Browns	1 Serving	57	170	1	14	12	2	64.29	0	250	1	0	10	0.18	0	0
Stuffed Jalapenos	7 Jalapenos	168	530	14	46	31	12	53.76	60	1730	3	5	300	1.44	1000	21
Onion Rings	1 Serving	125	410	6	45	23	5	50.36	0	1010	4	0	40	2.70	200	18
Potato, Bacon Cheddar Wedges	1 Serving	265	800	20	49	58	16	65.41	55	1470	4	2	350	1.44	500	9
Jack In The Box – Chicken and Seafood																
Chicken Breast Pieces	5 Pieces	150	360	27	24	17	3	42.86	80	970	1	0	20	1.80	200	1.20
Chicken Teriyaki Bowl	1 Serving	502	670	26	128	4	1	5.52	15	1730	3	27	100	4.50	6500	24
Fish & Chips	1 Serving	281	780	19	86	39	9	45.53	45	1740	6	2	20	2.70	100	15
Jack In The Box – Burgers																
Cheeseburger	1 Burger	115	320	14	30	16	6	45	40	720	2	5	150	3.60	300	1.20
Cheeseburger, Bacon Ultimate	1 Burger	302	1020	58	37	71	26	62.71	210	1740	1	7	300	7.20	750	0.60
Cheeseburger, Double Patty	1 Burger	165	460	24	32	27	12	52.03	80	1090	2	5	200	4.50	500	2.40
Cheeseburger, Jumbo Jack	1 Burger	282	680	31	39	45	16	59.12	115	1130	2	9	250	4.50	1000	9
Hamburger	1 Burger	103	280	12	30	12	4	39.13	30	490	2	5	100	3.60	100	1.20
Hamburger, Jumbo Jack	1 Burger	267	590	27	39	37	11	55.78	90	670	2	10	150	4.50	500	9
Hamburger, Sourdough Jack	1 Burger	233	690	34	37	45	15	58.78	105	1180	2	3	200	4.50	750	9
Jack In The Box – Sandwiches																
Chicken Fajita Pita Sandwich	1 Sandwich	187	280	24	25	9	4	29.24	75	840	3	5	150	2.70	1250	0

Source: CyberSoft, Inc. *The NutriBase Nutrition Facts Desk Reference*. 2nd ed. Avery, a member of Penguin Putnam, Inc. © 2001 by CyberSoft

Name	Serving Size	Gram weight	Calories	Protein (g)	Carb. (g)	Total Fat (g)	Sat Fat. (g)	% Calories from Fat	Chol. (mg)	Sodium (mg)	Fiber (g)	Sugar (g)	Calcium (mg)	Iron (mg)	Vit. A (IU)	Vit. C (mg)
Chicken Sandwich	1 Sandwich	184	420	16	39	23	4	48.48	40	950	2	4	100	2.70	200	4.80
Croissant, Sausage	1 Sandwich	187	700	21	38	51	20	66.04	240	1000	0	6	100	1.80	400	0.60
Grilled Chicken Fillet Sandwich	1 Sandwich	242	480	27	39	24	6	45	65	1110	4	6	200	4.50	400	9
Philly Cheesesteak Sandwich	1 Sandwich	234	580	33	56	16	8	28.80	80	1860	1	3	200	2.70	400	3.60
Jack In The Box – Deserts And Snacks																
Iced Tea, Regular	20 Fl Oz	600	0	0	0	0	0	0	0	0	0	0	0	0	0	0
Minute Maid® Lemonade, Regular,	20 Fl Oz	560	190	0	65	0	0	0	0	100	0	65	0	0	0	0
Barq's® Root Beer, Regular,	20 Fl Oz	627	180	0	50	0	0	0	0	40	0	50	0	0	0	0
Strawberry Ice Cream, Regular	16 Fl Oz	473	640	10	85	28	15	39.87	85	300	0	67	350	0	750	0
Jack In The Box – Mexican																
Taco	1 Serving	82	170	7	12	10	4	54.22	20	460	2	1	100	1.08	300	1.20
Taco, Monster	1 Serving	125	270	12	19	17	6	55.23	30	670	4	2	200	1.44	400	1.20
Jack In The Box – Salads																
Salad, Chicken Garden	1 Salad	253	200	23	8	9	4	39.51	65	420	3	4	200	0.72	3500	12
Jack In The Box – Desserts and Snacks																
Cake, Carrot	1 Serving	99	370	3	54	16	3	38.71	40	340	2	28	20	1.44	5350	0.60
Cake, Double Fudge	1 Serving	85	300	3	50	10	2	29.80	50	320	1	25	40	1.98	300	0.60
Cheesecake	1 Serving	103	320	7	32	18	10	50.94	65	220	1	22	50	0.18	700	3
Turnover, Hot Apple	1 Serving	107	340	4	41	18	4	47.37	0	510	2	12	10	1.80	100	10.20
KFC																
KFC – Sides																
Barbecue Baked Beans	5.5 Oz	156	190	6	33	3	1	14.75	5	760	6	13	80	1.80	400	**
Cole Slaw	5 Oz	142	232	2	26	13.50	2	52.03	8	284	3	20	30	**	450	34.20
Corn On The Cob	5.7 Oz	162	150	5	35	1.50	0	7.78	0	20	2	8	**	**	100	3.60
Macaroni & Cheese	5.4 Oz	153	180	7	21	8	3	39.13	10	860	2	2	150	**	1000	**
Potato Salad	5.6 Oz	160	230	4	23	14	2	53.85	15	540	3	9	20	2.70	500	**
Potato Wedges	4.8 Oz	135	280	5	28	13	4	46.99	5	750	5	1	20	1.80	**	1.20
Potato, Mashed w/Gravy	4.8 Oz	136	120	1	17	6	1	42.86	1	440	2	0	**	0.36	**	**
KFC – Chicken																
Chicken Wing, Honey Barbecue	6 Pieces	189	607	33	33	38	10	56.44	193	1145	1	18	40	1.44	400	4.80
Chicken Wing, Hot	6 Pieces	135	471	27	18	33	8	62.26	150	1230	2	0	40	1.44	**	**
Chicken, Breast, Extra Crispy	1 Breast	168	470	39	17	28	8	52.94	160	874	1	0	20	1.08	**	**

** Contains less than 2 % of the Daily Value of these nutrients.

Name	Serving Size	Gram weight	Calories	Protein (g)	Carb. (g)	Total Fat (g)	Sat Fat. (g)	% Calories from Fat	Chol. (mg)	Sodium (mg)	Fiber (g)	Sugar (g)	Calcium (mg)	Iron (mg)	Vit. A (IU)	Vit. C (mg)
Chicken, Breast, Original Recipe	1 Breast	153	400	29	16	24	6	54.55	135	1116	1	0	40	1.08	**	**
Chicken, Drumstick, Extra Crispy	1 Drumstick	67	195	15	7	12	3	55.10	77	375	1	0	**	0.72	**	**
Chicken, Drumstick, Original Recipe	1 Drumstick	61	140	13	4	9	2	54.36	75	422	0	0	**	0.72	**	**
Chicken, Popcorn, Larger	6.0 Oz	170	620	30	36	40	10	57.69	73	1046	0	0	20	0.72	0	0
Chicken, Thigh, Extra Crispy	1 Thigh	118	380	21	14	27	7	63.45	118	625	1	0	20	1.08	**	**
Chicken, Thigh, Original Recipe	1 Thigh	91	250	16	6	18	4.50	64.80	95	747	1	0	20	0.72	**	**
Chicken, Whole Wing, Extra Crispy	1 Wing	55	220	10	10	15	4	62.79	55	415	1	0	**	0.36	**	**
Chicken, Whole Wing, Original	1 Wing	47	140	9	5	10	2.50	61.64	55	414	0	0	**	0.36	**	**
Crispy Chicken Strips	3 Strips	115	300	26	18	16	4	45	56	1165	1	1	**	1.08	100	**
Pot Pie, Chunky Chicken	13 Oz	368	770	29	69	42	13	49.09	70	2160	5	8	100	1.80	4000	1.20

KFC – Sandwiches

Name	Serving Size	Gram weight	Calories	Protein (g)	Carb. (g)	Total Fat (g)	Sat Fat. (g)	% Calories from Fat	Chol. (mg)	Sodium (mg)	Fiber (g)	Sugar (g)	Calcium (mg)	Iron (mg)	Vit. A (IU)	Vit. C (mg)
Chicken Sandwich, Tender Roast w/o Sauce	1 Sandwich	177	270	31	26	5	1.50	16.48	65	690	1	1	40	1.80	**	**
Chicken Sandwich, Triple Crunch w/o Sauce	1 Sandwich	176	390	25	39	15	4.50	34.53	50	650	2	0	40	2.70	**	**

KFC – Bread

Name	Serving Size	Gram weight	Calories	Protein (g)	Carb. (g)	Total Fat (g)	Sat Fat. (g)	% Calories from Fat	Chol. (mg)	Sodium (mg)	Fiber (g)	Sugar (g)	Calcium (mg)	Iron (mg)	Vit. A (IU)	Vit. C (mg)
Biscuit	1 Biscuit	56	180	4	20	10	2.50	48.39	0	560	0	2	20	1.08	**	**

KFC – Desserts and Snacks

Name	Serving Size	Gram weight	Calories	Protein (g)	Carb. (g)	Total Fat (g)	Sat Fat. (g)	% Calories from Fat	Chol. (mg)	Sodium (mg)	Fiber (g)	Sugar (g)	Calcium (mg)	Iron (mg)	Vit. A (IU)	Vit. C (mg)
Cake, Double Chocolate Chip	1 Serving	76	320	4	41	16	4	44.44	55	230	1	28	40	1.80	0	0
Little Bucket Parfait, Chocolate Creme	1 Serving	113	290	3	37	15	11	45.76	15	330	2	25	40	1.08	**	0
Little Bucket Parfait, Fudge Brownie	1 Serving	99	280	3	44	10	3.50	32.37	145	190	1	35	20	1.08	100	0
Little Bucket Parfait, Lemon Creme	1 Serving	127	410	7	62	14	8	31.34	20	290	4	50	200	0.72	100	2.40
Pie, Apple	1 Slice	113	310	2	44	14	3	40.65	0	280	0	23	0	1.08	0	0
Pie, Pecan	1 Slice	113	490	5	66	23	5	42.16	65	510	2	31	20	1.44	200	0
Pie, Strawberry Creme	1 Slice	78	280	4	32	15	8	48.39	15	130	2	22	0	0.72	100	2.40

** Contains less than 2% of the Daily Value of these nutrients.

Source: CyberSoft, Inc. *The NutriBase Nutrition Facts Desk Reference*. 2nd ed. Avery, a member of Penguin Putnam, Inc. © 2001 by CyberSoft

McDonald's

McDonald's – Breakfast

Name	Serving Size	Gram weight	Calories	Protein (g)	Carb. (g)	Total Fat (g)	Sat Fat. (g)	% Calories from Fat	Chol. (mg)	Sodium (mg)	Fiber (g)	Sugar (g)	Calcium (mg)	Iron (mg)	Vit. A (IU)	Vit. C (mg)
Biscuit, Bacon Egg & Cheese	1 Sandwich	168	540	21	36	34	10	57.30	250	1550	1	4	200	2.70	500	*
Biscuit, Sausage w/Egg	1 Sandwich	178	550	18	35	37	10	61.10	245	1160	1	3	100	2.70	300	*
Burrito, Breakfast	1 Serving	117	320	13	21	20	7	56.96	195	660	1	2	150	1.80	500	9
Egg McMuffin	1 Sandwich	136	290	17	27	12	4.50	38.03	235	790	1	3	200	2.70	500	1.20
Hotcakes w/ Margarine & Syrup	1 Serving	228	600	9	104	17	3	25.29	20	770	3	40	100	4.50	400	*
Hotcakes, Plain	1 Serving	156	340	9	58	8	1.50	21.18	20	630	3	9	100	4.50	*	*
Hash Browns	1 Serving	53	130	1	14	8	1.50	54.55	0	330	1	0		0.36	*	2.40
Sausage w/Egg McMuffin®	1 Sandwich	162	440	19	27	28	10	57.80	255	890	1	3	250	2.70	500	*
Spanish Omelette Bagel	1 Sandwich	258	690	27	59	38	14	49.85	275	1560	10	10	250	4.50	750	15
Ham, Egg & Cheese Bagel	1 Sandwich	218	550	26	58	23	8	38.12	255	1490	9	10	200	4.50	750	*
Steak, Egg & Cheese Bagel	1 Sandwich	245	660	36	57	31	11	42.86	285	1300	9	9	200	5.40	750	*

McDonald's – Chicken

Name	Serving Size	Gram weight	Calories	Protein (g)	Carb. (g)	Total Fat (g)	Sat Fat. (g)	% Calories from Fat	Chol. (mg)	Sodium (mg)	Fiber (g)	Sugar (g)	Calcium (mg)	Iron (mg)	Vit. A (IU)	Vit. C (mg)
Chicken McNuggets®	6 Piece	108	290	15	20	17	3.50	52.22	55	540	2	0	20	0.72	*	*

McDonald's – Sandwiches

Name	Serving Size	Gram weight	Calories	Protein (g)	Carb. (g)	Total Fat (g)	Sat Fat. (g)	% Calories from Fat	Chol. (mg)	Sodium (mg)	Fiber (g)	Sugar (g)	Calcium (mg)	Iron (mg)	Vit. A (IU)	Vit. C (mg)
Crispy Chicken Sandwich	1 Sandwich	234	550	23	54	27	4.50	44.10	50	1180	2	7	200	3.60	300	6
Filet-O-Fish Sandwich	1 Sandwich	156	470	15	45	26	5	49.37	50	890	1	5	200	1.80	200	*

McDonald's – Beverages And Shakes

Name	Serving Size	Gram weight	Calories	Protein (g)	Carb. (g)	Total Fat (g)	Sat Fat. (g)	% Calories from Fat	Chol. (mg)	Sodium (mg)	Fiber (g)	Sugar (g)	Calcium (mg)	Iron (mg)	Vit. A (IU)	Vit. C (mg)
McFlurry, Oreo®	1 Serving	337	570	15	82	20	12	31.69	70	280	0	69	450	1.08	1250	2.40
Milkshake, Chocolate, Large	22 Fl Oz	458	582	15.57	93.89	16.95	10.59	25.64	59.54	444	3.66	81	518	1.42	425.94	1.83
Milkshake, Vanilla, Large	22 Fl Oz	458	508	16.03	81.98	13.74	8.51	23.78	50.38	375	1.83	80	558	0.41	595.40	3.66

McDonald's – Burgers

Name	Serving Size	Gram weight	Calories	Protein (g)	Carb. (g)	Total Fat (g)	Sat Fat. (g)	% Calories from Fat	Chol. (mg)	Sodium (mg)	Fiber (g)	Sugar (g)	Calcium (mg)	Iron (mg)	Vit. A (IU)	Vit. C (mg)
Cheeseburger	1 Burger	121	320	16	35	13	6	36.45	40	830	2	7	250	2.70	300	2.40
Cheeseburger, Quarter Pounder	1 Burger	200	530	28	38	30	13	50.56	95	1310	2	9	350	4.50	500	2.40
Hamburger	1 Burger	107	270	13	35	8	3.50	27.27	30	600	2	7	200	2.70	500	2.40
Hamburger, Big Mac	1 Burger	216	570	26	45	32	10	50.35	85	1100	3	8	250	4.50	300	3.60
Hamburger, Quarter Pounder	1 Burger	172	430	23	37	21	8	44.06	70	840	2	8	200	4.50	100	2.40
French Fries, Medium	1 Serving	147	450	6	57	22	4	44	0	290	5	0	20	1.08	*	18

* Values Unavailable.

Name	Serving Size	Gram weight	Calories	Protein (g)	Carb. (g)	Total Fat (g)	Sat Fat. (g)	% Calories from Fat	Chol. (mg)	Sodium (mg)	Fiber (g)	Sugar (g)	Calcium (mg)	Iron (mg)	Vit. A (IU)	Vit. C (mg)
McDonald's – Salads																
Salad, Shaker, Chef	1 Salad	206	150	17	5	8	3.50	45	95	740	2	2	150	1.44	1500	15
Salad, Shaker, Garden	1 Salad	149	100	7	4	6	3	55.10	75	120	2	1	150	1.08	1500	15
Salad, Shaker, Grilled Chicken Caesar	1 Salad	163	100	17	3	2.50	1.50	21.95	40	240	2	1	100	1.08	1250	12
McDonald's – Desserts And Snacks																
Cinnamon Roll	1 Serving	95	390	6	50	18	5	41.97	65	310	2	24	60	1.44	400	*
Cookie, Chocolate Chip	1 Serving	35	170	2	22	10	6	48.39	20	120	1	13	20	1.08	200	*
Danish, Cheese	1 Serving	105	400	7	45	21	5	47.61	40	400	2	16	80	1.44	300	*
Ice Cream Cone, Vanilla, Lower Fat	1 Serving	90	150	4	23	4.50	3	27.27	20	75	0	17	100	0.36	300	1.20
Pie, Baked Apple	1 Serving	77	260	3	34	13	3.50	44.15	0	200	0	13	20	1.08	*	24
Sundae, Hot Fudge	1 Serving	179	340	8	52	12	9	31.03	30	170	1	47	250	0.72	500	1.20
Sundae, Strawberry	1 Serving	178	290	7	50	7	5	21.65	30	95	0	46	200	0.36	500	1.20
Pizza Hut																
Pizza Hut – Pasta																
Cavatini Pasta	1 Serving	357	480	21	66	14	6	26.58	8	1170	9	12	150	3.60	1250	*
Cavatini Supreme Pasta	1 Serving	396	560	24	73	19	8	30.59	10	1400	10	11	150	4.50	1500	*
Spaghetti w/ Marinara Sauce	1 Serving	473	490	18	91	6	1	11.02	0	730	8	10	150	3.60	1000	*
Spaghetti w/ Meat Sauce	1 Serving	467	600	23	98	13	5	19.47	8	910	9	10	100	3.60	1750	*
Pizza Hut – Pizza																
Cheese, Hand Tossed, Med.	1 Slice	103	309	14	43	9	4.80	26.21	11	848	3.40	8	190	1.26	450	2.40
Cheese, Pan, Med.	1 Slice	111	361	13	44	15	5.70	37.19	11	678	3.30	1	200	2.52	500	2.40
Cheese, Thin & Crispy, Med.	1 Slice	79	243	11	27	10	4.90	37.19	11	653	2.40	1	190	1.26	450	2.40
Chicken Supreme, Hand Tossed, Med.	1 Slice	116	291	15	44	6	3	18.62	17	841	3.50	9	120	1.26	400	6
Chicken Supreme, Pan, Med.	1 Slice	125	343	15	45	12	3.90	31.03	16	671	3.40	2	150	2.70	400	6
Chicken Supreme, Thin & Crispy, Med.	1 Slice	102	232	13	29	7	3.20	27.27	19	681	2.50	2	120	1.44	400	7.20
Meat Lover's, Thin & Crispy, Med.	1 Slice	107	339	15	28	19	7.80	49.85	35	970	2.60	1	140	1.80	450	2.40
Meat Lover's, Hand Tossed, Med.	1 Slice	121	376	17	44	15	6.40	35.62	30	1077	3.60	8	140	1.62	400	2.40

* Values Unavailable.

Source: CyberSoft, Inc. *The NutriBase Nutrition Facts Desk Reference.* 2nd ed. Avery, a member of Penguin Putnam, Inc. © 2001 by CyberSoft

Name	Serving Size	Gram weight	Calories	Protein (g)	Carb. (g)	Total Fat (g)	Sat Fat. (g)	% Calories from Fat	Chol. (mg)	Sodium (mg)	Fiber (g)	Sugar (g)	Calcium (mg)	Iron (mg)	Vit. A (IU)	Vit. C (mg)
Meat Lover's, Pan, Med.	1 Slice	129	428	16	45	21	7.30	43.65	29	607	3.40	1	140	2.88	450	2.40
Pepperoni, Hand Tossed, Med.	1 Slice	100	301	13	43	8	4	24.32	15	867	3.20	8	120	1.26	350	2.40
Pepperoni, Pan, Med.	1 Slice	106	353	12	44	14	4.80	36	14	697	3.10	1	130	2.52	350	2.40
Pepperoni, Thin & Crispy, Med.	1 Slice	74	235	10	27	10	4.10	37.82	14	672	2.10	1	120	1.26	350	2.40
Supreme, Hand Tossed, Med.	1 Slice	123	333	15	44	11	4.90	29.55	18	927	3.70	9	130	1.62	400	6
Supreme, Pan, Med.	1 Slice	130	385	14	45	17	5.70	39.33	18	757	3.60	1	140	2.88	400	6
Supreme Pizza, Thin & Crispy, Med.	1 Slice	110	284	13	29	13	5.50	41.05	20	784	2.80	2	130	1.62	400	16.80
Veggie Lover's, Hand Tossed, Med.	1 Slice	120	281	12	45	6	3	19.15	7	771	3.80	9	130	1.44	450	9.60
Veggie Lover's, Pan, Med.	1 Slice	125	333	11	46	12	3.90	32.14	7	601	3.60	2	130	2.88	450	9.60
Pizza Hut – Desserts and Snacks																
Apple Dessert Pizza	1 Slice	81	250	3	48	4.50	1	16.56	0	230	2	25	*	1.08	*	*
Cherry Dessert Pizza	1 Slice	81	250	3	47	4.50	1	16.84	0	220	3	24	*	1.44	450	*
Pizza Hut – Bread																
Bread Stick	1 Serving	38	130	3	20	4	1	28.13	0	170	1	1	*	1.08	*	*
Bread, Garlic	1 Slice	37	150	3	16	8	1.50	48.65	0	240	1	1	40	1.44	500	*
Taco Bell																
Taco Bell – Mexican																
Bean Burrito, 7 Oz	1 Burrito	198	370	13	54	12	3.50	28.72	10	1080	12	3	150	2.70	2250	0
Burrito Supreme, Beef, 8.75 Oz	1 Burrito	248	430	17	50	18	7	37.67	40	1210	9	4	150	2.70	2500	4.80
Burrito Supreme, Chicken, 8.75 Oz	1 Burrito	248	410	20	49	16	6	34.29	45	1120	8	4	150	1.80	2250	4.80
Burrito Supreme, Steak, 8.75 Oz	1 Burrito	248	420	21	48	16	6	34.29	35	1140	8	4	150	2.70	2250	3.60
Chalupa Supreme, Beef, 5.5 Oz	1 Chalupa	156	380	14	29	23	8	54.62	40	580	3	3	150	1.80	300	4.80
Chalupa Supreme, Chicken, 5.5 Oz	1 Chalupa	156	360	17	28	20	7	50	45	490	2	3	100	1.80	200	4.80
Chalupa Supreme, Steak, 5.5 Oz	1 Chalupa	156	360	17	27	20	7	50.56	35	500	2	3	150	2.70	100	3.60
Enchirito, Beef, 7.5 Oz	1 Enchirito	213	370	18	33	19	9	45.60	50	1300	9	2	300	1.80	5000	1.20
Enchirito, Chicken, 7.5 Oz	1 Enchirito	213	350	21	32	16	8	40.45	55	1210	7	2	250	1.80	5000	1.20

* Values Unavailable.

Name	Serving Size	Gram weight	Calories	Protein (g)	Carb. (g)	Total Fat (g)	Sat Fat. (g)	% Calories from Fat	Chol. (mg)	Sodium (mg)	Fiber (g)	Sugar (g)	Calcium (mg)	Iron (mg)	Vit. A (IU)	Vit. C (mg)
Enchirito, Steak, 7.5 Oz	1 Enchirito	213	350	22	31	16	8	40.45	45	1220	7	2	250	2.70	4500	0
Gordita Supreme, Beef, 5.5 Oz	1 Gordita	156	300	17	27	14	5	41.72	35	550	3	4	150	1.80	100	3.60
Gordita Supreme, Chicken, 5.5 Oz	1 Gordita	156	300	16	28	13	5	39.93	45	530	3	4	150	1.44	200	3.60
Gordita Supreme, Steak, 5.5 Oz	1 Gordita	156	300	17	27	14	5	41.72	35	550	3	4	150	1.80	100	3.60
Grilled Stuft Burrito, Beef, 10.3 Oz	1 Burrito	292	730	27	75	35	11	43.57	65	2090	11	4	350	5.40	1500	9
Grilled Stuft Burrito, Chicken, 10.3 Oz	1 Burrito	292	690	33	73	29	8	38.10	70	1900	8	4	300	5.40	1250	9
Grilled Stuft Burrito, Steak, 10.4 Oz	1 Burrito	295	690	30	72	30	8	39.82	60	1970	8	4	300	6.30	1250	6
Mexican Pizza, 6.75 Oz	1 Pizza	191	390	18	28	25	8	55.01	45	930	8	2	250	2.70	1750	6
Mexican Rice, 4.75 Oz	1 Order	135	190	5	23	9	3.50	41.97	15	750	1	1	150	1.44	5000	1.20
Nachos, 3.5 Oz	1 Order	99	320	5	34	18	4	50.94	5	560	3	2	100	0.72	300	0
Nachos Bellgrande, 11 Oz	1 Order	312	760	20	83	39	11	46	35	1300	17	4	200	3.60	500	4.80
Nachos Mucho Grande, 18 Oz	1 Order	510	1320	31	116	82	25	55.66	75	2670	18	6	250	5.40	1000	12
Nachos Supreme, 7 Oz	1 Order	198	440	14	44	24	7	48.21	35	800	9	3	150	2.70	0	3.60
Pintos 'n Cheese, 4.5 Oz	1 Order	128	180	9	18	8	4	40	15	640	10	1	150	1.80	2250	0
Quesadilla, Cheese, 4.25 Oz	1 Quesadilla	170	350	16	31	18	9	46.29	50	860	3	2	350	0.72	400	0
Quesadilla, Chicken, 6 Oz	1 Quesadilla	170	400	25	33	19	9	42.43	75	1050	3	2	350	0.72	500	1.20
Seven-Layer Burrito, 10 Oz	1 Burrito	283	520	16	65	22	7	37.93	25	1270	13	4	200	3.60	1500	6
Soft Taco Supreme, Beef, 5 Oz	1 Taco	142	260	11	22	13	6	46.99	40	590	3	3	100	1.08	400	3.60
Soft Taco Supreme, Chicken, 4.75 Oz	1 Taco	135	240	14	21	11	5	41.42	45	490	2	3	100	0.72	300	3.60
Soft Taco Supreme, Steak, 4.75 Oz	1 Taco	135	240	15	20	11	5	41.42	35	510	2	2	100	1.08	200	3.60
Soft Taco, Beef, 3.5 Oz	1 Taco	99	210	11	20	10	4	42.06	30	570	3	1	80	1.08	400	0
Soft Taco, Chicken, 3.5 Oz	1 Taco	99	190	13	19	7	2.50	32.98	35	480	2	1	80	0.72	200	1.20

Source: CyberSoft, Inc. *The NutriBase Nutrition Facts Desk Reference.* 2nd ed. Avery, a member of Penguin Putnam, Inc. © 2001 by CyberSoft

Name	Serving Size	Gram weight	Calories	Protein (g)	Carb. (g)	Total Fat (g)	Sat Fat. (g)	% Calories from Fat	Chol. (mg)	Sodium (mg)	Fiber (g)	Sugar (g)	Calcium (mg)	Iron (mg)	Vit. A (IU)	Vit. C (mg)
Soft Taco, Steak, 3.5 Oz	1 Taco	99	190	14	18	7	3	32.98	25	490	1	1	100	1.08	200	0
Double Decker Taco, 7 Oz	1 Taco	198	330	14	37	15	5	39.82	30	740	9	2	100	1.80	400	0
Double Decker Taco Supreme, 7 Oz	1 Taco	200	380	15	39	18	7	42.86	40	760	9	3	150	1.80	400	3.60
Taco Supreme, 4 Oz	1 Taco	113	210	9	14	14	6	57.80	40	350	3	2	100	1.08	400	3.60
Taco Salad w/Salsa, 19 Oz	1 Salad	539	850	30	69	52	14	54.17	70	2250	16	12	300	6.30	1450	30
Taco, 2.75 Oz	1 Taco	78	170	9	12	10	4	51.72	30	330	3	1	80	0.72	400	0
Tostada, 6.25 Oz	1 Tostada	177	250	10	27	12	4.50	42.19	15	640	11	2	150	1.80	2500	1.20
Taco Bell – Dessert and Snacks																
Cinnamon Twists, 1.25 Oz	1 Order	35	150	1	27	4.50	1	26.56	0	190	1	13	0	0.36	0	0

Source: CyberSoft, Inc. *The NutriBase Nutrition Facts Desk Reference*. 2nd ed. Avery, a member of Penguin Putnam, Inc. © 2001 by CyberSoft

GLOSSARY

accident Sequence of events producing unintended injury, death, or property damage; refers to the event and not the consequences of the event.

acclimatize Refers to the physiological adaptations that occur to assist the body in adjusting to environmental extremes. Exercise in a hot or even moderately hot environment will cause the body to adapt to these conditions.

acute muscle soreness This condition may develop during or immediately following an exercise bout that has been too long or too intense. Acute muscle soreness is likely caused by alterations in the chemical balance within muscle, increased fluid accumulation in muscle, or injury to muscle tissue.

addiction A compulsive psychological need for a drug or behavior.

adenosine triphosphate (ATP) A high-energy compound that is synthesized and stored in small quantities in muscle and other cells. The breakdown of ATP results in a release of energy that can be used to fuel muscular contraction. ATP is the only compound in the body that can provide this immediate source of energy.

aerobic Means "with oxygen"; as pertains to energy-producing biochemical pathways in cells that use oxygen to produce energy.

aerobics A common term to describe all forms of low-intensity exercise designed to improve cardiorespiratory fitness (e.g., jogging, walking, cycling, and swimming). Because aerobic exercise has proved effective in promoting weight loss and reducing the risk of cardiovascular disease, many exercise scientists consider cardiorespiratory fitness to be one of the most important components of health-related physical fitness.

AIDS A fatal disease that develops from infection by the human immunodeficiency virus, or HIV.

amino acids The basic structural unit of proteins. Twenty different amino acids exist and can be linked end to end in various combinations to create different proteins with unique functions.

anabolic steroids Hormones produced by the body that enhance muscle growth. Usually refers to the synthetic form of the hormone testosterone.

anaerobic threshold The work intensity during graded, incremental exercise at which there is a rapid accumulation of blood lactic acid. This usually occurs at 50% to 60% of $\dot{V}O_2$ and contributes to muscle fatigue.

anaerobic Means "without oxygen"; as pertains to energy-producing biochemical pathways in cells that do not require oxygen to produce energy.

anorexia nervosa A common eating disorder that is unrelated to any specific physical disease. The end result of extreme anorexia nervosa is a state of starvation in which the individual becomes emaciated due to a refusal to eat.

antagonist The muscle on the opposite side of the joint.

antioxidants Substances that remove free radicals (also called oxygen radicals) from cells and thus prevent DNA damage. Although free radicals are constantly produced by the body, excess production of these compounds has been implicated in cancer, lung disease, heart disease, and even the aging process.

arteries The blood vessels that transport blood away from the heart.

arteriosclerosis A group of diseases characterized by a narrowing or "hardening" of the arteries. The end result of any form of arteriosclerosis is that blood flow to vital organs may be impaired due to a progressive blockage of the artery.

arthroscopic surgery A common type of surgery that can repair joint injuries without causing undue trauma to the joint.

asthma A disease that reduces the size of airways leading to the lungs and can result in a sudden difficulty in breathing. It is promoted by a number of factors, such as air pollution, pollen, and exercise.

atherosclerosis A special type of arteriosclerosis that results in arterial blockage due to collection of a fatty deposit (called *atherosclerotic plaque*) inside the blood vessel.

behavior modification A technique used in psychological therapy to promote desirable changes in behavior.

body composition The relative amounts of fat and lean body tissue (muscle, organs, bone) found in the body.

body mass index (BMI) A useful technique for categorizing people with respect to their degree of body fat. The body mass index is simply the ratio of the body weight (kilograms; kg) divided by the height squared (meters^2).

Borg rating of perceived exertion A subjective way of estimating exercise intensity based on a numerical scale of 6–20.

breathing exercises A simple means of achieving relaxation.

bulimia An eating disorder that involves overeating (called *binge eating*) followed by vomiting (called *purging*).

caffeine A stimulant found in a wide variety of common foods such as coffee, tea, and chocolate.

calorie The unit of measure used to quantify food energy or the energy expended by the body. Technically, a calorie is the amount of energy necessary to raise the temperature of 1 gram of water 1°C.

cancer A class of over 100 different diseases that can influence almost every body tissue. Cancer is caused by the uncontrolled growth and spread of abnormal cells.

capillaries Thin-walled vessels that permit the exchange of gases (oxygen and carbon dioxide) and nutrients to occur between the blood and tissues.

carbohydrates One of the macronutrients that is especially important during many types of physical activity because they are a key energy source for muscular contraction. Dietary sources of carbohydrates are breads, cereals, fruits, and vegetables.

carbon monoxide A gas produced during the burning of fossil fuels such as gasoline and coal; also contained in cigarette smoke. This pollutant binds to hemoglobin in the blood and reduces the blood's oxygen carrying capacity.

carcinogens Cancer-causing agents, which include radiation, chemicals, drugs, and other toxic substances.

cardiac output The amount of blood the heart pumps per minute.

cardiovascular disease Any disease that affects the heart or blood vessels.

cartilage A tough, connective tissue that forms a pad on the end of bones in certain joints, such as the elbow, knee, and ankle. Cartilage act as a shock absorber to cushion the weight of one bone on another and to provide protection from the friction due to joint movement.

cellulite The "lumpy" hard fat that often gives skin a dimpled look. Cellulite is just plain fat and not a special category of fat.

chancre A sore that appears at the site of infection in stage one syphilis.

chemical dependency A term for drug addiction.

chlamydia The most common sexually transmitted disease among heterosexuals in the United States. The disease is caused by a bacterial infection within the reproductive organs and is spread through vaginal, anal, and oral sex.

cholesterol A type of derived fat in the body that is necessary for cell and hormone synthesis. Can be acquired through the diet or can be made by the body.

chondromalacia Sometimes called "runner's knee"; it is a common exercise-induced injury that is manifest as pain behind the knee cap. In sports injury clinic, chondromalacia may account for almost 10% of all visits, or 20% to 40% of all knee problems.

cocaine Cocaine is a powerful stimulant derived from the leaves of the South American coca shrub, which grows primarily in the Andes mountains. Cocaine is extracted from the coca leaves using a multistep process to produce a white powder.

complete proteins Contain all the essential amino acids and are found only in foods of animal origin (meats and dairy products).

complex carbohydrates A term that refers to carbohydrates that provide both micronutrients and the glucose necessary for producing energy. They are contained in starches and fiber.

concentric contractions Isotonic muscle contractions that result in muscle shortening.

concepts The primary elements or major components of a theory.

construct A concept that has been developed or adopted for use within a specific theory.

contributory risk factors Also called secondary risk factors. Factors that increase the risk of CHD, but their direct contribution to the disease process has not been precisely determined.

convection Heat loss by the movement of air (or water) around the body.

cool-down The cool-down (sometimes called a *warm-down*) is a 5- to 15-min period of low-intensity exercise that immediately follows the primary conditioning period.

coronary artery disease See *coronary heart disease*.

coronary heart disease (CHD) Also called *coronary artery disease*. CHD is the result of atherosclerotic plaque forming a blockage of one or more coronary arteries (the blood vessels supplying the heart).

cortisol A hormone secreted by the outer layer (cortex) of the adrenal gland.

creeping obesity A slow increase in body fat collected over a period of several years.

cross training The use of a variety of activity modes for training the cardiorespiratory system.

cryokinetics A relatively new rehabilitation technique that is implemented after the acute injury and healing period have been completed. It incorporates varying periods of treatment using ice, rest, and exercise.

curl-up test A field test to evaluate abdominal muscle endurance.

cycle ergometer fitness test A submaximal exercise test designed to evaluate cardiorespiratory fitness.

delayed-onset muscle soreness (DOMS) This condition develops within 24 to 48 hours after a bout of exercise that is excessive in duration or intensity. It is common following new or unique physical activities that use muscle groups unaccustomed to exercise.

derived fats A class of fats that does not contain fatty acids but are classified as fat because they are not soluble in water.

diabetes A metabolic disorder characterized by high blood glucose levels. Chronic elevation of blood glucose is associated with increased incidence of heart disease, kidney disease, nerve dysfunction, and eye damage.

diastolic blood pressure The pressure of the blood in the arteries at the level of the heart during the resting phase of the heart (diastole).

duration of exercise The amount of time invested in performing the primary workout.

dynamic Means "movement"; in reference to muscle contractions, dynamic is synonymous with isotonic contraction.

eccentric contractions Isotonic contractions in which the muscle exerts force while the muscle lengthens (also called *negative contractions*).

epinephrine A hormone secreted by the inner core (medulla) of the adrenal gland; also called adrenaline.

ergogenic aid A drug or nutritional product that improves physical fitness and exercise performance.

essential amino acids Amino acids that cannot be manufactured by the body and, therefore, must be consumed in the diet.

eustress A stress level that results in improved performance.

evaporation The conversion of water (or sweat) to a gas (water vapor). The most important means of removing heat from the body during exercise.

exercise metabolic rate (EMR) The energy expenditure during any form of exercise.

exercise prescription The dosage of exercise that effectively promotes physical fitness. Exercise prescriptions should be tailored to meet the needs of the individual and include fitness goals, mode of exercise, a warm-up, a primary conditioning period, and a cool-down.

exercise stress test A diagnostic test designed to determine if the patient's cardiovascular system has a normal response to exercise. The test is generally performed on a treadmill while a physician monitors heart rate, blood pressure, and EKG.

fartlek training *Fartlek* is a Swedish word meaning "speed play," and it refers to a popular form of training for long-distance runners. It is much like interval training, but it is not as rigid in its work-to-rest interval ratios. It consists of "free-form" running done out on trails, roads, golf courses, and so on.

fast-twitch fibers Muscle fibers that contract rapidly but fatigue quickly. These fibers are white and have a low aerobic capacity, but they are well equipped to produce ATP anaerobically.

fat An efficient storage form for energy, because each gram of fat holds over twice the energy content of either carbohydrate or protein. Excess fat in the diet is stored in fat cells (called *adipose tissue*) located under the skin and around internal organs.

fatty acids The basic structural unit of triglycerides that are important nutritionally, not only because of their energy content, but also because they play a role in cardiovascular disease.

fiber A stringy, nondigestible carbohydrate found in whole grains, vegetables, and fruits in its primary form, cellulose.

flexibility The ability to move joints freely through their full range of motion.

frequency of exercise The number of times per week that one intends to exercise.

fructose Also called *fruit sugar*; a naturally occurring sugar found in fruits and in honey.

galactose A simple sugar found in the breast milk of humans and other mammals.

general adaptation syndrome A pattern of responses to stress that consists of an alarm stage, a resistance stage, and an exhaustion stage.

glucose The most noteworthy of the simple sugars because it is the only sugar molecule that can be used by the body in its natural form. All other carbohydrates must first be converted to glucose to be used for fuel.

glycogen The storage form of glucose in the liver and skeletal muscles.

gonorrhea A common sexually transmitted disease. The infection can be transmitted through vaginal, anal, and oral sex. Gonorrhea is caused by a bacterial infection and is curable by antibiotics.

heart attack Also called *myocardial infarction.* Stoppage of blood flow to the heart, resulting in the death of heart cells.

heart rate Number of heart beats per minute.

heat injuries Also called *heat illness.* Bodily injury that can occur when the exercise heat load exceeds the body's ability to regulate body temperature. They are serious and can result in damage to the nervous system and, in extreme cases, death.

hepatitis B A viral infection that attacks the liver. Hepatitis B can be transmitted by sexual intercourse with an infected person and at present, no cure exists for this disease.

herpes A general term for a family of diseases that are caused by viral infections. Herpes is highly contagious and can be transmitted through any form of sexual contact (e.g., hand-to-genital contact, oral sex, or intercourse).

high-density lipoproteins (HDL) A combination of protein, triglycerides, and cholesterol in the blood, composed of relatively large amounts of protein. Protects against fatty plaque accumulation in the coronary arteries of the heart that leads to heart disease. Research has shown individuals with high blood HDL-cholesterol levels have less risk of CHD. Often called "good cholesterol."

homeotherms Animals that regulate their body temperature around a constant level; that is, body temperature is regulated around a set point. Humans regulate their body temperature around the set point of 98.6°F or 37°C.

humidity The amount of water vapor in the air. If the relative humidity is high, meaning the air is relatively saturated with water, and the air temperature is high, evaporation is retarded and body heat loss is drastically decreased.

hydrostatic weighing A method of determining body composition that involves weighing the individual both on land and in a tank of water.

hyperplasia An increase in the number of muscle fibers.

hypertension (high blood pressure) Usually considered to be a blood pressure of greater than 140 for systolic or 100 for diastolic.

hypertrophy An increase in muscle fiber size.

incomplete proteins Proteins that are missing one or more of the essential amino acids; can be found in numerous vegetable sources.

intensity of exercise The amount of physiological stress or overload placed on the body during exercise.

intermediate fibers Muscle fibers that possess a combination of the characteristics of fast- and slow-twitch fibers. They contract rapidly and are fatigue resistant due to a well-developed aerobic capacity.

interval training Repeated bouts or intervals of relatively intense exercise. The duration of the intervals can be varied, but a 1- to 5-minute duration is common. Each interval is followed by a rest period, which should be equal to or slightly greater than the interval duration.

isocaloric balance Food energy intake that equals energy expenditure.

isokinetic contractions A muscle contraction that is a subtype of isotonic contraction; isokinetic contractions are concentric or eccentric isotonic contractions performed at a constant speed.

isometric Refers to muscle contractions in which muscular tension is developed but no movement of body parts takes place.

isotonic Refers to muscle contractions in which there is movement of a body part. Most exercise or sports skills use isotonic contractions.

lactic acid A by-product of glucose metabolism. Produced primarily during intense exercise (i.e., greater than 50%–60% of maximal aerobic capacity.). Results in inhibition of muscle contraction and, therefore, fatigue.

lactose A simple sugar found in milk products; it is composed of galactose and glucose.

layering Dressing for exercise in the cold by using layers of clothes to trap air.

ligaments Connective tissue within the joint capsule that holds bones together.

lipoproteins Combinations of protein, triglycerides, and cholesterol in the blood that are important because of their role in promoting heart disease.

long, slow distance training The term used to indicate continuous exercise that requires a steady, submaximal exercise intensity (i.e., the intensity is generally around 70% HRmax).

low-density lipoproteins (LDL) A combination of protein, triglycerides, and cholesterol in the blood, composed of relatively large amounts of cholesterol. Promotes the fatty plaque accumulation in the coronary arteries of the heart that leads to heart disease. The association between elevated total blood cholesterol and the increased risk of CHD is due primarily to LDL cholesterol. Research has shown that individuals with high blood LDL cholesterol levels have an increased risk of CHD. Because of this relationship, LDL cholesterol has been labeled "bad cholesterol."

macronutrients Carbohydrates, fats, and proteins, which are necessary for building and maintaining body tissues and providing energy for daily activities.

major risk factors Also called *primary risk factors.* Risk factors considered to be directly related to the development of CHD and stroke.

maltose A simple sugar found in grain products; it is composed of two glucose molecules linked together.

marijuana A plant mixture (stems, leaves, or seeds) from either the *Cannabis sativa* or *Cannabis indica* (hemp) plants. The active chemical in marijuana that produces physical effects is tetrahydrocannabinol (THC); the higher the THC concentration in marijuana, the greater the effect.

meditation A method of relaxation that has been practiced for ages in an effort to produce relaxation and achieve inner peace. There are many types of meditation, and there is no scientific evidence that one form is superior to another.

micronutrients Nutrients in food, such as vitamins and minerals, that regulate the functions of the cells.

minerals Chemical elements (e.g., sodium and calcium) that are required by the body for normal functioning.

mode of exercise The specific type of exercise to be performed. For example, to improve cardiorespiratory fitness, one could select from a wide variety of exercise modes, including running, swimming, or cycling.

model A subclass of theory.

motor unit A motor nerve and each of the muscle fibers that it innervates.

muscular endurance The ability of a muscle to generate force over and over again.

muscular strength The maximal ability of a muscle to generate force.

myocardial infarction (MI) Damage to the heart due to a reduction in blood flow, resulting in the death of heart muscle cells.

negative caloric balance Expending more calories than are consumed.

nicotine The addictive and psychoactive drug in tobacco plants.

nonessential amino acids Eleven amino acids that the body can make and are therefore not necessary in the diet.

norepinephrine A hormone secreted by the inner core (medulla) of the adrenal gland.

nutrients Substances contained in food that are necessary for good health.

obesity A term applied to individuals with a high percentage of body fat, generally over 25% for men and over 30% for women.

omega-3 fatty acid A type of unsaturated fatty acid that lowers both blood cholesterol and triglycerides and is found primarily in fresh or frozen mackerel, herring, tuna, and salmon.

1-mile walk test A fitness test designed to evaluate cardiorespiratory fitness. The objective of the test is to complete a 1 walking mile distance (preferably on a track) in the shortest possible time.

1.5-mile run test A fitness test designed to evaluate cardiorespiratory fitness. The objective of the test is to complete a 1.5-mile distance (preferably on a track) in the shortest possible time.

one-repetition maximum (1 RM) test Measurement of the maximum amount of weight that can be lifted one time.

organic Refers to foods that are grown without pesticides.

osteoporosis The loss of bone mass and strength, which increases the risk of bone fractures.

overload principle A basic principle of physical conditioning. The overload principle states that in order to improve physical fitness, the body or specific muscles must be stressed. For example, for a skeletal muscle to increase in strength, the muscle must work against a heavier load than normal.

overtraining Failure to get enough rest between exercise training sessions. Overtraining may lead to chronic fatigue and/or injuries.

overtraining syndrome A phenomenon resulting from improper training techniques that results in exercise-related injuries. Overtraining results from too much exercise and not enough recovery time between workouts. The symptoms may include increased resting heart rate, reduced appetite, weight loss, irritability, disturbed sleep, elevated blood pressure, frequent injuries, increased incidence of infectious, and chronic fatigue.

ozone A gas produced by a chemical reaction between sunlight and the hydrocarbons emitted from car exhausts. This form of pollution is extremely irritating to the lung and airways. It causes tightness in the chest, coughing, headaches, nausea, throat and eye irritation, and, worst of all, bronchoconstriction.

palpation Touching the skin in order to feel the pulse.

passive exercise Movement performed on a motor-driven device designed to move or vibrate the body without any muscular activity. Passive exercise devices come in many forms, including rolling machines, vibrating belts, pillows, and passive motion tables. Passive exercise devices do not improve physical fitness or promote weight loss.

patella-femoral pain syndrome (PFPS) A common exercise-induced injury that is manifest as pain behind the knee cap (patella).

pelvic inflammatory disease An inflammatory infection of the lining of the abdominal and pelvic cavities. Common symptoms of pelvic inflammatory disease include pain in the lower abdominal cavity, fever, and menstrual irregularities.

positive caloric balance Consuming more calories than are expended.

principle of progression A principle of training that dictates that overload should be increased gradually during the course of a physical fitness program.

principle of recuperation The body requires recovery periods between exercise training sessions in order to adapt to the exercise stress. Therefore, a period of rest is essential to achieve maximal benefit from exercise.

principle of reversibility The loss of fitness due to inactivity.

principle of specificity The exercise training effect is specific to those muscles involved in the activity.

progressive resistance exercise (PRE) The application of the overload principle applied to strength and endurance exercise programs. Even though the overload principle and PRE can be used interchangeably, PRE is preferred when discussing weight training.

proprioceptive neuromuscular facilitation (PNF) Combines stretching with alternating contracting and relaxing of muscles to improve flexibility. There are two common types of PNF stretching. One is called contract-relax (CR) stretching, while the second is called contract-relax/antagonist contract (CRAC) stretching.

pulmonary circuit The blood vascular system that circulates blood from the right side of the heart, through the lungs, and back to the left side of the heart.

push-up test A fitness test designed to evaluate muscular endurance of shoulder and arm muscles.

R.I.C.E. An acronym representing a treatment protocol for exercise-related injuries. It stands for a combination of rest-*R*, ice-*I*, compression-*C*, and elevation-*E*.

recovery index Measurement of heart rate during three 30-second recovery periods following a submaximal step test.

recruitment The process of involving more muscle fibers to produce increased muscular force.

repetition maximum (RM) The measure of the intensity of exercise in both isotonic and isokinetic weight training programs. The RM is the maximal load that a muscle group can lift a specified number of times before tiring. For example, 6 RM is the maximal load that can be lifted six times.

resting metabolic rate (RMR) The amount of energy expended during all sedentary activities.

saturated fatty acid A type of fatty acid that comes primarily from animal sources (meat and dairy products) and is solid at room temperature.

scabies Scabies is caused by a parasite (i.e., tiny mite) that can infect skin between the fingers, on the wrist, under the breasts, and the pubic area.

set The number of repetitions performed consecutively without resting.

set point theory A theory of weight regulation that centers around the concept that body weight is controlled at a set point by a weight-regulating control center within the brain.

sexually transmitted diseases (STDs) A group of more than 20 diseases that are generally spread through sexual contact.

sit and reach test A fitness test that measures the ability to flex the trunk (i.e., stretching the lower back muscles and the muscles in the back of the thigh).

sit-up test A field test to evaluate abdominal muscles endurance.

skinfold test A field test to estimate body composition. The test works on the principle that over 50% of the body fat lies just beneath the skin. Therefore, measurement of representative samples of subcutaneous fat provides a means of estimating overall body fatness.

slow-twitch fibers Muscle fibers that contract slowly and are highly resistant to fatigue. Red in appearance, they have the capacity to produce large quantities of ATP aerobically, making them ideally suited for low-intensity, prolonged exercise like walking or slow jogging.

specificity of training That development of muscular strength and endurance, as well as cardiorespiratory endurance, is specific to the muscle group that is exercised and the training intensity.

SPF Abbreviation for "sun protection factor." A sunscreen with an SPF of 15 provides you with 15 times more protection than unprotected skin.

spot reduction The false notion that exercise applied to a specific region of the body will result in fat loss in that region.

sprain Damage to a ligament that occurs if excessive force is applied to a joint.

starches Long chains of sugars commonly found in foods such as corn, grains, potatoes, peas, and beans. Starch is stored in the body as glycogen and is used for that sudden burst of energy often needed during physical activity.

static Stationary; in reference to muscle contractions, static is synonymous with isometric contraction.

static stretching Stretching that slowly lengthens a muscle to a point where further movement is limited.

step test A submaximal exercise test designed to evaluate cardiorespiratory fitness. The step test works on the principle that individuals with a high level of cardiorespiratory fitness will have a lower heart rate during recovery from 3 minutes of standardized exercise (bench stepping) than less-conditioned individuals.

strain Damage to a muscle that can range from a minor separation of fibers to a complete tearing of fibers.

stress A physiological and mental response to something in the environment that causes people to become uncomfortable.

stress fractures Tiny cracks or breaks in bone. Although stress fractures can occur in any leg bone, the long bones of the foot extending from the ankle to the toes are especially susceptible.

stressor A factor that produces stress.

stretch reflex Involuntary contraction of muscle that occurs due to rapid stretching of a muscle.

stroke Brain damage that occurs when the blood supply to the brain is reduced for a prolonged period of time.

stroke volume The amount of blood pumped per heart beat (generally expressed in milliliters).

substance abuse Abuse of any drug such as alcohol, tobacco, and cocaine.

sucrose Also called *table sugar*. A molecule composed of glucose and fructose.

syphilis A sexually transmitted disease that can be transmitted through direct sexual contact. Syphilis is caused by a bacterial infection and can be cured by antibiotics.

systemic circuit The blood vascular system that circulates blood from the left side of the heart, throughout the body, and back to the right side of the heart.

systolic blood pressure The pressure of the blood in the arteries at the level of the heart during the contractile phase of the heart (systole).

target heart rate (THR) The range of heart rates that corresponds to an exercise intensity of approximately 50%–85% $\dot{V}O_{2max}$. This is the range of training heart rates that results in improvements in aerobic capacity.

tendonitis Inflammation or swelling of a tendon. One of the most common exercise-related injuries.

tendons Connective tissue that connects muscles to bones.

ten percent rule A rule of training that states that the training intensity or duration of exercise should not be increased more than 10% per week.

theory A systematic arrangement of fundamental principles that provide a basis for explaining why certain things happen.

threshold for health benefits The minimum level of physical activity required to achieve some of the health benefits of exercise.

training threshold The training intensity above which there is an improvement in cardiorespiratory fitness. This intensity is approximately 50% of $\dot{V}O_{2max}$.

trans fatty acid A type of fatty acid that increases cholesterol in the blood and is a major contributor to heart disease.

trichomoniasis (trick) A vaginal infection caused by a one-celled protozoan called *Trichomonas vaginalis*.

triglycerides The form of fat that is broken down and used to produce energy to power muscle contractions during exercise. Triglycerides constitute approximately 95% of the fats in the diet and are the storage form of body fat.

tumor A group of cancer cells.

unintentional injury Injury resulting from unplanned actions; preferred term for accidental injury.

unsaturated fatty acid A type of fatty acid that comes primarily from plant sources and is liquid at room temperature.

valsalva maneuver Breath holding during an intense muscle contraction that can reduce blood flow to the brain and cause dizziness and fainting.

veins Blood vessels that transport blood toward the heart.

venereal warts Also known as *genital warts*. Warts caused by a small group of viruses called *human papilloma viruses*. Infection generally occurs through sexual contact with an infected individual; after exposure, the virus penetrates the skin or mucous membranes of the genitals or anus, and warts appear within 6 to 8 weeks.

visualization Also called *imagery*. A relaxation technique that uses mental pictures to reduce stress. The idea is to create appealing mental images that promote relaxation and reduce stress.

vitamins Small molecules that play a key role in many body functions, including the regulation of growth and metabolism. They are classified according to whether they are soluble in water or fat.

$\dot{V}O_{2max}$ The highest oxygen consumption achievable during exercise. Practically speaking, $\dot{V}O_{2max}$ is a laboratory measure of the endurance capacity of both the cardiorespiratory system and exercising skeletal muscles.

waist-to-hip circumference ratio An index for determining the risk of disease associated with high body fat. The rationale for this technique is that a high percentage of fat in the abdominal region is associated with an increased risk of disease (e.g., heart disease or hypertension). Therefore, an individual with a large fat deposit in the abdominal region would have a high waist-to-hip ratio and would have a higher risk of disease than someone with a lower waist-to-hip ratio.

warm-up A brief (5 to 15 minute) period of exercise that precedes the workout. The purpose of a warm-up is to elevate muscle temperature and increase blood flow to those muscles that will be engaged in the workout.

wellness A state of healthy living. This state is achieved by the practice of a healthy lifestyle, which includes regular physical activity, proper nutrition, eliminating unhealthy behaviors, and maintaining good emotional and spiritual health.

PHOTO CREDITS

INDEX

Note: A *t* following a page number indicates tabular material, an *f* following a page number indicates an illustration, and a *b* following a page number indicates a boxed feature.

omega-3 fatty acid affecting, 178
reducing intake of, 193, 193t
Cholesterol/saturated fat index (CSI), 193
Choline, 183t, 187b
RDA for, 189t
Chondroitin, joint health and, 153b
Chondromalacia ("runner's knee"/patella-femoral pain syndrome), 359–360, 359b, 360f
Chromium, RDA for, 189t
Chromium picolinate, 203t
Cigarette smoking. See Smoking
Circulatory system, 87–89
exercise affecting, 89–90, 90f
endurance training and, 103
"Clap." See Gonorrhea
Clarity (ecstasy/MDMA/methylenedioxymeth-amphetamine), 408b
"Club drugs," 408b
Cobalamin (vitamin B$_{12}$), 183t
RDA for, 188t
Cocaine (coke), 411–412, 411b, 412f
addiction risk and, 407f
Coenzyme Q-10, 203t
Coke. See Cocaine
Cold/cold weather, exercise in, 323f, 324b, 327–329, 328b, 329b
clothing for, 327f, 328–329, 328b, 329b
Complete proteins, 179, 179b
Complex carbohydrates, 176, 176b, 186
physical fitness and, 199
Compound fats, 178
Concentric contraction, 125, 125b, 125f
Concepts, theoretical, 291, 291b
Conditioning. See Conditioning period, primary; Exercise training
Conditioning period, primary (workout), 73f, 75–76, 76f
for cardiorespiratory exercise program, 92–95, 92t
individualization of, 76
for cardiorespiratory exercise program, 97–99, 98t, 99t, 100t
Condoms, STI risk reduction and, 399
Constructs, theoretical, 291, 291b
Consumer issues
fitness products and, 425–427, 425b, 426f, 439
evaluating, 439
fitness-testing software and, 35b
Contemplation stage, of behavior change, 292
Continuous training (long, slow distance training), 100–102, 100b
Contract-relax (CR) stretching, 154, 154b
Contract-relax/antagonist contract (CRAC) stretching, 154, 154b, 155f
Convection, heat loss by, 320, 320b
Cool-down, 73f, 76, 76b, 76f
for cardiorespiratory exercise program, 96
Cooper, Kenneth, 21, 84
Copper, 185t
Coronary arteries, atherosclerotic blockage of, 261, 262f. See also Coronary heart (coronary artery) disease

Coronary heart (coronary artery) disease, 261, 261b. See also Heart attack
genetic/hereditary factors and, 265f, 267, 269t
risk assessment and, 279–280
risk of, 264–269, 265f, 269t
assessment of, 275–277
contributory risk factors and, 264b, 265f, 267–269, 269t
modification of, 269t, 271
exercise affecting, 6, 6f, 7b, 271
major risk factors and, 264–267, 264b, 265f, 269t
modification of, 269–271, 269t, 271b
omega-3 fatty acids affecting, 178
personality types and, 285–286, 285f
reducing, 269–272, 269t
stress and, 265f, 269, 269t, 285–286, 285f
Cortisol, 283, 283f
CR stretching. See Contract-relax (CR) stretching
Crabs (pubic lice), 398
CRAC stretching. See Contract-relax/antagonist contract (CRAC) stretching
Crack cocaine, addiction risk and, 407f
Cramp (muscle), 124, 166b
Crank (methamphetamine), 408b
Creatine, 203t
Creeping obesity, 224, 224b, 225f
Cross training, 93, 93b, 100–102
Cryokinetics, 363–364, 363b, 363f
Crystal (methamphetamine), 408b
CSI. See Cholesterol/saturated fat index
Curl up, 164
Curl-up test, 35–37, 37b, 37f, 37t, 61
Cycle ergometer fitness test, 23–25, 23b, 23f, 23t, 24b, 24t, 25f, 25t, 55
Cytomegalovirus infection, in HIV infection/AIDS, 391t

Dairy products, weight control and, 236b
Deep knee bends, 163, 171
Dehydration
adverse effects of, 327b
cardiorespiratory fitness tests affected by, 27b
Delayed-onset muscle soreness (DOMS), 355, 355b
Dependency (chemical), 406, 406b
Derived fats, 178, 178b
Dermatologist, 430b
Diabetes, 6, 6b, 339–341
coronary heart disease risk and, 265f, 268, 269t
nutrition/exercise and, 269t, 271
diet and exercise affecting blood glucose levels in, 340b
exercise affecting risk of, 6, 6f
exercise prescription for individuals with, 339–341, 340b
type I diabetes and, 340–341
type II diabetes and, 341

Diastole, 88
Diastolic blood pressure, 88, 88b
exercise affecting, 90, 90f, 117
Diet, 173–222. See also Nutrition
aging and, 429
analysis of, 190–192, 213–215
balanced, 174, 174f, 176f
blood glucose levels and, 340b
cancer risk and, 377, 380, 380b, 380f, 381b
fast food and, 197b
fitness products and, 425–427, 425b
food selection for, 194–196, 195t, 219
goals for, 217
guidelines for, 186–198, 187b, 188–189t, 190f, 195t
low carb foods in, 196b
special considerations and, 196–198
in weight loss, 234–237, 235t, 236b. See also Weight control
questions about, 236b
Diet pills, 240, 240b
Dietary supplements, 201–204, 201f, 203t, 204b, 205b
ergogenic aids, 425–426, 425b
fraud detection and, 207b
government regulation of, 202
in healthful diet, 202, 203t, 204b
joint health and, 153b
stress reduction and, 293b
Disability
cardiorespiratory exercise for person with, 103b
sports participation and, 345b
Dishman, Rod, 422b
Distance training, long, slow (continuous training), 100–102, 100b
Distress (negative stress), 284, 285f
DNA, damage to, cell transformation in cancer and, 375, 376f
DOMS. See Delayed-onset muscle soreness
Donkey kick, 165
Dr. Atkins Diet Revolution (book), 196b
Drinking water, contaminated, environmental health and, 3
"Drip." See Gonorrhea
Driving stress, 283f
aggressive driver assessment and, 317–318
road rage and, 296b
tips for reducing, 286t
Drug addiction, 406, 406b. See also Substance use/abuse
DSHEA (Office of Nutritional Products, Labeling, and Dietary Supplements), 202
Duration of exercise, 76, 76b, 76f
for cardiorespiratory exercise program, 95, 95f
for flexibility/stretching, 156, 156t
Dynamic (isotonic) contraction, 124, 124b, 124f
Dynamic (ballistic) stretching, 153

EAR. See Estimated Average Requirement
Eating disorders, 242–243
"Eating right pyramid," 186–190, 190f
Eccentric (negative) contraction, 125, 125b, 125f